Nutritional and Integrative Strategies in Cardiovascular Medicine

T0176310

Nutritional and Integrative Strategies in Cardiovascular Medicine

Second Edition

Edited by
Stephen T. Sinatra and Mark C. Houston

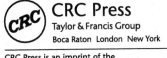

CRC Press
Taylor & Francis Group
Boca Raton London New York

CRC Press is an imprint of the
Taylor & Francis Group, an **informa** business

Second edition published 2022
by CRC Press
6000 Broken Sound Parkway NW, Suite 300, Boca Raton, FL 33487-2742

and by CRC Press
2 Park Square, Milton Park, Abingdon, Oxon, OX14 4RN

CRC Press is an imprint of Taylor & Francis Group, LLC

© 2022 Taylor & Francis Group, LLC

First edition published by CRC Press 2015

Library of Congress Cataloging-in-Publication Data
Names: Stephen T. Sinatra, editor. | Mark C. Houston, editor.
Title: Nutritional and integrative strategies in cardiovascular medicine /
edited by Stephen T. Sinatra, Mark C. Houston.
Description: Second edition. | Boca Raton: CRC Press, 2022. | Includes bibliographical references and index. |
Summary: "Building upon its predecessor, this new edition focuses on important cardiovascular risk factors and highlights recent discoveries and developments that can have a positive impact on cardiovascular disease"—Provided by publisher.
Identifiers: LCCN 2021049596 (print) | LCCN 2021049597 (ebook) |

ISBN: 9780367685003 (hbk)
ISBN: 9780367685010 (pbk)
ISBN: 9781003137849 (ebk)

DOI: 10.1201/9781003137849

Typeset in Times
by codeMantra

Contents

Introduction...vii
Editors..ix
Contributors xi

Chapter 1   Nutrition, the Mediterranean Diet and Selected Supplements for the Prevention
and Treatment of Coronary Heart Disease..1

Mark C. Houston

Chapter 2   Coronary Artery Disease: The Impact of the Mediterranean Cuisine, Targeted
Nutritional Supplements and Their Relationship to Autophagy/mTOR 31

Stephen T. Sinatra

Chapter 3   Naturopathic Medicine and the Prevention and Treatment
of Cardiovascular Disease...45

Drew Sinatra and Michael Murray

Chapter 4   Marine-Derived Omega-3 Fatty Acids and Cardiovascular Disease 77

Thomas G. Guilliams and Jørn Dyerberg

Chapter 5   Nutrition and Nutritional Supplements in the Management of Dyslipidemia and
Dyslipidemia-Induced Cardiovascular Disease 97

Mark C. Houston

Chapter 6   The Role of Nitric Oxide Supplements and Foods in Cardiovascular Disease........ 131

Nathan S. Bryan and Ernst R. von Schwarz

Chapter 7   The Treatment of Hypertension with Nutrition, Nutritional Supplements,
Lifestyle and Pharmacologic Therapies 143

Mark C. Houston

Chapter 8   Metabolic Cardiology: Management of Congestive Heart Failure 189

Stephen T. Sinatra

Chapter 9   Cardiovascular Disease in Women... 217

Stephen T. Sinatra and Sara Gottfried

Chapter 10 Hormones and Cardiovascular Disease.. 231

Sara Gottfried and Myles Spar

Chapter 11 The Heartbreak of Wheat-Related Disorders: Wheat, Gluten and
Cardiovascular Disease 249

Thomas O'Bryan

Chapter 12 The Role of the Gut Microbiome in Cardiovascular Disease 265

Jill C. Carnahan

Chapter 13 Environmental Toxins and Cardiovascular Disease 281

Joseph Pizzorno

Chapter 14 Dental Disease, Inflammation, Cardiovascular Disease, Nutrition and
Nutritional Supplements...293

Douglas G. Thompson, Gregori M. Kurtzman, and Chelsea Q. Watkins

Chapter 15 COVID-19: An Evidence-Based Integrative Approach to Disease Management....335

Douglas S. Harrington

Chapter 16 Lymphstasis, Inflammation and Atherogenesis – Connecting the Dots 349

Gerald M. Lemole

Chapter 17 Vitamin G. Grounding as Energetic Nutrition and Its Role in Oxidative
Defense and Cardiovascular Disease 359

Stephen T. Sinatra, Gaetan Chevalier, and Drew Sinatra

Chapter 18 The Role of Botanicals in Cardiovascular Health...................................369

Tieraona Low Dog

Chapter 19 Depression, Anxiety, Stress, and Spirituality in Cardiovascular Disease 381

Erminia Guarneri and Shyamia Stone

Index..405

Introduction

The first edition of *Nutritional and Integrative Strategies in Cardiovascular Medicine* was published in 2015. Now several years later, our second edition has not only been updated but also reflects several themes and attributes of the rapidly changing medical environment. The last few years with the advent of antibiotic-resistant organisms, killer-type viruses and increasing environmental toxicities have indeed pushed our medical system to the limits with cardiovascular disease still being the number one cause of death and disability in the world. This textbook will not only address the zeitgeist of the times but will offer numerous multiple strategies into the investigation and treatment of cardiovascular disease.

The authors have their own way of telling their stories while offering valuable information at the same time. Some chapters are conversational, others are like reading a scientific journal, and still others reflect personal observations in the care of their patients. Multiple styles of writing offer the reader creative ways of assimilating the information. Although there is some duplication of content, the reader is offered multiple interventions in the search for treatments and solutions.

Targeted nutraceuticals are not a good substitute for good nutrition, but they do provide support that can help prevent inflammatory pathology while bolstering energy production in the body at the same time. For example, knowing which nutrients are suitable and are designed to facilitate and stimulate energy substrate production is the basis of my chapter on Metabolic Cardiology.

The combination of targeted supplements and a healthy diet has been the cornerstone of the nutritional strategy that I applied for decades to assist my patients with heart disease and in many other pathological situations. I use this approach therapeutically as well as preventively to assist and create optimum health. Although pharmaceutical drugs do work in restoring blood flow, many times surgeons may be called to perform lifesaving bypasses or even cardiovascular transplants when a pharmaceutical approach is not optimal. Indeed, conventional medicine works! However, in integrative medicine, we use or recommend many methodologies to help support our patients. But we have learned to do something extra, something normally ignored, and absolutely simplistic and sometimes bargain-based cheap compared to the dazzling big ticket technology. We optimize nutritional status with vitamins, minerals, herbs, antioxidants, and other natural substances – by doing so, we optimize your health and healing. In the fight against disease, we use many weapons. We use what works best, whether the interventions are conventional, natural, or complementary. It doesn't matter as we all want our patients to get well and thrive.

In this book, a group of talented authors will offer multiple discussions and therapeutic options highlighting their expertise in cardiovascular disease. Cardiologists, thoracic surgeons, internists, dentists, chiropractors, naturopaths, doctors of osteopathy, PhDs, and more will discuss their individual, sophisticated approach to cardiovascular disease. In the final analysis, we physicians and healthcare professionals want to reduce the suffering of our patients while extending quality of life at the same time. This second edition is a testimony to the balanced and insightful integrative care of the patient.

I personally want to thank all the authors for assisting me in this publication with their hard work and contribution. I would also like to thank the American Nutrition Association for their genuine support.

Stephen T. Sinatra, M.D., F.A.C.C.
Editor

Editors

Dr. Stephen T. Sinatra is a board-certified cardiologist and an Assistant Clinical Professor of Medicine at the University of Connecticut School of Medicine in Farmington, Connecticut. He is the founder of www.heartmdinstitute.com, an informational website dedicated to promoting public awareness of integrative medicine as well as www.vervana.com a website focused on high vibrational living and foods.

His expertise is grounded in more than fifty years of clinical practice, research, and study beginning as an attending physician at Manchester Memorial Hospital. His career included nine years as Chief of Cardiology and nineteen years as Director of Medical Education.

Today, Dr. Sinatra is active primarily as an author, speaker, and advisor for the research and development of targeted nutritional supplements at Healthy Directions. In addition to his board certifications in internal medicine and cardiology, Dr. Sinatra is a Fellow of the American College of Cardiology, a Certified Nutrition Specialist (CNS) and American Board of Nutrition Fellow at the American College of Nutrition, Certified Bioenergetic Psychotherapist, and Certified by the American Board of Anti-aging Medicine.

He has authored over 20 books including The Great Cholesterol Myth, The Sinatra Solution – Metabolic Cardiology, Earthing: The most important health discovery ever, Heartbreak and Heart Disease, Health Revelations from Heaven and Earth, etc. He just completed his most recent book entitled "Get Grounded, Get Well" which will be released in the fall/winter of 2022.

Dr. Sinatra has also appeared on many TV shows including Dr. Oz, The Doctors, The Today Show, The 700 Club, Fox on Health, MSNBC, and Your Health. He is also the recipient of numerous awards in the integrative medical field including Excellence in Health Journalism. He feels his most significant legacy is his contribution to metabolic cardiology.

Dr. Mark C. Houston is director of the Hypertension Institute and Vascular Biology, Medical Director of the Division of Human Nutrition, and Medical Director of Clinical Research at the Hypertension Institute in Nashville, TN. He is a Clinical Instructor in the Department of Physical Therapy and Health Care Sciences at George Washington University (GWU) School of Medicine and Health Science. He served as an Assistant Professor of Medicine then as an Associate Professor of Medicine from 1978–1990 at Vanderbilt University School of Medicine and was an Associate Clinical Professor of Medicine at Vanderbilt University School of Medicine, (VUMS) (1990–2012). He has four board certifications from the American Board of Internal Medicine (ABIM), the American Society of Hypertension (ASH) (FASH-Fellow), the American Board of Anti-Aging and Regenerative Medicine (ABAARM, FAARM), and the American Board of Cardiology (ABC) Certification in Hypertensive Cardiovascular Disease (DABC).

Contributors

Nathan S. Bryan
Department of Molecular and Human Genetics
Baylor College of Medicine
Houston, Texas

Jill Carnahan
Flatiron Functional Medicine
Boulder, Colorado

Gaetan Chevalier
California Institute for Human Sciences
Encinitas, California

Tieraona Low Dog
Medicine Lodge Academy
Pecos, New Mexico

Jørn Dyerberg
University of Copenhagen
Charlottenlund, Copenhagen, Denmark

Sara Gottfried
Department of Integrative Medicine and
    Nutritional Sciences
Sidney Kimmel Medical College, Thomas
    Jefferson University
Philadelphia, Pennsylvania
and
Department of Precision Medicine
Marcus Institute of Integrative Health
Villanova, Pennsylvania

Erminia Guarneri
President Academy Integrative Health
    and Medicine
Medical Director Guarneri Integrative Health
Clinical Associate UCSD

Thomas G. Guilliams
University of Wisconsin School of Pharmacy
Madison, Wisconsin
and

Douglas S. Harrington
Predictive Health Diagnostics Company
Irvine, California
and
MUSE Microscopy, LLC
Irvine, California
and
Oncocyte
Irvine, California
and
Morningstar Laboratories
Irvine, California
and
Change Healthcare
Nashville, Tennessee

Mark C. Houston
Department of Medicine (1990–2012)
Vanderbilt University Medical School
Nashville, Tennessee
and
Hypertension Institute and Vascular Biology
St. Thomas West Hospital
Nashville, Tennessee
and
Division of Human Nutrition
Saint Thomas Medical Group, Saint Thomas
    Hospital and Health Services
Nashville, Tennessee
and
Department of Physical Therapy and Health
    Care Sciences
George Washington University (GWU) School
Washington, District of Columbia

Gregori M. Kurtzman
Private General Dental Practice
Silver Spring, Maryland

Gerald M. Lemole
Lewis Katz School of medicine
Temple University
Philadelphia, Pennsylvania
and
Thomas Jefferson Medical College
Woodbury, New Jersey

Michael Murray

Thomas O'Bryan
Institute for Functional Medicine
Seattle, Washington, District of Columbia
and
National University Health Services
Lombard, Illinois

Joseph Pizzorno
Bastyr University
Kenmore, Washington, District of Columbia

Drew Sinatra
Inspire Naturopathic Medicine
Mill Valley, California

Stephen T. Sinatra
Department of Medicine
University of Connecticut School of Medicine
Farmington, Connecticut

Myles Spar
Vault Health
Integrative Internal Medicine
New York, New York

Shyamia Stone
Stone Naturopathic Medicine, President

Douglas G. Thompson
Private General Dental Practice
Bloomfield Hills, Michigan
and
Wellness Dentistry Network
Bloomfield Hills, Michigan
and
Kois Center
Seattle, Washington, District of Columbia

Ernst R. von Schwarz
Department of Medicine
Cedars Sinai Medical Center
David Geffen School of Medicine at UCLA
Los Angeles, California
and
University of California Riverside
Riverside, California
and
Southern California Hospital Heart Institute
Culver City, California
University of California Los Angeles (UCLA)
Culver City, California

Chelsea Q. Watkins
Private General Dental Practice
Bloomfield Hills, Michigan

1 Nutrition, the Mediterranean Diet and Selected Supplements for the Prevention and Treatment of Coronary Heart Disease

Mark C. Houston

CONTENTS

Introduction 2
Revolutionizing the Treatment of Coronary Heart Disease and Interrupting the Finite Pathways 2
Atherosclerosis, Endothelial Dysfunction and Arterial Stiffness 2
Nutrition and CHD 3
Specific Diets and Coronary Heart Disease 3
      Mediterranean Diet (TMD: Traditional Mediterranean Diet) (PREDIMED Diet) 3
Dietary Approaches to Stop Hypertension (DASH) Diets (DASH 1 and 2) 7
Dietary Fats 8
      Omega 3 Fatty Acids (PUFA) 8
Monounsaturated Fats 9
Saturated Fatty Acids 9
Conclusions and Summary on SFA [14,28,31–56] 10
Trans Fatty Acids 11
Coconut Oil 12
Milk, Milk Products and Peptides 12
Whey Protein 12
Eggs 12
Refined Carbohydrates, Sugars and Sugar Substitutes 13
Advanced Glycation End Products (AGEs) 14
Protein 14
      Vegetarian Diets and Plant-Based Nutrition 14
Animal Protein Diets 15
      Soy Protein 15
      Fish 15
Dietary Acid Load and Protein 16
Specific Dietary and Nutritional Components and Caloric Restriction 16

DOI: 10.1201/9781003137849-1

Caffeine...17
Caloric Restriction 17
Alcohol..17
Gluten..18
Nuts...18
Dietary Sodium, Potassium and Magnesium...19
Summary and Conclusions 20
References..20

INTRODUCTION

Cardiovascular disease (CVD) remains the number one cause of morbidity and mortality in the United States [1,2]. The annual cost (direct and indirect) of treatment of CVD is over $320 billion USD [2]. One in every three deaths is a result of CVD, and over 2200 US citizens die from stroke or myocardial infarction (MI) each day [2–5]. More than 400 coronary heart disease (CHD) risk factors have been defined [2]. Most CVDs can be prevented by addressing behavioral risk factors such as tobacco use, optimal nutrition, obesity, physical inactivity and harmful use of alcohol using population-wide strategies. People with CVD or who are at high risk of CVD (due to the presence of one or more risk factors such as hypertension, diabetes, hyperlipidemia or already-established disease) need early detection and management. Approximately 80% of CHDs can be prevented by optimal nutrition, regular aerobic and resistance exercise, ideal body weight and composition, limited alcoholic intake and avoiding all tobacco products [1]. There are numerous insults to the cardiovascular system, but there are only three finite vascular responses which include inflammation, oxidative stress and vascular immune dysfunction which lead to the atherosclerotic process and plaque, CHD and MI.Coronary heart disease (CHD) remains the cause of the highest mortality in industrialized societies. About 80% of CHDs can be prevented with optimal nutrition, proper exercise, weight management, limited alcohol intake and smoking cessation. Among all of these factors, nutrition provides the basic foundation for the prevention and treatment of CHD in numerous prospective nutrition clinical trials. As nutritional science, nutrigenomic and metabolomic research continues, we will develop a better personalized and precision-based nutritional program to reduce the risk of CHD and myocardial infarction (MI) (Figure 1.1).

REVOLUTIONIZING THE TREATMENT OF CORONARY HEART DISEASE AND INTERRUPTING THE FINITE PATHWAYS

Interaction of various insults with cell membranes and endothelial vascular receptors (pattern recognition receptors (PRRs), NOD-like receptors (NLRs), toll-like receptors (TLRs) and caveolae, which contain endothelial nitric oxide synthase (eNOS) and nitric oxide (NO)) determines the cellular internal signaling and vascular responses [2,6–8] (Figure 1.2).

Chronic insults of any type induce inflammatory, oxidative stress and immune responses which become dysregulated and produce damage to the vascular system. In this scenario, the blood vessel becomes an "innocent bystander" to the pathogenic mechanisms, which eventually leads to functional and structural cardiovascular injuries [2]. Numerous scientifically validated nutritional or dietary components and nutraceutical supplements have great promise to reduce the vascular damage [4,8].

ATHEROSCLEROSIS, ENDOTHELIAL DYSFUNCTION AND ARTERIAL STIFFNESS

Atherosclerosis, endothelial dysfunction (the earliest vascular abnormality) and arterial stiffness of small arteries begin early in life [9–12] (Figure 1.3).

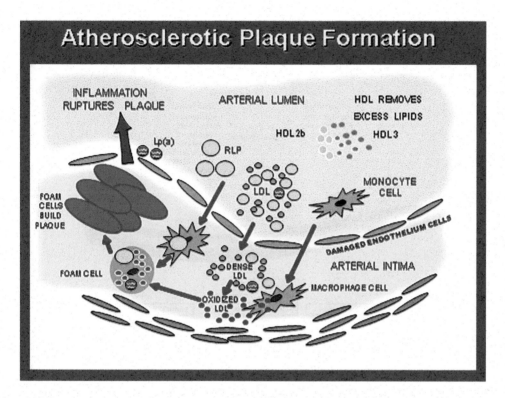

FIGURE 1.1 The pathogenesis atherosclerotic plaque formation.

The consumption of excessive dietary sodium chloride (NaCl), refined carbohydrates (CHO), sugars, starches, trans fatty acids (TFAs) and some, but not all, saturated fatty acids (SFAs) will promote glucotoxicity, triglyceride toxicity, vascular metabolic endotoxemia, inflammation, oxidative stress and vascular immune dysfunction that may persist long after the initial insult. This may also result in exaggerated responses (through metabolic memory) with repeated or chronic nutritional insults [6,9–12].

NUTRITION AND CHD

Targeted nutrition in combination with other lifestyle changes is a foundational recommendation for the reduction of CHD risk. National and international nutritional guidelines are still evolving as new science, nutrigenomic and metabolomic studies are published. There are many recent clinical trials that demonstrate improved CHD outcomes related to nutrition (Table 1.1) [13,14].

SPECIFIC DIETS AND CORONARY HEART DISEASE

MEDITERRANEAN DIET (TMD: TRADITIONAL MEDITERRANEAN DIET) (PREDIMED DIET)

In a 4.8-year primary prevention by following PREDIMED (PREvención con DIeta MEDiterránea) diet, the rate of major cardiovascular events from MI, cerebrovascular accidents (CVA) and total CV deaths was reduced by 28% with nuts and 30% with extra-virgin olive oil (EVOO) [16]. The reduction in CVA was 39% overall ($p < 0.003$) with a 33% reduction from EVOO and a 46% reduction from nuts. The reduction in MI was 23% overall ($p = 0.25$) with a 20% reduction with EVOO and a 26% reduction from nuts. Total CV deaths were reduced by 17% ($p = 0.8$) [15–18]. New onset of type 2 diabetes mellitus (T2DM) was decreased by 40% with EVOO and 18% with mixed nuts

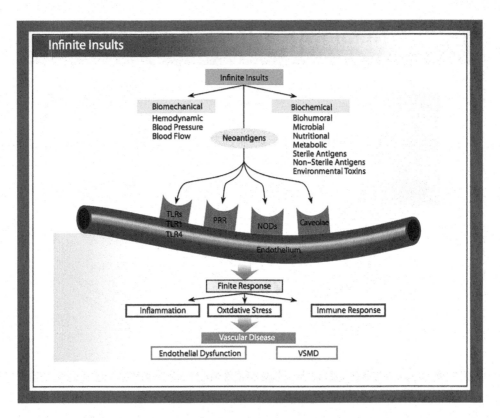

FIGURE 1.2 Biochemical and biomechanical insults that interact with vascular receptors (pattern recognition receptors, PRRs; NOD-like receptors, NLRs; toll-like receptors, TLRs; and caveolae) to induce the three finite responses of vascular inflammation, oxidative stress and vascular immune dysfunction which lead to endothelial dysfunction and vascular smooth muscle and cardiac dysfunction.

[18]. This reduction was associated with decreases in high-sensitivity C-reactive protein (hsCRP) and interleukin (IL-6).

The high content of nitrate (NO_3) that is converted to nitrite (NO_2) (average of 400 mg/day) and the increased amount of omega 3 fatty acids, good omega 6 fatty acids, and polyphenols (such as quercetin, resveratrol and catechins) in grapes and wine provide many of the beneficial outcomes in CHD [17]. The Lyon Heart study [19] of post-MI secondary prevention demonstrated significant reductions in all events including cardiac death, nonfatal MI, unstable angina, CVA, congestive heart failure (CHF) and hospitalization by following the Mediterranean-style diet supplemented with alpha-linolenic acid (ALA) for 4 years compared to a prudent Western diet. Compared to the control, the Mediterranean-style diet with ALA demonstrated a 73% lower risk of cardiac death and nonfatal MI during the study period [19]. Olive oil was associated with a decreased risk of overall mortality and a significant reduction in CVD mortality in a large Mediterranean cohort of 40,622 subjects [20]. For each increase in olive oil by 10 grams, there was a 13% decrease in CV mortality. In the highest quartile of olive oil intake, there was a 44% decrease in CV mortality [20].

One of the mechanisms by which the TMD, particularly if supplemented with EVOO at 50 g/day, can exert CV health benefits is through changes in the transcriptomic response of genes related to cardiovascular risk that include genes for atherosclerosis, inflammation, oxidative stress vascular immune dysfunction, T2DM and hypertension [16,17,21–23]. This includes genes such as ADR-B2 (adrenergic beta 2 receptor), IL7R (interleukin 7 receptor), IFN gamma (interferon), MCP1 (monocyte chemotactic protein), TNFα (tumor necrosis factor alpha), interleukin 6 (IL-6) and hsCRP [16,17,20–23]. In summary, the TMD has been shown to have the following effects [15–17,21–23]:

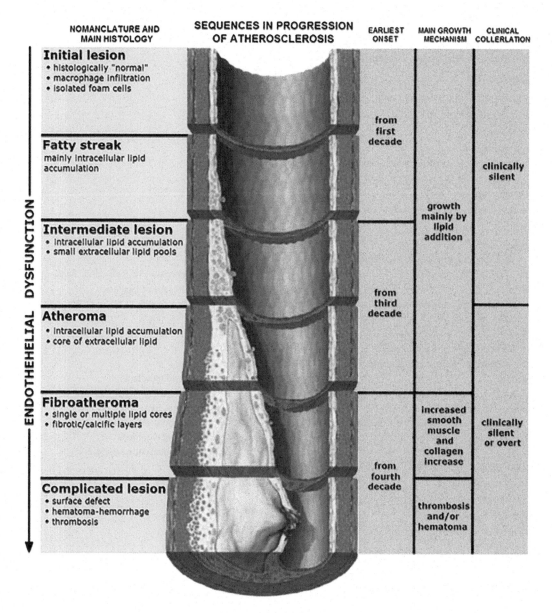

FIGURE 1.3 Atherosclerosis progression. The initial lesion progresses to a fatty streak, and then to an intermediate lesion, atheroma, and fibroatheroma, a complicated lesion prone to rupture and thrombosis.

- Lowers blood pressure.
- Improves serum lipids: lowers total cholesterol (TC), low-density lipoprotein (LDL) and triglycerides (TG); increases high-density lipoprotein (HDL); lowers oxidized LDL (oxLDL) and lipoprotein a (Lp(a)); and improves LDL size and decreases the LDL particle number (LDL P) to a less atherogenic profile.
- Improves T2DM and dysglycemia.
- Improves oxidative defense and reduces oxidative stress: F-2 isoprostanes and 8-Oxo-2′-deoxyguanosine (8OHDG).
- Reduces inflammation: lowers hsCRP, interleukin-6 (IL6), soluble vascular cell adhesion molecule (sl-VCAM) and soluble cell adhesion molecule (sl-CAM).
- Reduces thrombosis and factor VII after meals.

TABLE 1.1

Summary of Nutrition, Nutrients and Daily Intake

Nutrient	Daily Intake
Diets that benefit cardiovascular health	
Mediterranean diet and MD+ALA	
DASH 1 and 2	
Vegetarian diet	
• Potential for nutrient deficiencies, including vitamin B12, vitamin D, omega 3 fatty acids, iron, calcium, carnitine, zinc and protein	
Paleolithic diet	
Caloric restriction and intermittent fasting	
Low ages	
Alkaline diet	
• No definitive results but appears in line with DASH and TMD	
Fats	Less than 35% total caloric intake
SFA	<7%–9% of total diet
• LCFA and MCFA have variable effects, with LCFA having a higher risk; SCFA are neutral	Replace with PUFA or MUFA
Coconut oil	
• No recommendation for prevention or treatment of CHD or CVD, but it is a possible substitute for high glycemic carbohydrates in low amounts	
Trans fat	Avoid trans fat
PUFA	Omega 3 to omega 6 ratio at 4:1
Omega 3 fatty acids	>1g of EPA+DHA per day
• Opt for balanced formulation with DHA, EPA, GLA, and gamma-delta tocopherols	1.1 g/day for women
	1.6 g/day for men
	~2% total daily calories
MUFA [165]:	
Extra-virgin olive oil	50 g/day
Diet elements	
Animal protein	
• Avoid processed red meat	
• Aim for lean cuts	
Fish	1–2 servings/week
• Choose fish with high omega-3 content and low mercury levels	20 g/day
Nuts	>5 servings/week; 28 g/day
Vegetables and fruits	200 g–800 g/day
• Dark leafy greens have the strongest effect on CHD risk	
Milk and milk products	
• Intake has an inverse association with CVD	
Eggs	*6–12 eggs per week as part of a healthy cardiovascular diet*
• No association with increased risk, except possibly for diabetics	
Special recommendation for diabetics	
Refined carbs, sugar and sugar substitutes	Reduce or eliminate from diet
Alcohol	1–2 drinks/day for women
	2–4 drinks/day for men
Isolated nutrients and nutraceutical supplements	
Curcumin	
Cinnamaldehyde (cinnamon)	
Sulforaphane (broccoli)	

(Continued)

TABLE 1.1 (*Continued*)
Summary of Nutrition, Nutrients and Daily Intake

Nutrient	Daily Intake
Resveratrol	
Luteolin	
Quercetin	
Caffeine	Caffeinated coffee for slow metabolizers
• Different effect on fast metabolizers compared to slow metabolizers	59 and younger <2–3 cups
	Older than 59 < 1 cup
Soy protein	15–30 g/day
Whey protein	20 g/day
Gluten	
• No link even in those with celiac disease	
• Choose 100% whole grains	
Sodium	Low sodium–potassium ratio
Potassium	4.7 g/day, preferably from food
Magnesium	

- Decreases brain natriuretic peptide (BNP).
- Increases nitrates/nitrites.
- Improves membrane fluidity.
- Reduces risks of MI, CHD and CVA.
- Reduces homocysteine.

DIETARY APPROACHES TO STOP HYPERTENSION (DASH) DIETS (DASH 1 AND 2)

The DASH diets reduce blood pressure (BP) and CHD. Both DASH 1 and DASH 2 diets empha-size increased daily intake of fruits, vegetables, whole grains, beans, fiber, low-fat dairy prod-ucts, poultry, fish, seeds and nuts, but limiting red meat, sweets and sugar-containing beverages. The intake of potassium, magnesium and calcium is increased but with a variable restriction in dietary sodium [24,25]. Borderline or stage 1 hypertension (<160 to 80–95 mmHg) was evaluated in 379 non-medicated subjects following DASH diets over 8 weeks. A control diet was prescribed for 3 weeks, and then the study subjects were randomized to the control diet, a fruit and vegetable diet with 8.5 servings or a combined fruit and vegetable diet with 10 servings and low-fat dairy. The contents of sodium, potassium, magnesium, calcium and fiber were the same in the two diets. The control diet had less potassium, magnesium and calcium by 50%, less fiber by 22 g and only 4 servings of fruits and vegetables but was otherwise the same as the other. Both DASH diets reduce BP within 4 weeks by approximately 10/5 mmHg. The BP remains stable as long as there is good adherence to the diets.

The results of the various types of DASH 1 and DASH 2 diets are summarized below:

1. DASH 1 overall combination diet vs. control diet: 5/3 mmHg.
2. DASH 1 hypertensive patients. Combination diet vs. control diet: 10.7/5.2 mmHg.
3. DASH 2 overall combination vs. low-sodium DASH diet: 8.9/4.5 mmHg vs. control high-sodium diet.
4. DASH 2 hypertensive patients. Combination low-sodium DASH diet: 11.5/6.8 mmHg vs. control high-sodium diet.

Limiting refined carbohydrates, despite an increased dietary SFAs, improves the lipid profile with both of the DASH diets. The DASH diets are as effective in BP reduction as one anti-hypertensive medication and also decrease the levels of hsCRP and serum lipids. In the Nurses' Health Study (NHS), the DASH dietary pattern was associated with a lower risk of CHD by 14% in those with the highest adherence to the diet [26].

The DASH diets provide various mechanisms for improvement in all the cardiovascular risk factors and CHD risk that are based on specific genetic influences including:

1. Increased nitric oxide and increased plasma nitrate
2. Natriuresis
3. Decreased oxidative stress and increased oxidative defense
4. Reduced urinary F2-isoprostanes
5. Improved endothelial function
6. Decreased pulse wave velocity (PWV) and augmentation index (AI) with reduced arterial stiffness.

DIETARY FATS

OMEGA 3 FATTY ACIDS (PUFA)

The role of fats in CHD has been evaluated in numerous clinical trials [14,27–71]. A large meta-analysis of omega 3 fatty acids [30] reviewed 18 randomized controlled trials (RCTs) (93,000 subjects) and 16 prospective cohort studies (732,000 subjects) and examined EPA+DHA (eicosapentaenoic acid and docosahexaenoic acid) from foods and supplements and their relationship to CHD, MI, sudden cardiac death, coronary death and angina in primary and secondary preventions. Among RCTs, there was a non-statistically significant 6% reduction in CHD risk with EPA+DHA. Subgroup analyses of data from RCTs indicated a statistically significant 14%–16% CHD risk reduction with EPA+DHA among higher-risk populations including participants with elevated triglyceride levels over 150 mg/dL and elevated LDL cholesterol above 130 mg/dL. Meta-analysis of data from prospective cohort studies resulted in an 18% significant reduction of CHD risk for higher intakes of EPA+DHA over 1 g/day and risk of any CHD event. The sudden cardiac death (SCD) rate was reduced 47%. The greatest reduction in CHD (25%) occurred in those with high TG over 150 mg/dL and doses of omega 3 fatty acids over 1 g/day. These results and others indicate that EPA+DHA may be associated with a reduction of CHD risk, with the greatest benefit observed among higher-risk populations in RCTs and those taking higher doses of EPA and DHA. Omega 3 fatty acids reduce ventricular arrhythmias [60] and decrease cardiovascular and total mortality [58]. Omega 3 fatty acids are typically found in cold-water fish such as salmon, mackerel and others as well as plant-based products like algae, flax, chia, and hemp seeds, but as fatty fish eat algae, they serve as a supply for these essential fats. Omega 3 fatty acids decrease risks of MI and CHD 18% more with concomitant use of statins [61]; reduce stent restenosis [59]; reduce post-MI mortality [62], coronary artery bypass graft (CABG) occlusion [63,64], plaque formation [65,66], coronary artery calcification [65,66], and atherosclerosis [65,66]; improve the lipid profile [10,67]; lower glucose; improve insulin resistance [68–70]; and reduce BP [2,4,11,71]. A total of 40 studies with a combined 135,267 participants [70] showed that s supplementation was associated with reduced risk of MI (relative risk [RR], 0.87; 95% CI, 0.80–0.96), high certainty number needed to treat (NNT) of 272; CHD events (RR, 0.90; 95% CI, 0.84–0.97), high certainty NNT of 192; fatal MI (RR, 0.65; 95% CI, 0.46–0.91]), moderate certainty NNT = 128; and CHD mortality (RR, 0.91; 95% CI, 0.85–0.98), low certainty NNT = 431, but not CVD events (RR, 0.95; 95% CI, 0.90–1.00). The effect is dose dependent for CVD events and MI. Cardiovascular disease remains the leading cause of death worldwide. Supplementation with EPA and DHA is an effective lifestyle strategy for CVD prevention, and the protective effect probably increases with dosage.

The dose prescribed will depend on the condition being treated as well as age, body weight and use of concomitant medications and other nutritional supplements. It is best to use a balanced formulation with DHA, EPA, GLA and gamma-delta tocopherols. This will prevent oxidation in the cell membranes and reduce depletions of the EPA and DHA by GLA and vice versa [10,67,71].

MONOUNSATURATED FATS

The effects of cis-monounsaturated fatty acids (cis-MUFAs) on the risk of CHD and on CHD mortality have not been firmly established [72]. In addition, dietary recommendations for cis-MUFA from various organizations do not agree. The effects of cis-MUFA on serum lipids, lipoproteins and endothelial vascular function are favorable [49,72,73]. There are no RCTs with CHD events as endpoints, but several large prospective cohort studies have been published on the relationship between cis-MUFA and CHD risk [15–18,43,49,51,73,74]. Partial replacement of SFA with MUFA improves the blood lipid and lipoprotein profile and reduces the risk of CHD [49]. The NHS and the Health Professionals Follow-up Study followed over 84,000 patients for 24–30 years [51]. Replacing 5% of energy from SFA with equivalent energy intake from MUFA was associated with a 15% lower risk of CHD (hazard ratio (HR): 0.85, 95% CI: 0.74–0.97; $p=0.02$) [51]. Isocaloric replacement of 1% energy from 12:0 to 18:0 SFA combined showed a HR of CHD for MUFA of 0.94 (0.91–0.97; $P<0.001$), and for 16:0, the HR was 0.90 (0.83–0.97; $P=0.01$) [43]. A recent review of the literature of randomized controlled clinical trials (RCCTs) that used a four-step cost-of-illness analysis estimated the success rate, disease biomarker reduction, disease incidence reduction and cost savings of incorporating MUFA into the diet [73]. Improvements were seen in CHD biomarkers' incidence of CHD and T2DM, in addition to annualized healthcare and societal cost savings for the daily MUFA intake [73].

In the PREDIMED diet, the rate of major cardiovascular events from MI, cerebrovascular accidents (CVA) or total CV deaths was reduced by 28% with nuts and 30% with EVOO [16].

In a prospective study of Dutch patients with cardiac disease (Alpha Omega Cohort) [74], the risk of CVD and CHD mortality was evaluated over 7 years and the sum of SFAs and TFAs was theoretically replaced by PUFAs or cis-MUFAs in a group of drug-treated patients with a history of MI. In continuous analyses, replacement of SFAs and TFAs with MUFAs (per 5% of energy) was associated with significantly lower risks of CVD mortality (HR 0.75) and CHD mortality (HR 0.70) [74]. Nutrition guidelines for dietary fats are now shifting to recommend higher intakes of MUFA such as EVOO and nuts [15–18,49,72–74].

SATURATED FATTY ACIDS

Clinical trials offer conflicting conclusions regarding the role of SFA in the risk of CHD [14,18,27,28,-31–56]. The source of the confusion lies within the complexity, accuracy and the coordination of the results and conclusions in basic science, clinical epidemiology and prospective clinical trials. Some of the misconceptions and improper interpretations are related to the source of the SFA, carbon length absorption, the replacement nutrient(s), the genotypic expression to dietary SFAs, metabolism and the composition and chemical expressions within the microbiome [31–35].

SFA also have variable effects on serum lipids and lipid subfractions, hepatic LDL receptor activity, nonalcoholic liver disease (NAFLD), thrombosis, release of tissue plasminogen activator, macrophage foam cell formation and growth, TLRs (TLR 2 and TLR 4) interactions, nuclear factor (NF-kB) cytokine gene expression, NADPH oxidase, detoxification of radical oxygen species (ROS), activity of catalase, glutathione peroxidase (GPx), superoxide dismutase (SOD 1), thioredoxin reductase (TxNRD1) and the genetic ability to desaturate SFA to monounsaturated fatty acids (MUFA) [31–41]. Stearate (C-18) has minimal effect on CHD risk and serum lipids due to its rapid desaturation to MUFA by stearoyl-CoA Δ-9-desaturase (SCD), which is genetically determined [31–33]. The dietary SFA intake may not correlate with the measured SFA content in serum cholesterol esters and erythrocytes, resulting in a discrepancy in the ability to accurately predict CHD risk based on the "real" SFA status of an individual [31,36–38]. High SFA content in serum cholesterol esters and erythrocytes, not high SFA intake, more accurately predicts CHD risk [36]. Endogenous SFA synthesis, especially that of palmitic acid (16:0) from carbohydrates, contributes to the SFA status. Increased dietary intake of refined carbohydrates with low dietary consumption of SFA spares SFA due to the de novo synthesis of SFA from refined carbohydrates. A diet with reduced carbohydrate intake allows SFA to be utilized directly for energy production. Long-chain fatty acids (LCFA) enhance gastrointestinal growth of gram negative bacteria (GNB) and lipo-polysaccharide (LPS) uptake, inflammation and immune activation of T-cells which will increase gastrointestinal permeability, the risk of endotoxemia and infection from a variety of pathobionts at a dysfunctional microbial-epithelial interface [31,36–40].

Published clinical trials and reviews have provided more accurate insights into the relationship between SFA and CHD [27,28,42–48]. A meta-analysis of 32 trials with over 600,000 subjects included 17 observational studies of fatty acid biomarkers, 32 observational studies of fatty acid intake and 27 RCCTs of fatty acid supplementation [27]. The results of this meta-analysis are at variance with other studies perhaps due to the heterogeneity of the populations, selection bias, quality of the studies selected, self-reporting of diet and other confounders due to unmeasured dietary factors, and other lifestyle factors. Despite the size of this meta-analysis, the results and conclusions drawn need to be interpreted with caution.

The largest meta-analysis of three large cohort studies (Health Professionals Follow-Up Study (HPFS), Nurses' Health Study 1 (NHS 1) and Nurses' Health Study 2 (NHS 2)) utilizing a 5% isoca-loric (ISC) energy replacement of SFA with polyunsaturated fatty acids (PUFA) or vegetable fat, was associated with 24% and 10% reductions in CHD risk, respectively [43]. The reduction in CHD with ISC energy replacement of SFA with PUFA, monounsaturated fatty acids (MUFA), TFAs, omega-6 fatty acids, whole grains, vegetable or plant proteins, refined carbohydrates, high-fructose corn syrup or starches depends on the percent of energy that is substituted [43,44]. Replacement of 1% of energy from SFAs with PUFAs lowers LDL-cholesterol which predicts a 2%–8% reduction in CHD [43].

SFA intake and CHD were positively associated in the prospective, longitudinal cohort studies of over 115,000 men and women in the HPFS and the NHS over a 34–38 years follow-up [44]. SFAs were mostly lauric acid (12:0), myristic acid (14:0), palmitic acid (16:0) and stearic acid (18:0) at 9.0%–11.3% of energy intake. Comparing the highest versus the lowest groups of individual SFA intakes, CHD increased 7% for 12:0, 13% for 14:0, 18% for 16:0, 18% for 18:0, and 18% for all four SFAs combined ($p=0.05$–0.001). The reduction in CHD after 1% energy ISC replacement of SFA 12:0–18:0 was 8% for PUFA, 5% for MUFA, 6% for whole grains and 7% for plant proteins [45].

The PREDIMED was a 6-year prospective study of 7,038 subjects with a high CVD risk that included MI, CVA or death from CV causes [28]. The dietary consumption of SFA and TFA from the highest to the lowest quintiles increased overall CVD by 81% and 67%, respectively. The intake of PUFAs and MUFAs reduced the risk of CVD and death. The ISC replacement of SFAs and TFA with MUFAs and PUFAs reduced CVD [28]. SFA from processed foods increased CVD [28].

CONCLUSIONS AND SUMMARY ON SFA [14,28,31–56]

SFA are diverse compounds that cannot be "lumped" into a single category and have variable effects on CHD. It is prudent to replace LCFA with PUFA, MUFA, short-chain fatty acids (SCFA), whole grains, plant proteins and perhaps medium-chain fatty acids (MCFA). The daily recommended grams per day or percent of SFA relative to total fat or total calories cannot be accurately determined at this time. Some studies suggest that the SFA dietary intake should be well below 9% of the total caloric intake. The overall relationship of the human diet to CHD should include the totality of our nutrition and avoid reductionist evaluations of single macronutrients. New nutritional guidelines should promote dietary patterns that improve CHD based on validated science. Refined carbohydrates, high-fructose corn syrup, starches and TFA increase the risk of CHD.

Omega 6 fatty acids appear to be neutral or improve CHD risk, whereas omega 3 fatty acids (PUFA), MUFA, fermented foods, fiber, fruits and vegetables, and the PREDIMED diet reduce the risks of CHD and CVD.

Conclusions:

1. Dietary SFA intake is associated with an increased CHD risk, and reducing dietary SFA in isocaloric (ISC) replacement with PUFA, MUFA, omega 6 fatty acids, whole grains and plant proteins decreases CHD risk.
2. The source of SFAs is associated with the risk of CHD. Dietary intake of meat and animal fat has the greatest risk with a range of 6%–48%.
3. LCFA are the most likely SFAs associated with CHD risk. SCFAs are not associated with CHD risk, but additional studies are needed to confirm this.
4. The carbon chain number of the SFA, as odd or even, may be associated with CHD risk.
5. Replacement of SFA with PUFA reduces CHD risk.
6. Replacement of SFA with MUFA reduces CHD risk.
7. Replacement of SFA with omega 6 fatty acids decreases CHD risk.
8. Replacement of SFA with refined CHO increases CHD risk.

TRANS FATTY ACIDS

A study of 126,233 participants from the NHS and the HPFS analyzed the relationship between choices of dietary fats and overall mortality [75]. During the follow-up, 33,304 deaths were documented. Dietary TFA had the most significant adverse impact on health. Every 2% higher intake of TFA was associated with a 16% higher chance of premature death and a 25% increase in CHD death and nonfatal MI during the study period [75]. A panel of experts in cardiovascular nutrition recently reported on trending controversies and provided some recommendations regarding fat intake [14]. The overall recommendations were to reduce omega 6 fatty acids, increase omega 3 fatty acids and the ratio of omega 3 to omega 6 fatty acids, and reduce SFA in addition to the elimination of TFA. The cardiovascular adverse effects of industrialized produced TFAs are listed below [76,77]:

1. Dyslipidemia
   A.   Increase TC 8%
   B.   Increase LDL-C 9%
   C.   Increase TG and VLDL 9%
   D.   Lower HDL-C 2%–3%
   E.   Increase TC/HDL ratio 11%
   F.   Increase apolipoprotein B 8%
   G.   Increase lipoprotein (a) [Lp(a)] 4%
2. Increase in adipose tissue TFA levels
3. Increase in TG and phospholipid TFA levels
4. Increase insulin resistance, glucose and T2DM risk
5. Increase thrombogenic risk and plaque vulnerability
6. Increase risk of CHD and MI
7. Increase the risk of primary cardiac arrhythmias and sudden death
8. Increase in all-cause mortality by 25% from the lowest to the highest quintile
9. Increase of 2% in energy in total TFA intake results in 25% increase in CHD (CHD death and nonfatal MI)
10. Hypertension
11. Endothelial dysfunction
12. Obesity
13. Increased inflammation.

COCONUT OIL

Coconut oil has been inappropriately promoted for a reduction in CHD and other CV events with no evidence to support it in human clinical trials. In a meta-analysis of 21 studies with 8 clinical trials and 13 observational studies, coconut oil increased TC and LDL more than PUFA, but less than butter, and increased HDL and TG with no change in the TC/HDL ratio. There was no change in CV events [78]. Coconut oil is 92% SFA, mostly lauric acid C12:0 (MCFA) and myrisitc acid (C14:0), which acts mostly like an LCFA. MCFA have rapid absorption, hepatic uptake and immediate oxidation for energy production [79]. Both lauric and myristic acids increase LDL-C similar to other MCFA and LCFA, but increase HDL-C more [80]. MCT (medium-chain triglycerides) which are C-10 or less have direct portal vein absorption and are more water soluble. Only 4% of coconut oil is MCT of C-10 or less fatty acids. Coconut oil should not be recommended at this time for prevention and treatment of CHD and CVD due to the lack of prospective studies on CV outcomes, the mixed effects on serum lipids, the content of LCFA, and the fact that replacement of coconut oil with PUFA and MUFA reduces CHD risk.

However, as a substitute for cane sugar in one's coffee, coconut oil just makes sense as sugar should be minimized in the prevention of inflammation which may lead to cardiovascular risk.

MILK, MILK PRODUCTS AND PEPTIDES

Recent clinical studies indicate that milk, milk peptides and milk products reduce BP, CHD, DM, CVA and atherosclerosis [81–83]. In a recent meta-analysis of 27 studies, there was an inverse association between total dairy intake and CVD (RR=0.90, 95% CI: 0.81–0.99), while no association was observed between total dairy intake and CHD [82]. Milk and milk products improve insulin resistance, control postprandial hyperglycemia, lower BP, increase nitric oxide, improve endothelial function, and decrease inflammation and oxidative stress [81,83]. All of these effects may reduce the risk of CHD [81–83]. Milk proteins, both caseins and whey proteins, and buttermilk with MFGM (milk fat globule membrane) are rich sources of angiotensin-converting enzyme (ACE) inhibitory peptides that significantly reduce BP [81–83]. Val-Pro-Pro (VPP) and Ile-Pro-Pro (IPP) from *Lactobacillus helveticus* in fermented milk given at 12 g/day reduce BP about 11.2/6.5 mmHg. The pooled data from the meta-analysis indicate an average reduction in BP of 4.8/2.2 mmHg with milk peptides [81–83]. Although milk products appear innocuous, they are pro-inflammatory for some individuals, and caution is advised especially in intolerant subjects.

WHEY PROTEIN

Several studies show that chronic intake of several grams (typically 20 g) of whey protein significantly reduces BP [84–87], decreases TG and cholesterol levels [88], and lowers inflammation in patients with CVD [85,89]. These benefits may come from chronic consumption rather than a single dose [90]. The type of whey protein may have impact on the results. Clinical trial data indicate that whey protein must be hydrolyzed to ACE inhibitor peptides for it to have anti-hypertensive properties [84–86,91,92]. In addition, certain whey protein preparations may result in a relatively higher insulin response relative to other protein sources [93,94] which may or may not be beneficial in some patient populations.

EGGS

The effect of egg consumption on serum cholesterol and CHD risk has been a contentious argument over the past few decades, but recent studies have provided scientific guidance. A retrospective review of 17 studies with 556 subjects found that for each 100 mg of dietary cholesterol per day in eggs, the TC increased 2.2 mg %, low-density cholesterol (LDL-C) increased 1.9 mg %, high-density cholesterol (HDL-C) increased 0.3 mg % and the TC/HDL ratio increased 0.2 units [95]. A 50 g egg contains about 200 mg of cholesterol, 6 g of protein, and 5 g of fat (36% SFA, 48% MUFA and 16% PUFA) [95].

Subjects with metabolic syndrome or type 2 diabetes mellitus (T2DM) consuming three whole eggs per day on a carbohydrate-restricted diet of less than 30% energy compared to an egg substitute, had reductions in tumor necrosis alpha (TNF alpha) and triglycerides (TG), increases in HDL-C with no change in TC, LDL, or other inflammatory markers, and a lower risk of T2DM or its progression [96,97]. In the HPFS and NHS studies with almost 18,000 subjects followed for 8–14 years, there was no evidence of any significant association between egg consumption and risk of CHD with the possible exception of T2DM [98]. However, in another study, egg consumption was not associated with any CVD outcome in individuals with T2DM [99]. In a prospective cohort study over 13 years of 37,766 men (Cohort of Swedish Men) and 32,805 women (Swedish Mammography Cohort) who were free of CVD, egg consumption was assessed at baseline with a food-frequency questionnaire [99]. There was no statistically significant association between egg consumption and risk of MI in either men or women. In the Kuopio Ischaemic Heart Disease Risk Factor Study of 1,032 men, egg and cholesterol intakes were not associated with increased CHD risk, even in ApoE4 carriers [100]. A meta-analysis of 22 independent cohorts from 16 studies, including participants ranging in number from 1.600 to 90,735 and a follow-up time from 5.8 to 20.0 years, evaluated the effect of egg consumption on CHD risk [101]. Comparison of the highest category (≥1 egg/day) of egg consumption with the lowest (<1 egg/week or none) resulted in a pooled HR of 0.96 (0.88, 1.05) for overall CVD, 0.97 (0.86, 1.09) for ischemic heart disease and 0.98 (0.77, 1.24) for ischemic heart disease mortality. This meta-analysis suggests that egg consumption is not associated with the risk of CVD and cardiac mortality in the general population. However, egg consumption may be associated with an increased incidence of T2DM among the general population and CVD comorbidity among diabetic patients of up to 42% for CHD mortality. Nevertheless, results from RCTs suggest that consumption of 6–12 eggs per week, in the context of a diet that is consistent with guidelines on cardiovascular health promotion, has no adverse effect on major CHD risk factors in individuals at risk for developing diabetes or in those with T2DM. However, heterogeneities in study design, population included and interventions prevent firm conclusions from being drawn.

REFINED CARBOHYDRATES, SUGARS AND SUGAR SUBSTITUTES

Refined carbohydrates are associated with an increased risk of CHD in prospective clinical trials and cohort studies [31,51,102,103]. Sugars, refined carbohydrates, high-fructose corn syrup (HFCS) and starches confer significant risk for dyslipidemia, nonalcoholic fatty liver disease (NAFLD) and CHD compared to omega 3 fatty acids, MUFA, fermented foods, fiber, fruits and vegetables, dairy, the TMD and DASH 2 diets [32]. A prospective study of 117,366 Chinese women and men (40–74 years of age) without history of diabetes, CHD and stroke examined intakes of carbohydrates and staple grains, glycemic index and glycemic load in relation to CHD using validated food-frequency questionnaires over a median of 7.6 years [102]. Carbohydrate intake (70% from white rice and 17% from refined wheat products) accounted for about 68% of the total energy intake. Carbohydrate intake and CHD was highly associated with hazard ratios for the lowest to highest quartiles of carbohydrate intake, respectively, were 1.00, 1.38, 2.03, and 2.88 (95% confidence interval: 1.44, 5.78; P for trend = 0.001). The combined hazard ratios comparing the highest quartile with the lowest were 1.80 (95% confidence interval: 1.01, 3.17) for refined grains and 1.87 (95% confidence interval: 1.00, 3.53) for glycemic load (both P for trend = 0.03). Prior to this Chinese study, Keller at al. [103] performed a review of intervention and longitudinal studies on the intake of sugar-sweetened beverages related to changes in BP, blood lipids and glucose levels, or CVD events such as stroke or MI. Two of the four prospective studies noted direct associations between consumption of sugar-sweetened beverages and CHD. All included studies examining vascular risk factors found direct associations between consumption of sugar-sweetened beverages and change in BP, and blood lipids and glucose levels [103]. In the NHS and HPFS, carbohydrates from refined starches and added sugars were positively associated with the risk of CHD (HR: 1.10, 95% CI: 1.00–2.1; p trend=0.04) [51]. Replacing SFA with carbohydrates from refined starches and added sugars was not significantly associated with CHD risk ($p > 0.10$) [51].

In a population-based cohort study of 39,786 subjects over 18 years, consumption of soft drink in daily diet increased the risk of total CVA by 21% and the risk of all vascular events by 43%, which includes ischemic CVA, CHD, MI and vascular death [104]. The Japan Public Health Center study showed both sugar-sweetened and low-calorie sodas significantly increased the risk of stroke by 16% per one serving a day and CHD by 20% per one serving a day [105]. Sugar substitutes increase the risk for obesity, weight gain, metabolic syndrome, T2DM and CHD. The sugar substitutes interfere with learned responses that normally contribute to glucose and energy homeostasis, negatively alter the microbiome, alter leptin levels and decrease satiety [106,107].

ADVANCED GLYCATION END PRODUCTS (AGES)

Food preparation needs to be discussed in relation to nutrition and cardiovascular health. Advanced glycation end products (AGEs) are a group of oxidant and inflammatory compounds known to play a role in the pathogenesis of chronic diseases including CVD. They are formed during the Maillard reaction in which sugars and free amino groups of proteins, lipids or nucleic acids come together through metabolism while cooking in the presence of heat. Several modern cooking methods, including industrial heat processing, grilling, broiling, roasting, searing, and frying, significantly increase dietary AGE formation and exposure [108]. A low-AGE diet may decrease endogenously circulating AGE levels, impair endothelial function, lower inflammatory mediators and reduce atherosclerosis development [109,110]. A 6-week human intervention study in diabetics fed a low-AGE diet demonstrated a marked reduction in inflammation and oxidative stress compared to a standard diet [111]. Dietary intake of AGEs can be reduced by avoiding foods known to be high in AGEs such as full-fat cheeses, meats, and highly processed foods, while increasing the consumption of fish, grains, low-fat milk products, fruits and vegetables. Boiling, poaching and stewing as well as steaming and slower cooking at a lower heat can reduce dietary AGE exposure [108].

PROTEIN

VEGETARIAN DIETS AND PLANT-BASED NUTRITION

Vegetarian diets significantly reduce CVD, CHD and coronary artery calcium (CAC) score that is proportional to the dietary intake [32,103–115]. In the European Prospective Investigation into Cancer and Nutrition (EIPC) Study of 44,561 subjects in England and Scotland followed for 11.6 years, the body mass index (BMI), blood lipid level and BP were all reduced in the vegetarian group, and there was a 32% lower incidence of CHD after adjustment for other CHD risk factors [112]. A study of 96,469 Seventh-Day Adventist men and women from 2002 to 2007 demonstrated a 12% decrease in total mortality, 15% in vegans, 9% in lacto-ovo vegetarians, 19% in pesco-vegetarians and 8% in semi-vegetarians which was primarily related to decreases in CVD [113]. The CAC score is also reduced with chronic dietary intake of fruits and vegetables [114].

A meta-analysis of nine cohort studies of 2,22,081 men and women found that the overall reduction in CHD risk was 4% for each additional portion of fruit and vegetable intake per day ($p=0.0027$) and by 7% for each additional serving of fruit ($p=0.0001$) [115]. The association between vegetable intake and CHD risk was heterogeneous ($p=0.0043$), more marked for cardiovascular mortality (0.74, $p<0.0001$) than for fatal and nonfatal MI (0.95, $p=0.0058$) [115]. Dark green-leafy vegetables had the most dramatic reduction in CHD risk. In a meta-analysis of 95 studies, for fruits and vegetables combined, the overall RR per 200 g/day was 0.92 (95% confidence interval (CI): 0.90–0.94) for CHD, 0.84 (95% CI: 0.76–0.92) and for cardiovascular disease, 0.97 (95% CI: 0.95–0.99). Similar associations were observed for fruits and vegetables separately. Reductions in risk were observed for up to 800 g/day for all outcomes. Inverse associations were observed between CHD risk and the intake of apples and pears, citrus fruits, green-leafy vegetables, cruciferous vegetables and salads [116]. Some vegetarian diets may be deficient in many nutrients which require supplemental B12, vitamin D, omega 3 fatty acids, iron, calcium, carnitine, zinc and some high-quality amino acids and protein [117]. Other studies suggest several other problems such as decreased sulfur amino acid intake with a low elemental sulfur, increased homocysteine and oxidative stress, and lower cysteine (33% of control) and glutathione (63% of controls). In addition, lean muscle mass was 10% lower, and there may be an increased risk of subclinical malnutrition and CVD [117].

ANIMAL PROTEIN DIETS

Recent studies show either no correlation or an inverse correlation of grass-fed beef, wild game, organically fed animals and other sources of protein with CHD [118–123]. The Paleolithic diet has also shown reductions in total mortality of 23% and CV mortality of 22% in a cohort study of 21,423 subjects [118]. All meats (including red meat, fish, seafood and poultry) had an inverse relationship to CVD mortality in men in Asian countries [120]. Other meta-analyses showed no association between red-meat consumption and CHD but found that processed red meat increased risk of hypertension, total mortality, CHD and T2DM [118–123]. A recently published study of over a half a million subjects answering food questionnaires that were followed for 16 years did identify a significant association between all forms of red-meat consumption, all-cause and cardiovascular mortality (https://www.ncbi.nlm.nih.gov/pubmed/28487287). In the **BOLD** (Beef in an Optimal Lean Diet Study) trial, a heart healthy diet containing lean beef with a low dietary SFA elicited a favorable effect on CHD, serum lipids and lipoproteins compared to the DASH diet [119]. This may be related to the content of certain amino acids in meat and vegetables such as lysine and arginine.

Soy Protein

A meta-analysis [124] found that soy protein intake at 15–30 g daily had favorable impacts on LDL-cholesterol, HDL-cholesterol and TG compared to non-soy controls. Data indicate that soy protein reduces LDL-cholesterol and increases HDL-cholesterol compared with milk proteins [125]. Despite the positive studies, there has been a debate about the inclusion of soy protein in the diet and whether the health claim on soy protein and heart health should be reconsidered [126,127]. Most likely, the variability in results may also be due to the heterogeneity of available soy products and their degree of processing, resulting in a variety of byproducts formed such as fermentation complexes. Thus, not all soy is equal, and the more processed it is, the more it should be avoided. Organic tofu, tempeh, and miso edamame are important sources of soy protein that one may consider.

Fish

Studies largely support fish consumption for cardiovascular health [128–141]. Park et al. [128] found that eating fish one to two times weekly, especially higher omega 3 fatty acid-containing fish, reduces risk of coronary death by 36% and total mortality by 17%. They advised eating a variety of seafood with limited intake of high mercury-containing fish with greater fish consumption (≥ 5 servings/week). Findings of a meta-analysis confirmed positive results for heart health and fish consumption. Li et al. [130] reported that fish intake reduces the risk of CHF by 6% for each 20 g of daily fish. Chowdhury et al. [132] identified a similar, yet moderate, inverse association between fish consumption and cerebrovascular risk. Gender differences may also be responsible, as a large prospective trial with 20,069 men and women followed over 8–13 years [133] found that increased fish intakes were associated with reduced stroke incidence in women, while the same association was absent in men. Active ingredients in bonito and other cold-water fish may contribute to its cardio-protective qualities, such as the presence of ACE inhibitory peptides [134–136]. Intake of sardine muscle protein, which contains Valyl–Tyrosine (Val–Tyr), by mildly hypertensive volunteers led to 9.7/5.3 mmHg reduction in BP in one week [137].

It is important to consider the type of fish and their relative methylmercury levels as well as the degree to which individuals can transport mercury based on polymorphisms for the metallothio-nein protein [138]. Methylmercury has detrimental effects that increase the risk of CHD, MI and hypertension [139–141]. Thus, larger fish such as tilefish, shark, swordfish, large grouper, and tuna may contain higher mercury levels, and consideration to caution and even omission are advised. However, the benefits of smaller fish consumption likely outweigh the risks from the potential tox-ins it contains [129].

DIETARY ACID LOAD AND PROTEIN

Diet-induced 'low-grade' metabolic acidosis is thought to play an important role in the development of cardiovascular disease, hypertension, dyslipidemia and obesity [142,143]. Vegetables, fruits, and alkali-rich beverages (red wine and coffee) are considered alkaline, while fats and oils are neutral. Meats, especially red meat, has a high acid load, and also dairy products and cereal grains are acid-producing [142,143]. Dietary acid load can be improved by increasing intake of fruits and veg-etables and decreasing excessively high dietary animal protein intake [144]. A ten-day intervention with an alkaline Paleolithic-style diet led to a marked increase in potassium levels and improve-ments in vascular reactivity, BP, glucose tolerance, insulin sensitivity and lipid profiles [144]. While the definitive effects of dietary acid load on cardiovascular health are not yet clear, it is apparent that such dietary changes are in line with the DASH and TMD.

SPECIFIC DIETARY AND NUTRITIONAL COMPONENTS AND CALORIC RESTRICTION

Several dietary and nutritional components have been shown to interrupt the inflammatory vas-cular receptors such as PRRs, nucleotide-binding oligomerization domain-like receptors, NOD-like receptors (NLRs, (NOD) and TLRs [8]. These include:

- Curcumin (from turmeric) blocks TLR 4, NOD 1, and NOD 2.
- Cinnamaldehyde (from cinnamon) blocks TLR 4.
- Sulforaphane (from broccoli) blocks TLR 4.
- Resveratrol (from nutritional supplement, red wine and grapes) blocks TLR 1.
- Epigallocatechin gallate (EGCG) (from green tea) blocks TLR 1.
- Luteolin (from celery, green pepper, rosemary, carrots, oregano, oranges and olives) blocks TLR 1.
- Quercetin (from tea, apples, onion, tomatoes and capers) blocks TLR 1.

These interactions of food groups or supplements with the vascular membrane receptors may initi-ate improved vascular responses, decreased vascular inflammation, and reduced oxidative stress and vascular immune responses that reduce CHD risk.

A prospective study of 42 subjects over 2 years showed a significant reduction in the progres-sion of CHD as assessed by CAC compared to historical controls using a phytonutrient concentrate containing a high amount of fruit and vegetable extracts. The change in the CAC score was signifi-cantly less in the treated patients compared to the control patients (19.6% vs. a 34.7%, respectively ($p < 0.009$, a 15.1% difference) [145].

CAFFEINE

The cytochrome P-450-CYP1A2 genotype modifies the association between caffeinated coffee intake and the risk of hypertension, CVD, CHD and MI in a linear relationship [146–153]. Caffeine is exclusively metabolized by CYP1A2 to paraxanthine, theobromine and theophylline [146]. The gene lies on chromosome 15q24.1, and the SNP is rs7762551 A to C [146]. The C SNP decreases enzymatic activity [146]. Caffeine also blocks vasodilating adenosine receptors [153]. The rapid metabolizers of caffeinated coffee IA/IA allele have an average BP reduction of 10/7 mm Hg and a reduced risk of MI by 17%–52% [151]. This SNP represents about 40%–45% of the population [146–151]. The slow metabolizers of caffeine IF/IF or IA/IF allele have a higher BP of 8.1/5.7 mmHg lasting >3 hours after consumption, tachycardia, increased aortic stiffness, higher PWV, vascular inflammation and increased catecholamines [146–151]. Hypertension risk is increased (1.72–3.00 RR) [147]. Based on age and consumption, the risk of MI will vary. At age 59, there was a 36% increase in MI with 2–3 cups/day and a 64% increase with 4 cups/day or more. Under the age of 59, MI increased by 24% (1 cup/day), 67% (2 cups/day) and 233% (4 or more cups/day) [151,152]. This SNP represents about 55%–60% of the population.

CALORIC RESTRICTION

Caloric restriction refers to reduction of energy intake at the individualized level that is sufficient to maintain a slightly low to normal body weight (i.e. BMI < 21 kg/m^2) without causing malnutrition [154]. Findings from long-term calorie restriction in animal models have revealed improvements in metabolic health, offsetting chronic disease and consequently extending life span [155].

Animal studies on caloric restriction at 40% have identified cardiovascular benefits, including reductions in oxidative stress and inflammation in the heart and vasculature, beneficial effects on endothelial function and arterial stiffness, protection against atherosclerosis and less detrimental age-related changes in the heart [156]. Limited evidence from human data suggests some of these effects translate to human caloric restriction [157]. Fasting mimicking diet (FMD), alternate-day intermittent fasting (ADF) and 14-hour overnight fasting are good approaches with cardiovascular benefit. Typically, ADF involves consuming 25% of energy needs on the fast day and ad libitum food intake on the following day [158]. Results indicate weight loss and improvements in cardio-metabolic health such as reductions in aortic vascular smooth muscle cell proliferation, C-reactive protein, adiponectin, leptin, TC, LDL-cholesterol, triacylglycerol concentrations and systolic BP and increases in LDL particle size in a relatively short time period [159]. Caloric restriction could be implemented by constructing a personalized diet based on nutrient-dense, low-energy foods such as vegetables, fruits, whole grains, nuts, fish, low-fat dairy products and lean meats [160].

ALCOHOL

The connection between alcohol consumption and CHD is based on a U-shaped curve such that over- or underconsumption is not as likely to reduce CHD as the base of the U-shaped curve is associated with the lowest risk of CHD [161–163]. A drink in most research studies is 14 g of ethanol or 0.6 fluid ounces of pure alcohol. This equates to a 12 oz beer, a 5 oz glass of table wine, or 1.5 oz of hard liquor [161]. "Light to moderate" drinking (defined as 1 drink a day for women and 2 drinks a day for men) is associated with lower rates of total mortality, CHD morbidity and mortality, diabetes mellitus, heart failure and strokes especially in people over 50 years of age [161–163]. This was confirmed in an analysis of studies combining data on over 1 million people and overall death rates where the U-shaped curve was best at 1–2 drinks/day for women and 2–4 drinks/day for men [162]. There are many beneficial effects of alcohol, including enhancing insulin action, raising HDL-cholesterol, reducing inflammation, and improving arterial function. Red wine, in particular, is rich in polyphenols, with antioxidant, anti-inflammatory, and antiplatelet actions [161,162].

In a recent review and meta-analysis of alcohol consumption and cardiovascular disease, light to moderate alcohol consumption [163], the reduction in risk for CHD 29% and all-cause mortality was also reduced by 13%. Pinot noir is generally credited with having the highest concentration of the potent polyphenol resveratrol, and the grape cannonau from the island of Sardinia, Italy, has been associated with the exceptional longevity in those communities [161–163].

GLUTEN

About 1% of the public has celiac disease, and perhaps another 6%–7% have verified gluten sensitivity with dramatic changes in the appearance of their gastrointestinal tract [164]. A key consequence of the damage to the intestinal wall lining is that the normally tight junctions that bind cells lining the gastrointestinal (GI) tract become loose. When these junctions are loose, the contents of the GI tract can enter the wall of the bowels and then enter into the bloodstream. Many studies have shown that after a fatty meal, a wave of inflammation and endotoxins enter the bloodstream and may remain present for hours [6,9,10]. When gliadin, a component of gluten-containing foods like bread, is present in the intestines of those with celiac or gluten sensitivity, a newly discovered protein called zonulin is released into the gut [164]. Zonulin is now thought to have a potential role not only in celiac disease but also in type 1 diabetes, obesity and other immune illnesses [164]. Zonulin has been shown to be the "crowbar" that opens tight junctions and leads to autoimmune responses such as a leaky GI tract [164]. The ability to measure blood levels of zonulin may revolutionize our understanding of GI, autoimmune, and other systemic diseases. A pharmaceutical molecule that is a zonulin blocker (AT-1001) is being developed to determine if a patient with celiac disease can consume wheat products without damage.

There are little data linking gluten and CHD. In an analysis of patients who had suffered an MI in Sweden, those with celiac disease had similar outcomes to those without celiac disease [165]. There are case reports of cardiomyopathy being associated with gluten sensitivities that respond to withdrawal foods [166]. In another case report, a review of gluten antibodies and proven celiac disease was reported in nine additional cases of cardiomyopathy [167].

Generally, 100% whole grains, as opposed to processed white flour-based foods, are to be encouraged to patients with CHD. A meta-analysis that examined whole grain consumption and the risk of developing CHD and MI in more than 400,000 participants found that the highest consumption of whole grains reduced the risk by about 25% [168]. The authors indicated that whole grain foods contain fiber, vitamins, minerals, phytoestrogens and phenolic compounds, and also have a favorable effect on measures of cholesterol, blood glucose, inflammation and arterial function. In a 26-year follow-up of 64,714 women in the NHS and 45,303 men in the HPFS, dietary gluten intake was not associated with the risk of CHD (fatal or nonfatal MI) [169]. After adjustment for known risk factors, participants in the highest fifth of estimated gluten intake had a multivariable HR for CHD of 0.95 (95% confidence interval 0.88–1.02; P for trend=0.29). After additional adjustment for intake of whole grains, the multivariate HR was 1.00 (0.92–1.09; P for trend=0.77). In contrast, after additional adjustment for intake of refined grains, the estimated gluten consumption was associated with a lower risk of CHD (multivariate HR 0.85, 0.77–0.93; P for trend=0.002) [169].

NUTS

Nuts are high in MUFA and PUFA, but they may also contain some omega 6 fatty acids. The beneficial effects of nut consumption on cardiovascular disease, CV deaths, CHD and MI were well documented in the PREDIMED trial with a reduction in total CV death of 28% [15–18]. In the Adventist Health Study which examined obesity and metabolic syndrome in more than 800 people, there was a strong inverse relationship between tree nut consumption and developing both medical conditions [170]. Other studies suggest that eating tree nuts does not lead to weight gain and the high concentration of fiber and nutrients offsets the calories consumed. Nuts may reduce CHD deaths and all-cause mortality as well [15–18,171]. In a larger analysis of the Adventist Health Study examining death in residents aged over 84 years, consuming nuts >5 times a week had a 20% reduction in total mortality and 40% reduction in CHD mortality [171]. The impact of including nuts in the diet has been analyzed in a recent large meta-analysis [172]. The habit of eating 28 g of nuts/day reduced the risk for CHD by 0.71, for stroke, 0.93, for all cardiovascular disease and 0.79 for all-cause mortality. It was estimated that 4 million deaths could be avoided per year worldwide by eating a handful of nuts. In an even more recent analysis of dietary habits and outcome, inadequate nut intake was associated with increased cardiometabolic deaths as were the consumption of excess salt, excess sugar, sweetened beverages, inadequate vegetables and the consumption of processed meats [173]. In a study of 40 subjects comparing a walnut-enriched diet to a control diet over 8 weeks, the walnut diet reduced TC and apolipoprotein B [174]. Walnuts also significantly improve endothelial function [175].

DIETARY SODIUM, POTASSIUM AND MAGNESIUM

Increased dietary sodium is associated with an increased risk of hypertension, CHD, MI, CHF, CVA, renal insufficiency and proteinuria [176–182]. Approximately 75 million people in the United States and up to 1 billion worldwide have been diagnosed with hypertension [176–182]. Up to 50% cardiovascular-related deaths result from hypertension.

The sodium–potassium ratio may be more important that the actual dietary sodium and potassium intake and the association with CHD [176]. A number of population studies demonstrate that higher dietary potassium, as rated by urinary excretion or dietary recall, is generally associated with lower BP and CHD regardless of the level of sodium intake [176–182]. According to a report of the Institute of Medicine, adult recommendations are to consume at least 4.7 g of potassium daily to control BP and reduce dietary sodium intake to about 1.5–2 g/day [2,4,176–182]. The potassium–sodium ratio should be greater than 2.5–3.0 [2,4,176–182]. Foods high in potassium include bran, mushrooms, macadamia nuts and almonds, dark leafy greens, avocados, apricots, fruits and acorn squash.

The sodium–potassium ratio was evaluated recently in a South Korean study [177]. The study population was constructed by pooling the Korean National Health and Nutrition Examination Surveys between 2010 and 2014. The study groups were divided into quartiles based on the sodium–potassium ratio. The quartiles with the higher sodium–potassium ratio had greater hypertension prevalence rates. Significantly higher systolic and diastolic BPs were observed in the second quartiles compared to the first quartiles. A strong association was also detected between the sodium–potassium ratio and blood pressure even at a low level of sodium–potassium ratio.

The role of dietary magnesium in cardiovascular health is important and supported by many studies. It is estimated that nearly half of the US population consume less than the recommended amount of magnesium in their diets, and magnesium deficiency is a commonly overlooked risk factor for cardiovascular disease [178]. The lower the dietary intake of magnesium, the greater the risk of succumbing to cardiovascular disease. Magnesium supplementation can be therapeutic for a range of cardiovascular issues including arrhythmias, hypertension, atherosclerosis and endothelial dysfunction. Magnesium is critical for tissues that have electrical or mechanical activity, such as nerves, muscles (including the heart), and blood vessels [178]. In a 6-month study of patients with known ischemic heart disease, magnesium supplementation led to an impressive *decrease* in angina attacks and a *decrease* in the use of antianginal drugs such as nitroglycerin by improving endothelial function [179]. In patients on dialysis, magnesium supplements had improved arterial remodeling and elasticity [180].

In a recent analysis of a group of hypertensive women randomized to magnesium supplements or placebo, no change in measurements of carotid intimal medial thickening (IMT) occurred in the group given magnesium, while the carotid IMT worsened over 6 months in the placebo group [181]. There was also an improvement in flow-mediated dilation in the magnesium-treated group. In another study, researchers investigated the relationship between dietary magnesium intake and mortality from cardiovascular disease in a sample of Asian adults [182]. The Japan Collaborative Cohort (JACC) study assessed dietary intake in 58,615 healthy Japanese aged 40–79 years by food-frequency questionnaires with a median of 14.7-year follow-up. Overall, there were 2,690 deaths from cardiovascular disease, comprising 1,227 deaths from strokes and 557 deaths from CHD. Dietary magnesium intake was inversely associated with mortality from hemorrhagic stroke in men and with mortality from total and ischemic strokes, CHD, CHF and total cardiovascular disease in women. Increased dietary magnesium intake was associated with reduced mortality from cardiovascular disease in the population.

SUMMARY AND CONCLUSIONS

The role of nutrition in the prevention and treatment of CHD has been clearly demonstrated in published clinical trials. The top five cardiovascular risk factors, as presently defined, are not an adequate explanation for the current limitations to prevent and reduce CHD. Proper definition and analysis of the top five CV risk factors, evaluation of the three finite responses, and sound nutritional advice and evaluation based the scientific studies will be required to effect an improvement in the risk of CHD. Early detection of CHD coupled with aggressive prevention and treatment of all cardiovascular risk factors will diminish the progression of functional and structural cardiovascular abnormalities and clinical CHD. Utilization of targeted, personalized and precision treatments with optimal nutrition coupled with exercise, ideal weight and body composition and discontinuation of all tobacco use can prevent approximately 80% of CHD. The published nutritional studies provide evidence that CHD can be reduced with a weighted plant-based diet with ten servings of fruits and vegetables per day; intake of MUFA, PUFA, nuts, whole grains and cold-water fish; DASH diets; PREDIMED-TMD diet; reduction of refined carbohydrates and sugars; consumption of high glycemic load and index foods, sugar substitutes, HFCS, long-chain SFAs and processed foods; and elimination of all TFAs.

Eggs and dairy products are not associated with CHD with the possible exception eggs consumption on the risk of CHD in T2DM. Coconut oil is not recommended unless if used as substitute for cane sugar. Organic, grass-fed beef and wild game may reduce CHD. High intakes of potassium and magnesium are recommended in conjunction with sodium restriction. Caffeine intake should be adjusted depending on the genetic ability to metabolize it via the CYP 1A2 system. Alcohol is associated with a U-shaped curve and CHD. The role of gluten, soy and caloric restriction and CHD in humans will require more studies.

REFERENCES

1. Yusuf S, Hawken S, Ounpuu S, Dans T, Avezum A, Lanas F, McQueen M, Budaj A, Pais P, Varigos J, Lisheng L; Effect of potentially modifiable risk factors associated with myocardial infarction in 52 countries (the INTERHEART study)—case-control study. INTERHEART study investigators. *Lancet.* 2004;364(9438):937–52.
2. Houston Mark C. *What Your Doctor May Not Tell You About Heart Disease. The Revolutionary Book that Reveals the Truth Behind Coronary Illnesses and How You Can Fight Them. Grand Central Life and Style.* Hachette Book Group: New York. 2012.
3. O'Donnell CJ, Nabel EG. Genomics of cardiovascular disease. *N Engl J Med.* 2011;365(22):2098–109.
4. Houston MC. Nutrition and nutraceutical supplements in the treatment of hypertension. *Expert Rev Cardiovasc Ther.* 2010;8:821–33.
5. ACCORD Study Group, Gerstein HC, Miller ME, Genuth S, Ismail-Beigi F, Buse JB, Goff DC Jr, Probstfield JL, Cushman WC, Ginsberg HN, Bigger JT, Grimm RH Jr, Byington RP, Rosenberg YD, Friedewald WT. Long-term effects of intensive glucose lowering on cardiovascular outcomes. *N Engl J Med.* 2011;364(9):818–28.
6. Youssef-Elabd EM, McGee KC, Tripathi G, et al. Acute and chronic saturated fatty acid treatment as a key instigator of the TLR-mediated inflammatory response in human adipose tissue, in vitro. *J Nutr Biochem.* 2012;23:39–50.

7. El Khatib N, Génieys S, Kazmierczak B, Volpert V. Mathematical modelling of atherosclerosis as an inflammatory disease. *Philos Trans A Math Phys Eng Sci.* 2009;367(1908):4877–86.
8. Zhao L, Lee JY, Hwang DH. Inhibition of pattern recognition receptor-mediated inflammation by bioactive phytochemicals. *Nutr Rev.* 2011;69(6):310–20.
9. Mah E, Bruno RS. Postprandial hyperglycemia on vascular endothelial function—mechanisms and consequences. *Nutr Res.* 2012;32(10):727–40.
10. Houston MC. The role of nutraceutical supplements in the treatment of dyslipidemia. *J Clin Hypertens (Greenwich).* 2012;14(2):121–32.
11. Houston MC. *Handbook of Hypertension.* Wiley-Blackwell: Oxford. 2009.
12. Della Rocca DG, Pepine CJ. Endothelium as a predictor of adverse outcomes. *Clin Cardiol.* 2010;33(12):730–2.
13. Houston MC The role of cellular micronutrient analysis, nutraceuticals, vitamins, antioxidants and minerals in the prevention and treatment of hypertension and cardiovascular disease. *Ther Adv Cardiovasc Dis.* 2010;4(3):165–83.
14. Freeman AM, Morris PB, Barnard N, et al. Trending cardiovascular nutrition controversies. *J Am Coll Cardiol.* 2017 Mar 7;69(9):1172–87. doi: 10.1016/j.jacc.2016.10.086.
15. Sofi F, Abbate R, Gensini GF, Casini A. Accruing evidence on benefits of adherence to the Mediterranean diet on health—an updated systematic review and meta-analysis. *Am J Clin Nutr.* 2010;92(5):1189–96.
16. Estruch R, Ros E, Salas-Salvadó J, Covas MI, Corella D, Arós F, Gómez-Gracia E, Ruiz-Gutiérrez V, Fiol M, Lapetra J, Lamuela-Raventos RM, Serra-Majem L, Pintó X, Basora J, Muñoz MA, Sorlí JV, Martínez JA, Martínez-González MA, PREDIMED Study Investigators. Primary prevention of cardiovascular disease with a Mediterranean diet. *N Engl J Med.* 2013;368(14):1279–90.
17. Nadtochiy SM, Redman EK. Mediterranean diet and cardioprotection—the role of nitrite, polyunsaturated fatty acids, and polyphenols. *Nutrition.* 2011;27(7–8):733–44.
18. Salas-Salvadó J, Bulló M, Estruch R, Ros E, Covas MI, Ibarrola-Jurado N, Corella D, Arós F, Gómez-Gracia E, Ruiz-Gutiérrez V, Romaguera D, Lapetra J, Lamuela-Raventós RM, Serra-Majem L, Pintó X, Basora J, Muñoz MA, Sorlí JV, Martínez-González MA. Prevention of diabetes with Mediterranean diets—a subgroup analysis of a randomized trial. *Ann Intern Med.* 2014;160(1):1–10.
19. de Lorgeril M, Salen P, Martin JL, Monjaud I, Delaye J, Mamelle N. Mediterranean diet, traditional risk factors, and the rate of cardiovascular complications after myocardial infarction—final report of the Lyon Diet Heart Study. *Circulation.* 1999;99(6):779–85.
20. Buckland G, Mayén AL, Agudo A, Travier N, Navarro C, Huerta JM, Chirlaque MD, Barricarte A, Ardanaz E, Moreno-Iribas C, Marin P, Quirós JR, Redondo ML, Amiano P, Dorronsoro M, Arriola L, Molina E, Sanchez MJ, Gonzalez CA. Olive oil intake and mortality within the Spanish population (EPIC-Spain). *Am J Clin Nutr.* 2012;96(1):142–9.
21. Castañer O, Corella D, Covas MI, Sorlí JV, Subirana I, Flores-Mateo G, Nonell L, Bulló M, de la Torre R, Portolés O, Fitó M, PREDIMED Study Investigators. In vivo transcriptomic profile after a Mediterranean diet in high-cardiovascular risk patients—a randomized controlled trial. *Am J Clin Nutr.* 2013;98(3):845–5.
22. Konstantinidou V, Covas MI, Sola R, Fitó M. Up-to date knowledge on the in vivo transcriptomic effect of the Mediterranean diet in humans. *Mol Nutr Food Res.* 2013;57(5):772–83.
23. Corella D, Ordovás JM. How does the Mediterranean diet promote cardiovascular health? Current progress toward molecular mechanisms—gene-diet interactions at the genomic, transcriptomic, and epigenomic levels provide novel insights into new mechanisms. *Bioessays.* 2014;36(5):526–37.
24. Appel LJ, Moore TJ, Obarzanek E, Vollmer WM, Svetkey LP, Sacks FM, Bray GA, Vogt TM, Cutler JA, Windhauser MM, Lin PH, Karanja N, DASH Collaborative Research Group. A clinical trial of the effects of dietary patterns on blood pressure. *N Engl J Med.* 1997;336(16):1117–24.
25. Sacks FM, Svetkey LP, Vollmer WM, Appel LJ, Bray GA, Harsha D, Obarzanek E, Conlin PR, Miller ER 3rd, Simons-Morton DG, Karanja N, Lin PH, DASH-Sodium Collaborative Research Group. Effects on blood pressure of reduced dietary sodium and the dietary approaches to stop hypertension (DASH) diet. *N Engl J Med.* 2001;344(1):3–10.
26. Fung TT Chiuve SE, McCullough ML, Rexrode KM, Logroscino G, Hu FB. Adherence to a DASH-style diet and risk of coronary heart disease and stroke in women. *Arch Intern Med.* 2008;168(7):713–20.
27. Chowdhury R, Warnakula S, Kunutsor S, Crowe F, Ward HA, Johnson L, Franco OH, Butterworth AS, Forouhi NG, Thompson SG, Khaw KT, Mozaffarian D, Danesh J, Di Angelantonio E. Association of dietary, circulating, and supplement fatty acids with coronary risk—a systematic review and meta-analysis. *Ann Intern Med.* 2014;160(6):398–406.

28. Guasch-Ferré M, Babio N, Martínez-González MA, Corella D, Ros E, Martín-Peláez S, Estruch R, Arós F, Gómez-Gracia E, Fiol M, Santos-Lozano JM, Serra-Majem L, Bulló M, Toledo E, Barragán R, Fitó M, Gea A, Salas-Salvadó J, PREDIMED Study Investigators. Dietary fat intake and risk of cardiovascular disease and all-cause mortality in a population at high risk of cardiovascular disease. *Am J Clin Nutr.* 2015;102(6):1563–73.

29. Ravnskov U, DiNicolantonio JJ, Harcombe Z Kummerow FA, Okuyama H, Worm N. The questionable benefits of exchanging saturated fat with polyunsaturated fat. *Mayo Clin Proc.* 2014;89(4):451–3.

30. Alexander DD, Miller PE, Van Elswyk ME, Kuratko CN, Bylsma LC. A meta-analysis of randomized controlled trials and prospective cohort studies of eicosapentaenoic and docosahexaenoic long-chain omega-3 fatty acids and coronary heart disease risk. *Mayo Clin Proc.* 2017:92(1):15–29.

31. DiNicolantonio JJ, Lucan SC, O'Keefe JH. The evidence for saturated fat and for sugar related to coronary heart disease. *Prog Cardiovasc Dis.* 2016;58(5):464–72.

32. Siri-Tarino PW, Krauss RM. Diet, lipids, and cardiovascular disease. *Curr Opin Lipidol.* 2016;27(4):323–8.

33. Adamson S, Leitinger N. Phenotypic modulation of macrophages in response to plaque lipids. *Curr Opin Lipidol.* 2011;22(5):335–42.

34. Dow CA, Stauffer BL, Greiner JJ, DeSouza CA. Influence of dietary saturated fat intake on endothelial fibrinolytic capacity in adults. *Am J Cardiol.* 2014;114(5):783–8.

35. Santos S, Oliveira A, Lopes C. Systematic review of saturated fatty acids on inflammation and circulating levels of adipokines. *Nutr Res.* 2013;33(9):687–95.

36. Ruiz-Núñez B, Kuipers RS, Luxwolda MF, De Graaf DJ, Breeuwsma BB, Dijck-Brouwer DA, Muskiet FA. Saturated fatty acid (SFA) status and SFA intake exhibit different relations with serum total cholesterol and lipoprotein cholesterol—a mechanistic explanation centered around lifestyle-induced low-grade inflammation. *J Nutr Biochem.* 2014;25(3):304–12.

37. Forsythe CE, Phinney SD, Fernandez ML, Quann EE, Wood RJ, Bibus DM, Kraemer WJ, Feinman RD, Volek JS. Comparison of low fat and low carbohydrate diets on circulating fatty acid composition and markers of inflammation. *Lipids.* 2008;43(1):65–77.

38. Volek JS, Fernandez ML, Feinman RD, Phinney SD. Dietary carbohydrate restriction induces a unique metabolic state positively affecting atherogenic dyslipidemia, fatty acid partitioning, and metabolic syndrome. *Prog Lipid Res.* 2008;47(5):307–18.

39. Peña-Orihuela P, Camargo A, Rangel-Zuñiga OA, Perez-Martinez P, Cruz-Teno C, Delgado-Lista J, Yubero-Serrano EM, Paniagua JA, Tinahones FJ, Malagon MM, Roche HM, Perez-Jimenez F, Lopez-Miranda J. Antioxidant system response is modified by dietary fat in adipose tissue of metabolic syndrome patients. *J Nutr Biochem.* 2013;24(10):1717–23.

40. Devkota S, Wang Y, Musch MW, Leone V, Fehlner-Peach H, Nadimpalli A, Antonopoulos DA, Jabri B, Chang EB. Dietary-fat-induced taurocholic acid promotes pathobiont expansion and colitis in Il10−/− mice. *Nature.* 2012;487(7405):104–8.

41. Ma W, Wu JH, Wang Q, Lemaitre RN, Mukamal KJ, Djoussé L King IB, Song X, Biggs ML, Delaney JA, Kizer JR, Siscovick DS, Mozaffarian D. Prospective association of fatty acids in the de novo lipogenesis pathway with risk of type 2 diabetes—the cardiovascular health study. *Am J Clin Nutr.* 2015;101(1):153–63.

42. Praagman J, Beulens JW, Alssema M, Zock PL, Wanders AJ, Sluijs I, van der Schouw YT. The association between dietary saturated fatty acids and ischemic heart disease depends on the type and source of fatty acid in the European prospective investigation into cancer and nutrition-Netherlands cohort. *Am J Clin Nutr.* 2016;103(2):356–65.

43. Chen M, Li Y, Sun Q, Pan A, Manson JE, Rexrode KM, Willett WC, Rimm EB, Hu FB. Dairy fat and risk of cardiovascular disease in 3 cohorts of US adults. *Am J Clin Nutr.* 2016;104(5):1209–17.

44. Zong G, Li Y, Wanders AJ, Alssema M, Zock PL, Willett WC, Hu FB, Sun Q. Intake of individual saturated fatty acids and risk of coronary heart disease in US men and women—two prospective longitudinal cohort studies. *BMJ.* 2016 Nov 23;355:i5796.

45. Micha R, Mozaffarian D. Saturated fat and cardiometabolic risk factors, coronary heart disease, stroke, and diabetes—a fresh look at the evidence. *Lipids.* 2010;45(10):893–905.

46. de Souza RJ, Mente A, Maroleanu A, Cozma AI, Ha V, Kishibe T, Uleryk E, Budylowski P, Schünemann H, Beyene J, Anand SS. Intake of saturated and trans unsaturated fatty acids and risk of all-cause mortality, cardiovascular disease, and type 2 diabetes—systematic review and meta-analysis of observational studies. *BMJ.* 2015;351:h3978.

47. Ruiz-Núñez B, Dijck-Brouwer DA, Muskiet FA The relation of saturated fatty acids with low-grade inflammation and cardiovascular disease. J Nutr Biochem. 2016;36:1–20.

48. Chang LF, Vethakkan SR, Nesaretnam K, Sanders TA, Teng KT. Adverse effects on insulin secretion of replacing saturated fat with refined carbohydrate but not with monounsaturated fat—a randomized controlled trial in centrally obese subjects. *J Clin Lipidol*. 2016;10(6):1431–41.

49. Zock PL, Blom WA, Nettleton JA, Hornstra G. Progressing insights into the role of dietary fats in the prevention of cardiovascular disease. *Curr Cardiol Rep*. 2016 Nov;18(11):111.

50. Ros E, López-Miranda J, Picó C, Rubio MÁ, Babio N, Sala-Vila A, Pérez-Jiménez F, Escrich E, Bulló M, Solanas M, Gil Hernández A, Salas-Salvadó J. Consensus on fats and oils in the diet of S ISH adults; position paper of the Spanish Federation of Food, Nutrition and Dietetics Societies. *Nutr Hosp*. 2015 Aug 1;32(2):435–77.

51. Li Y, Hruby A, Bernstein AM, Ley SH, Wang DD, Chiuve SE, Sampson L, Rexrode KM, Rimm EB, Willett WC, Hu FB. Saturated fats compared with unsaturated fats and sources of carbohydrates in relation to risk of coronary heart disease—a prospective cohort study. *J Am Coll Cardiol*. 2015;66(14):1538–48.

52. Flock MR, Kris-Etherton PM. Diverse physiological effects of long-chain saturated fatty acids—implications for cardiovascular disease. *Curr Opin Clin Nutr Metab Care*. 2013;16(2):133–40.

53. Hooper L, Summerbell CD, Thompson R, Sills D, Roberts FG, Moore HJ, Smith GD. Reduced or modified dietary fat for preventing cardiovascular disease. *Sao Paulo Med J*. 2016;134(2):182–3.

54. Björck L, Rosengren A, Winkvist A, Capewell S, Adiels M, Bandosz P, Critchley J, Boman K, Guzman-Castillo M, O'Flaherty M, Johansson I. Changes in dietary fat intake and projections for coronary heart disease mortality in Sweden—a simulation study. *PLoS One*. 2016;11(8):e0160474. doi: 10.1371/journal.pone.0160474. eCollection 2016.

55. Williams CM, Salter A. Saturated fatty acids and coronary heart disease risk—the debate goes on. *Curr Opin Clin Nutr Metab Care*. 2016;19(2):97–102.

56. Dawczynski C, Kleber ME, März W, Jahreis G, Lorkowski S. Saturated fatty acids are not off the hook. *Nutr Metab Cardiovasc Dis*. 2015;25(12):1071–8.

57. Finzi AA, Latini R, Barlera S, Rossi MG, Ruggeri A, Mezzani A, Favero C, Franzosi MG, Serra D, Lucci D, Bianchini F, Bernasconi R, Maggioni AP, Nicolosi G, Porcu M, Tognoni G, Tavazzi L, Marchioli R. Effects of n-3 polyunsaturated fatty acids on malignant ventricular arrhythmias in patients with chronic heart failure and implantable cardioverter-defibrillators—a substudy of the Gruppo Italiano per lo Studio della Sopravvivenza nell'Insufficienza Cardiaca (GISSI-HF) trial. *Am Heart J*. 2011;161(2):338–43.

58. Mozaffarian D, Lemaitre RN, King IB, Song X, Huang H, Sacks FM, Rimm EB, Wang M, Siscovick DS. Plasma phospholipid long-chain ω-3 fatty acids and total and cause-specific mortality in older adults—a cohort study. *Ann Intern Med*. 2013;158(7):515–25.

59. Gajos G, Zalewski J, Rostoff P, Nessler J, Piwowarska W, Undas A. Reduced thrombin formation and altered fibrin clot properties induced by polyunsaturated omega-3 fatty acids on top of dual antiplatelet therapy in patients undergoing percutaneous coronary intervention (OMEGA-PCI clot). *Arterioscler Thromb Vasc Biol*. 2011;31(7):1696–702.

60. Davis W, Rockway S, Kwasny M. Effect of a combined therapeutic approach of intensive lipid management, omega-3 fatty acid supplementation, and increased serum 25 (OH) vitamin D on coronary calcium scores in asymptomatic adults. *Am J Ther*. 2009;16(4):326–32.

61. Nozue T, Yamamoto S, Tohyama S, Fukui K, Umezawa S, Onishi Y, Kunishima T, Sato A, Nozato T, Miyake S, Takeyama Y, Morino Y, Yamauchi T, Muramatsu T, Hibi K, Terashima M, Michishita I. Effects of serum n-3 to n-6 polyunsaturated fatty acids ratios on coronary atherosclerosis in statin-treated patients with coronary artery disease. *Am J Cardiol*. 2013;111(1):6–11.

62. Greene SJ, Temporelli PL, Campia U, Vaduganathan M, Degli Esposti L Buda S, Veronesi C, Butler J, Nodari S. Effects of polyunsaturated fatty acid treatment on postdischarge outcomes after acute myocardial infarction. *Am J Cardiol*. 2016;117(3):340–6.

63. Arnesen H. N-3 fatty acids and revascularization procedures. *Lipids*. 2001;36:S103–6.

64. Arnesen H, Seljeflot I. Studies on very long chain marine n-3 fatty acids in patients with atherosclerotic heart disease with special focus on mechanisms, dosage and formulas of supplementation. *Cell Mol Biol (Noisy-le-grand)*. 2010;56(1):18–27.

65. Sekikawa A, Miura K, Lee S, Fujiyoshi A, Edmundowicz D, Kadowaki T, Evans RW, Kadowaki S, Sutton-Tyrrell K, Okamura T, Bertolet M, Masaki KH, Nakamura Y, Barinas-Mitchell EJ, Willcox BJ, Kadota A, Seto TB, Maegawa H, Kuller LH, Ueshima H, ERA JUMP Study Group. Long chain n-3 polyunsaturated fatty acids and incidence rate of coronary artery calcification in Japanese men in Japan and white men in the USA—population based prospective cohort study. *Heart*. 2014;100(7):569–73.

66. Abedin M, Lim J, Tang TB, Park D, Demer LL, Tintut Y. N-3 fatty acids inhibit vascular calcification via the p38-mitogen-activated protein kinase and peroxisome proliferator-activated receptor-gamma pathways. *Circ Res.* 2006;98(6):727–9.

67. Jacobson TA, Glickstein SB, Rowe JD, Soni PN. Effects of eicosapentaenoic acid and docosa-hexaenoic acid on low-density lipoprotein cholesterol and other lipids—a review. *J Clin Lipidol.* 2012;6(1):5–18.

68. Jans A, Konings E, Goossens GH, Bouwman FG, Moors CC, Boekschoten MV, Afman LA, Müller M, Mariman EC, Blaak EE. PUFAs acutely affect triacylglycerol-derived skeletal muscle fatty acid uptake and increase postprandial insulin sensitivity. *Am J Clin Nutr.* 2012;95(4):825–36.

69. García-López S, Arriaga RE, Medina ON, López CP, Figueroa-Valverde L, Cervera EG, Skidmore OM, Rosas-Nexticapa M. One month of omega-3 fatty acid supplementation improves lipid profiles, glucose levels and blood pressure in overweight schoolchildren with metabolic syndrome. *J Pediatr Endocrinol Metab.* 2016;29(10):1143–50.

70. Bernasconi AA, Wiest MM, Lavie CJ, Milani RV, Laukkanen JA. Meta-analysis effect of omega-3 dosage on cardiovascular outcomes—an updated meta-analysis and meta-regression of interventional trials. *Mayo Clin Proc.* 2021 Feb;96(2):304–13.

71. Abdelhamid AS, Brown TJ, Brainard JS, Biswas P, Thorpe GC, Moore HJ, Deane KH, Summerbell CD, Worthington HV, Song F, Hooper L. Omega-3 fatty acids for the primary and secondary prevention of cardiovascular disease. *Cochrane Database Syst Rev.* 2020 Feb 29;3(2):1–34.

72. Joris PJ, Mensink RP. Role of cis-monounsaturated fatty acids in the prevention of coronary heart disease. *Curr Atheroscler Rep.* 2016;18(7):38.

73. Abdullah MM, Jew S, Jones PJ. Health benefits and evaluation of healthcare cost savings if oils rich in monounsaturated fatty acids were substituted for conventional dietary oils in the United States. *Nutr Rev.* 2017 Feb 1. doi: 10.1093/nutrit/nuw062 [Epub ahead of print].

74. Mölenberg FJ, de Goede J, Wanders AJ, Zock PL, Kromhout D, Geleijnse JM. Dietary fatty acid intake after myocardial infarction—a theoretical substitution analysis of the alpha omega cohort. *Am J Clin Nutr.* 2017 Aug 9. doi: 10.3945/ajcn.117.157826 [Epub ahead of print].

75. Wand DD, Li Y, Chiuve S, et al. Specific dietary fats in relation to total and cause-specific mortality. *JAMA Intern Med.* 2016;176(8):1134–45.

76. Trumbo PR, Shimakawa T. Tolerable upper intake levels for trans fat, saturated fat, and cholesterol. *Nutr Rev.* 2011;69(5):270–8.

77. Nestel P. Trans fatty acids—are its cardiovascular risks fully appreciated? *Clin Ther.* 2014;36(3):315–21.

78. Eyres L, Eyres MF, Chisholm A, Brown RC. Coconut oil consumption and cardiovascular risk factors in humans. *Nutr Rev.* 2016;74(4):267–80.

79. DeLany JP, Windhauser MM, Champagne CM, Bray GA. Differential oxidation of individual dietary fatty acids in humans. *Am J Clin Nutr.* 2000;72(4):905–11.

80. Feranil AB, Duazo PL, Kuzawa CW, Adair LS. Coconut oil is associated with a beneficial lipid profile in pre-menopausal women in the Philippines. *Asia Pac J Clin Nutr.* 2011;20(2):190–5.

81. Ballard KD, Bruno RS. Protective role of dairy and its constituents on vascular function independent of blood pressure-lowering activities. *Nutr Rev.* 2015;73(1):36–50.

82. Khoramdad M, Esmailnasab N, Moradi G, Nouri B, Safiri S, Alimohamadi Y. The effect of dairy consumption on the prevention of cardiovascular diseases—a meta-analysis of prospective studies. *J Cardiovasc Thorac Res.* 2017;9(1):1–11. doi: 10.15171/jcvtr.2017.01. [Epub 2017 Mar 18].

83. Chrysant SG, Chrysant GS. An update on the cardiovascular pleiotropic effects of milk and milk products. *J Clin Hypertens (Greenwich).* 2013;15(7):503–10.

84. FitzGerald RJ, Murray BA, Walsh DJ. Hypotensive peptides from milk proteins. *J Nutr.* 2004 Apr;134(4):980S–8S.

85. Pins JJ, Keenan JM. Effects of whey peptides on cardiovascular disease risk factors. *J Clin Hypertens (Greenwich).* 2006 Nov;8(11):775–82. Retraction in *J Clin Hypertens (Greenwich).* 2008 Aug;10(8):631.

86. Aihara K, Kajimoto O, Takahashi R, Nakamura Y. Effect of powdered fermented milk with Lactobacillus helveticus on subjects with high-normal blood pressure or mild hypertension. *J Am Coll Nutr.* 2005;24(4):257–65.

87. Sousa GT, Lira FS, Rosa JC, de Oliveira EP, Oyama LM, Santos RV, Pimentel GD. Dietary whey protein lessens several risk factors for metabolic diseases—a review. *Lipids Health Dis.* 2012 Jul 10;11:67.

88. Berthold HK, Schulte DM, Lapointe JF, Lemieux P, Krone W, Gouni-Berthold I. The whey fermentation product malleable protein matrix decreases triglyceride concentrations in subjects with hypercho-lesterolemia—a randomized placebo-controlled trial. *J Dairy Sci.* 2011 Feb;94(2):589–601.

89. de Aguilar-Nascimento JE, Prado Silveira BR, Dock-Nascimento DB. Early enteral nutrition with whey protein or casein in elderly patients with acute ischemic stroke—a double-blind randomized trial. *Nutrition*. 2011 Apr;27(4):440–4.

90. Pal S, Ellis V. Acute effects of whey protein isolate on blood pressure, vascular function and inflammatory markers in overweight postmenopausal women. *Br J Nutr*. 2011 May;105(10):1512–9.

91. Tavares T, Sevilla MÁ, Montero MJ, Carrón R, Malcata FX. Acute effect of whey peptides upon blood pressure of hypertensive rats, and relationship with their angiotensin-converting enzyme inhibitory activity. *Mol Nutr Food Res*. 2012 Feb;56(2):316–24.

92. Pins JJ, Geleva D, Keenan JM, Frazel C, O'Connor PJ, Cherney LM. Do whole-grain oat cereals reduce the need for antihypertensive medications and improve blood pressure control? *J Fam Pract*. 2002 Apr;51(4):353–9.

93. Mortensen LS, Holmer-Jensen J, Hartvigsen ML, Jensen VK, Astrup A, de Vrese M, Holst JJ, Thomsen C, Hermansen K. Effects of different fractions of whey protein on postprandial lipid and hormone responses in type 2 diabetes. *Eur J Clin Nutr*. 2012 Jul;66(7):799–805.

94. De Oliveira FC, Volp AP, Alfenas RC. Impact of different protein sources in the glycemic and insulinemic responses. *Nutr Hosp*. 2011 Jul–Aug;26(4):669–76.

95. Weggemans RM, Zock PL, Katan MB. Dietary cholesterol from eggs increases the ratio of total cholesterol to high-density lipoprotein cholesterol in humans—a meta-analysis. *Am J Clin Nutr*. 2001;73(5):885–91.

96. Blesso CN, Andersen CJ, Barona J, Volk B, Volek JS, Fernandez ML. Effects of carbohydrate restriction and dietary cholesterol provided by eggs on clinical risk factors in metabolic syndrome. *J Clin Lipidol*. 2013;7(5):463–71.

97. Virtanen JK, Mursu J, Tuomainen TP, Virtanen HE, Voutilainen S. Egg consumption and risk of incident type 2 diabetes in men—the Kuopio ischaemic heart disease risk factor study. *Am J Clin Nutr*. 2015;101(5):1088–96.

98. Hu FB, Stampfer MJ, Rimm EB, Manson JE, Ascherio A, Colditz GA, Rosner BA, Spiegelman D, Speizer FE, Sacks FM, Hennekens CH, Willett WC. A prospective study of egg consumption and risk of cardiovascular disease in men and women. *JAMA*. 1999;281(15):1387–94.

99. Larsson SC, Åkesson A, Wolk A. Egg consumption and risk of heart failure, myocardial infarction, and stroke—results from 2 prospective cohorts. *Am J Clin Nutr*. 2015;102(5):1007–13.

100. Virtanen JK, Mursu J, Virtanen HE, Fogelholm M, Salonen JT, Koskinen TT, Voutilainen S, Tuomainen TP. Associations of egg and cholesterol intakes with carotid intima-media thickness and risk of incident coronary artery disease according to apolipoprotein E phenotype in men—the Kuopio ischaemic heart disease risk factor study. *Am J Clin Nutr*. 2016.;103(3):895–901.

101. Shin JY, Xun P, Nakamura Y, He K. Egg consumption in relation to risk of cardiovascular disease and diabetes—a systematic review and meta-analysis. *Am J Clin Nutr*. 2013;98(1):146–59.

102. Yu D, Shu XO, Li H, Xiang YB, Yang G, Gao YT, Zheng W, Zhang X. Dietary carbohydrates, refined grains, glycemic load, and risk of coronary heart disease in Chinese adults. *Am J Epidemiol*. 2013;178(10):1542–9.

103. Keller A, Heitmann BL, Olsen N. Sugar-sweetened beverages, vascular risk factors and events—a systematic literature review. *Public Health Nutr*. 2015;18(7):1145–54.

104. Bernstein AM, de Koning L, Flint AJ, Rexrode KM, Willett WC. Soda consumption and the risk of stroke in men and women. *Am J Clin Nutr*. 2012;95(5):1190–9.

105. Eshak ES, Iso H, Kokubo Y, Saito I, Yamagishi K, Inoue M, Tsugane S. Soft drink intake in relation to incident ischemic heart disease, stroke, and stroke subtypes in Japanese men and women—the Japan Public Health Centre-based study cohort I. *Am J Clin Nutr*. 2012;96(6):1390–7.

106. Swithers SE. Artificial sweeteners produce the counterintuitive effect of inducing metabolic derangements. *Trends Endocrinol Metab*. 2013;24(9):431–41.

107. Shankar P, Ahuja S, Sriram K. Non-nutritive sweeteners—review and update. *Nutrition*. 2013;29(11–12):1293–9.

108. Uribarri J, Woodruff S, Goodman S, Cai W, Chen X, Pyzik R, Yong A, Striker GE, Vlassara H. Advanced glycation end products in foods and a practical guide to their reduction in the diet. *J Am Diet Assoc*. 2010 Jun;110(6):911–6.

109. Lin RY, Choudhury RP, Cai W, Lu M, Fallon JT, Fisher EA, Vlassara H. Dietary glycotoxins promote diabetic atherosclerosis in apolipoprotein E-deficient mice. *Atherosclerosis*. 2003 Jun;168(2):213–20.

110. Uribarri J, Stirban A, Sander D, Cai W, Negrean M, Buenting CE, Koschinsky T, Vlassara H. Single oral challenge by advanced glycation end products acutely impairs endothelial function in diabetic and nondiabetic subjects. *Diabetes Care*. 2007 Oct;30(10):2579–82.

111. Luévano-Contreras C, Garay-Sevilla ME, Wrobel K, Malacara JM, Wrobel K. Dietary advanced glycation end products restriction diminishes inflammation markers and oxidative stress in patients with type 2 diabetes mellitus. *J Clin Biochem Nutr.* 2013 Jan;52(1):22–6.
112. Crowe FL Appleby PN, Travis RC, Key TJ. Risk of hospitalization or death from ischemic heart disease among British vegetarians and nonvegetarians—results from the EPIC-Oxford cohort study. *Am J Clin Nutr.* 2013;97(3):597–603.
113. Orlich MJ, Singh PN, Sabaté J, Jaceldo-Siegl K, Fan J, Knutsen S, Beeson WL, Fraser GE. Vegetarian dietary patterns and mortality in Adventist health study 2. *JAMA Intern Med.* 2013;173(13):1230–8.
114. Miedema MD, Petrone A, Shikany JM, Greenland P, Lewis CE, Pletcher MJ, Gaziano JM, Djousse L. Association of fruit and vegetable consumption during early adulthood with the prevalence of coronary artery calcium after 20 years of follow-up—the coronary artery risk development in young adults (CARDIA) study. *Circulation.* 2015;132(21):1990–8.
115. Dauchet L, Amouyel P, Hercberg S, Dallongeville J. Fruit and vegetable consumption and risk of coronary heart disease—a meta-analysis of cohort studies. *J Nutr.* 2006;136(10):2588–93.
116. Aune D, Giovannucci E, Boffetta P Fadnes LT, Keum N, Norat T Greenwood DC, Riboli E, Vatten LJ, Tonstad S. Fruit and vegetable intake and the risk of cardiovascular disease, total cancer and all-cause mortality—a systematic review and dose-response meta-analysis of prospective studies. *Int J Epidemiol.* 2017 Feb 22. doi: 10.1093/ije/dyw319 [Epub ahead of print].
117. Ingenbleek Y, McCully KS. Vegetarianism produces subclinical malnutrition, hyperhomocysteinemia and atherogenesis. *Nutrition.* 2012;28(2):148–53.
118. Whalen KA, Judd S, McCullough ML, Flanders WD, Hartman TJ, Bostick RM Paleolithic and Mediterranean diet pattern scores are inversely associated with all-cause and cause-specific mortality in adults. *J Nutr.* 2017 Feb 8. doi: 10.3945/jn.116.241919 [Epub ahead of print].
119. Roussell MA, Hill AM, Gaugler TL, West SG, Heuvel JP, Alaupovic P, Gillies PJ, Kris-Etherton PM. Beef in an optimal lean diet study—effects on lipids, lipoproteins, and apolipoproteins. *Am J Clin Nutr.* 2012;95(1):9–16.
120. Lee JE, McLerran DF, Rolland B, Chen Y, Grant EJ, Vedanthan R, Inoue M, Tsugane S, Gao YT, Tsuji I, Kakizaki M, Ahsan H, Ahn YO, Pan WH, Ozasa K, Yoo KY, Sasazuki S, Yang G, Watanabe T, Sugawara Y, Parvez F, Kim DH, Chuang SY, Ohishi W, Park SK, Feng Z, Thornquist M, Boffetta P, Zheng W, Kang D, Potter J, Sinha R. Meat intake and cause-specific mortality—a pooled analysis of Asian prospective cohort studies. *Am J Clin Nutr.* 2013;98(4):1032–41.
121. Micha R, Wallace SK, Mozaffarian D. Red and processed meat consumption and risk of incident coronary heart disease, stroke, and diabetes mellitus—a systematic review and meta-analysis. *Circulation.* 2010;121(21):2271–83.
122. Bellavia A, Larsson SC Bottai M, Wolk A, Orsini N. Differences in survival associated with processed and with nonprocessed red meat consumption. *Am J Clin Nutr.* 2014;100(3):924–9.
123. Lajous M, Bijon A, Fagherazzi G, Rossignol E, Boutron-Ruault MC, Clavel-Chapelon F. Processed and unprocessed red meat consumption and hypertension in women. *Am J Clin Nutr.* 2014;100(3):948–52.
124. Anderson JW, Bush HM. Soy protein effects on serum lipoproteins—a quality assessment and meta-analysis of randomized, controlled studies. *J Am Coll Nutr.* 2011 Apr;30(2):79–91.
125. Rebholz CM, Reynolds K, Wofford MR, Chen J, Kelly TN, Mei H, Whelton PK, He J. Effect of soybean protein on novel cardiovascular disease risk factors—a randomized controlled trial. *Eur J Clin Nutr.* 2013 Jan;67(1):58–63.
126. Campbell SC, Khalil DA, Payton ME, Arjmandi BH. One-year soy protein supplementation does not improve lipid profile in postmenopausal women. *Menopause.* 2010 May–Jun;17(3):587–93.
127. Roughead ZK, Hunt JR, Johnson LK, Badger TM, Lykken GI. Controlled substitution of soy protein for meat protein—effects on calcium retention, bone, and cardiovascular health indices in postmenopausal women. 2005 Jan;90(1):181–9 [Epub 2004 Oct 13].
128. Park K, Mozaffarian D. Omega-3 fatty acids, mercury, and selenium in fish and the risk of cardiovascular diseases. *Curr Atheroscler Rep.* 2010 Nov;12(6):414–22.
129. Mozaffarian D, Rimm EB. Fish intake, contaminants, and human health—evaluating the risks and the benefits. *JAMA.* 2006 Oct 18;296(15):1885–99. Review. Erratum in *JAMA.* 2007 Feb 14;297(6):590.
130. Li YH, Zhou CH, Pei HJ, Zhou XL, Li LH, Wu YJ, Hui RT. Fish consumption and incidence of heart failure—a meta-analysis of prospective cohort studies. *Chin Med J (Engl).* 2013 Mar;126(5):942–948.
131. Watanabe Y, Tatsuno I. Omega-3 polyunsaturated fatty acids for cardiovascular diseases—present, past and future. *Expert Rev Clin Pharmacol.* 2017 Aug;10(8):865–73.

132. Chowdhury R, Stevens S, Gorman D, Pan A, Warnakula S, Chowdhury S, Ward H, Johnson L, Crowe F, Hu FB, Franco OH. Association between fish consumption, long chain omega 3 fatty acids, and risk of cerebrovascular disease—systematic review and meta-analysis. *BMJ*. 2012 Oct 30;345:e6698.

133. de Goede J, Verschuren WM, Boer JM, Kromhout D, Geleijnse JM. Gender-specific associations of marine n-3 fatty acids and fish consumption with 10-year incidence of stroke. *PLoS One*. 2012;7(4):e33866

134. Curtis JM, Dennis D, Waddell DS, MacGillivray T, Ewart HS. Determination of angiotensin-converting enzyme inhibitory peptide Leu-Lys-Pro-Asn-Met (LKPNM) in bonito muscle hydrolysates by LC-MS/MS. *J Agric Food Chem*. 2002 Jul 3;50(14):3919–25.

135. Qian ZJ, Je JY, Kim SK. Antihypertensive effect of angiotensin in converting enzyme-inhibitory peptide from hydrolysates of Bigeye tuna dark muscle, Thunnus obesus. *J Agric Food Chem*. 2007 Oct 17;55(21):8398–403 [Epub 2007 Sep 26].

136. Otani L, Ninomiya T, Murakami M, Osajima K, Kato H, Murakami T. Sardine peptide with angiotensin I-converting enzyme inhibitory activity improves glucose tolerance in stroke-prone spontaneously hypertensive rats. *Biosci Biotechnol Biochem*. 2009 Oct;73(10):2203–9. [Epub 2009 Oct 7].

137. Kawasaki T, Seki E, Osajima K, Yoshida M, Asada K, Matsui T, Osajima Y. Antihypertensive effect of valyl-tyrosine, a short chain peptide derived from sardine muscle hydrolyzate, on mild hypertensive subjects. *J Hum Hypertens*. 2000 Aug;14(8):519–23.

138. Schläwicke Engström K, Strömberg U, Lundh T, Johansson I, Vessby B, Hallmans G, Skerfving S, Broberg K. Genetic variation in glutathione-related genes and body burden of methylmercury. *Environ Health Perspect*. 2008 Jun;116(6):734–9.

139. Valera B, Dewailly E, Poirier P. Association between methylmercury and cardiovascular risk factors in a native population of Quebec (Canada)—a retrospective evaluation. *Environ Res*. 2013 Jan;120:102–8.

140. Choi AL, Weihe P, Budtz-Jørgensen E, Jørgensen PJ, Salonen JT, Tuomainen TP, Murata K, Nielsen HP, Petersen MS, Askham J, Grandjean P. Methylmercury exposure and adverse cardiovascular effects in Faroese whaling men. *Environ Health Perspect*. 2009 Mar;117(3):367–72.

141. Roman HA, Walsh TL, Coull BA, Dewailly É, Guallar E, Hattis D, Mariën K, Schwartz J, Stern AH, Virtanen JK, Rice G. Evaluation of the cardiovascular effects of methylmercury exposures—current evidence supports development of a dose-response function for regulatory benefits analysis. *Environ Health Perspect*. 2011 May;119(5):607–14.

142. Zhang L, Curhan GC, Forman JP. Diet-dependent net acid load and risk of incident hypertension in United States women. *Hypertension*. 2009 Oct;54(4):751–5.

143. Engberink MF, Bakker SJ, Brink EJ, van Baak MA, van Rooij FJ, Hofman A, Witteman JC, Geleijnse JM. Dietary acid load and risk of hypertension—the Rotterdam Study. *Am J Clin Nutr*. 2012 Jun;95(6)---1438–44.

144. Pizzorno J, Frassetto LA, Katzinger J. Diet-induced acidosis—is it real and clinically relevant? *Br J Nutr*. 2010 Apr;103(8):1185–94.

145. Houston MC, Cooil B, Olafsson BJ, Raggi P. Juice powder concentrate and systemic blood pressure, progression of coronary artery calcium and antioxidant status in hypertensive subjects—a pilot study. *Evid Based Complement Alternat Med*. 2007;4(4):455–62.

146. Palatini P, Ceolotto G, Ragazzo F, Dorigatti F, Saladini F, Papparella I, Mos L, Zanata G, Santonastaso M. CYP1A2 genotype modifies the association between coffee intake and the risk of hypertension. *Hypertension*. 2009 Aug;27(8):1594–601.

147. Hu G, Jou Ilahti P, Nissinen A, Bidel S, Antikainen R, Tuomilehto J. Coffee consumption and the incidence of antihypertensive drug treatment in Finnish men and women. *Am J Clin Nutr*. 2007; 86(2):457–64.

148. Vlachopoulos CV, Vyssoulis GG, Alexopoulos NA, Zervoudaki AI, Pietri PG, Aznaouridis KA, Stefanadis CI. Effect of chronic coffee consumption on aortic stiffness and wave reflections in hypertensive patients. *Eur J Clin Nutr*. 2007;61(6):796–802.

149. Mesas AE, Leon-Muñoz LM, Rodriguez-Artalejo F, Lopez-Garcia E. The effect of coffee on blood pressure and cardiovascular disease in hypertensive individuals—a systematic review and meta-analysis. *Am J Clin Nutr*. 2011;94(4):1113–26.

150. Cornelis MC, El-Sohemy A. Coffee, caffeine, and coronary heart disease. *Curr Opin Lipidol*. 2007;18(1):13–9.

151. Cornelis MC, El-Sohemy A, Kabagambe EK, Campos H. Coffee, CYP1A2 genotype, and risk of myocardial infarction. *JAMA*. 2006;295(10):1135–41.

152. Liu J, Sui X, Lavie CJ, Hebert JR, Earnest CP, Zhang J, Blair SN. Association of coffee consumption with all-cause and cardiovascular disease mortality. *Mayo Clin Proc*. 2013;88(10):1066–74.

153. Renda G, Zimarino M, Antonucci I, Tatasciore A, Ruggieri B, Bucciarelli T, Prontera T, Stuppia L, De Caterina R. Genetic determinants of blood pressure responses to caffeine drinking. *Am J Clin Nutr.* 2012;95(1):241–8.
154. Omodei D, Fontana L. Calorie restriction and prevention of age-associated chronic disease. *FEBS Lett.* 2011 Jun 6;585(11):1537–42.
155. Fontana L. Modulating human aging and age-associated diseases. *Biochim Biophys Acta.* 2009 Oct;1790(10):1133–8.
156. Weiss EP, Fontana L. Caloric restriction—powerful protection for the aging heart and vasculature. *Am J Physiol Heart Circ Physiol.* 2011 Oct;301(4):H1205–19.
157. Longo VD, Antebi A, Bartke A, Barzilai N, Brown-Borg HM, Caruso C, Curiel TJ, de Cabo R, Franceschi C, Gems D, Ingram DK, Johnson TE, Kennedy BK, Kenyon C, Klein S, Kopchick JJ, Lepperdinger G, Madeo F, Mirisola MG, Mitchell JR, Passarino G, Rudolph KL, Sedivy JM, Shadel GS, Sinclair DA, Spindler SR, Suh Y, Vijg J, Vinciguerra M, Fontana L. Interventions to slow aging in humans—are we ready? *Aging Cell.* 2015 Aug;14(4):497–510.
158. Varady KA, Hellerstein MK. Alternate-day fasting and chronic disease prevention—a review of human and animal trials. *Am J Clin Nutr.* 2007 Jul;86(1):7–13.
159. Varady KA, Bhutani S, Church EC, Klempel MC. Short-term modified alternate-day fasting—a novel dietary strategy for weight loss and cardioprotection in obese adults. *Am J Clin Nutr.* 2009 Nov;90(5):1138–43. doi: 10.3945/ajcn.2009.28380 [Epub 2009 Sep 30].
160. Jakicic JM, Tate DF, Lang W, Davis KK, Polzien K, Rickman AD, Erickson K, Neiberg RH, Finkelstein EA. Effect of a stepped-care intervention approach on weight loss in adults—a randomized clinical trial. *JAMA.* 2012 Jun 27;307(24):2617–26.
161. O'Keefe JH, Bhatti SK, Bajwa A, et al. Alcohol and cardiovascular health—the dose makes the poison…or the remedy. *Mayo Clin Proc.* 2013;89(3):382–93.
162. Di Castelnuevo A, Costanzo S, Bagnardi V, et al. Alcohol dosing and total mortality in men and women—an updated meta-analysis of 34 prospective studies. *Arch Intern Med.* 2006;166 (22):2437–45.
163. Ronksley PE, Brien SE, Turner BJ, et al. Association of alcohol consumption with selected cardiovascular disease outcomes—a systematic review and meta-analysis. *BMJ.* 2011 Feb 22;342:d671.
164. Sturgeon C, Fasano A. Zonulin, a regulator of epithelial and endothelial barrier functions, and its involvement in chronic inflammatory diseases. *Tissue Barriers.* 2016 Oct 21;4(4):e1251384.
165. Emilsson L Carlsson R, James S, et al. Follow-up of ischaemic heart disease in patients with coeliac disease. *Eur J Prev Cardiol.* 2015 Jan;22(1):83–90.
166. McGrath S, Thomas A, Gorard DA. Cardiomyopathy responsive to gluten withdrawal in a patient with coeliac disease. *BMJ Case Rep.* 2016 Mar 14;2016:bcr2015213301.
167. Milisavljević N, Cvetković M, Nikolić G, et al. Dilated cardiomyopathy associated with celiac disease—case report and literature review. *Srp Arh Celok Lek.* 2012 Sep–Oct;140(9–10):641–3.
168. Tang G, Wang D, Long J, et al. Meta-analysis of the association between whole grain intake and coronary heart disease risk. *Am J Cardiol.* 2015 Mar 1;115(5):625–9.
169. Lebwohl B, Cao Y, Zong G, Hu FB, Green PHR, Neugut AI, Rimm EB, Sampson L, Dougherty LW, Giovannucci E, Willett WC Sun Q, Chan AT. Long term gluten consumption in adults without celiac disease and risk of coronary heart disease—prospective cohort study. *BMJ.* 2017 May 2;357:j1892. doi: 10.1136/bmj.j1892.
170. Jaceldo-Siegel K, Haddad E, Fraser GE, et al. Tree nuts are inversely associated with metabolic syndrome and obesity—the Adventist health study-2. *PLoS One.* 2014 Jan 8;9(1):e85133.
171. Fraser GE, Shavlik DJ. Risk factors for all-cause and coronary heart disease mortality in the oldest-old. The Adventist health study. *Arch Intern Med.* 1997 Oct 27;157(19):2249–58.
172. Aune D, Keum N, Giovannucci E, et al. Nut consumption and risk of cardiovascular disease, total cancer, all-cause and cause-specific mortality—a systematic review and dose-response meta-analysis of prospective studies. *BMC Med.* 2016 Dec 5;14(1):207.
173. Micha R, Peñalvo JL, Cudhea F, et al. Association between dietary factors and mortality from heart disease, stroke, and type 2 diabetes in the United States. *JAMA.* 2017 Mar 7;317(9):912–24.
174. Wu L, Piotrowski K, Rau T et al. Walnut-enriched diet reduces fasting non-HDL cholesterol and apolipoprotein B in healthy Caucasian subjects—a randomized controlled cross-over clinical trial. *Metabolism.* 2014 Mar;63(3):382–91.
175. Xiao Y, Huang W, Peng C, Zhang J, Wong C, Kim JH, Yeoh EK, Su X. Effect of nut consumption on vascular endothelial function—a systematic review and meta-analysis of randomized controlled trials. *Clin Nutr.* 2017 Apr 20:pii-S0261-5614(17)30150-4. doi: 10.1016/j.clnu.2017.04.011 [Epub ahead of print].

176. McDonough AA, Veiras LC, Guevara CA, et al. Cardiovascular benefits associated with higher dietary K$^+$ vs. lower dietary Na$^+$—evidence from population and mechanistic studies. *Am J Physiol Endocrinol Metab.* 2017 Apr 1;312(4):E348–56.
177. Park J, Kwock CK, Yang YJ. The effect of the sodium to potassium ratio on hypertension prevalence—a propensity score matching approach. *Nutrients.* 2016 Aug 6;8(8):pii-E482.
178. Cunha AR, Umbelino B, Correia ML, et al. Magnesium and vascular changes in hypertension. *Int J Hypertens.* 2012;2012:75425.
179. Pokan R, Hofmann P, von Duvillard SP, et al. Oral magnesium therapy, exercise heart rate, exercise tolerance, and myocardial function in coronary artery disease patients. *Br J Sports Med.* 2006 Sep;40(9):773–8.
180. Turgut F, Kanbay M, Metin MR, et al. Magnesium supplementation helps to improve carotid intima media thickness in patients on hemodialysis. *Int Urol Nephrol.* 2008;40(4):1075–82.
181. Cunha AR, D'El-Rei J, Medeiros F, et al. Oral magnesium supplementation improves endothelial function and attenuates subclinical atherosclerosis in thiazide-treated hypertensive women. *J Hypertens.* 2017 Jan;35(1):89–97.
182. Zhang W, Iso H, Ohira T, et al. Associations of dietary magnesium intake with mortality from cardiovascular disease—the JACC study. *Atherosclerosis.* 2012 Apr;221(2):587–95. doi: 10.1016/j.atherosclerosis.2012.01.034. [Epub 2012 Jan 28].

2 Coronary Artery Disease

The Impact of the Mediterranean Cuisine, Targeted Nutritional Supplements and Their Relationship to Autophagy/mTOR

Stephen T. Sinatra

CONTENTS

Takeaways and Key Concepts..31
What Is So Powerful about Polyphenols?...33
    Cocoa and Dark Chocolate 33
Extra Virgin Olive Oil – The King of Polyphenols...34
    How Do You Know Your Olive Is Premium?...35
    How to Select Your Olive Oil..36
    The Nutritional Benefits of Artichokes...36
    Artichoke Health Benefits..37
Lycopene – The Carotenoid of Tomatoes 37
    Tomato Nutrition...37
Nattokinase and Lumbrokinase...38
    Astaxanthin – My Discovery in Japan...39
    Omega-3s...40
    NMN/Autography/mTOR..40
The Body Heals Itself 41
mTOR...41
References...42

TAKEAWAYS AND KEY CONCEPTS...

1. The Mediterranean diet, in conjunction with four tablespoons of olive oil or approximately 4 oz of nuts, leads to a 30% reduction in cardiovascular events when compared to the American Heart Association (AHA) low-fat diet.
2. Mediterranean diet improves multiple biochemical parameters while reducing coronary heart disease (CHD), cerebral vascular accident (CVA) and myocardial infraction (MI) at the same time.
3. Mediterranean cuisine is abundant in multiple polyphenols including constituents of extra virgin olive oil – the secret sauce of the Mediterranean diet that favorably changes gene expression.
4. Cocoa flavonoids prevent CHD.
5. Amazing health benefits of onion, artichoke, tomato, broccoli, and citrus bergamot found in the Mediterranean region.

DOI: 10.1201/9781003137849-2

6. Nattokinase and lumbrokinase – powerful blood-thinning agents that reduce CHD risk.
7. Astaxanthin – a darling carotenoid with major cardiovascular (CV) benefits.
8. Omega 3 essential fatty acids – the medicinal debate continues, but advantages still greatly outweigh possible risks.
9. NMN (nicotinamide mononucleotide) – a new nutraceutical in mitigating age-associated physiological decline.
10. Autophagy and mTOR – a new and vital vocabulary for the next-generation health professional.

Coenzyme Q10, the benchmark of metabolic cardiology, was discussed in Chapter 8. This nutrient is also prominent in the Mediterranean and Okinawan diets, which are considered the best longevity styles of eating on the planet. Spain[1] will became the premiere country in longevity, outliving the Okinawans, in the next two decades. The Mediterranean cuisine is perhaps the world's best diet in supporting and promoting health and longevity while stifling heart disease at the same time. In fact, the average Mediterranean person lives approximately 7 years longer than the average American. In this section, I'll focus on some of the specific foods in the Mediterranean diet that will not only ameliorate heart disease, but hopefully improve your longevity at the same time.

Years ago, when I was writing *Heartbreak and Heart Disease*, Keats Publishing, 1996,[2] literature came out praising the Mediterranean way of living as being the most supportive in not only preventing the ravages of aging but mitigating heart disease as well. In fact, on the island of Crete,[3] there was a period of approximately 10 years when a documented heart attack was not even reported on the island. This fact indeed is remarkable, and years later, the most scientific study of the Mediterranean way of eating was published as the well-known PREDIMED Study.[4] The PREDIMED analysis was reported among several journals with criticisms as well as rebuttals of efficacy. This well-known trial demonstrated that the Mediterranean diet, in conjunction with four tablespoons of olive oil or utilizing a couple of handfuls of nuts, led to a 30% reduction in major cardiovascular events when compared to an AHA low-fat diet.[4]

In short, the Mediterranean diet had a wide application of improvements. For example, in our review article on the diet, we observed that it:[5]

- Improves type 2 diabetes and hyperglycemia.
- Lowers blood pressure.
- Improves serum lipids: lowers total cholesterol, LDL and triglycerides; increases HDL; and lowers Lp(a). Small-particle LDL-P is transposed to a lesser atherogenic profile.
- Improves oxidative defense.
- Reduces inflammation: lowers hs-CRP, interleukin 6 (IL-6), and vascular cell adhesion molecules.
- Decreases brain natriuretic peptide.
- Improves membrane fluidity.
- Reduces homocysteine.
- Reduces CHD, cerebral vascular accident (CVA) and myocardial infarction.

So why is this characteristic way of eating so supportive to the cardiovascular system, and especially the brain and the heart? And what is the Mediterranean diet? The traditional Mediterranean diet has the following characteristics:[4]

Olive oil – the main dietary fat (and what I consider the "secret sauce") of the Mediterranean diet.

- Plant-based (fruits, vegetables, legumes, seeds and nuts).
- Moderately high intakes of precious omega 3 fatty acids found in fish and seafood.

- Adequate consumption of poultry, eggs, cheeses (containing metaquinone-7) and yogurt. Metaquinone-7 assists in transporting calcium out of blood vessels where it does not belong and places it back in bones.
- Relatively low consumption of red meats with exception of lamb, which is the best source of L-carnitine in the diet.
- Red wine and some white wines during mealtimes.

The French paradox[6] is a real phenomenon that strongly suggests that inhabitants that consume red wine tend have lower CHD, even though their level of serum cholesterols is higher. For example, the average cholesterol in France is approximately 275; however, the French have perhaps the lowest incidence of CHD in Western Europe. Researchers and well-known French physicians, such as Dr. de Lorgeril,[6] have attributed the intake of wine as being a primary consideration why the French have a lower incidence of CHD. Red wine and its potent polyphenol activity suggest that this component to the diet – when not abused – proves fruitful over time. Such polyphenols, as well as many nitric oxide-supporting foods such as kale, broccoli, and migratory fish, are widely abundant in the culture.

WHAT IS SO POWERFUL ABOUT POLYPHENOLS?

Polyphenols are natural phytochemicals made by plants to protect themselves from various stressors, including pathogens, environmental assaults, ultraviolet radiation, and even insects and other pests. When we add polyphenols in the diet, these same protective compounds help to safeguard our health. Polyphenolic compounds alleviate oxidative stress by sequestering and clearing the superoxide and hydroxyl radicals by increasing the level of glutathione peroxidase.

Polyphenols also gives plants their distinctive aromas and flavors. You can find polyphenols in many types of fruits and vegetables – including grapes, olives, spinach, red onions, and berries, as well as nuts, which are serious components of the Mediterranean diet. Although all grapes contain polyphenols, red grapes provide a richer source as opposed to the green. Herbs and spices like cloves, peppermint, and rosemary are also high in polyphenols. Beverages like black and green teas, coffee and red wine, as well as cocoa, contain these remarkable antioxidants.

COCOA AND DARK CHOCOLATE

Whether chocolate offers health benefits depends on how it is made. Specifically, the healthiest chocolate contains the most cocoa, as cocoa is a special gift from the nature. You can say that chocolate grows on trees, since cocoa in its unprocessed form actually does. The seeds are inside the fruits of the Theobroma cacao tree. To make chocolate, cocoa seeds or beans are extracted from the cacao tree fruit, fermented, dried, and then roasted to remove the hulls. What remains is the "nib" which gets ground down and processed to produce the chocolate we are all familiar with. During processing, different types of chocolates are created: dark, milk and white. Dark chocolate contains between 50% and 90% cocoa solids, cocoa butter and sugar. Milk chocolate contains 10%–50% cocoa solids, cocoa butter, sugar and milk in some form.

Milk and white chocolates do not deliver any of the same benefits as dark chocolate. Milk chocolate contains milk and a much higher sugar content than its dark counterpart, and so forget white chocolate completely as it has no antioxidants and no nutritional value at all. If you want to truly take advantage of the flavonoid aspects of health and healing, dark chocolate is the way to go. In fact, I am only comfortable in recommending at least 70% dark chocolate, and even then, you should eat it in small amounts – no more than a square or a few at a time – approximately 4–5 days per week. That said, eating in moderation, dark chocolate has some exciting health benefits.

Dark chocolate has antioxidant properties to fight free radical activity and thwart inflammation, perhaps the two most crucial factors in the development and progression of heart disease and other illness situations. Specifically, the flavonoids in these cocoa solids are quite similar to the anti-inflammatory power of wine, olive oil, herbs, spices, and other plant foods. In addition to fighting free radicals, the flavonoids and cocoa solids aid in the production of nitric oxide in the endothelium, assisting the relaxation of blood vessels, improving blood flow while reducing clotting risk, and lowering blood pressure at the same time. In a 2017 meta-analysis[7] that examined the results of 14 studies, researchers concluded that chocolate intake was associated with decreased risks of CHD, stroke and diabetes. Consuming chocolate in moderation (less than 6 servings per week) may be supportive in preventing these pathological situations.

Cocoa flavonoid intake in a meta-analysis of randomized controlled trials (RCTs) including 1,131 participants demonstrated improved markers of cardiac inflammation, including CRP as well as reduced insulin sensitivity.[8] An earlier review in *Circulation* (An AHA Journal) attests to the anti-inflammatory effect of cocoa flavonoids as well as activation of nitric oxide as mechanisms in attenuating cardiovascular risk.[9]

The largest and most recent randomized trial of 21,444 male and female participants is in progress to evaluate whether cocoa flavonoids will help prevent heart disease and strokes. The trial was completed in December 2020 with the results most likely available in 2021/2022. COSMOS will hopefully shed further light on the preventive aspects of cocoa flavanol supplements in the prevention of heart disease.[10] It is encouraging to note that an earlier issue (2020) of the European Society of Cardiology Research looked at a combined analysis of studies over the last 50 years, totaling 336,289 participants.[11] Chocolate consumption was reported with an 8% reduced risk of coronary artery disease when the participants were eating chocolate more than one time per week as opposed to less than one time a week. The most important fact of the study was that the dark flavonoid content of the chocolate was not evaluated as any type of chocolate was ingested.

It will be most enlightening to assess the COSMOS data as it appears from previous research that dark chocolate does contain more cardiovascular risk-reducing constituents such as steric acid, flavonoids and precious polyphenols.

EXTRA VIRGIN OLIVE OIL – THE KING OF POLYPHENOLS

Olive oil is the primary fat in the Mediterranean basin, and it comes with an unimpeachable reputation as one of the healthiest fats for the heart and brain. PREDIMED[4] confirmed that olive oil, as well as the monounsaturated fats found in nuts, has demonstrated a significant reduction in mortality among those who have been diagnosed with heart disease. Olive oil even lowers high blood pressure. When compared to sunflower oil, an omega 6 oil used in Western diets, extra virgin olive oil demonstrated a credible reduction in blood pressure medications when compared to sunflower oil.[12]

Olive oil's "secret sauce" is probably related to its antioxidant activity, particularly oleocanthal. This polyphenol is extremely important, as its antioxidant and anti-inflammatory activities are most likely the source of its antiaging benefits. Other polyphenols such as oleuropein (OL) and hydroxytyrosol (HT) represent molecules of extreme interest for their favorable biological and pharmacological properties. Oleuropein and hydroxytyrosol not only serve as potent antioxidants, but they also exhibit antimicrobial and anti-inflammatory activities while promoting healthy blood vessel dilation and reducing the risk of blood clotting. A 2018 rodent study[13] evaluated oleuropein and concluded that this phenolic compound prevents oxidation and protects against strokes. Hydroxytyrosol bestows equally remarkable benefits, including the prevention of plaque buildup in arteries. In an animal study,[14] rabbits given HT for 1 month ended up with improved cholesterol profiles and elevated blood antioxidant status, as well as reduction of atherosclerotic lesions in their arteries.

Another exciting genetic study on olive oil was performed by researchers in Spain.[15] According to this study out of Cordoba, consuming olive oil high in phenols helps to reduce the expression of pro-inflammatory genes. For the 6-week trial, researchers recruited 20 men and women with metabolic syndrome, standardized their diets, and then had them consume an olive oil-based breakfast that was either high in phenols or low in phenols. After each meal, blood samples were analyzed. In total, 98 genes were identified as being affected by the amount of phenols the participants consumed. Most importantly, there was a reduction in pro-inflammatory genes associated with NF-kappaB. Since inflammation is the etiology of heart disease, a suppression of pro-inflammatory mediators with reversing genes back to a non-inflammatory state is indeed noteworthy. Olive oil may just be the ticket and is a simple intervention to protect yourself.

Years later, in a 2017 rodent model,[16] researchers found that extra virgin olive oil (EVOO) had a protective effect against Alzheimer's disease. Since the brain and heart have such specialized tissues and cells, this makes a lot of sense. This promising clinical investigation also supported data that link olive oil consumption with the prevention of age-related cognitive decline. In this study, the researchers suggested that EVOO activates a vital component defined as autophagy, or the body's unique detoxification process. In a 2020 investigation in another mouse model, investigators demonstrated that EVOO improved synaptic activity and short-term memory. Their results strengthened the health benefits of EVOO as a possible dietary potential for protecting against Alzheimer's disease and other primary Tauopathies.[17]

How Do You Know Your Olive Is Premium?

One of the most important considerations regarding olive oil is to make certain that it is 100% extra virgin. The problem is that many olive oils coming from Western Europe are "adulterated" with canola oil. Although many physicians may embrace canola oil, this is certainly not my position. Honestly, I believe that canola oil is good for using in machines but not for human consumption. While canola is shown as if it has health benefits on papers and is made extremely popular, it's my opinion that canola's benefits are more hype than science. Although many nutritionists and those in the mainstream medicine may strongly suggest that canola oil is healthy as it is high in healthy monounsaturated fat and low in saturated fat, it is high in omega-6 essential fatty acids. I especially do not like an overabundance of omega-6 fatty acids in the diet. Omega-6's, like omega-3's, are essential fatty acids which must be taken through the diet. Although we need some minimal amounts of omega-6's, the problem is that the American diet has an extreme overabundance of it, thus throwing off the critical balance which results in increased inflammation in the body. Ideally, the ratio of omega-6 to omega-3 should be maintained as close to 2:1 as possible. In reality, most people are closer to 15:1 and even as high as 30:1, which results in insidious chronic inflammation which could lead to heart disease. Another aspect of canola oil that is disturbing is that 90% of all the canola grown in the United States is genetically modified. Canola plants are genetically modified to be resistant to the herbicide Roundup, allowing the plants to be endlessly sprayed yet not die. This means the crops are continuously exposed to glyphosate (the primary ingredient in Roundup), which has been linked to disruption of sex hormones, fertility problems, miscarriages, thyroid and neurological concerns, and ironically, heart disease.

One final disturbing reason is the processing of canola oil. Canola and other vegetable oils are extracted from seeds by crushing them and heating them along with chemical solvents, such as hexane. Hexane is derived from petroleum and crude oil; it is used as a cleaning agent in furniture industries, and as an additive in glue and varnishes. The EPA classifies hexane as an air pollutant, and the CDC says it is a neurotoxin. Although vegetable oil manufacturers may suggest that hexane is completely safe, honestly, I am a little skeptical. I prefer an oil that is not heated at high temperatures or goes through a procedure of deodorization. When it comes to oils, I like cold-pressed EVOOs, as no chemical solvents are used and there is minimal processing. So, the question is – what do you cook with? Firstly, I am not a big fan of high-heat frying with any oil as high heat can cause the oil to oxidize, which tends to enhance inflammatory status. If I do use olive oil or organic butter, I prefer a quick sauté in a minimal heat. If higher heats are required, I prefer coconut oil. If you do not like the taste of coconut oil, avocado oil could be another option. Although I tend to keep olive oil away from the frying pan, I use it for "finishing" meals. It is outstanding when it is sprinkled over thinly sliced grass-fed beef, sautéed veggies like broccoli and asparagus, and certainly salads.

To summarize, I prefer olive oil over canola oil because it tastes better, is not genetically modified nor is it highly processed. Besides, when you see the aging peoples of the Mediterranean Basin, the daily use of olive oil may be that secret sauce in their health and longevity.

How to Select Your Olive Oil

Several years ago, when I toured the olive groves in California and picked and smelled the olives, I was amazed by how quickly the olives went from the trees to the olive oil mill facility. The process of making olive oil, especially when it is cold-pressed, is quite an education. I learned that EVOO is derived from the first pressing of the olives, making it more deeply hued, thicker and tastier than refined olive oils. If you are purchasing a flavored olive oil, make sure that it is cold-pressed and remember that flavored oils cannot be called extra virgin because of the addition of the flavor. You certainly want a minimally processed oil because research demonstrates up to 80% of the phenolic compounds are destroyed in the refining process. Always remember that EVOO can be used in marinades or dressings of vegetables and salads, and to reiterate, excessive heat can create uncertain compounds. Another important point is to make sure that your olive oil is purchased in dark glass bottles. I especially prefer to consume olive oil within 1–2 months' time after opening the bottle. Unfortunately, many of us store olive oils in our cabinets, and over time light and oxygen eventually deteriorate its health-promoting qualities. Over time, its freshness is compromised and its protective properties are reduced.

Also remember, an olive oil's flavor can give you some idea about its polyphenol content. I'll never forget the moment when I was sitting down on a chair and slurping and tasting various olive oils out of small cups on a table in my visit to vineyards in California. While holding the olive oil in your mouth, you tend to suck in your cheeks a bit, and if the oil goes down smooth without much of a "bite," it is probably not very potent on the polyphenol side. On the other hand, if the taste is strong, spicy or – even better – "peppery," or if your throat feels a little tingly after you swallow and you have an urge to cough, you've selected a good oil. These are the hallmarks of a polyphenol-rich olive oil. Although the polyphenol "bite" may take a little getting used to, at least you know that you have a potent antioxidant polyphenol oil. I'll never forget how the day I was tasting various olive oils in California left me coughing and tired after trying several batches. The moral of the story is, a high-quality extra virgin olive oil is not only good for your heart, but it may also add years to your life! This leads me to another potent Mediterranean food that delights with olive oil, and that is the artichoke.

The Nutritional Benefits of Artichokes

Back in the BC 300 era, the Greek philosopher Theophrastus described that artichokes were not only a delicacy but strangely an aphrodisiac as well. Artichokes were not introduced to America until the early 1800s when French immigrants brought them over when they settled in the Louisiana territory. Today, however, nearly all artichokes are mostly grown commercially in California. Though widely considered a vegetable, an artichoke is actually an edible immature flower bud from a plant in the thistle family.

Since they are native to the Mediterranean region, artichokes are enjoyed by those living in the Mediterranean basin. They are low in calories and sodium, free of cholesterol and a great source of fiber (averaging approximately 5–6 g per artichoke). They are an excellent source of potassium, magnesium, folate and vitamin C to mention a few. The antioxidants and phytonutrients in artichokes include cynarine, silymarin, rutin, gallic acid, and my most favorite bioflavonoid of all, quercetin.

As a cardiologist, quercetin is one of my top-ten nutraceuticals. Even in this age of Covid-19, quercetin has been effective in helping to ameliorate viral inflammatory illnesses.[18] One aspect of quercetin reminds me of when I was a young cardiologist in my mid-30s and first discovered the Zutphen Elderly Study,[19] which blew me away. It was an exciting study, and like the Framingham

Study, it lasted for decades; they looked at quercetin in the bloodstream of elderly Dutchman, and the endpoint of the study was death. In other words, the researchers were not concerned about how participants met their demise. They evaluated not only how long they lived, but also the quercetin content in their blood. The bottom line was simple: the higher the blood levels of quercetin, the longer these Dutchman lived! They looked at foods such as onions, green apples, and black tea, which are all foods and beverages containing significant quantities of the bioflavonoid. As a young cardiologist, when I reviewed the study and continued to follow the results, I started adding raw onions to my salads and always cooked my pasta sauces with chopped onions. It is no wonder that onions and artichokes are in my top-ten foods. Now back to artichokes....

ARTICHOKE HEALTH BENEFITS

Artichokes contain lots of heart-healing antioxidants which may impact circulation. A 2018 meta-analysis[20] that looked at data from nine trials concluded that supplementation with artichoke extract was associated with a significant reduction in total and LDL cholesterols, as well as tri-glycerides. Artichoke also contains the vital mineral potassium which is certainly excellent for heart health. One aspect of artichoke that needs to be embellished is the supporting impact it has on the liver. The antioxidants cynarine and silymarin play the greatest role in the liver-supporting benefits. In patients with liver disease, artichoke has also been shown to improve the scenario of non-alcoholic steatohepatitis (NASH). In fact, one of my best recipes for supporting liver dysfunc-tion or even fatty liver is the combination of coenzyme Q10 and artichoke.

There is only one minor consideration or caveat I have with artichokes: since they are thistle, they are closely related to ragweed, daisies and marigolds. If you have any allergies to these plants, you may want to eat artichokes with caution or strictly avoid them.

One of my favorite ways of combining flavonoids and carotenoids in salads doused with extra virgin oil is the use of artichoke heart, diced onions and garlic while especially using tomato as a nutritional powerhouse.

LYCOPENE – THE CAROTENOID OF TOMATOES

Tomatoes haven't always been viewed in a positive light. Yes, they are part of the nightshade fam-ily which contains a list of toxic plants, including belladonna known for its use as a poison. In fact, in colonial America, although gardeners grew tomatoes for their beauty, they were afraid to eat them because of their probable connection with belladonna. It was really the Europeans in the 16th century who began to accept them as a popular staple. Although there are numerous inedible night-shades, the list of non-toxic nightshades includes potatoes, peppers, tomatoes and eggplant. While most people can eat these nightshades without any consequence, those with autoimmune diseases, especially rheumatoid arthritis, may find that these foods can exacerbate their symptoms.

TOMATO NUTRITION

One thing about tomatoes is they are an excellent source of nutrition. They are also low in calories (a medium-sized tomato approximates 25 calories) and high in vitamins, minerals and phytonutrients. Vitamins A, C, K, and various B vitamins are part of the phytonutrient nature. Tomatoes are rich in minerals like potassium, manganese, magnesium, chromium and copper. They also are a good source of fiber, but perhaps the best health benefit of tomatoes is courtesy of a phytonutrient called lycopene.

Lycopene is part of a family of carotenoids, compounds that offer colorful pigmentations to plants and even to animals that eat plants such as salmon and shrimp. There are hundreds of carot-enoids in nature, but only a few of them have been thoroughly researched like beta-carotene, lutein, lycopene and astaxanthin. Lycopene is really the pigment that is responsible for the rich red color of tomatoes, as well as the bright pink seen in watermelon, pink grapefruit and papaya. Lycopene is an extraordinary compound and perhaps the most well-featured for cardiovascular health. There are multiple studies that strongly suggest that tomato-based products such as tomato paste and tomato sauce may be beneficial for reducing inflammation and cardiovascular risk, especially endothelial dysfunction while decreasing blood lipids, preventing the oxidation of LDL and controlling blood pressure at the same time.[21–23] The benefits of lycopene also extend to supporting other vital tissues and organs.

In a study published in 1995 that followed nearly 50,000 men, those with the highest levels of lycopene had a 20% reduction in prostate cancer compared to the men with the lowest levels.[24] There was also a meta-analysis that looked over 26 studies totaling more than 560,000 men.[25] Researchers found that higher levels of lycopene significantly lowered prostate cancer risk, and the greater the consumption, the greater the protection.

Keeping this preventive cancer impact in mind, there is a family story I would like to share. One of my young relatives developed breast cancer, and because she was so young with small children in the household, I did an extensive literature search trying to bring natural healing modalities to the table and discovered the sulforaphane/lycopene connection. When it comes to cancer prevention, especially breast cancer in a female or prostate cancer in a male, you want to eat tomatoes and broccoli at the same time. Eaten together, this dynamic duo acts synergistically, offering greater protection against cancer than when each is eaten alone.[26] The sulforaphane in broccoli and the lycopene in tomatoes consumed at the same time are synergistic. In fact, recent research demonstrates that sulforaphane is a powerful inducer of Nrf2 which regulates expression of cytoprotective genes in pairing viral reproduction. This consideration is especially important in aging people. Indeed, sulforaphane, as a modulator of epigenetic pathways, may be both prophylactic and curative in the fight against SAR-CoV-2 as well.[27–30]

To summarize, just like lycopene can be the king of the carotenoids, sulforaphane is perhaps the king of the flavonoids, and both are expressed in the antiaging Mediterranean diet. And when taken together at the same meal, the cardioprotective and cancer-protective activities through the antioxidant functions are superior. One of the advantages of flavonoids is that even consuming relatively small amounts of such flavonoid-containing foods may create a beneficial effect. Another flavonoid such as citrus bergamot may also help to reduce cardiovascular risk.

Citrus bergamot is a fruit that is endemic to the Calabrian region in Sicily, as well as other sections in southern Italy. I've personally used citrus bergamot in my patients for several years, and one of the most interesting aspects is the reduction in the risk of metabolic syndrome. In fact, when a typical patient came into my office with slightly elevated systolic and diastolic pressures, weight gain around the middle, and laboratory evidence of higher blood sugars, triglycerides, and lower HDLs, the syndrome of insulin resistance popped into my mind. In addition to a low-carbohydrate diet and some degree of weight loss, I believe that citrus bergamot had played a role in lowering blood sugar, triglycerides, and possibly even blood pressure. At doses of 500–1000 mg, I saw many favorable changes in my patients.

NATTOKINASE AND LUMBROKINASE

Lp(a), in my opinion, is the most devastating small inflammatory and thrombotic LDL particle that enhances the progression of inflammatory coronary artery disease. Since the biogenome project was discovered more than two decades ago, more and more people are being evaluated with abnormal levels of this exceedingly small-particle LDL. Unfortunately, to my knowledge, there have been no pharmaceutical drugs that can play a favorable role in lowering Lp(a), including statins. Statins at times actually increased laboratory values of Lp(a), which made me question again the reported efficacious effects. On occasion, I saw lowering of Lp(a) numbers in both men and women taking testosterone and estrogen therapies as part of their hormonal replacement therapy regimen.

So, what helps Lp(a), especially if it is in your genetic profile and is significantly elevated? This is where nattokinase and lumbrokinase have been extremely helpful. In the 21st century, hyperviscosity blood syndrome refers to sticky, sludgy blood. When blood thickens, it moves through blood vessels slowly, allowing platelets to stick together and clump. Electromagnetic forces such as wireless devices, cordless phones, cellular phones, etc. may enhance this process. The problem with rising blood sugars in the 21st century is due to the overdependence on carbohydrates in the diet, and the outbreak of multiple EMF-emitting devices throughout the planet. Essentially, we are creating the perfect storm for sticky blood which has a propensity for hypercoagulation. Even if we consider the cardiac risk factors of a decade ago – high cholesterol, high blood sugar, cigarette smoking, high fibrinogen and homocysteine, ferritin, etc. – we must ask ourselves, are these components the forerunners of sticky blood syndrome? In my practice of cardiology, I've used nattokinase and lumbrokinase to help thin the blood while attempting to neutralize the toxic inflammatory and thrombotic effects of Lp(a).

Nattokinase is extracted from the traditional fermented soy food called natto. It was believed by many to contribute to the low incidence of CHD in Japan. It makes sense since nattokinase not only helps to eliminate clots, but also reduces the tendency to form thick, sludgy blood and thus decreases the incidence of heart attack and stroke.

Lumbrokinase developed in Asia comes from the extract of earthworm, a traditional source of healing in both Japan and China.[31] I first came across lumbrokinase more than a decade ago, after I realized that increasing blood levels of Lp(a) was perhaps the most significant risk factor in coronary artery disease. I was lecturing at a conference in Canada when a naturopath approached me, asking if I have ever used lumbrokinase before. He gave me some literature and samples. The positive impact it had in reducing some of my patients' Lp(a) numbers was noteworthy, and many of my patients who were riddled with coronary artery disease felt better on lumbrokinase.

Lumbrokinase and, to a lesser degree, nattokinase are natural blood-thinning agents that may tend to break down excessive fibrin in the blood vessels.[31–32] Nattokinase and lumbrokinase may also enhance blood flow in critically narrowed blood vessels. It just makes sense to consider these agents in people with unsatisfactory quality-of-life issues resulting from shortness of breath or angina. Another nutraceutical supplement that I stumbled upon by accident, just like lumbrokinase, was astaxanthin.

ASTAXANTHIN – MY DISCOVERY IN JAPAN

Ten years ago, I was in Japan lecturing on Metabolic Cardiology. Just like American symposiums, the Japanese had multiple exhibitors, and after my lecture, I visited the exhibit hall. Unfortunately, I didn't speak Japanese, so I ended up just walking at a pace and not stopping at any of the booths. But by a stroke of fate, someone went to my lecture who was at an astaxanthin booth and spoke English. He told me that their product was something that I needed to learn about, and he was right! Ever since that encounter in Japan, while working for Healthy Directions, I lobbied to find a good source of astaxanthin. While the investigation went on, I searched the medical literature and was amazed at how many articles on astaxanthin were published, demonstrating antiaging and antioxidant aspects in not only supporting the heart but also brain function, the retina of the eye, and the complexion of the skin.[33–35] But what is astaxanthin?

Astaxanthin is an orange-red carotenoid that gives the color to migratory salmon, shrimp, lobster and crab to mention a few. It is an incredible antioxidant demonstrating superior function to popular nutrients like vitamin C and pycnogenol. Astaxanthin will continue to get the notoriety it needs.

Remember, astaxanthin is in migratory fish with red color. Many of these fish, as well as other omega-3 varietals found in the Mediterranean basin, include red snapper, sardines and Alistado red shrimp, to mention a few. One of the best cardiovascular reviews on astaxanthin was published in the *International Journal of Molecular Medicine* in 2021.[36] A virulent and dangerous free radical causing oxidized LDL is the peroxynitrite free radical. Astaxanthin not only neutralizes this horrific free radical, but it also converts it to the 15-N nitro astaxanthin that helps to support further antioxidant action. The powerful antioxidant and inflammatory effects of astaxanthin extend to stimulating reverse cholesterol transport, thus attenuating the formation of foam cells. In addition, favorable rheological properties create better blood flow while reducing blood transit time as well. Precious omega-3 essential fatty acids also support the circulatory system.

Omega-3s

The debate concerning the attractive health benefits of omega-3 essential fatty acids has been a controversial and contested focus over my career as a cardiologist for decades. In my day-to-day practice, omega-3s are not only supportive, but they are lifesaving as well. For example, one recent pooled analysis from 17 prospective cohort studies[37] examined the association of blood levels of omega-3 and all risk mortality. There was an amazing 15%–18% lower risk of total mortality comparing the top to bottom quintiles of omega-3. Reductions in mortality were also seen from cancer. The extensive cohort analysis suggested that higher levels of marine omega essential fatty acids were associated with a lower risk of death. Interestingly, in an extensive study conducted in the United Kingdom including over 427,000 participants, the reported use of fish oil supplements demonstrated a lower risk of death from any cause.[38] There are multiple benefits regarding omega-3s such as antihypertensive, antiplatelet and hypotriglyceridemic, as well as positive effects on endothelial function and autonomic balance.

However, investigators recently reported that there may be a caveat to omega-3 essential fatty acids. In the *European Heart Journal*,[39] researchers suggest that there may be an increased risk of atrial fibrillation in patients who are at elevated risk of cardiovascular disease and have high triglycerides at the same time.[39] Indeed, omega-3 essential fatty acids require more research regarding this possible relationship.

Omega-3 essential fatty acids have also been reported to be mTOR inhibitors which extend lifespans in many species.[40] Thus, it makes sense to improve our blood levels of DHA and EPA, as higher blood levels are not only inversely associated with all-cause mortality, but higher levels are also attributed to a slower rate of telomere shortening.[41] Taking omega-3 essential fatty acids in the diet suggests slowing of the aging process. The same is true for curcumin, resveratrol and other newer antiaging nutraceuticals like NMN (nicotinamide mononucleotide).

NMN/Autography/mTOR

One of the greatest advantages of being a physician for more than 50 years is that you gain insight into what targeted nutraceuticals really do for patients. Attending conferences on a regular basis has often validated nutraceutical efficacy and has opened many other doors of introspection. Let me give you an example.

One of the newer antiaging molecules is referred to NMN (nicotinamide mononucleotide). This metabolite of vitamin B3 is found throughout our bodies and in some healthy foods like broccoli, which is a popular vegetable in the Mediterranean diet. NMN is a precursor to the vitally important molecule NAD+ which not only supports multiple metabolic functions but also healthy aging. The problem is that NAD+ levels decline by as much as 50% as we reach middle age. Several of my colleagues, including myself, have taken NMN in supplemental form to help bolster the natural production of NAD+ which ameliorates the inexorable decline of aging. In the mouse model, the administration of NMN at extremely high doses was found to be safe and well-tolerated while mitigating age-associated physiological decline.[42] This is one substance you should keep on your radar as many targeted nutritional supplement suppliers will probably market this vital compound. Such science-based genetic nutraceuticals like NMN and others will be highlighted at future medical symposiums and conferences as targeted genetic supports are gaining momentum in the scientific community.

As a heart specialist, I've written about toxic blood syndrome in many of my previous books, discussing about the APOE 2 allele, homocysteine, Lp(a), fibrinogen and ferritin, to mention a few. Many of these undesirable blood components are genetically endowed. The Earth Biogenome Project has now identified dozens and dozens of other markers of inflammation. In retrospect, several years ago I was looking at the tip of the iceberg. In 2022 and beyond, health professionals will be utilizing the interplay between genetic markers and inflammation to assist them in determining common as well as bizarre pathological conditions.

The doctors of the future will be more in touch with such genetic considerations, especially since the Earth Biogenome Project revolutionized the future of medicine more than two decades ago. For example, the vocabulary of autophagy and mTOR will be frequently utilized in the discussions of health, wellness and aging by the healing professionals. Although the phenomenon of autophagy has been explored for over five decades, in 2016 the Nobel Prize was awarded to the Japanese researcher Yoshinori Ohsumi, which exploded the awareness of its genetic basis and description.

THE BODY HEALS ITSELF

Autophagy is the natural body's wisdom of detoxifying itself. When you improve autophagy, you are ameliorating inflammation and healing the body at the same time. In essence, when your body recycles and supports the process of apoptosis or getting rid of old or tired cells, the body's protoplasm and cellular components are strengthened. Since the body is constantly trying to heal itself or achieve homeostasis in this increasingly toxic environment, it makes sense to support autophagy. You will be taking the old, tired, vulnerable, and infected cells out and recharging the body with new stronger cells.

Since the mitochondrial theory of aging is the most popular attribute of optimum health, autophagy helps to eliminate tired and dysfunctional mitochondria while supporting the body in its growth and development. Although the Mediterranean diet contains multiple nutraceuticals, flavonoids and carotenoids to enhance autography, weight reduction and fasting are other methodologies to help foster the body's wisdom of detoxification.

mTOR

The definition of mTOR is a complex varietal of terms. Simply stated, mTOR regulates mammalian metabolism of various complex tissues in the body. As a protein enzyme, mTOR regulates cellular division,[43] survival, protein synthesis and autophagy. As a regulator of physiology, the mTOR pathway plays an important role in the brain.[44] It is not a coincidence that an over-activation of mTOR could lead to Alzheimer's disease[45] as well as cancer. Thus, inhibitors of mTOR may become instrumental in supporting health and longevity. If the mTOR pathway can be decreased, this alteration in complex metabolic pathways perhaps will increase lifespan.

For example, quercetin, discussed previously, is a premier component of autophagy while inhibiting mTOR at the same time. The Zutphen Elderly Study now makes even more sense. Onions containing the quercetin bioflavonoid are not only an antagonist to mTOR but also a component of autophagy – a perfect antiaging strategy.

Other mTOR inhibitors include curcumin and resveratrol which are major nutraceuticals of the Mediterranean basin. Green tea, a typical beverage of Okinawa, is also a cardinal mTOR inhibitor. Citrus bergamot, mentioned previously, is also a cheerleader for autophagy and has a favorable impact on cholesterol and sugar metabolism. Berberine, a component of several plants, has shown great promise in lowering blood sugar. In fact, Metformin, the darling of many antiaging physicians in supporting metabolism while lowering blood sugar, is now being replaced by berberine. Berberine makes even more sense as it drives AMP-activated protein kinase (AMPK) in a preferential direction, thus supporting metabolic pathways. AMPK or 5' adenosine monophosphate-activated protein kinase is a unique enzyme that plays a crucial role in energy homeostasis by activating glucose and fatty acid oxidation when cellular energy reserves are low.

To summarize, constituents in the Mediterranean diet such as quercetin, curcumin, resveratrol and occasional green tea are all inhibitors of mTOR while supporting autophagy at the same time. Perhaps utilizing all these nutraceuticals in combination with olive oil as well as fresh fruits and vegetables containing multiple carotenoids and flavonoids, gives even more credibility that the Mediterranean way of eating is the best way to improve health and longevity.

In conclusion, the PREDIMED Study overwhelmingly demonstrated reductions in illness, disease and improvement in longevity. However, there is even something more special and more provocative about the Mediterranean diet. Since the Mediterranean diet offers several foods that benefit autography while decreasing mTOR at the same time, perhaps researchers in the near future will dissect the Mediterranean dietary compounds even more. What needs to be brought into the discussion is how the endogenous diet of a region helps to support the genetic foundations that every individual person possesses. The Earth Biogenome Project may unlock even more secrets of longevity. This new style with an emphasis on genetic thinking will perhaps alter the way doctors practice medicine. In other words, the doctors of the future will use phytonutrients and nutraceuticals to help eliminate metabolic and physiological weaknesses while improving genetic strengths at the same time. This new medicine of the future will have a solid genetic base to work from. The doctors of the future will have an enormous advantage in reducing illness, pathology, and human suffering while probably improving longevity at the same time.

REFERENCES

1. Minder R. 2019. Spain's formula to live forever. https://foreignpolicy.com/2019/07/04/spains-formula-to-live-forever/.
2. Sinatra ST. 1999. *Heartbreak and Heart Disease*. Keats Publishing, New Canaan, CT.
3. Simopoulos AP. 2001. The Mediterranean diets: what is so special about the diet of Greece? The scientific evidence. *J Nutr* 131(11):3065S–3073S.
4. Martinez-Gonzalez MA, Salas-Salvado J, Estruch R, et al. 2015. Benefits of the Mediterranean diet: insights from the PREDIMED study. *Prog Cardiovasc Dis* 58(1):50–60.
5. Houston M, Minich D, Sinatra ST, et al. 2018. Recent science and clinical application of nutrition to coronary heart disease. *J Am Coll Nutr* 37(3):169–187.
6. Renaud S, de Lorgeril M. 1992. Wine, alcohol, platelets, and the French paradox for coronary heart disease. *Lancet* 339(8808):1523–1526.
7. Yuan S, Li X, Jin Y, et al. 2017. Chocolate consumption and risk of coronary heart disease, stroke, and diabetes: a meta-analysis of prospective studies. *Nutrients* 9(8):852.
8. Lin X, Zhang I, Li A, et al. 2016. Cocoa flavanol intake and biomarkers for cardiometabolic health: a systemic review and meta-analysis of randomized controlled trials. *J Nutr* 146(11):2325–2333.
9. Corti R, Flammer AJ, Hollenberg NK, et al. 2009. Cocoa and cardiovascular health. *Circulation* 119(10):1433–1441.
10. COSMOS Trial. To be completed 2021. Brigham and Women's Hospital.
11. Krittanawong C, Narasimhan B, Wang Z, et al. 2020. Association between chocolate consumption and risk of coronary artery disease: a systematic review and meta-analysis. *Eur J Prev Cardiol*. Doi: 10.1177/2047487320936787.
12. Ferrara LA, Raimondi AS, d'Episcopo L, et al. 2000. Olive oil and reduced need for antihypertensive medications. *Arch Intern Med* 160(6):837–842.
13. Zhang W, Liu X, Li Q. 2018. Protective effects of oleuropein against cerebral ischemia/reperfusion by inhibiting neuronal apoptosis. *Med Sci Monit* 24:6587–6598.
14. Gonzalez-Santiago M, Martin-Bautista E, Carrero JJ, et al. 2006. One-month administration of hydroxytyrosol, a phenolic antioxidant present in olive oil, to hyperlipemic rabbits improves blood lipid profile, antioxidant status and reduces atherosclerosis development. *Atherosclerosis* 188(1):35–42.
15. Camargo A, Ruano J, Fernandez JM, et al. 2010. Gene expression changes in mononuclear cells in patients with metabolic syndrome after acute intake of phenol-rich virgin olive oil. *BMC Genom* 11:253.
16. Lauretti E, Iuliano L, Pratico D. 2017. Extra-virgin olive oil ameliorates cognition and neuropathology of the 3xTg mice: role of autophagy. *Ann Clin Transl Neurol* 4(8):564–574.
17. Luretti E, Nenov M, Dincer O, et al. 2020. Extra virgin olive oil improves synaptic activity, short-term plasticity, memory, and neuropathology in autopathy model. *JAN* 19(1):e13076.

18. Wu W, Li R, Li X, et al. 2016. Quercetin as an antiviral agent inhibits influenza A virus (IAV) entry. *Viruses* 8(1):6.

19. Hertog MG, Feskens EJ, Hollman PC, et al. 1993. Dietary antioxidant flavonoids and risk of coronary heart disease: the Zutphen Elderly Study. *Lancet* 342(8878):1007–1011.

20. Sahebkar A, Pirro M, Banach M, et al. 2018. Lipid-lowering activity of artichoke extracts; A systematic review and meta-analysis. *Crit Rev Food Sci Nutr* 58(15):2549–2556.

21. Story EN, Kopec RE, Schwartz SJ, et al. 2010. An update on the health effects of tomato lycopene. *Annu Rev Food Sci Technol* 1:189–210.

22. Ried K, Fakler P. 2011. Protective effect of lycopene on serum cholesterol and blood pressure: meta-analyses of intervention trials. *Maturitas* 68(4):299–310.

23. Cheng HM, Koutsidis G, Lodge JK, et al. 2017. Tomato and lycopene supplementation and cardiovascular risk factors: a systemic review and meta-analysis. *Atherosclerosis* 257:100–108.

24. Giovannucci E, Ascherio A, Rimm EB, et al. 1995. Intake of carotenoids and retinol in relation to risk of prostate cancer. *National Cancer Inst* 87(23):1767–1776.

25. Chen P, Zhang W, Wang X, et al. 2015. Lycopene and risk of prostate cancer: a systematic review and meta-analysis. *Meta-Anal Med (Baltimore)* 94(33):e1260.

26. Langner E, Lemieszek MK, Rzeski W. 2019. Lycopene, sulforaphane, quercetin, and curcumin applied together show improved antiproliferative potential in colon cancer cells in vitro. *J Food Biochem* 43(4):e12802.

27. Hyun TK. 2020. A recent overview on sulforaphane as a dietary epigenetic modulator. *EXCLI J.* 19:131–134.

28. Houghton CA. 2019. Sulforaphane: its "coming of age" as a clinically relevant nutraceutical in the prevention and treatment of chronic disease. *Oxid Med Cell Longev.* 2716870. https://www.ncbi.nlm.nih.gov/pubmed/31737167.

29. Wyler E, Franke V, Menegatti J, et al. 2019. Single-cell RNA sequencing of herpes simplex virus 1-infected cells connected NRF2 activation to an antiviral program. *Nat Commun* 10:4878. https://www.ncbi.nlm.nih.gov/pubmed/31653857.

30. Mller L, Meyer M, Bauer RN, et al. 2016. Effect of broccoli sprouts and live attenuated influenza virus on peripheral blood natural killer cells: a randomized, double-blind study. *PLoS One* 11(1):e0147742. https://www.ncbi.nlm.nih.gov/pubmed/26820305.

31. Akazawa S, Tokuyama H, Sato S, et al. 2018. High-pressure tolerance of earthworm fibrinolytic and digestive enzymes. *J Biosci Bioeng* 125(2):155–159.

32. Chen H, McGowan E, Ren N, et al. 2018. Nattokinase: a promising alternative in prevention and treatment of cardiovascular diseases. *Biomark Insights* 13:1177271918785130.

33. Nakagawa K, Kiko T, Miyazawa T, et al. 2011. Antioxidant effect of astaxanthin on phospholipid peroxidation in human erythrocytes. *Br J Nutr* 105(11):1563–1571.

34. Yoshida H, Yanai H, Ito K, et al. 2010. Adminstration of natural astaxanthin increases serum HDL-cholesterol and adiponectin in subjects with mild hyperlipidemia. *Atherosclerosis* 209(2):520–523.

35. Hashimoto H, Arai K, Hayashi S, et al. 2016. The effect of astaxanthin on vascular endothelial growth factor (VEGF) levels and peroxidation reactions in the aqueous humor. *J Clin Biochem Nutr* 59(1):10–15.

36. Martins Pereira CP, Remondi Souze AC, Rodrigues Vasconcelos A, et al. 2021. Antioxidant and anti-inflammatory mechanisms of action of astaxanthin in cardiovascular diseases (Review). *Int J Mol Med* 47(1):37–48.

37. Harris WS, Tintle NL, Imamura F, et al. 2021. Blood n-3 fatty acid levels and total and cause-specific mortality from 17 prospective studies. *Nat Commun.* Doi: 10.1038/s41467-021-22370-2.

38. Li Z-H, Zhong W-F, Liu S, et al. 2020. Associations of habitual fish oil supplementation with cardiovascular outcomes and all cause mortality: evidence from a large population based cohort study. *Br Med J.* 368:m456.

39. Lombardi M, Carbone S, Del Buono MG. 2021. Omega-3 fatty acids supplementation and risk of atrial fibrillation: an updated meta-analysis of randomized controlled trials. *Eur Heart J Cardiovasc Pharmacother*:pvab008. Doi: 10.1093/ehjcvp/pvab008.

40. Papadopoli D, Boulay K, Kazak L, et al. 2019. mTOR as a central regulator of lifespan and aging. *F1000Research* 8:F1000.

41. Farzaneh-Far R, Lin J, Epel ES, et al. 2010. Association of marine omega-3 fatty acids with telomeric aging in patients with coronary artery disease. *JAMA* 303(3):250–257.

42. Mills KF, Yoshida S, Stein LR, et al. 2016. Long-term administration of nicotinamide mononucleotide mitigates age-associated physiological decline in mice. *Cellular Metab* 24(6):795–806.

43. Liss MA, Rickborn L, DiGiovanni J, et al. 2018. mTOR inhibitors for treatment of low-risk prostate cancer. *Med Hypotheses* 117:63–68.
44. Liang H, Nie J, Van Skike CE, et al. 2019. Mammalian target of rapamycin at the crossroad between Alzheimer's disease and diabetes. *Adv Exp Med Biol* 1128:185–225.
45. Chang YF, Hu WM. 2019. Roles of mammalian target of rapamycin signaling and autophagy pathway in Alzheimer's disease. *Acta Academiae Medicinae Sinicae* 41(2):248–255.

3 Naturopathic Medicine and the Prevention and Treatment of Cardiovascular Disease

Drew Sinatra

Michael Murray

CONTENTS

Introduction...46
Vegetarian, Paleolithic, and Mediterranean Diets – Food as Medicine 47
The Standard Western Diet and Refined Sugar...48
Wheat (gluten), Blood Sugar, and Inflammation 49
Know Thy Food Source 50
Understanding Atherosclerosis 50
The Vascular Lining – A Key Target for Nutritional Therapies...51
The Role of Nutrition and Endothelial Function 52
Berberine...53
Garlic...53
Pantethine 54
Bergamot...54
The Naturopathic Approach to Treating Hypertension..54
Diet, Lifestyle, and Hypertension 56
Special Foods to Lower Blood Pressure 56
The DASH Diet...57
Fluids, Salt, and Hypertension 57
Exercise and Hypertension...58
Stress, Breathing, and Hypertension...59
Targeted Nutritional Supplements, Botanical Medicines, and Acupuncture and Hypertension 60
Fasting and Hypertension 62
Grounding and Hypertension...63
    Monitor Your Blood Pressure 63
Concise Recommendations for High Blood Pressure...63
The Importance of Detoxification in Supporting the Cardiovascular System 64
The Effects of Environmental Toxins on Blood Pressure and the Cardiovascular System.............64
    Introduction...64
Reducing Toxic Exposure with Simple and Easy Interventions 65
    Sauna Therapy 65
    High-Fiber, Phytonutrient-Rich, Organic Fruits and Vegetables 66
    Liver and Gastrointestinal Supportive Foods and Botanical Medicines.........................67
    Skin Brushing 68
    Contrast Hydrotherapy..68

DOI: 10.1201/9781003137849-3

Therapeutic Fasting..68
Electromagnetic Radiation (EMR) 68
Summary 69
Conclusion 69
References 70

INTRODUCTION

As specialists in integrative and functional medicine, naturopathic doctors (NDs) offer many treatment options for patients with cardiovascular disease. Since our visits are typically longer than most primary care providers, we provide enough time to educate patients about dietary and lifestyle practices that serve as the fundamental pillars for optimal health. We acknowledge and support the body's inherent healing mechanisms and use nutrition, herbal and nutraceutical medicines, hydrotherapy, acupuncture, detoxification, stress management therapies, and counseling to help shift disease back into health. We recognize when the body requires additional support through medications and surgery, and utilize these modalities when necessary. Above all, we work with cardiologists and other specialists to provide the best care for the patient.

We know that most cases of cardiovascular disease (CVD) are preventable through proper diet and lifestyle modification. Many physicians, however, do not provide enough time during office visits to give specific nutritional advice or to discuss healthy living habits with their patients. A visit with a naturopathic doctor typically lasts 30–60 minutes, and plenty of time is allocated to discussing which diet is appropriate for a particular cardiovascular condition. Awareness of healthy eating options is essential for proper meal planning, so we strive to empower patients by teaching them which foods to eat and which foods to avoid. As discussed below, a seemingly healthy vegetarian diet, touted by many to be heart healthy, may do more harm than good if improper food choices are made.

Learning to identify and address the root cause of cardiovascular dysfunction, such as high blood pressure, is essential for healing to occur. Hypertension can be due to many factors including stress, hormone imbalance, environmental toxin exposure, lack of exercise, medications, obesity, and/or nutritional deficiencies. Lowering a surrogate marker such as blood pressure using diuretics, ACE inhibitors, beta-blockers, or other medications never truly addresses the cause, which if left unchecked can result in additional physiological change and damage. Moreover, putting patients on medications is a lot easier than taking them off! Therefore, when addressing CVD, physicians must look at all causative factors before recommending treatment options and start with the safest therapies first.

Some statistics show that 60%–90% of doctor visits are stress related. What can we do for patients to help minimize stress in their lives? What treatments or techniques can we offer for quick and easy stress reduction? What effect can yoga, slowed breathing, meditation, or biofeedback have on cardiovascular endpoints? We will always have stress in our lives because mortgages, demanding jobs, sick family members, and living in a constant fear or worry are difficult to avoid. Learning how to manage these stressors is critical for sound health. Asking your patients about the stress in their lives and teaching them methods to reduce it are extremely important considerations in naturopathic medicine.

In this chapter, we will investigate the multidisciplinary role a naturopathic doctor plays in the prevention and treatment of CVD, specifically endothelial dysfunction and hypertension. Lifestyle optimization through diet, mind-body medicines, targeted nutritional supplements, exercise, fasting, grounding, and detoxification techniques will be discussed as appropriate adjunctive therapies in not only the prevention of endothelial dysfunction and hypertension, but also in the overall management. First, we will take a deep dive into how certain diets and food choices can impact the cardiovascular system.

VEGETARIAN, PALEOLITHIC, AND MEDITERRANEAN DIETS – FOOD AS MEDICINE

Epidemiological research has looked into the cardioprotective benefits of vegetarian, Mediterranean, and Paleolithic diets.[1–7] These diets all focus on the consumption of fresh fruits and vegetables, nuts, and heart-healthy oils. They differ in how much, or little, meat, fish, grains, legumes, dairy, and eggs are consumed. In this section, modified vegetarian, Paleolithic, and Mediterranean diets are recommended as medically appropriate diets for preventing and treating heart disease. They all are very practical diets that not only improve the health of the cardiovascular system, but vitality in general. It's very important to know how to implement and eat a healthy vegetarian or Paleolithic diet, as unhealthy versions are quite common without proper guidance.

The definition of a vegetarian is one who eats most foods except meat products. There are varying levels of vegetarianism, however, as some vegetarians choose to eat fish (pesco-vegetarians) and/or dairy products and eggs (lacto-ovo vegetarians). There is a wide range of health-promoting vegetarian diets, as some vegetarians may choose to avoid fish and dairy products, but eat in abundance highly refined, processed, and sugary foods that may promote inflammation in the body. As we'll discuss later in this chapter, avoiding processed, high-sugar, and high-glycemic foods is key for supporting cardiovascular health outcomes.

Studies show that eating a vegetarian diet does lead to a reduction in CVD. A cohort study comparatively looked at 67 vegetarians and 134 omnivores (consumers of plant and animal origins), and assessed the risk of CVD. The vegetarians had a marked reduction in the following measures: blood pressure, body mass index (BMI), waist to hip ratio, fasting blood glucose, and elevated total cholesterol. In the Oxford Vegetarian Study, 6,000 vegetarians and vegans were compared with 5,000 omnivores. The authors proposed that eating a lifelong vegetarian diet reduced the incidence of ischemic heart disease by as much as 24%, while the incidence was 57% lower among lifelong vegans, who strictly avoid all animal products including dairy and eggs. The vegans in this study had the lowest LDL cholesterol, and the fish eaters the highest HDL cholesterol.[8]

It is important to note that high consumption of fruits, vegetables, and fiber is the foundation of a healthy vegetarian diet, and thus contributes to lowered risk of heart disease.[9] Eating a vegetarian diet high in fruits and vegetables, and moderately high in fish, eggs, nuts, oils, and gluten-free grains is conducive to superior heart health. For patients who want to eat a whole foods diet and consume animal products, high-quality lean meats such as grass-fed beef, buffalo, bison, and pasture-raised chicken are healthy options. This type of gluten- and dairy-free diet that promotes high-quality meats is known as the Paleolithic or hunter-gatherer diet.

The Paleolithic diet is based on what our ancestors ate before the agricultural revolution 10,000 years ago. Genetically, we are practically identical to our Paleolithic ancestors, yet the Western diet is drastically different in macro and micronutrients, phytonutrients, electrolytes, and composition of fats, proteins, and particularly carbohydrates. Some say that the pre-agricultural diet should be the standard for contemporary human nutrition considering the genetic similarity to our Paleolithic ancestors.[10]

The typical hunter-gatherer culture consumed sweet and ripe fruits and berries, shoots, flowers, buds and young leaves, meat, bone marrow, organ meats, fish, shellfish, insects, larvae, eggs, roots, bulbs, nuts, and non-grass seeds.[5] These hunter-gatherers relied on finding food rather than cultivating it. Grains and dairy were not available, and thus were not consumed. It is thought that hunter-gatherers had greater metabolic output due to their mobile nature, and greater caloric intake compared to modern humans.[10] The high nutrient content of wildly harvested foods and game helped sustain their greater metabolic needs. Considering the high carbohydrate intake of modern humans coupled with no to minimal exercise, it's no wonder why the obesity epidemic is out of control. Low-fat diets rarely seem to work well for weight loss, as more carbohydrates (sugars) are consumed in place of fats. The Paleolithic diet selects low-sugar carbohydrates and allows consumption of high-quality fats.

Traditional hunter-gatherers that eat a Paleo-type diet have shown exceptionally favorable levels of serum cholesterol, blood pressure, and other cardiovascular risk factors.[5] In a 12-week study where pigs were fed a Paleo-type diet or cereal diet, the pigs eating Paleo had lower C-reactive protein, lower blood pressure, and higher insulin sensitivity. The authors of this study suggest that diseases of affluence may be attributable to insufficient evolutionary adaptation to grains.[11] In a recent systematic review and meta-analysis looking at the Paleo diet and CVD makers, the authors reported that eating the Paleo diet led to significant reductions in body weight, waist circumference, BMI, body fat percentage, systolic and diastolic blood pressures (SBP and DBP, respectively), total cholesterol, LDL cholesterol, CRP, and an elevated HDL. The authors also concluded, however, that some of these markers including CRP, lipid profile, and blood pressure may have been influenced by removing some studies, so the results must be interpreted with caution.[12]

If we compare the Paleolithic diet to the standard Western diet, we see stark differences in nutrient composition, antioxidants, fiber, and sugar intake. Overall, hunter-gatherers consumed less sodium, and more potassium, riboflavin, folate, thiamin, carotene, vitamin A, vitamin C, and vitamin E. They also consumed more fiber (100–150 vs 24 g/day) and fewer carbohydrates (22%–46% vs 50% total calories).[13]

The Mediterranean diet, which reflects food patterns typical of some Mediterranean regions in the early 1960s, such as Crete, parts of the rest of Greece, and southern Italy, is the most well-documented heart-healthy diet and is one that we routinely recommend to our patients.[14]

A large body of epidemiological and clinical evidence indicates that adherence to the Mediterranean diet is associated with lower risk CVD and overall mortality. These benefits are due to multiple underlying effects including reduction of blood lipids, inflammatory and oxidative stress markers, improvement of insulin sensitivity, enhancement of endothelial function, and antithrombotic function.[15]

One important point regarding the Mediterranean diet the research clearly shows is that there is a significant synergy among all the components of the diet rather than one specific factor responsible for all of the benefits. That said, the PREDIMED (PREvención con DIeta MEDiterránea) study, one of the most important dietary studies ever conducted, has provided some refinements on the composition and benefits of the Mediterranean diet; in particular, the importance of nut consumption. In the study, 7,447 men and women aged 50–80 years who had a high risk for a heart attack or stroke were assigned to one of the three interventions: a Mediterranean diet enriched with extra virgin olive oil, a Mediterranean diet supplemented with mixed nuts, or advice on a low-fat diet (control diet). The results were quite significant.

Compared to those who did not eat nuts, those subjects who reported consuming greater than 3 servings of nuts per week before the study started had a significant 39% lower risk of all-cause mortality when the study was completed nearly 5 years later. When subjects were then randomized into one of the three treatment groups, the results were even more conclusive. The participants following a Mediterranean diet who consumed nuts greater than 3 servings per week at the beginning of the study had a whopping 63% reduced risk of mortality compared to those consuming the low-fat diet and less than 3 servings of nuts per week. A reduced risk of mortality means a reduced risk of dying from any cause.[16]

THE STANDARD WESTERN DIET AND REFINED SUGAR

One of most shocking differences between a diet like the Paleolithic or Mediterranean diet and standard Western diet is the consumption of refined sugar. Since refined sugar did not exist in hunter-gatherer societies, 0 kg/year were consumed compared to 69.1 kg/year in the United States in the year 2000![13] This translates to 152 lbs of refined sugar consumed by Americans every year. According to Dr. Staffan Lindeberg, "roughly three-fourths of the calories in Western countries is today provided by foods that were practically unavailable during human evolution: wheat and other cereal grains, dairy foods, refined fats, and sugar."[5]

When you consider the pro-inflammatory nature of refined sugar, it comes as no surprise why chronic disease is rising steadily, and why CVD is the number one cause of mortality in the United States. As a culture, Americans are consuming too much sugar and too many refined carbohydrate calories. According to a small randomized clinical trial, consuming sugar-sweetened beverages for 3 weeks led to increases in waist to hip ratio, fasting blood glucose, and hs-CRP levels. The researches also noted a decrease in LDL particle size.[17] People need to be aware that sugar is very toxic for the body even in socially acceptable portion sizes (i.e., 12 oz soda), and that drinking these sugar beverages regularly can increase the risk for CVD.

Underlying chronic inflammation is emerging as the pivotal risk factor in the genesis of CVD. Sugar and highly refined foods are thought to cause inflammation in the body particularly in the endothelial lining (or innermost membrane) of blood vessels. To say it bluntly, sugar and subsequent insulin surges are the most endothelial-unfriendly components that promote oxidative stress. As a rise in blood sugar leads to inflammation in the endothelial lining, the body reacts by depositing cholesterol along the walls of the blood vessels as a protective mechanism to stabilize and strengthen the vessel. This is the inflammatory cascade that leads to atherosclerosis, one of the most common contributors to heart disease. By removing or at least dramatically decreasing sugar from a diet, you are eliminating a key player in the inflammatory response to heart disease.

WHEAT (GLUTEN), BLOOD SUGAR, AND INFLAMMATION

One of the biggest players responsible for this inflammation is a grain hidden in almost all packaged or processed foods: wheat. It's found in breads, bagels, pastas, pizzas, pastries, pretzels, wraps, crackers, candy bars, soy sauce, and other foods. For decades, the medical establishment has supported consuming a moderate intake of grains including wheat. If you browse grocery store isles and analyze the endless array of processed foods, you may see an endorsement from the American Diabetes Association or American Heart Association. We are taught from a very young age that grains including wheat are good for us.

Over the years, wheat has dominated the market in processed foods that are convenient, inexpensive, and long lasting. The wheat found in most foods these days, however, is not the same wheat that was around decades ago, nor is how it's processed healthy for you. We're really dealing with a Frankenstein food product, as wheat genes have been spliced over 50,000 times to make it more desirable (i.e., pest or drought resistant, higher gluten content, etc.), but in the process, a toxic form of wheat has been created. The gene splicing has transformed the wheat species into one of the highest glycemic index foods that humans consume, a glycemic index higher than even table sugar.

Higher glycemic index foods, like wheat, are broken down into sugar. Sugar raises insulin levels, and high insulin levels are pro-inflammatory, accelerating the aging process. Higher blood sugars in combination with proteins and lipids in the plasma create advanced glycation end products (AGEs).[18] AGEs not only accelerate aging but also cause enormous oxidative stress in the body at the same time. Never in the history of modern humans have diabetes, insulin resistance, and metabolic syndrome been expressed in the population at such an accelerating rate, largely due to our modern industrial food production. Flooding the body with sugar is only going to aggravate preexisting heart disease and make it more challenging to reverse.

Gluten consumption may not only contribute to inflammation in the arteries, but may lead to inflammation in the intestines as well. In a landmark study of *The Lancet*, Dr. Alessio Fasano discovered an intestinal protein called zonulin elevated in people with celiac disease. In the small intestine, regardless of if someone has celiac or non-celiac gluten sensitivity, zonulin induces tight junction disassembly, which leads to an increase in intestinal permeability.[19] In other words, gluten consumption can cause leaky gut syndrome. The intestines become inflamed, and "leaky" contents of the intestinal tract including bacterium and undigested food proteins are allowed to pass through the intestinal epithelium into the bloodstream. Chronically, this can lead to an overactivation of the immune system that may set the stage for auto-immune disease and other chronic inflammatory conditions.[20] Surprisingly, even individuals who do not have celiac disease are susceptible to zonulin elevations. Gliadin, one of the proteins found in gluten, can trigger zonulin release temporarily regardless of whether someone has celiac disease or not.[21] Therefore, all of us are susceptible to the increased intestinal permeability due to gluten consumption.

KNOW THY FOOD SOURCE

When choosing to eat a vegetarian diet, it is important to limit or completely eliminate processed foods (i.e., highly refined carbohydrates), and to make sure particular vitamins are replenished. Unhealthy vegetarians are those that typically consume high quantities of gluten and sugar products in place of meat products. They too suffer from most of the modern world's chronic diseases that are highly preventable through healthy eating. Many wheat-free (gluten-free) grains are beneficial to consume in their whole form, and these include quinoa, amaranth, millet, and buckwheat. Try to avoid processed gluten-free grains, however, as these too are high glycemic index foods products. Legumes such as lentils and beans can also be eaten in moderation to provide additional fiber, B vitamins, calcium, and iron.

Although vegetarian diets are high in fiber, vitamin C, vitamin E, folic acid, magnesium, and potassium, strict vegetarians and vegans have been known to be deficient in vitamin B12, vitamin D, zinc, and long-chain omega-3 fatty acids.[22,23] Low levels of vitamin B12, found in meat and eggs, cause an increase in plasma homocysteine, an amino acid linked with heart disease.[24] It is therefore important for vegetarians to supplement with vitamin B12, folate, and vitamin B6 to help metabolize methionine more efficiently, thus lowering homocysteine.[25] Since meat and eggs are consumed regularly on a Paleolithic diet, most Paleo followers do not need to take additional B vitamins, carnitine, alpha-lipoic acid, and coenzyme Q10 as these nutrients are found in abundance in the animal kingdom.

It can be challenging to find high-quality meat sources. The majority of red meat and chicken in the United States is factory farmed. Factory-farmed animals eat genetically modified soy and corn, are housed in extremely inhumane quarters, and fed and injected with antibiotics to treat and prevent infection. When choosing to eat a Paleolithic type diet, it is important to select the meats wisely. Typically, local farmer markets and health food stores sell grass-fed beef or pasture-raised chickens and eggs. Although the cost of pasture-raised meat is slightly higher compared to factory-farmed meats, its trans fat levels are lower, while omega-3 fatty acid levels are significantly higher.[26–28]

Choosing to eat a whole foods diet, whether vegetarian, Paleolithic, or Mediterranean, will help promote healthy eating habits and help reduce risk for CVD.[5,29] These three diets thrive on eating lots of fruits and vegetables (raw and cooked), and in moderation, nuts, seeds, eggs, and fish. Paleolithic diets include meats, and we recommend sourcing high-quality grass-fed or pasture-raised local meats, when possible, to optimize healthy fats. Vegetarian diets do include grains, but we suggest eliminating highly processed gluten-containing grains, particularly wheat, to minimize sugar intake. In summary, we recommend all three diets depending on one's personal preference.

Care should be taken in those with moderate to severe diabetes as blood sugar levels may drop when beginning one of these healthy diets. Make sure your diabetic patients are closely monitoring blood sugar, as hypoglycemia is not uncommon. Remember that radically shifting a diet from highly refined, processed, and sugary foods/drinks to one of healthy whole foods can dramatically affect body physiology, so be watchful and check in regularly with your patients.

UNDERSTANDING ATHEROSCLEROSIS

Arteries, the blood vessels that develop atherosclerosis, have three major layers. The innermost layer, the intima or the endothelium, is exposed to constant friction as blood and various particles flow by, often at high pressure. Glycosaminoglycans (GAGs) line the endothelial cells, protecting them from damage and promoting repair. Beneath the surface of endothelial cells is a protective membrane, which also contains GAGs.

The middle layer, or media, is mainly smooth muscle that allows the vessel to dilate or constrict in diameter, depending on the circulation needs of the moment. The outer layer, the adventitia, is an elastic membrane consisting of connective tissue. These layers also contain GAGs and other substances that provide support and elasticity.

Atherosclerosis begins when some factors damage the GAG layer that protects the endothelial cells. That factor might be oxidized LDL cholesterol, a virus or other organism, a drug or environmental toxin, physical damage due to high blood pressure, or the result of an immune response.

Even a small amount of damage to the inner lining can set a deadly chain of events in motion. One common triggering event is when LDL attaches to the GAGs lining the intima. When LDL binds to GAGs, it oxidizes and causes the release of other oxidants and free radicals, which further damages nearby cells. This is why elevated LDL cholesterol is such a major risk factor for heart disease. The more you have in your blood, the more likely it will set off this reaction to injury at the site of damage to the blood vessel.

Vessel damage causes endothelial cells to secrete growth factors and adhesion molecules, which furthers atherogenesis. The cells also release fibrinogen, the sticky stringy protein that collects platelets, so a clot can form to prevent blood from leaking out of the vessel. Monocytes arrive at the site, attach themselves to the vessel wall, and turn into macrophages and eventually into foam cells packed full of oxidized LDL and other damaged molecules.

The localized inflammatory milieu leads to migration of smooth muscle cells into the intima and replicating. Soon a fibrous cap appears in the surface of the artery lining, and an atherosclerotic plaque is formed. Over time, the plaque continues to grow until eventually it either ruptures and a clot breaks off or it blocks the entire artery.

Blood flow can be reduced by up to 90% before any symptoms of atherosclerosis appear. Most often, the first symptom is when vulnerable plaque characterized by a large lipid core breaks off to form an embolism that produces a myocardial infarction, pulmonary embolism, or stroke.

THE VASCULAR LINING – A KEY TARGET FOR NUTRITIONAL THERAPIES

What if we told you that your body has an internal medicine chest the size of a football field that is packed full of phenomenal and powerful remedies for inflammation, poor blood flow, high blood pressure, memory loss and virtually every other condition imaginable? Would you believe it? Well, it is true. This medicine chest is the vascular endothelium. From the heart to the smallest capillary, all vascular tissue has an endothelium. If all of the endothelial cells in the body were laid out flat, the endothelial surface area would be about the size of a football field. That is incredible to think about, isn't it? Even more incredible is the way that nutrition and dietary supplements can impact the vascular lining. Here is a brief look at some of the important and profound functions that the endothelium is responsible for:

- **Barrier Function**: the endothelium acts as a semi-selective barrier controlling the passage of materials and the transit of white blood cells into and out of the bloodstream. Excessive or prolonged increases in permeability of the endothelial layer are associated with inflammation and swelling.
- **Inflammation**: the endothelium helps to control inflammation in order to protect the deeper layers of blood vessels.
- **Blood Clotting (Thrombosis and Fibrinolysis)**: the surface of the endothelium normally possesses factors that prevent the formation of blood clots. When it lacks these protective factors, it can lead to the formation of blood clots that could lead to the buildup of plaque or the formation of a large clot that may break off and cause a heart attack or stroke.
- **The Constriction and Dilation of Blood Vessels**: hence, the endothelium plays a key role in controlling blood flow and blood pressure.

- In some organs, there are highly differentiated endothelial cells to perform specialized "filtering" functions. Examples of such unique endothelial structures include those found in the kidneys (the renal glomerulus) and those that protect the brain (the blood-brain barrier).

The loss of proper endothelial function is a hallmark for vascular diseases and the key early event in the development of atherosclerosis (hardening of the arteries). Impaired endothelial function is often seen in patients with diabetes, hypertension, and high cholesterol levels, as well as in smokers.

The main causes of endothelial dysfunction are high blood sugar levels and damage caused by free radicals and pro-oxidants. One of the key consequences of this damage is a diminished ability to manufacture nitric oxide, a key chemical messenger used by the endothelial cells to perform its duties.

THE ROLE OF NUTRITION AND ENDOTHELIAL FUNCTION

Virtually, all of the compounds that you have ever heard of that provides benefits to the vascular system, whether it is dark chocolate, pomegranate, olive oil, nuts and seeds, grape seed extract, arginine, coenzyme Q10 or fish oil, all impact endothelial function. One of the key benefits of the heart-healthy Mediterranean diet is that it greatly improves endothelial function.

The amazing thing about this barrier is that it is only one cell thick. It is kind of like shingles on a roof. If this barrier is damaged, it really sets in motion all of the factors that ultimately lead to the formation of the arterial plaque that is the hallmark feature of atherosclerosis. The endothelial cells can be damaged by free radicals and pro-oxidants as well as by immune, viral, chemical, and various drugs. Therefore, it is absolutely critical to support healthy endothelial function.

One of the keys to eating a diet high in antioxidant activity is focusing on flavonoids, a type of plant pigment and a member of the larger polyphenol family. As a class of compounds, flavonoids are often called "nature's biological response modifiers" because of their anti-inflammatory, anti-allergic, anti-viral, and anticancer properties. Many of the super foods like cacao, acai, goji, blueberries, etc. owe their benefits to their flavonoid content. While different flavonoids have different effects in the body, the key factor may not be a high intake of any one particular flavonoid, but rather a high total flavonoid intake that also provides a high variety of flavonoids rather than any one particular flavonoid class. There are more than 8,000 different types of flavonoids out there in nature.

What the research also shows is that it does not seem to matter where the flavonoids come from, e.g., through dietary sources such as legumes, fruit, green tea, coffee, chocolate or through flavonoid-rich extracts (grape seed, ginkgo, milk thistle, pine bark, bilberry, etc.), as long as an effective dosage is being taken. The caveat is that the proanthocyanidin flavonoids must be a major part of the flavonoid intake. Good dietary sources of these compounds are found in red or black grapes (especially the seeds), apples, cacao, cocoa, dark chocolate, berries (especially blueberries, cranberries, and black currants), certain nuts (e.g., hazelnuts, pecans, and pistachios), and red wine. So, with this caveat of the importance of proanthocyanidins in mind, what is an effective dosage of flavonoids? There has been an explosion of good scientific studies on a wide variety of flavonoid sources that help answer this question. For example, there are fantastic studies with proanthocyanidin-rich extracts from grape seed, cocoa, pomegranate, and pine bark, as well as flavonoid-rich extracts from citrus, soy, and green tea all showing significant clinical benefits, including in the following cardiovascular conditions:

- Atherosclerosis
- Cerebral vascular insufficiency
- High blood pressure
- High cholesterol levels
- Varicose veins, venous insufficiency and capillary fragility
- Visual function, retinopathy and macular degeneration.

There have also been a large number of studies with flavonoid-rich sources looking at immediate effects on blood vessel function, blood flow, or antioxidant capacity. Most of the studies with the aforementioned flavonoid-rich extracts have used an average dosage of about 300 mg/day to show an effect. Longer-term studies show even more benefit. For example, one of the best examples of the practical effect seen by normalizing endothelial function is with grape seed extract (standardized to contain 95% procyanidolic oligomers) in people with high blood pressure (discussed below). Similar studies exist with pine bark (pycnogenol), pomegranate, hibiscus, and hawthorn extracts—all are natural products rich in procyanidins. And, all are used in a dosage close to 300 mg/day in order to see a clinical effect.[30–32]

BERBERINE

Berberine has been extensively studied in clinical trials for lowering blood sugar, lipids, and blood pressure. There have been over 30 clinical studies with berberine in these disorders. In regard to its effects on blood lipids, not only does it lower total and LDL cholesterols (typically 20%–30%), unlike statins, berberine also lowers blood triglycerides (–20%) and raises beneficial HDL cholesterol (7%–12%). Berberine has also been shown to lower apolipoprotein B by 13%–15%, which is another very important risk factor to reduce heart disease. Studies also supported that berberine combined with conventional drugs in these conditions is safe and can produce better results than the drugs used alone. Side effects with berberine occurred at much lower rates and were milder than prescription drugs.[33–35]

Results have also shown quite convincing that in the treatment of type 2 diabetes, berberine (500 mg two to three times daily) lowered the level of fasting blood sugar levels, after-meal blood sugar levels, and glycosylated hemoglobin (HbA1c). In fact, when berberine was compared to oral hypoglycemic drugs used in type 2 diabetes like metformin, glipizide, and rosiglitazone, there was no statistical significance between treatment of berberine and these drugs. In other words, the clinical results seen with berberine are on par with the drugs, but with no significant side effects.[36]

Berberine produces these metabolic effects through various mechanisms. For example, berberine activates AMP-activated protein kinase (AMPk), an enzyme involved in regulating the body's energy levels. By targeting this pathway, berberine induces the uptake of glucose into cells, where it is converted into energy. Activating AMPk is also key to berberine's function in regulating blood lipids, such as LDL cholesterol, total cholesterol, and triglycerides. This enzyme acts as a master switch, regulating energy production and storage as well as lipid metabolism. It helps burn fatty acids within cells, stabilizes the receptors for LDL cholesterol, and inhibits the formation of lipids by the liver.

GARLIC

Garlic appears to be an important protective factor against heart disease and stroke via its ability to affect the process of atherosclerosis at so many steps. A major area of focus on garlic's ability to offer significant protection against heart disease and strokes has been the evaluation of its ability to lower blood cholesterol levels, even in apparently healthy individuals. According to the results from numerous double-blind, placebo-controlled studies in patients with initial cholesterol levels greater than 200, supplementation with commercial preparations providing a daily dose of at least 10 mg allicin or a total allicin potential of 4,000 mcg can lower total serum cholesterol levels by about 10%–12%, LDL cholesterol decreases by about 15%, HDL cholesterol levels usually increase by about 10%, and triglyceride levels typically drop by 15%. However, most trials not using products that can deliver this dosage of allicin fail to produce a lipid-lowering effect.[37–39]

Although the effects of supplemental garlic preparations on cholesterol levels are modest, the combination of lowering LDL and raising HDL can greatly improve the HDL-to-LDL ratio, a significant goal in the prevention of heart disease and strokes. Garlic preparations have also demonstrated blood pressure-lowering effects, inhibition of platelet aggregation, reduction of plasma viscosity, promotion of fibrinolysis, prevention of LDL oxidation, and an ability to exert positive effects on endothelial function, vascular reactivity, and peripheral blood flow.

PANTETHINE

Pantethine is the stable form of pantetheine, the active form of vitamin B_5 or pantothenic acid. Pantothenic acid is the most important component of coenzyme A (CoA). This enzyme is involved in the transport of fats to and from cells, as well as to the energy-producing compartments within the cell. Without coenzyme A, the cell's fats cannot be metabolized to energy.

Pantethine has significant lipid-lowering activity, while pantothenic acid has little (if any) effect in lowering cholesterol and triglyceride levels due to pantethine's ability to be converted to cysteamine. Pantethine administration (standard dose 900 mg/day) has been shown to significantly reduce serum triglyceride (32%), total cholesterol (19%), and LDL cholesterol (21%) levels while increasing HDL cholesterol (23%) levels. It appears to be especially useful in diabetics.[40–43]

The lipid-lowering effects of pantethine are most impressive when its toxicity (virtually none) is compared with conventional lipid-lowering drugs. Its mechanism of action is due to inhibited cholesterol synthesis and acceleration of the use of fat as an energy source.

BERGAMOT

Bergamot is a bitter, yellowish-orange citrus fruit native to southern Italy. It is cultivated mainly for an essential oil from the colored peel that is used to scent foods, cosmetic products, and perfumes. It is also what gives Earl Grey tea its distinctive taste (Table 3.1).

Bergamot has also historically been used to improve cardiovascular function. Multiple clinical trials have now shown evidence that bergamot can reduce total and LDL cholesterols. Like berberine, flavonoids and other polyphenols from the bergamot enhance AMPk activity. They also exert antioxidant and anti-inflammatory effects. The typical dosage of bergamot polyphenol fraction extract is 1,000–1,500 mg/day.[44,45]

THE NATUROPATHIC APPROACH TO TREATING HYPERTENSION

In the United States, nearly half of all Americans have elevated blood pressures in the prehypertensive (SBP 120–139 or DBP 80–89) to hypertensive (SBP > 140 or DBP > 90) range. This statistic is alarming considering the deleterious effects of high blood pressure and negative sequela including

TABLE 3.1

Comparative Effects on Blood Lipids of Several Natural Compounds in Patients with High Cholesterol and Triglyceride Levels[a]

	Niacin	Berberine	Garlic	Pantethine	Bergamot
Total cholesterol (% decrease)	−18%	−24%	−10%	−19%	−24%
LDL cholesterol (% decrease)	−23%	−30%	−15%	−21%	−28%
HDL cholesterol (% increase)	+32%	+20%	+31%	+23%	+26%
Triglycerides (% decrease)	−26%	−20%	−13%	−35%	−25%

[a] Typically, lipid-lowering agents will show a greater percentage reduction when cholesterol or triglyceride levels are high. The effects noted in this table are not entirely accurate as the results are displayed in a range of elevated levels in the studies included in this illustration.

stroke, CVD, and kidney disease. Although antihypertensive medications are effective in the reduction of blood pressure, adherence is often poor and cost can be high.[46] Additionally, side effects are common with antihypertensive medications and include hypokalemia, insomnia, depression, dry mouth, bronchospasm, impotence, and headaches.[47] It is therefore suggested that prehypertensive and hypertensive patients pursue complementary therapies including diet and lifestyle modifications, and mind-body medicines, to assist in blood pressure control.[46]

There is overwhelming evidence supporting the use of lifestyle measures to reduce blood pressure. Health care in the United States is more like disease care, with an emphasis on drugs and surgery for treating symptoms and diseases with a lack of attention for prevention. A naturopathic doctor's goal is to help change prescription pad readiness into education and self-responsibility. Patients need to be exposed to the most up-to-date evidence-based medicines possible, and to be able to make informed decisions about their treatment plan. In this section on hypertension, evidence-based diet and lifestyle modifications including nutraceuticals that reduce blood pressure without the use of pharmaceuticals will be addressed.

One of the foundations of medicine is learning how to identify and treat the cause of disease. Often we focus too much attention on treating the symptom, which will only alleviate the problem temporarily. For acute conditions like a myocardial infarction, treating the symptom such as acute coronary syndrome or unstable angina with nitroglycerine is necessary to reduce pain and perfuse blood-starved heart muscle. It's certainly not the ideal time or place for dietary recommendations or stress-reduction management. Knowing how and when to address the cause is a fine art, and it takes time and effort to uncover. Help your patients learn WHY they have a symptom or disease.

For most patients with essential hypertension, there is an underlying cause that can be identified with proper questions and insight. If we think of hypertension like an alarm going off in a burning building, prescribing a diuretic, ACE inhibitor, beta-blocker, or ARB is analogous to turning off the alarm without addressing the fire. We need to know where the alarm is going off, why it's making noise, and how to turn it off. Once we investigate the source of the fire, then we can treat it using proper lifestyle measures like a non-inflammatory diet, stress control, and targeted nutraceuticals. Occasionally, the fire is burning out of control and requires immediate attention with medication. This is usually a hypertensive crisis where blood pressure is higher than 180/110 mmHg, or when renal function is impaired.

Many factors go into deciding whether a medication is required to lower blood pressure. The most important ones are blood pressure levels, family and past medical history, age, exercise, diet, stress level, smoking, environmental toxin exposure, oxidative stress, co-morbidities (e.g., diabetes, auto-immune disease), medications, and the degree of motivation to make changes. Unfortunately, there is no simple algorithm to help you decide whether to use medication or not. There are over a dozen recommendations in this section for natural ways to lower blood pressure. Although some interventions only lower blood pressure modestly, cumulatively these treatments can have a profound impact on the cardiovascular system.

Identifying and treating the etiology of hypertension can be challenging as many causes can overlap and create confusion. For instance, the following commonly contribute to hypertension cases: nutritional deficiencies, stress, endocrine dysfunction (e.g., hyperthyroidism), obesity, lack of exercise, smoking, alcohol, and prescription medications (e.g., NSAIDS, birth control). Other causes need to be ruled out as well such as renal disease, hyperaldosteronism, Cushing's disease, coarctation of the aorta, and white-coat hypertension.

As naturopathic doctors, we cannot emphasize the importance of spending ample time questioning our patient about their current and past health. Without hesitation, ask your patients about their diet and nutrient intake, weight, exercise, lifestyle (i.e., smoking, alcohol intake), stress, and prescription drug use. What foods and fluids are they regularly consuming? What's their home and work life like? Are they shift workers? What's their level of emotional stress? Are they unhappy or unfulfilled? Asking these types of questions cannot only help unravel a complex case, but also build a strong patient-doctor relationship, which is an important step for healing to occur. If there is no obvious cause after an in-depth intake, basic labs (CBC, TSH, BUN, GFR, CR, aldosterone, cortisol) and imaging (renal ultrasound, echocardiogram) may help to determine the cause.

The bottom line is spend time with your patients, ask appropriate questions, and thoroughly investigate their case. Even if the cause is very challenging to determine and treat, always address diet and lifestyle. You may learn from reviewing a simple diet diary that your hypertensive patient eats a bag of potato chips at night because she is angry with a co-worker. The high sodium and trans fat intake coupled with sustained cortisol release from chronic stress is setting the stage for CVD including hypertension. Instead of prescribing a diuretic, talk about the patient's stress and offer suggestions to alleviate emotional toxicity, and thus emotional eating.

DIET, LIFESTYLE, AND HYPERTENSION

How many times have you heard that healthy eating, exercise, restricted salt intake, and stress reduction are supportive for blood pressure control? Why are these therapies often overlooked? Is it because we don't have the time during visits to teach our patients this valuable information? We believe it's important to know quantitatively how much these lifestyle factors can influence SBP and DBP. One of the roles of a physician is to educate patients about the risk/benefit ratio of a treatment plan, and this includes lifestyle changes as well as medications. In medicine, it's easy to get caught up in treating numbers (blood pressure) when ultimately we are treating people, and when treating people, laying the foundation with diet and lifestyle factors is essential.

For hypertensive patients, we generally recommend a whole food diet similar to the modified Paleolithic and vegetarian diets discussed earlier, or the Mediterranean diet – which we know from many studies are heart healthy.[6,7] These types of diets all include fresh fruits, vegetables, nuts, seeds, heart-healthy oils (e.g., olive, avocado, macadamia nut), pasture-raised eggs, fish, and legumes (lentils, beans). This means eating little to no processed and fast foods, as these "foods" contain mainly sugar, toxic fats, GMOs, preservatives, food colorings, and a whole list of other chemicals. Hippocrates, the father of Western medicine, once said that "let food be thy medicine and medicine be thy food." In other words, eat real foods to support, nourish, and heal the body.

SPECIAL FOODS TO LOWER BLOOD PRESSURE

Special foods for people with high blood pressure include beet juice, celery, garlic and onions, nuts and seeds or their oils for their essential fatty acid content, cold-water fish (salmon, mackerel, etc.), or fish oil supplements concentrated for EPA+DHA (dosage 1,000–3,000 mg/day), green leafy vegetables as a rich source of calcium and magnesium, legumes for their fiber, and foods rich in vitamin C like broccoli and citrus fruits.

Ground flaxseeds are also helpful in high blood pressure. In a study conducted at the St. Boniface Hospital Research Centre in Winnipeg, Canada, the effects of daily ingestion of ground flaxseed on SBP and DBP in patients with peripheral artery disease was studied. While individuals with normal BP showed no effect with 6 months of flaxseed ingestion (two tablespoons daily), those patients who entered the trial with a SBP ≥ 140 mmHg at baseline obtained an average reduction of 15 mmHg in SBP and 7 mmHg in DBP. In other words, this major antihypertensive effect was achieved selectively in hypertensive patients. Flaxseeds can be purchased either whole or already ground or sliced. We prefer purchasing ground/milled flaxseeds as it enhances their digestibility and therefore their nutritional value. Most of the beneficial research has focused on the use of ground flaxseeds. Ground flaxseeds have also been shown to be helpful in improving blood lipid profiles.[48]

Celery is another particularly interesting food for lowering blood pressure. A celery seed extract standardized to contain 85% 3-n-butylphthalide (3nB) has been shown to help improve blood pressure control. 3nB is a compound that is unique to celery and is responsible for the characteristic flavor and odor of celery. It was discovered as the active component of celery in response to investigations by researchers seeking to explain some of the traditional effects of celery, including lowering of blood pressure and relief of joint pain. The dosage of the extract is 75–150 mg twice daily. This amount would translate to about 12 ribs of celery, probably too high of an amount of whole celery to eat, but easily done by juicing.[49]

To prove the effects of dietary flavonoids in lowering blood pressure, let's take a look at a study conducted at Florida State University. In the study, 48 postmenopausal women with mild hypertension were enrolled to evaluate the effects of daily blueberry consumption for 8 weeks. The women were randomly assigned to receive either 22 g freeze-dried blueberry powder or 22 g control powder daily. Approximately 22 g freeze-dried blueberry powder is equal to 1 cup fresh blueberries, an attainable dosage for people to consume on a daily basis. After 8 weeks, SBP and DBP (131 and 75 mmHg, respectively) were significantly lower than baseline levels (138 mmHg and 80 mmHg, respectively). Blueberry consumption was also associated with improved elasticity within the arteries as noted by improvements in brachial-ankle pulse wave velocity compared to baseline levels. Nitric oxide levels were also greater in the blueberry powder group at 8 weeks compared with baseline values. There were no changes in any parameters in the control group.[50]

THE DASH DIET

The Dietary Approach to Stop Hypertension (DASH) diet, a very common diet for those suffering from hypertension, is rich in fruits, vegetables, and low-fat dairy foods, and low in saturated fat. It is also low in cholesterol, high in dietary fiber, potassium, calcium, and magnesium, and moderately high in protein. Research shows it can lower SBP and DBP by 5.5 and 3.3 mmHg, respectively.[51] Some large randomized controlled trials (RCTs) looking at the DASH diet show even greater reductions in SBP of approximately 11 mmHg and DBP of 5 mmHg.[52] These results are clinically significant and indicate that a sodium intake below 1,500 mg daily can significantly and quickly lower blood pressure.

For reducing blood pressure, we do support a DASH-type diet. Overall, we believe that it's a very healthy diet and very similar to the Mediterranean diet.

On the DASH diet, low-fat dairy products are recommended. There is moderate research suggesting an inverse relationship between dairy consumption and blood pressure, although more clinical research is needed to delineate a causal relationship.[53] If choosing to consume dairy, try to buy organic full-fat products instead, as low-fat products typically contain more sugar and other additives which may not be conducive to optimal blood pressure control. Studies show that cows fed grass instead of grains have higher levels of omega-3s in their milk.[54] If available, consume organic grass-fed dairy products as the fatty acid profile is more desirable.[29] Also, organic dairy products should not contain any hormone byproducts, which may lead to oxidative stress in the body.

The DASH diet suggests consuming 2–3 servings a day of fats and oils including vegetable oil and/or margarine. We do not recommend these oils because they may contain trans fats, and may promote free radical oxidation in the body, particularly in the blood vessels. Instead, we like olive, avocado, and coconut oils for supporting cardiovascular health. Studies on olive oil show promising reductions in blood pressure when consumed in upwards of 60 g (4 Tbsp) a day.[55] The oleic acid present in olive oil may be responsible for the blood pressure-lowering effect. Coconut oil is a very stable oil and great to use for high-heat cooking. In one study, virgin coconut oil fed to rats helped prevent blood pressure elevation, which the authors suggest may be due to a reduction in vasoconstriction of the endothelium.[56] Therefore, when used in moderation, these oils can exert cardioprotective qualities.

FLUIDS, SALT, AND HYPERTENSION

In regard to fluids, we recommend consuming mainly filtered water, and avoiding excessive alcohol and caffeine intake. In a meta-analysis of 15 RCTs, reducing alcohol intake lowered SBP and

DBP by 3.31 and 2.04 mmHg, respectively.[57] Caffeine intake mainly from coffee elicits very minor increases in blood pressure, so we suggest coffee in moderation.[58] Remember, blood sugar swings can contribute to fluctuations in blood pressure. Minimally consume desserts and highly refined carbohydrates and sugary foods, as sugar will also trigger a neurohormonal response leading to an elevation in blood pressure.

In addition to consuming filtered water, some studies show promising reductions in blood pressure with the use of hibiscus tea. Hibiscus flowers contain anthocyanins, which are thought to exhibit blood pressure-lowering effects through mild ACE inhibitor and diuretic actions. In a randomized, double-blinded, placebo-controlled trial, 3 240 mL servings per day of hibiscus tea were administered for 6 weeks to pre and mildly hypertensive adults. Compared to placebo, those consuming hibiscus tea had lower SBP and DBP by 7.2 and 3.1 mmHg, respectively.[59] In two other RCTs (one of them double-blinded), hibiscus tea was almost comparable to the ACE inhibitors lisinopril and captopril in lowering BP with a wide margin of tolerability and safety.[60,61]

Patients commonly ask us about salt and whether they can add it to meals. Excessive salt intake is associated with an elevation in blood pressure, and an increased risk for CVD, renal disease, and stroke.[62,63] In a meta-analysis of 34 trials, researchers found that a reduction in salt intake of 4 g/day led to reductions in SBP and DBP of 4.18 and 2.06 mmHg, respectively, in normotensive and hypertensive individuals. They propose that reducing salt intake to 4–5 g/day can have a major effect on blood pressure, and that lowering it to 3 g/day offers the most cardioprotective benefits.[64] As reference, 3 g of sodium a day is just over 1 tsp of salt.

Numerous studies have shown that sodium restriction alone does not improve blood pressure control in most people, and it must be accompanied by a high potassium intake. Most Americans have a potassium-to-sodium ratio of less than 1:2, meaning that they ingest more than twice as much sodium as potassium. Researchers recommend a dietary potassium-to-sodium ratio of greater than 5:1 to maintain health. The easiest way to lower sodium intake is to avoid prepared foods and table salt.

The main source of salt in the standard American diet is processed food products such as canned goods, fast foods, pickles, chips, candies, and processed meats. If the above foods are consumed infrequently, it's okay in moderation to add high-quality sea salt (a "pinch") to meals as this can actually benefit digestion and provide essential trace minerals.

It should be noted that increasing potassium in the diet or via a supplement can lower the risk of stroke, and help reduce blood pressure.[65,66] According to research, if 4.7 g/day of dietary potassium is consumed, SBP and DBP decrease by 8.0 and 4.1 mmHg, respectively. A potassium-induced reduction in blood pressure can offer other cardiovascular benefits including a reduction in myocardial infarction and coronary heart disease.[67] In a large prospective study of 43,738 men, greater potassium intake through diet resulted in a lowered incidence of stroke.[65] If supplemental potassium is administered, care should be taken in those patients taking potassium-sparing medications or with renal disease.[67]

EXERCISE AND HYPERTENSION

Regular exercise can reduce blood pressure in hypertensive and normotensive individuals. In a meta-analysis of 54 RCTs, aerobic exercise lowered SBP and DBP by 3.84 and 2.58 mmHg, respectively.[68] One study had participants exercise 3–4 times per week for 1 hour at 75%–85% of their initial HR reserve, and then compared this group to an exercise and weight management group. The participants in the exercise and weight management group had the greatest reductions in SBP and DBP of 7 and 5 mmHg, respectively.[69] The lesson to learn from this study is exercise coupled with weight loss promotes greater blood pressure control than exercise alone.

Research reports that modest increases in exercise of 61–90 minutes per week can decrease BP in a sedentary hypertensive population.[70] One study indicated that 10,000 steps per day, regardless of duration or intensity, is effective in lowering blood pressure and reducing sympathetic nerve activity.[71] Walking for most people is a simple form of exercise that can benefit the cardiovascular system. We recommend exercise that is practical, convenient, and enjoyable, and for most people a daily 20-minute walk in the neighborhood will suffice. It also provides time to walk with a loved one, pet, or enjoy the quiet solitude of nature.

STRESS, BREATHING, AND HYPERTENSION

One of the most important, and often neglected, lifestyle measures to address with your patients is stress. Stress exists in many forms and may include situational (e.g., car accident), mental (e.g., anxiety), emotional (e.g., fear, guilt), physical (e.g., chronic back pain), chemical (e.g., pesticides), oxidative (e.g., heavy metals, electromagnetic radiation), and psychospiritual (e.g., relationship, career) factors. Everyone manages stress on a daily basis whether it's paying bills, waiting in traffic, caring for a sick family member, or constantly connecting through social media. These stressors have a cumulative effect that can result in chronic stimulation of the sympathetic nervous system.

An overactive sympathetic nervous system may lead to chronically elevated vasoconstrictive stress hormones that set the stage for hypertension.[72] When under chronic stress, the hypothalamic-pituitary-adrenal axis overproduces glucocorticoid and catecholamine hormones. These fight-or-flight hormones include cortisol, epinephrine, and norepinephrine, and can elevate blood sugar and blood pressure causing significant neurohormonal changes including immune system dysfunction. *Acutely* activating this "fight-or-flight" system is advantageous because heart rate, respiratory rate, and blood flow increase, and our ability to react to stimuli is enhanced. We desperately need these hormones to survive, but balancing them in a chronically stressful environment is key to supporting cardiovascular health.

One method to calm an overactive sympathetic nervous system is to increase parasympathetic tone. Many mind-body therapies including Tai chi, Qi gong, Yoga, biofeedback, and meditation and/or slow belly breathing help reduce stress by activating parasympathetic pathways. When practiced regularly, these therapies can have a profound impact on the quality of life, and can reduce blood pressure as well. These mind-body therapies have a common denominator: meditation through habitual breathing. Learning how to breathe, and building awareness around breathing exercises, is likely why these therapies are beneficial for lowering blood pressure; breathing encourages parasympathetic tone in the body which in turn supports heart rate variability. Increasing heart rate variability is a major prognosticator in protecting cardiovascular health.[73]

Biofeedback can be used to slow breathing rate, and therefore, help lower blood pressure. In a small RCT, 22 menopausal women with pre-hypertension were assigned to either a control group (slow abdominal breathing) or an experimental group. The experimental group performed ten 25-minute sessions of slow abdominal breathing (6 cycles per minute) combined with frontal electromyographic biofeedback training and daily home practice. The biofeedback training involved muscle relaxation techniques and guided imagery. The experimental group showed the greatest reductions in SBP and DBP of 8.4 and 3.9 mmHg, respectively. The control group experienced a small drop in SBP of 4.3 mmHg, but no significant drop in DBP. The researchers conclude that slow breathing at 6 cycles a minute coupled with biofeedback training is an effective intervention to manage pre-hypertension.[74]

In addition to biofeedback, breathing devices can also help regulate blood pressure. In a randomized, double-blinded, placebo-controlled study, participants were able to lower their blood pressure using a Breathe with Interactive Music (BIM) device for 10 minutes every evening. The BIM device guided users how to breathe slowly and regularly using sound patterns. A control group listened to a Walkman with a soft music. At the end of the 8-week study, BIM participants' SBP and DBP lowered by 15.2 and 10 mmHg, respectively, and control group's SBP and DBP by 11.3 and 5.6 mmHg, respectively. These findings suggest that a calming cardiovascular response opposite to that caused by mental stress is responsible for the decrease in BP in both groups. The lower BP in the BIM group is further attributed to breathing modulation.[75] These BIM devices produced reductions in BP similar to those found by commonly prescribed anti-hypertensives.

In a RCT of 79 patients using Device-Guided-Breathing-Exercises (DGBE), hypertensive medicated participants spent 15 minutes per day practicing deep breathing at home. Blood pressures were measured at home and in office over an 8-week period. By the end of the study, the participants using DGBE had a reduction in SBP of 5.5 mmHg and DBP of 3.6 mmHg.[76] These results from the previous two studies show that breathing devices, commonly available to patients, can help lower blood pressure by assisting with deep-breathing exercises. Moreover, reductions in blood pressure can be seen weeks after cessation of treatment.

Many of the abovementioned studies use machines to guide breathing. Other practices such as yoga or Tai chi focus on the breath as well. It's important to understand that it's not the machine that's lowering blood pressure, but the habitual practice of breathing! One of the reasons why yoga is so popular is because the practice not only supports the musculoskeletal system with stretching and posture alignment, but it also teaches people to breathe properly. Effectively learning how to breathe can take time and practice. Fortunately, biofeedback and breathing machines, breathing exercises, teachers, or group work can help develop awareness around the breath.

Out of all the meditation practices, transcendental meditation (TM) seems to offer the greatest blood pressure-lowering effect. TM is a non-religious meditation technique that focuses on mantra repetition for 20 minutes 2 times a day. It is thought to promote relaxation, and can bring the meditator into a deeper state of consciousness. In a meta-analysis of nine RCTs looking at TM and its effect on blood pressure, regular practice of TM has the potential to approximately lower SBP and DBP by 4.7 and 3.2 mmHg, respectively.[77] In one RCT, 298 university students were assigned to a TM program or wait list control. The students in the TM program exhibited lower SBP and DBP, and improvements were noted in total psychological stress, anxiety, depression, anger/hostility, and coping.[78]

For an excellent discussion and analysis of the science of breathing, the author James Nester recently wrote a book appropriately titled *Breath*. From this book, you will learn the importance of breathing through the nostrils, how slow structured breathing is optimal for your health, and the role that carbon dioxide tolerance plays in retraining your body how to breathe properly.[79]

TARGETED NUTRITIONAL SUPPLEMENTS, BOTANICAL MEDICINES, AND ACUPUNCTURE AND HYPERTENSION

While there is no question that hypertensive medications significantly lower blood pressure, and reduce CVD events and stroke, side effects are common and cost can be prohibitive. Many patients these days are searching for a more holistic approach to treating hypertension, and demand alternatives for drug therapy. When blood pressure elevation is mild to moderate (pre to stage I hypertension), diet and lifestyle interventions should be addressed first as these treatments are fundamental to sound health. In addition to diet and lifestyle changes (e.g., exercise, fasting, meditation), targeted nutritional supplements, botanical medicines, and acupuncture can further lower blood pressure. These natural medicine treatments may be necessary to get blood pressure under control quickly while diet and lifestyle measures take effect, and can help wean patients off certain hypertensive medications. Although there are multiple targeted supplements to choose from, we have had the most success with coenzyme Q10, magnesium, omega-3 fatty acids, garlic, grape seed extract, and berberine to name a few.

Coenzyme Q10 (which is discussed in detail in other chapters of this textbook) is a powerful antioxidant found in all human cells. It also helps to support ATP turnover in the mitochondria, is a membrane stabilizer, and can help reduce inflammatory markers.[80,81] Although the exact mechanism is unknown in humans for reducing blood pressure, CoQ10 does reduce peripheral resistance through nitric oxide preservation, and acts as a potent free radical scavenger helping reduce free radical stress.[82] While some studies show mixed results with CoQ10 for blood pressure control, other studies show a moderate reduction in blood pressure. One randomized, double-blinded, placebo-controlled trial found a mean reduction of 17.8 mmHg in SBP.[83] In a Cochrane meta-analysis of three double-blinded, placebo-controlled studies, mean decreases in SBP and DBP were 11 and

7 mmHg, respectively. It should be noted that the authors of this analysis were concerned about quality of blinding, and author credibility.[84] The typical dose for CoQ10 supplementation is 100–200 mg a day. Side effects are rarely seen.

Magnesium is a mineral involved in over 300 enzymatic reactions in the body. It may help reduce blood pressure due to the mild smooth muscle relaxation and Ca^{2+} ion antagonizing effects. A meta-analysis of 22 trials showed that 410 mg (mean dosage) of magnesium can reduce SBP by 3–4 mmHg and DBP by 2–3 mmHg.[85]

The average intake of magnesium by healthy adults in the United States ranges from 143 to 266 mg/day. This level is well below even the recommended daily allowance (RDA) of 350 mg for men and 300 mg for women. Food choices are the main reason. Because magnesium occurs abundantly in whole foods, most nutritionists and dietitians assume that most Americans get enough magnesium in their diets. But most Americans are not eating whole, natural foods. They are consuming large quantities of processed foods. Because food processing refines a large portion of magnesium, most Americans are not getting the RDA for magnesium.

We recommend a magnesium bound to citrate, aspartate, or malate over the popular magnesium oxide. A good daily dose is 250–300 mg. Side effects may include diarrhea or abdominal cramping if dosed too high, and magnesium should not be given to patients with renal insufficiency.

There are many studies on fish oil supplementation and increased fish intake for the treatment of blood pressure for medicated and unmedicated hypertensive patients. Some studies show modest reductions in blood pressure. In a recent meta-analysis of 17 studies, researchers concluded that reductions in SBP of 2.56 mmHg and DBP of 1.47 mmHg were found with fish oil supplementation. Varying doses of fish oil including DHA and EPA were used in this analysis. Although a small reduction in blood pressure was found, the researchers state that a 2 mmHg reduction in SBP can lower mortality by 10% for strokes and mortality by 7% for ischemic heart disease.[86] Typical doses for fish oil are to provide a dosage of EPA+DHA of 1,000–2,000 daily. Side effects may include burping and abdominal discomfort.

Garlic as mentioned earlier as a food-based supplement is very helpful for reducing blood pressure. In one meta-analysis of ten trials, participants with hypertension (SBP > 140 mmHg) experienced reductions in SBP and DBP by 16.3 and 9.3 mmHg, respectively. There was no clinically significant drop in SBP or DBP in normotensive participants, however.[87] Similar results were found in another meta-analysis of hypertensive participants where reductions in SBP of 8.4 mmHg and in DBP of 7.3 mmHg were observed.[88] These findings suggest that garlic supplementation may help reduce blood pressure in hypertensive individuals. It should be noted that many forms of garlic were used in these studies and that the average dose was 600–900 mg a day providing 3.6–5.4 mg of allicin, the active compound in garlic.[88] As a side note, garlic cloves generally contain 5–9 mg of allicin, so they may be used in cooking to achieve some hypotensive benefits. Garlic may interact with some pharmaceuticals such as coumadin, so make sure you look up possible herb/drug interactions before initializing treatment.

There are many other food-based supplements and nutraceuticals that help reduce blood pressure. For example, four clinical studies have also shown grape seed extract (standardized to contain 95% procyanidolic oligomers) to normalize high blood pressure in patients with initial blood pressure in the range of 150/95 mmHg. Significant improvements were also noted in various markers of vascular function such as stiffness, distensibility, elasticity, and pulse wave velocity (PWV).[89] The dosage was 300 mg daily (Table 3.2).

The benefits noted with grape seed extracts and other flavonoid-rich extracts (e.g., olive, pomegranate, hibiscus) may also be achieved through dietary means by focusing on proanthocyanidin-rich foods such as berries. Even something as simple as consuming the equivalent of 8 oz of blueberries per day has shown benefit (discussed above).[89–92]

Studies have shown that extracts rich in olive polyphenols lower blood pressure and cholesterol levels. In the largest trial to date, 232 patients with high blood pressure were given either an olive leaf extract (500 mg twice daily) or the conventional antihypertensive drug captopril (12.5 mg twice

TABLE 3.2

Olive Extract vs. Captopril in Patients with High Blood Pressure

Group	Beginning Blood Pressure	Blood Pressure at 8 Weeks
Olive extract	149.3/93.9	137.8/89.1
Captopril	148.4/93.8	134.7/87.4

daily) for 8 weeks. Results showed that the olive extract was clinically as effective in lowering blood pressure as the drug, but without side effects.[93,94]

In addition to lowering blood pressure, olive polyphenols have been shown to lower LDL cholesterol while increasing HDL cholesterol. Researchers were unsure exactly how this effect was accomplished until a recent study showed that olive polyphenols exert a very complex action on the expression of genes that made LDL and HDL cholesterols. In other words, the olive compounds blocked the expression of the DNA that would lead to the making of LDL cholesterol while simultaneously assisting the expression of DNA for making HDL cholesterol. It also modulates the expression of blood pressure-related genes.[95,96]

The following can also assist with blood pressure control: taurine, L-arginine, vitamins E, C, D, and B6, alpha-lipoic acid, N-acetyl cysteine, melatonin, and flavonoid-rich extracts such as pomegranate, black and green teas, and chocolate.[97] Many of these vitamins and nutrients can be found in whole foods, which brings us back to the notion of food as medicine. They can also be taken in supplement form as well.

Traditionally, botanical medicines have been used to lower blood pressure and support the heart. Many naturopathic physicians and herbalists compound antihypertensive botanical formulas that may contain the following herbs: hawthorn, rauwolfia, rosemary, dandelion leaf, mistletoe, *Coleus forskohlii*, and arjuna. While there is some research to support their use, a physician must intensely study these herbs and interactions to feel confident enough to prescribe them. Most herbal medicines are very safe to use, but caution must be taken particularly if patients are taking multiple hypertensive pharmaceuticals concurrently.

Naturopathic doctors often use botanical formulas to wean a patient off a pharmaceutical while addressing diet and lifestyle changes. The above herbs, especially rauwolfia, have been used with great success. When prescribing rauwolfia, however, you must be careful about potential drug interactions including MAO inhibitors. Severe depression and Parkinson's disease are contraindications. Since rauwolfia contains the alkaloid reserpine, side effects are not uncommon, so care needs to be taken when prescribing this herb.

Acupuncture is a system of medicine that has been around for thousands of years that can help treat hypertension. Although research does support its use for reducing blood pressure, many of the trials have unclear methodological quality and most are in other languages other than English (i.e., Chinese, Russian). In a recent meta-analysis of 35 studies, acupuncture significantly reduced SBP by 7.47 mmHg and DBP by 4.22 mmHg. The authors of this analysis conclude, however, that the results are limited by methodological flaws in the studies. They suggest further large-scale studies be done to confirm these results.

FASTING AND HYPERTENSION

Fasting has been shown to lower blood pressure and reduce the prevalence of coronary artery disease.[98,99] In one study, 174 hypertensive adults participated in extended water-only fasting, which averaged 10–11 days in length. At the end of the study, 90% of the participants were normotensive with an average reduction in SBP and DBP of 37 and 13 mmHg, respectively. The greatest reduction in blood pressure occurred in those with Stage III hypertension with an average reduction of

60/17 mmHg (systolic/diastolic). This study suggests that medically supervised water-only fasting is a safe and effective treatment for hypertension.[99]

GROUNDING AND HYPERTENSION

There is research emerging showing a positive cardiovascular benefit from connecting our bodies to the surface of the earth. This technique is known as grounding or earthing and can improve heart rate variability, reduce blood viscosity, lower nighttime cortisol, reduce pain, increase zeta potential, and increase parasympathetic activity.[100–102] The simplest way to ground our bodies is to walk barefoot on the grass. For most of our existence, humans have walked barefoot or with conductive footwear (e.g., leather), and have slept close to the earth. With the introduction of rubber and plastic sole shoes, however, people are rarely in contact with the earth. When the skin touches the earth's electron-rich surface, there is a free flow of negative charge into the body, which may help neutralize free radicals or reactive oxygen species. This may be a possible mechanism of action for the physiological benefits attributed through grounding. Although there are case reports of grounding lowering blood pressure, more research needs to be done to suggest this as a treatment for hypertension.[102]

MONITOR YOUR BLOOD PRESSURE

You will know if these recommendations are working by monitoring your blood pressure. As a reminder, high blood pressure must not be taken lightly. By keeping your blood pressure in the normal range, you will not only lengthen your life, but you will also improve the quality of your life.

CONCISE RECOMMENDATIONS FOR HIGH BLOOD PRESSURE

- General lifestyle, dietary, and supplement recommendations
  - Reduce excess weight
  - Follow a healthy lifestyle: avoid alcohol, caffeine, and smoking, exercise and use stress-reduction techniques especially deep-breathing exercises
  - Eat a high-potassium diet rich in whole plant foods
  - Increase dietary consumption of celery, garlic, and onions
  - Reduce or eliminate the intake of animal fats while increasing the intake of olive oil and omega-3 fatty acids
  - Eliminate salt (sodium chloride) intake and use PerfeKt Sea Salt instead
  - Supplement the diet with all of the following:
    - High-potency multiple vitamin and mineral formula
    - Grape seed or pine bark extract: 300 mg daily
    - Fish oil: 1,000–3,000 mg of EPA+DPA+DHA daily
    - Vitamin C: 500–1,000 mg two to three times daily
    - Magnesium: 250 mg two to three times daily
    - Coenzyme Q10 (CoQ10): ubiquinone form dosage is 300 mg daily, and ubiquinol form dosage is 100 mg daily.

NOTE: If you have severe hypertension, you will need to work with a physician to select the most appropriate medication. If a prescription drug is necessary, ACE inhibitors alone or in combination with a diuretic appear to be the safest. If your blood pressure has not dropped below 140/105 after following the above recommendations for 2 months, you may also need to be on prescription medication. When satisfactory control over the high blood pressure has been achieved, work with the physician to taper off the medication.

- Additional recommendations if needed, choose one or more of the following:
  - Berberine: 500 mg three times daily before meals
  - Celery seed extract standardized to contain 85% 3-n-butylphthalide (3nB): 75–150 mg twice daily
  - Hibiscus tea or extracts have demonstrated blood pressure-lowering properties in clinical trials. In double-blind studies, hibiscus extract showed similar blood pressure-lowering effects to popular antihypertensive drugs. But unlike the drugs, which carry a significant side effect profile, hibiscus has a 100% tolerability and safety response. Typical reductions in SBP are 15–20 mmHg in subjects with initial readings of 140 mmHg. Dosage: for the tea, three 240 mL servings per day, and for an extract, take enough to supply 10–20 mg anthocyanidins daily
  - Olive leaf extract has been shown in clinical trials to work as effective as the conventional antihypertensive drug captopril in lowering blood pressure, but without the side effects. Dosage: 500 mg (17%–23% oleuropein content) twice daily.

THE IMPORTANCE OF DETOXIFICATION IN SUPPORTING THE CARDIOVASCULAR SYSTEM

Considering the enormous toxin burden we are facing today, detoxification must become of way of life, or toxin accumulation will inadvertently affect our health, and more importantly the health of future generations. Since the industrial revolution and the introduction of chemical fertilizers and pesticides, the level of toxins present in the air, water, and soil has skyrocketed to unprecedented levels. Heavy metals such as mercury, pesticides such as DDT, and xenoestrogens such as phthalates found in plastics have infiltrated the environment and ultimately our bodies. The amount of chemicals used for agriculture alone has increased tremendously over the last half decade, and some of these pesticides originally deemed as safe are proving to be carcinogenic.[103] This massive increase in environmental toxins has put tremendous strain on our cell's detoxification mechanisms, and consequently, toxins are being stored rather than properly excreted.

THE EFFECTS OF ENVIRONMENTAL TOXINS ON BLOOD PRESSURE AND THE CARDIOVASCULAR SYSTEM

INTRODUCTION

Many studies have looked at the effects of environmental toxins on blood pressure and CVD. It is known that heavy metals including mercury, arsenic, cadmium, and lead, cigarette smoke, and pesticides can cause elevations in blood pressure.[104,105] In one study looking at residents living near a Monsanto chemical plant, those with high polychlorinated bisphenyl exposure had elevations in SBP and DBP. Polychlorinated biphenyls (PCBs) are manmade chemicals banned in the United States in 1979 due to their high level of toxicity. Although the exact mechanism for how PCBs affect blood pressure is unclear, it is thought that they promote endothelial dysfunction through their pro-inflammatory nature. PCBs have been shown to induce oxidative stress in endothelial cells, which may be an underlying mechanism for the development of atherosclerosis and hypertension.[106] Sadly, PCBs are still showing up in our food supply, and subsequently our bodies, as they continue to be dumped into the environment, and have a considerably long half-life (EPA.gov).

There is speculation that exposure to pesticides before birth may lead to greater susceptibility to hypertension in adulthood. DDT (dichlorodiphenyltrichloroethane) is a pesticide banned in the United States decades ago, but still used worldwide for indoor malaria vector control, and as a pesticide in countries outside the United States. Today, DDT is still found in our soil and indoor air samples, and continues to infiltrate our bodies due to its long half-life and semivolatility. In a birth cohort study following women into their fifth decade of life, prenatals exposed to DDT were at higher risk for developing hypertension in adulthood.[107] The implications of this study are enormous considering the plethora of toxins found in prenatals today.

In a recent monumental study looking at environmental chemical levels in 268 pregnant women, many chemicals known to have detrimental effects on health (e.g., carcinogenic compounds) were positively identified. In fact, some of these chemicals were found in 99%–100% of the samples tested, and they included PCBs, organochlorine pesticides, perfluoroalkyl chemicals (PFCs), phenols, polybrominated diphenyl ethers (PBDEs), phthalates, polycyclic aromatic hydrocarbins, and perchlorate.[108] According to research, exposure to PCBs, PBDEs, PFCs, and phthalates leads to an increased risk of developing hypertension and other CVDs.[109–113] When you consider the ubiquitous nature of some of these chemicals, such as phthalates, found in food and commercial plastics, it's no surprise that exposure is increasing.

Considering the high level of prenatal exposure to chemicals in the womb, including the ones listed above, physicians should implement detoxification into every parent's pre-conception plan. Detoxification treatments for future parents may develop into a specialty in the future. Health professionals must protect the unborn and newborn from the onslaught of chemicals in the environment. Ideally, detoxification should be prioritized as important as prenatal vitamins and folate support. Treating disease does not begin once a symptom or disease develops, but starts before the fertilization of an egg.

The Woodruff study above elucidates that we are all vulnerable to toxin exposure even before birth! What happens to physiological processes in the body after years of exposure? In one study looking at the biological mechanisms of ambient air pollution on cardiovascular health, chronic exposure to air pollution can increase rates of hypertension, CAD, CVD, and thromboembolism.[114–118] It is thought that particulate matter in air pollution activates inflammatory pathways and hemostasis factors, produces reactive oxygen species due to elevated oxidative stress, alters vascular tone, and decreases heart rate variability.[114] Normally, healthy endothelial cells secrete endothelial-derived relaxing factor (EDRF), which helps relax vascular smooth muscle. Oxidative stress via exposure to particulate matter is thought to damage endothelial cells, thus preventing the release of EDRF, which could contribute to systemic hypertension. Additionally, white blood cells adhere to the endothelium in response to tissue damage from oxidative stress, which sets the stage for atherosclerosis to develop. Atherosclerotic disease can be a sequela of hypertension.[118]

Research shows that reductions in particulate matter exposure over a few years lower cardiovascular mortality rates.[116] Although many of us live in urban centers and are exposed to ever-increasing levels of particulate matter and air pollution, we can reduce our risk of CVD by reducing exposure. The best way to reduce our exposure to toxins is avoidance of them in the first place. Additionally, we can support the body's detoxification pathways by helping mobilize and eliminate toxins that have been stored. Working in concert together, the organ systems are able to effectively remove toxins that we accumulate through the air, water, and soil.

Detoxification is a systematic lifestyle practice to enhance optimal functioning of body physiology. It is absolutely necessary to detoxify on a daily basis considering the overabundance of environmental toxins, and our increasing levels of exposure. Toxins are natural and foreign substances found in the environment, and are normal byproducts of cell metabolism. Below we present a general overview of detoxification therapies, and how they can be utilized every day to minimize toxin exposure and accumulation. While the emphasis is on supporting overall health, additional benefits for the cardiovascular system are discussed as well.

REDUCING TOXIC EXPOSURE WITH SIMPLE AND EASY INTERVENTIONS

SAUNA THERAPY

Any method to increase circulation will support detoxification pathways. For basic detoxification support, try walking at least 20 minutes each and every day. If walking or light exercise is not an option due to arthritis or injury, sauna therapy is another great method to increase circulation. Finnish saunas have been studied the most because of their extensive use in Europe, and popularity in North America. A Finnish sauna is usually constructed of wood walls and benches, and uses radiant heat to warm the air from 176°F to 194°F.[119] Infrared saunas are another option for sauna therapy. They are typically heated to 110°F–130°F using infrared rays, and some patients fare better in infrared saunas due to the lower temperature and humidity. Both the Finnish and infrared saunas can be used for detoxification purposes.

Saunas can improve hemodynamics through vasodilation of arteries, which can support the mobilization of fat-soluble xenobiotics.[119] Although there are few studies looking at heavy metal removal with sauna therapy, we do know that mercury, cadmium, antimony, lead, and nickel are released through sweat. Sauna therapy can increase left ventricular ejection fraction in patients with heart failure, and increase peripheral circulation by 5%–10% accounting for 50%–70% of cardiac output. Also, some studies report moderate reductions in blood pressure with sauna therapy.[119,120]

Most people, including cardiac patients with stable coronary heart disease or history of myocardial infarction, can safely use saunas. Contraindications include unstable angina, aortic stenosis, and recent myocardial infarction. Relative contraindications include heart arrhythmias and decompensated heart failure.[120] If the goal of sauna therapy is to lower blood pressure, only 15-minute sessions are recommended. If optimizing detoxification is the primary outcome, longer sessions at lower temperatures (140°F) are recommended.[121] Remember to drink plenty of fluids and electrolytes before, during, and after treatment to help mobilize toxins and prevent dehydration. Ginger/yarrow tea is another drink commonly consumed before saunas to increase vasodilation, and thus diaphoresis.

If saunas are not an option, hot yoga is another excellent form of detoxification therapy to promote toxin release via sweating. Typically, rooms are heated at 104°F with 40%–60% humidity. Practicing yoga in this temperature and humidity promotes profuse sweating, and improves flexibility and strength.[122] In a pilot study on Bikram yoga, a popular form of hot yoga, older obese adults who practiced three times per week for 90 minutes had improved insulin sensitivity by the end of the 8-week study.[123] We recommend that patients go 1–2 times per week to a sauna for general detoxification and musculoskeletal support.

HIGH-FIBER, PHYTONUTRIENT-RICH, ORGANIC FRUITS AND VEGETABLES

Eating a high-fiber, predominately plant-based diet of organic vegetables and fruits provides protection for the cardiovascular system. Fruits and vegetables are loaded with antioxidants, vitamins, and minerals that can neutralize free radical stress, and contain high levels of fiber to move toxins out of the digestive tract. The average American consumes 11–18 g of fiber a day,[124] but we should consume greater than 50 g a day to maintain optimal colon health. Eating a combination of raw and cooked vegetables is best. If buying organic foods is not an option, at the very least try to avoid the "dirty dozen" fruits and vegetables known to have higher levels of pesticides: celery, peaches, strawberries, apples, hot peppers, sweet bell peppers, nectarines, spinach, cherry tomatoes, potatoes, cherries, and grapes. Avoiding these "dirty dozen" foods will decrease your pesticide exposure tremendously.

The fruits and vegetables with the lowest levels of pesticide residues include onion, avocado, sweet corn, pineapple, mango, sweet peas, asparagus, kiwi, cabbage, eggplant, cantaloupe, mushrooms, papaya, grapefruit, and sweet potato. You can print out a handy, wallet-sized chart of the least and most toxic fruits and vegetables at http://www.foodnews.org/fulllist.php. The dirty dozen can fluctuate over time, so it's a good idea to update your list regularly. More useful information about the Environmental Working Group, which strives to educate the public about environmental toxicants, may be found at www.ewg.org and www.foodnews.org.

Children who eat organic fruits and vegetables have lower detectable levels of organophosphorus pesticides in their urine. This finding came out of a study conducted in Mercer Island, WA. Children were fed conventional foods for 4 days, then all organic foods for 5 days, and then back to conventional foods for 6 days. Malathion and chlorpyrifos were the organophosphorus pesticides detected in daily urine samples. Median levels of these two pesticides significantly dropped to non-detectable levels immediately after the introduction of the organic diets, and remained non-detectable until the conventional foods were reintroduced again.[125]

Consuming organic fruits and vegetables is important because pesticides may damage the cardiovascular system. Pesticides including organophosphates have been shown to induce lipid peroxidation, stimulate free radical production, and disturb the total antioxidant capability of the body.[126] In a study where rats were exposed to varying levels of the organophosphate pesticide chlorpyrifos (the same pesticide tested for in the WA study above), blood pressure elevations were recorded and strongly correlated with increasing doses of the pesticide. The authors of this study propose that chlorpyrifos, which is an irreversible acetylcholinesterase inhibitor, causes cholinergic stimulation.[127] Acute CNS stimulation can lead to elevations in SBP and DBP.

LIVER AND GASTROINTESTINAL SUPPORTIVE FOODS AND BOTANICAL MEDICINES

We can alleviate the burden that toxins put on our cardiovascular system by supporting two very important elimination pathways (organs): the liver and gastrointestinal tract. The liver is responsible for metabolizing drugs, toxins, hormones, and other endogenous and exogenous substances into metabolites that are then excreted through the skin, kidneys, or gastrointestinal tract. Any substance (food, vitamin, nutraceutical, etc.) that supports liver detoxification pathways will enhance removal of toxins. Once these toxins enter the small intestine, they need support getting out properly, and this is where a healthy gastrointestinal tract comes into play. There is a saying in medicine that when in doubt treat the liver and gastrointestinal tract; if detoxification pathways are impaired the body literally becomes too toxic to function optimally.

There are various foods that you can eat on a daily basis to support the liver and gastrointestinal tract. Root vegetables (artichokes, carrots, dandelion, beets), sulfur-containing foods (eggs, garlic, and onions), water-soluble fibers (pears, oat bran, apples, and beans), and cabbage family vegetables (broccoli, brussels sprouts, and cabbage) all optimize healthy liver and intestine function. You can also juice many of the abovementioned fruits and vegetables, which also aids in the detoxification process by supplying live enzymes. Avoiding sugary foods will also help your body detox, which may help you think twice about reaching for that mid-afternoon cookie. Instead, eat a handful of raisins and almonds, or dip an apple slice into a freshly made hummus.

Other foods that you should try to implement into your diet to support the liver and gastrointestinal tract include fermented foods and drinks. Fermented foods and drinks include kimchi, sauerkraut, pickled ginger, beet kvass, kombucha, miso, tempeh, natto, yogurt, raw cheese, and kefir. There are many other foods and drinks including high-quality beers and wines that are considered fermented. Fermented foods and drinks supply a natural source of probiotics to the gastrointestinal tract, which help digest foods, improve immune function, and prevent "bad" microorganisms (*Escherichia coli*) from causing infection. Many cultures around the world consume fermented foods and drinks with every meal. When looking for a high-quality fermented food or drink, check to see if excess heating has been used, which destroys the natural fermentation process. We highly recommend making these foods and drinks at home, as quality is increased with smaller production. Check out the book, *Wild Fermentation*, by Sandor Ellix Katz for more information and home recipes.

There are many botanical medicines that support liver function, and therefore augment liver detoxification pathways. Some of these botanicals include milk thistle seed, schisandra seed, dandelion root, burdock root, turmeric root, and artichoke leaf. These herbs can be ingested in foods, tinctures, teas, or in pills. They have different functions (e.g., hepatoprotective, antioxidant, alterative) depending on how they are prescribed, and can be combined in formulas to create synergistic effects. Generally, they are very safe in lower doses; however, consult with an experienced practitioner before using these botanicals.

SKIN BRUSHING

To improve the functioning of the skin and lymphatic system, try incorporating skin brushing into a daily routine. Skin brushing has been practiced in many cultures over the years to improve skin hygiene. By keeping the skin free from dry, dead skin cells, waste removal from the body is greatly enhanced, blood flow is increased, and buildup of bacteria is decreased. The best time to skin brush is before a shower or before bed. Using a natural vegetable bristle or loofa brush, start at the feet using gentle, quick strokes, and move upward toward the heart covering most of the body. This is the direction of lymph and venous blood flow. It is completely normal for the skin to feel slightly tingly, but be sure to avoid harsh brushing, and brushing over open wounds, the face, or over any lymphatic malignancies.

CONTRAST HYDROTHERAPY

Contrast hydrotherapy has been used for centuries to improve circulation, immune system function, and remove toxins. Ever visit a spa and notice that a cold pool for immersion is usually next to a sauna or whirlpool? When the body is exposed to heat, blood vessels vasodilate to improve nutrient/waste transfer and blood flow. This is what causes us to sweat. Quickly jumping into a cold plunge causes vasoconstriction, which drives the oxygen rich blood to the vital organs. Research shows that hydrotherapy tonifies the immune system by increasing migration of white blood cells.[128] In one study, men who were submerged in warm baths or exercised prior to cold immersion showed an increase in migration of leukocytes, monocytes, and granulocytes.[129] Most of us do not have cold plunges in our homes, but contrast hydrotherapy can be practiced in the shower. After taking a warm shower, try ending with a 30-second cool water spray starting with the extremities and ending with the abdominal area and low back.

THERAPEUTIC FASTING

One of the most ancient, powerful, and cost-effective methods of cleansing is fasting. Historically, religious and spiritual peoples have fasted to cleanse the body, mind, and spirit of impurities. From a purely physical perspective, fasting enables the body to rest and work more efficiently. Fasting induces metabolic and hormonal changes by improving insulin sensitivity, enhancing enzyme status, recalibrating taste sensation (e.g., salt), promoting weight loss, and reducing leaky gut. Though fasting is indicated for loss of appetite, acute illness, chronic illness, to accelerate healing, change behaviors (e.g., quit smoking), and its psychospiritual effect, not everyone is a candidate for fasting.[99] Please consult with a healthcare professional before choosing to do a fast.

ELECTROMAGNETIC RADIATION (EMR)

There is another environmental toxicant that is slowly emerging as a threat to our health, and it's not a heavy metal, chemical, or pesticide. This invisible toxin is the increasing expansion and use of wireless technologies that emit radio frequencies. Electromagnetic radiation (EMR), or wireless radiation, is a frequency that we cannot see, feel, hear, taste, or smell, and as such, we don't realize when we are exposed. These devices include cell phones and cell phone antennas, cordless phones, Wi-Fi routers, microwave ovens, smart meters, baby monitors, tablets, computers, and any other device that utilizes wireless technology. Unfortunately, radio frequency devices were not rigorously tested before market release, and some say our safety regulations are obsolete.

There are many harmful non-thermal biological effects caused by wireless radiation that have emerged via recent research, but standards continue to stay the same.[130] For instance, we do know that wireless radiation induces oxidative damage,[131] but the magnitude of oxidative damage caused by radio frequencies is unknown. Also, there have been no long-term studies on radio frequency safety, or analysis of the cumulative effect of using multiple wireless technologies at once over an extended period of time. The best way to reduce exposure to these technologies is to avoid them. This entails talking on cellular speakerphone, using wires instead of wireless whenever possible (i.e., corded phone, Ethernet), and refusing to use a "smart meter" for your electrical utility meter. There are radio frequency protective clothing, fabrics, and devices available as well if wireless use is necessary.

Be particularly careful if you are pregnant or carrying a young one as their tiny bodies and developing brains are more susceptible to radiation exposure. Remember, we shouldn't sacrifice safety for convenience, and the effect of lifelong exposure to these frequencies is unknown. Any couple trying to conceive should avoid using wireless devices. A study showed that men who use laptops with Wi-Fi had a significant decrease in sperm motility and an increase in sperm DNA fragmentation.[132,133] Since Wi-Fi is currently used in many homes and businesses, avoidance is tricky, but can be done. It should be noted that many public libraries in France have removed Wi-Fi due to health concerns, and Germany has warned its citizens to use corded connections (Ethernet) as often as possible.

SUMMARY

It is important to remember that although we live in a toxic world where exposure to chemicals, industry byproducts, and pollution is common, our bodies are intelligently designed to protect us from toxin exposure. We can optimize organ function and detoxification mechanisms by following these simple-to-implement strategies: drink plenty of filtered water, consciously breathe, exercise, encourage sweating, eat foods that are low in pesticide residue, are fermented and support the liver and gastrointestinal tract, apply castor oil packs, practice skin brushing and hydrotherapy, and reduce wireless radiation exposure. Try incorporating some or all of these suggestions into your daily regimen and see how you feel.

A word of caution when starting to detoxify is you may feel worse before you feel better particularly if you have a history of toxin exposure. Moreover, when beginning to eat healthier foods, the body may begin detoxifying more efficiently, so detoxification reactions are common. Symptoms may include headaches, nausea, joint pain, fatigue, insomnia, irritability, anxiety, depression, and changes in bowel habits. These reactions may happen because you are eliminating toxins that have been stored in your body for years.

There are many techniques and treatments discussed above to minimize adverse reactions by optimizing the body's detoxification pathways. Special care and support need to be given to the key organs of elimination, which include the liver, intestines, lungs, kidneys, skin, and lymphatic system. After implementing some of the abovementioned detoxification strategies for a couple of weeks/months, you may notice increased vitality, improved sleep and energy, elevated mood, and fewer signs and symptoms. These changes indicate that your organs of elimination are functioning well and properly detoxifying your body. It may take some time and effort to feel better though. For many NDs, detoxification therapies are one of the most important modalities offered to patients. If we could visibly see what we are exposed to on a daily basis, detoxification would become the standard of care for every person on this planet.

CONCLUSION

In medicine, there are many ways to achieve an outcome. We find that practicing individualized medicine is the foundation for optimal health. Every patient is different due to genetics, diet and lifestyle choices, co-morbidities, stress, overall toxic burden, gender, age, and other factors. Empower your patients by increasing their awareness and consciousness about health. Teach your patients about healthy diet and lifestyle measures, mind-body medicines including breathing and meditation, nutraceuticals, botanical medicines, therapeutic fasting, detoxification techniques, and grounding. All of these modalities will strengthen your practice as more and more people are searching for non-pharmacological ways to stay healthy. Remember to spend time with your patients, ask questions about their current and past health, listen to their concerns, and investigate the true cause of their suffering.

REFERENCES

1. Kok F.J., D. Kromhout. 2004. Atherosclerosis—epidemiological studies on the health effects of a Mediterranean diet. *Eur J Nutr.* 43(Suppl 1):i2–5.
2. Lindeberg S., M. Eliasson, B. Lindahl, B. Ahren. 1999. Low serum insulin in traditional Pacific Islanders—the Kitava Study. *Metabolism* 48(10):1216–9.
3. Lindeberg S., P. Nilsson-Ehle, A. Terent, B. Vessby, B. Schersten. 1994. Cardiovascular risk factors in a Melanesian population apparently free from stroke and ischaemic heart disease: the Kitava study. *J Intern Med.* 236(3):331–40.
4. Huang T., B. Yang, J. Zheng, G. Li, M.L. Wahlgvist, D. Li. 2012. Cardiovascular disease mortality and cancer incidence in vegetarians: a meta-analysis and systematic review. *Ann Nutr Metab.* 60(4):223–40. doi: 10.1159/000337301.
5. Lindeberg S. 2012. Paleolithic diets as a model for prevention and treatment of Western disease. *Am J Hum Biol.* 24(2):110–5.
6. Solas-Solvado J., N. Becerra-Tomas, J.F. Garcia-Gavilan, M. Bullo, L. Barrubes. 2018. Mediterranean Diet and cardiovascular disease prevention: what do we know? *Prog Cardiovasc Dis.* 61(1):62–7.
7. Minelli P., M.R. Montinari. 2019. The Mediterranean Diet and cardioprotection: historic overview and current research. *J Multidiscip Healthc.* 12:805–15.
8. Appleby P.N., M. Thorogood, J.I. Mann, T.J. Key. 1999. The Oxford Vegetarian Study: an overview. *Am J Clin Nutr.* 70(3 Suppl):525S–31S.
9. Segasothy M., P.A. Phillips. 1999. Vegetarian diet: panacea for modern lifestyle diseases? *QJM* 92(9):531–44.
10. Eaton S.B., S.B. 3rd Eaton, M.J. Konner. 1997. Paleolithic nutrition revisited: a twelve-year retrospective on its nature and implications. *Eur J Clin Nutr.* 51(4):207–16.
11. Jonsson T., B. Ahren, G. Pacini, F. Sundler, N. Wierup, S. Steen, T. Sjoberg, M. Ugander, J. Frostegard, L. Goransson, S. Lindeberg. 2006. A Paleolithic diet confers higher insulin sensitivity, lower C-reactive protein and lower blood pressure than a cereal-based diet in domestic pigs. *Nutr Metab (Lond).* 2(3):39.
12. Ghaedi E., M. Mohammadi, H. Mohammadi, N. Ramezani-Jolfaie, J. Malekzadeh, M. Hosseinzadeh, A. Salehi-Abargouei. 2019. Effects of a Paleolithic diet on cardiovascular disease risk factors: a systematic review and meta-analysis of randomized controlled trials. *Adv Nutr.* 10(4):634–46.
13. Neustadt J. 2006. Western diet and inflammation. *Integr Med* 5(4):14–8.
14. Shen J, Wilmot KA, Ghasemzadeh N, et al. 2015 Mediterranean Dietary Patterns and Cardiovascular Health. *Annu Rev Nutr.* 35:425–49.
15. Schwingshackl L, J. Morze, G. Hoffmann. 2020. Mediterranean diet and health status: active ingredients and pharmacological mechanisms. *Br J Pharmacol.* 177(6):1241–57.
16. Guasch-Ferré M, M. Bulló, M.Á. Martínez-González, et al. 2013. Frequency of nut consumption and mortality risk in the PREDIMED nutrition intervention trial. *BMC Med.* 11:164.
17. Aeberli I., P.A. Gerber, M. Hochuli, S. Kohler, S.R. Haile, I. Gouni-Berthold, H.K. Berthoid, G.A. Spinas, K. Berneis. 2011. Low to moderate sugar-sweentened beverage consumption impairs glucose and lipid metabolism and promotes inflammation in healthy young men: a randomized controlled trial. *Am J Clin Nutr.* 94(2):479–85. doi: 10.3945/ajcn.111.013540.
18. Goldin A., J.A. Beckman, A.M. Schmidt, M.A. Creager. 2006. Advanced glycation end products: sparking the development of diabetic vascular injury. *Circulation* 114(6):597–605.
19. Fassano A., T. Not, W. Wang, S. Uzzau, I. Berti, A. Tommasini, S. Goldblum. 2000. Zonulin, a newly discovered modulator of intestinal permeability, and its expression in coeliac disease. *The Lancet* 335(9214):1518–9.
20. Fasano A. 2020. All disease begins in the (leaky) gut: role of zonulin mediated gut permeability in the pathogenesis of chronic inflammatory diseases. *F1000research.* Doi: 10.12688/f1000research.20510.1.
21. Visser J., J. Rozing, A. Sapone, K. Lammers, A. Fasano. 2009. Tight junctions, intestinal permeability, and autoimmunity: celiac disease and type I diabetes paradigms. *Ann NY Acad Sci.* 1165:195–205. doi: 10.1111/j.1749-6632.2009.04037.x.
22. Craig W.J. 2009. Health effects of vegan diets. *Am J Clin Nutr.* 89(5):1627S–33S.

23. Key T.J., P.N. Abbleby, M.S. Rosell. 2006. Health effects of vegetarian and vegan diets. *Proc Nutr Soc.* 65(1):35–41.
24. Humphrey L.L, R. Fu, K. Rogers, M. Freeman, M. Helfand. 2008. Homocysteine level and coronary heart disease incidence: a systematic review and meta-analysis. *Mayo Clin Proc.* 83(11):1203–12. doi: 10.4065/83.11.1203.
25. Schnyder G., M. Roffi, Y. Flammer, R. Pin, O.M. Hess. 2002. Effect of homocysteine-lowering therapy with folic acid, vitamin B12, and vitamin B6 on clinical outcome after percutaneous coronary intervention: the Swiss Heart study: a randomized controlled trial. *JAMA* 288(8):973–9.
26. Cordain L., B.A. Watkins, G.L. Florant, M. Kelher, L. Rogers, Y. Li. 2002. Fatty acid analysis of wild ruminant tissues: evolutionary implications for reducing diet-related chronic disease. *Eur J Clin Nutr.* 56:181–91.
27. Ponnampalam E.N., N.J. Mann, A.J. Sinclair. 2006. Effect of feeding systems on omega-3 fatty acids, conjugated linoleic acid and trans fatty acids in Australian beef cuts: potential impact on human health. *Asia Pac J Clin Nutr.* 15(1):21–9.
28. Daley C.A., A. Abbott, P.S. Doyle, G.A. Nader, S. Larson. 2010. A review of fatty acid profiles and antioxidant content in grass-fed and grain-fed beef. *Nutr J.* 9:10. doi: 10.1186/1475-2891-9-10.
29. Teixeira R.C., C. Molina Mdel, E. Zandonade, J.G. Mill. 2007. Cardiovascular risk in vegetarians and omnivores: a comparative study. *Arg Bras Cardiol.* 89(4):237–44.
30. Khan J, P.K. Deb, S. Priya, K.D. Medina, R. Devi, S.G. Walode, M. Rudrapal. 2021. Dietary flavonoids: cardioprotective potential with antioxidant effects and their pharmacokinetic, toxicological and therapeutic concerns. *Molecules* 26(13):4021.
31. Yamagata K, Y. Yamori. 2020. Inhibition of endothelial dysfunction by dietary flavonoids and preventive effects against cardiovascular disease. *J Cardiovasc Pharmacol.* 75(1):1–9.
32. Ciumărnean L, M.V. Milaciu, O. Runcan, Ş.C. Vesa, A.L. Răchişan, V. Negrean, M.G. Perné, V.I. Donca, T.G. Alexescu, I. Para, G. Dogaru. 2020. The effects of flavonoids in cardiovascular diseases. *Molecules* 25(18):4320.
33. Ju J, J. Li, Q. Lin, H. Xu. 2018. Efficacy and safety of berberine for dyslipidaemias: a systematic review and meta-analysis of randomized clinical trials. *Phytomedicine* 50:25–34.
34. Xu X, H. Yi, J. Wu, T. Kuang, J. Zhang, Q. Li, H. Du, T. Xu, G. Jiang, G. Fan. 2021. Therapeutic effect of berberine on metabolic diseases: both pharmacological data and clinical evidence. *Biomed Pharmacother.* 133:110984.
35. Fatahian A, S.M. Haftcheshmeh, S. Azhdari, et al. 2020. Promising anti-atherosclerotic effect of berberine: evidence from in vitro, in vivo, and clinical studies. *Rev Physiol Biochem Pharmacol.* 178:83–110.
36. Liang Y, X. Xu, M. Yin, Y. Zhang, L. Huang, R. Chen, J. Ni. 2019. Effects of berberine on blood glucose in patients with type 2 diabetes mellitus: a systematic literature review and a meta-analysis. *Endocr J.* 66(1):51–63
37. Varshney R, M.J. Budoff. 2016. Garlic and heart disease. *J Nutr.* 146(2):416S–21S.
38. Xiong X.J., P.Q. Wang, S.J. Li, et al. 2015. Garlic for hypertension: a systematic review and meta analysis of randomized controlled trials. *Phytomedicine* 22(3):352–61.
39. Sainani G.S., Desai DB, Gohre NH, et al. 1979. Effect of dietary garlic and onion on serum lipid profile in Jain community. *Ind J Med Res.* 69:776–80.
40. Evans M, J.A. Rumberger, I. Azumano, J.J. Napolitano, D. Citrolo, T. Kamiya. 2014. Pantethine, a derivative of vitamin B5, favorably alters total, LDL and non-HDL cholesterol in low to moderate cardiovascular risk subjects eligible for statin therapy: a triple-blinded placebo and diet-controlled investigation. *Vasc Health Risk Manag.* 10:89–100.
41. Arsenio L, P. Bodria, G. Magnati, et al. 1986. Effectiveness of long-term treatment with pantethine in patients with dyslipidemias. *Clin Ther.* 8:537–45.
42. Gaddi A, G.C. Descovich, P. Noseda, et al. 1984. Controlled evaluation of pantethine, a natural hypolipidemic compound, in patients with different forms of hyperlipoproteinemia. *Atherosclerosis* 50:73–83.
43. Donati C, R.S. Bertieri, G. Barbi. 1989. Pantethine, diabetes mellitus and atherosclerosis. Clinical study of 1045 patients. *Clin Ter.* 128:411–22.
44. Cicero A.F.G., F. Fogacci, M. Bove, M. Giovannini, C. Borghi. 2019. Three-arm, placebo-controlled, randomized clinical trial evaluating the metabolic effect of a combined nutraceutical containing a bergamot standardized flavonoid extract in dyslipidemic overweight subjects. *Phytother Res.* 33(8):2094–101.
45. Cappello A.R., V. Dolce, D. Iacopetta, et al. 2016. Bergamot (Citrus bergamia Risso) flavonoids and their potential benefits in human hyperlipidemia and atherosclerosis: an overview. *Mini Rev Med Chem.* 16(8):619–629.
46. Goldstein C.M., R. Josephson, S. Xie, J.W. Hughes. 2012. Current perspectives on the use of meditation to reduce blood pressure. *Int J Hypertens*:11. doi: 10.1155/2012/578397.

47. Ram C.V. 2002. Antihypertensive drugs: an overview. *Am J Cardiovasc Drugs* 2(2):77–9.
48. Maddaford T.G., B. Ramjiawan, M. Aliani, R. Guzman, G.N. Pierce. 2013. Potent antihypertensive action of dietary flaxseed in hypertensive patients. *Hypertension* 62(6):1081–9.
49. Madhavi D, D. Kagan, V. Rao, M. Murray. 2013. A pilot study to evaluate the antihypertensive effect of a celery extract in mild to moderate hypertensive patients. *Nat Med J.* 4(4):1–3.
50. Johnson S.A., A. Figueroa, N. Navaei, et al. 2015. Daily blueberry consumption improves blood pressure and arterial stiffness in postmenopausal women with pre- and stage 1-hypertension: a randomized, double-blind, placebo-controlled clinical trial. *J Acad Nutr Diet.* pii: S2212-2672(14)01633-5.
51. Bacon S.L., A. Sherwood, A. Hinderliter, J.A. Blumenthal. 2004. Effects of exercise, diet and weight loss on high blood pressure. *Sports Med.* 34(5):307–16.
52. Conlin P.R., D. Chow, E.R. 3rd Miller, L.P. Svetkev, P.H. Lin, D.W. Harsha, T.J. Moore, F.M. Sacks, L.J. Appel. 2000. The effect of dietary patterns on blood pressure control in hypertensive patients: results from the Dietary Approaches to Stop Hypertension (DASH) trial. *Am J Hypertens.* 13(9):949–55.
53. Park K.M., C.J. Cifelli. 2013. Dairy and blood pressure: a fresh look at the evidence. *Nutr Rev.* 71(3):149–57.
54. Hebeisen D.F., F. Hoeflin, H.P. Reusch, E. Junker, B.H. Lauterburg. 1993. Increased concentrations of omego-3 fatty acids in milk and platelet rich plasma of grass-fed cows. *Int J Vitam Nutr Res.* 63(3):229–33.
55. Perona J.S., J. Canizares, E. Montero, et al. 2004. Virgin olive oil reduces blood pressure in hypertensive elderly subjects. *Clin Nutr.* 23(5):1113–21.
56. Badlishah S., Y. Kamisah, J. Kamsiah, H.M. Oodriyah. 2013. Virgin coconut oil prevents blood pressure elevation and improves endothelial functions in rats fed with repeatedly heated palm oil. *Evid Based Complementary Altern Med:*7. doi: 10.1155/2013/629329.
57. Xin X., J. He, M.G. Frontini, L.G. Ogden, O.I Motsamai, P.K. Whelton. 2001. Effects of alcohol reduction on blood pressure: a meta-analysis of randomized controlled trials. *Hypertension* 38(5):1112–7.
58. Noordzij M., C.S. Uiterwaal, L.R. Arends, F.J. Kok, D.E. Grobbee, J.M. Geleijnse. 2005. Blood pressure response to chronic intake of coffee and caffeine: a meta-analysis of randomized controlled trials. *J Hypertens.* 23(5):921–8.
59. McKay D.L., C.Y. Chen, E. Saltzman, J.B. Blumberg. Hibiscus sabdariffa L. tea (tisane) lowers blood pressure in prehypertensive and mildly hypertensive adults. *J Nutr.* 140(2):298–303.
60. Herrera-Arellano A., J. Miranda-Sanchez, P. Avila-Castro, S. Herrera-Alverez, J.E. Jimenez-Ferrer, A. Zamipa, R. Roman-Ramos, H. Ponce-Monter, J. Tortoriello. 2007. Clinical effects produced by a standardized herbal medicinal product of Hibiscus sabdariffa on patients with hypertension: a randomized, double blind, lisinopril controlled clinical trial. *Plana Med.* 73(1):6–12.
61. Herrera-Arellano A., S. Flores-Romero, M.A. Chavez-Soto, J. Tortoriello. 2004. Effectiveness and tolerability of a standardized extract from Hibiscus sabdariffa in patients with mild to moderate hypertension: a controlled and randomized clinical trial. *Phytomedicine* 11(5):375–82.
62. He F.J., G.A. MacGregor. 2007. Salt, blood pressure and cardiovascular disease. *Curr Opin Cardiol.* 22(4):298–305.
63. Kotchen, T.A., D.A. McCarron. 1998. Dietary electrolytes and blood pressure: a statement for healthcare professionals from the American Heart Association Nutrition Committee. *Circulation* 98(6):613–7.
64. He F.J., J. Li, G.A Macgregor. 2013. Effect of longer-term modest salt reduction on blood pressure. *Cochrane Database Syst Rev.* 346:CD004937. doi: 10.1002/14651858.CD004937.pub2.
65. Ascherio A., E.B. Rimm, M.A. Hernan, E.L Giovannucci, I. Kawachi, M.J. Stampfer, W.C. Willett. 1998. Intake of potassium, magnesium, calcium, and fiber and risk of stroke among US men. *Circulation* 98(12):1198–204.
66. Whelton P.K., J. He, J.A. Cutler, F.L. Brancati, L.J. Appel, D. Follmann, M.F. Klag. 1997. Effects of oral potassium on blood pressure. Meta-analysis of randomized controlled clinical trials. *JAMA* 28(20):1624–32.
67. Houston M. 2013. Nutrition and nutraceutical supplements for the treatment of hypertension: part II. *J Clin Hypertens (Greenwich).* 15(11):845–51. doi: 10.1111/jch.12212.
68. Whelton S.P., A. Chin, X. Xin, J. He. 2002. Effect of aerobic exercise on blood pressure: a meta-analysis of randomized, controlled trials. *Ann Intern Med.* 136(7):493–503.
69. Blumenthal J.A, A. Sherwood, E.C Gullette, M. Babyak, R. Waugh, A Georgiades, L.W. Craighead, D. Tweedy, M. Feinglos, M. Appelbaum, J. Hayano, A. Hinderliter. 2000. Exercise and weight loss reduce blood pressure in men and women with mild hypertension: effects on cardiovascular, metabolic, and hemodynamic functioning. *Arch Intern Med.* 160(13):1947–58.

70. Ishikawa T.K., T. Ohta, H. Tanaka. 2003. How much exercise is required to reduce blood pressure in essential hypertensives: a dose-response study. *Am J Hypertens.* 16(8):629–33.
71. Iwane M., M. Arita, S. Tominoto, O. Satnai, M. Matsumoto, K. Miyashita, I. Nishio. Walking 10,000 steps/day or more reduces blood pressure and sympathetic nerve activity in mild essential hypertension. *Hypertens Res.* 23(6):573–80.
72. Kulkarni S., I. O'Farrell, M. Erasi, M.S. Kochar. 1998. Stress and hypertension. *WMJ* 97(11):34–8.
73. Thayer J.F., S.S. Yamamoto, J.F Brosschot. 2010. The relationship of autonomic imbalance, heart rate variability and cardiovascular disease risk factors. *Int J Cardiol.* 141(2):122–31.
74. Wang S.Z., S. Li, X.Y. Xu, G.P. Lin, L. Shao, Y. Zhao, T.H. Wang. 2010. Effect of slow abdominal breathing combined with biofeedback on blood pressure and heart rate variability in prehypertension. *J Altern Complement Med.* 16(10):1039–45.
75. Schein M.H., B. Gavish, M. Herz, D. Rosner-Kahana, P. Naveh, B. Knishkowy, E. Zlotnikov, N. Ben-Zyi, R.N. Melmed. 2001. Treating hypertension with a device that slows and regularizes breathing: a randomized, double-blind controlled study. *J Hum Hypertens.* 15(4):271–8.
76. Meles E., C. Giannattasio, M. Failla, G. Gentile, A. Capra, G. Mancia. 2004. Nonpharmacologic treatment of hypertension by respiratory exercise in the home setting. *Am J Hypetens.* 17(4):370–4.
77. Anderson J.W., C. Liu, R.J. Kryscio. 2008. Blood pressure response to transcendental meditation: a meta-analysis. *Am J Hypertens.* 21(3):310–6.
78. Nidich S.I., M.V. Rainforth, D.A. Haaga, J. Hagelin, J.W. Salerno, E. Travis, M. Tanner, C. Gaylord-King, S. Grosswald, R.H. Schneider. 2009. A randomized controlled trial on effects of the Transcendental Meditation program on blood pressure, psychological distress, and coping in young adults. *Am J Hypertens.* 22(12):1326–31. doi: 10.1038/ajh.2009.184.
79. Nester J. 2020. Breath: the new science of a lost art. Riverhead books.
80. Lee B.J., Y.C. Huang, S.J. Chen, P.T. Lin. 2012. Effects of coenzyme Q10 supplementation on inflammatory markers (high-sensitivity C-reactive protein, interleukin-6, and homocysteine) in patients with coronary artery disease. *Nutrition* 28(7–8):767–72. doi: 10.1016/j.nut.2011.11.008.
81. Greenberg S., W.H. Frishman. 1990. Co-Enzyme Q10: a new drug for cardiovascular disease. *J Clin Pharmacol.* 30(7):596–608.
82. Salvatore P., S.F. Marasco, S.J. Haas, F.L. Sheeran, H. Krum, F.L. Rosenfeldt. 2012. Coenzyme Co$_{10}$ in cardiovascular disease. *Mitrochondrion* 7:154–67.
83. Burke B.E., R. Neuenschwander, R.D. Olson. 2001. Randomized, double-blind, placebo-controlled trial of coenzyme Q10 in isolated systolic hypertension. *South Med J.* 94(11):1112–7.
84. Ho M.J, A. Bellusci, J.M. Write. 2009. Blood pressure lowering efficacy of coenzyme Q10 for primary hypertension. *Cochrane Database Syst Rev.* CD007435. doi: 10.1002/14651858. CD007435.pub2.
85. Kass L., J. Weekes, L. Carpenter. 2012. Effect of magnesium supplementation on blood pressure: a meta-analysis. *Eur J Clin Nutr.* 66(4):411–8. doi: 10.1038/ejcn.2012.4.
86. Campbell F., H.O. Dickinson, J.A. Critchlev, G.A. Ford, M. Bradburn. 2013. A systematic review of fish-oil supplements for the prevention and treatment of hypertension. *Eur J Prev Cardiol.* 20(1):107–20. doi: 10.1177/2047487312437056.
87. Reinhart K.M., C.I. Coleman, C. Teevan, P. Vachhani, C.M. White. 2008. Effects of garlic on blood pressure in patients with and without systolic hypertension: a meta-analysis. *Ann Pharmacother.* 42(12):1766–71. doi: 10.1345/aph.1L319.
88. Reid K., F.R. Oliver, N.P. Stocks, P. Fakler, T. Sullivan. 2008. Effect of garlic on blood pressure: a systematic review and meta-analysis. *BMC Cardiovasc Disord.* 8:13. doi: 10.1186/1471-2261-8-13.
89. Odai T, M. Terauchi, K. Kato, A. Hirose, N. Miyasaka. 2019. Effects of grape seed proanthocyanidin extract on vascular endothelial function in participants with prehypertension: a randomized, double-blind, placebo-controlled study. *Nutrients* 11(12):2844.
90. Ras R.T., P.L. Zock, Y.E. Zebregs, N.R. Johnston, D.J. Webb, R. Draijer. 2013. Effect of polyphenol rich grape seed extract on ambulatory blood pressure in subjects with pre- and stage I hypertension. *Br J Nutr.* 110(12):2234–41.
91. Park E, I. Edirisinghe, Y.Y. Choy, A. Waterhouse, B. Burton-Freeman. 2015. Effects of grape seed extract beverage on blood pressure and metabolic indices in individuals with pre-hypertension: a randomized, double-blinded, two-arm, parallel, placebo-controlled trial. *Br J Nutr.* 16:1–13.
92. Schön C, P. Allegrini, K. Engelhart-Jentzsch, A. Riva, G. Petrangolini. 2021. Grape seed extract positively modulates blood pressure and perceived stress: a randomized, double-blind, placebo-controlled study in healthy volunteers. *Nutrients* 13(2):654.

93. Perrinjaquet-Moccetti T, A. Busjahn, C. Schmidlin, et al. 2008. Food supplementation with an olive (Olea europaea L.) leaf extract reduces blood pressure in borderline hypertensive monozygotic twins. *Phytother Res.* 22(9):1239–42.
94. Susalit E, N. Agus, I. Effendi, R.R. Tjandrawinata, et al. 2011. Olive (Olea europaea) leaf extract effective in patients with stage-1 hypertension: comparison with Captopril. *Phytomedicine* 18(4):251–8.
95. Farràs M, R.M. Valls, S. Fernández-Castillejo, M. Giralt, R. Solà, I. Subirana, M.J. Motilva, V. Konstantinidou, M.I. Covas, M. Fitó. 2013. Olive oil polyphenols enhance the expression of cholesterol efflux related genes in vivo in humans. A randomized controlled trial. *J Nutr Biochem.* 24(7):1334–9.
96. Martín-Peláez S, O. Castañer, V. Konstantinidou, et al. 2015. Effect of olive oil phenolic compounds on the expression of blood pressure-related genes in healthy individuals. *Eur J Nutr.* 56(2):663–70.
97. Houston, M. 2013. Nutrition and Nutraceutical Supplements for the treatment of hypertension: part III. *J Clin Hypertens (Greenwich).* doi: 10.1111/jch.12212.
98. Horne B.D., J.B. Muhlestein, D.L. Lappe, H.T. May, J.F. Carlquist, O. Galenko, K.D. Brunisholz, J.L. Anderson. 2012. Randomized cross-over trial of short-term water-only fasting: metabolic and cardiovascular consequences. *Nutr Metab Cardiovasc Dis.* doi: 10.1016/j.numecd.2012.09.007.
99. Goldhamer, A., D. Lisle, B. Parpia, S.V. Anderson, T.C. Campbell. 2001. Medically supervised water-only fasting in the treatment of hypertension. *J Manipulative Physiol Ther.* 24(5):335–9.
100. Ghaly M., D. Teplitz. 2004. The biologic effects of grounding the human body during sleep as measured by cortisol levels and subjective reporting of sleep, pain, and stress. *J Altern Complement Med.* 10(5):767–76.
101. Chevalier, G., S.T. Sinatra, J.L Oschman, R.M. Delany. 2013. Earthing (grounding) the human body reduces blood viscosity-a major factor in cardiovascular disease. *J Altern Complement Med.* 19(2):102–10. doi: 10.1089/acm.2011.0820.
102. Chevalier G., S.T. Sinatra, J.L. Oschman, K. Sokal, P. Sokal. 2012. Earthing: health implications of reconnecting the human body to the Earth's surface electrons. *J Environ Public Health.* doi: 10.1155/2012/291541.
103. Alavanja M.C.R. 2009. Pesticides use and exposure extensive worldwide. *Rev. Environ Health* 24(4):303–9.
104. Goncharov A., M. Pavuk, H.R. Foushee, D.O. Carpenter. 2011. Blood pressure in relation to concentrations of PCB congeners and chlorinated pesticides. *Environ Health Perspect.* 119(3):319–25. doi: 10.1289/ehp.1002830.
105. Rahman, M., M. Tondel, S.A. Ahmad, I.A. Chowdhury, M.H. Faruquee, O. Axelson. 1999. Hypertension and arsenic exposure in Bangladesh. *Hypertension* 33(1):74–8.
106. Hennig B., P. Meerarani, R. Slim, M. Toborek, A. Daugherty, A.E. Silverstone, L.W. Robertson. 2002. Proinflammatory properties of coplanar PCB's: in vitro and in vivo evidence. *Toxicol Appl Pharmacol.* 181(3):174–83.
107. La Merrill M., P.M. Cirillo, M.B. Terry, N.Y. Krigbaum, J.D. Flom, B.A. Cohn. 2013. Prenatal exposure to the pesticide DDT and hypertension diagnosed in women before age 50: a longitudinal birth cohort study. *Environ Health Perspect.* 121(5):594–9. doi: 10.1289/ehp.1205921.
108. Woodruff T.J., A.R. Zota, J.M. Schwartz. 2011. Environmental chemicals in pregnant women in the United States: NHANES 2003–2004. *Environ Health Perspect.* 119(6):878–85. doi: 10.1289/ehp.1002727.
109. Everett C.J., A.G. 3rd Mainous, I.L. Frithsen, M.S. Player, E.M. Matheson. 2008. Association of polychlorinated biphenyls with hypertension in the 1999–2002 National Health and Nutrition Examination Survey. *Environ Res.* 108(1):94–7. doi: 10.1016/j.envres.2008.05.006.
110. Trasande L., S. Sathyanarayana, A.J. Spanier, H. Tractman, T.M. Attina, E.M. Urbina. 2013. Urinary phthalates are associated with higher blood pressure in childhood. *J Pediatr.* 163(3):747–53. doi: 10.1016/j.jpeds.2013.03.072.
111. Shankar A., J. Xiao, A. Ducatman. 2011. Perfluoralky chemicals and elevated serum uric acid in US adults. *Clin Epidemiol.* 3:251–8. doi: 10.2147/CLEP.S21677.
112. Gump B., Yun S., Kannan K. 2014. Polybrominated diphenyl ether (PBDE) exposure in children: possible associations with cardiovascular and psychological functions. *Environmental Research.* 142: 244–250. doi: 10.1016/j.envres.2014.04.009.
113. Min J.Y., K.J. Lee, J.B. Park, K.B Min. 2012. Perfluorooctanoic acid exposure is associated with elevated homocysteine and hypertension in US adults. *Occup Environ Med.* 69(9):658–62. doi: 10.1136/oemed-2011-100288.
114. Franchini M., P.M. Mannucci. 2011. Thrombogenicity and cardiovascular effects of ambient air pollution. *Blood* 118(9):2405–12. doi: 10.1182/blood-2011-04-343111.

115. Dyonch J.T., S. Kannan, A.J. Schultz, G.J. Keeler, G. Mentz, J. House, A. Benjamin, P. Max, R.L. Bard, R.D. Brook. Acute effects of ambient particulate matter on blood pressure: differential effects across urban communities. *Hypertension* 53(5):853–9. doi: 10.1161/HYPERTENSIONAHA.108.123877.

116. Brook R.D., S. Rajagopalan, C.A. 3rd Pope, J.R. Brook, A. Bhatnagar, A.V. Diez-Roux, F. Holguin, Y. Hong, R.V. Luepker, M.A. Mittleman, A. Peters, D. Siscovick, S.C. Smith, L. Whitsel, J.D. Kaufman. 2010. Particulate matter air pollution and cardiovascular disease: an update to the scientific statement from the American Heart Association. *Circulation* 121(21):2331–78. doi: 10.1161/CIR.0b013e3181dbece1.

117. Bhatnangar A. 2006. Environmental cardiology: studying mechanistic links between pollution and heart disease. *Circ Res.* 99:692–705.

118. Taylor A. 1996. Cardiovascular effects of environmental chemicals. *Otolaryngol Head Neck Surg.* 114(2):209–11.

119. Crinnion W. 2011. Sauna as a valuable clinical tool for cardiovascular, autoimmune, toxicant-induced and other chronic health problems. *Altern Med Rev.* 16(3):215–25.

120. Hannuksela M., E. Samer. 2001. Benefits and risks of sauna bathing. *Am J Med.* 110(2):118–26.

121. Crinnion W. 2007. Components of practical clinical detox programs—sauna as a therapeutic tool. *Altern Ther Health Med.* 13(2):S154–6.

122. Tracy B.L., C.E. Hart. 2013. Bikram yoga training and physical fitness in healthy young adults. *J Strength Cond Res.* 27(3):822–30. doi: 10.1519/JSC.0b013e31825c340f.

123. Hunter S., M. Dhindsa, E. Cunnngham, et al. 2013. Improvements in glucose tolerance with Bikram Yoga in older obese adults: a pilot study. *J BodyW Mov Ther.* 17(4): 404–7.

124. King D.E., A.G. 3rd Mainous, C.A. Labourne. 2012. Trends in dietary fiber intake in the United States, 1999–2008. *J Acad Nutr Diet.* 112(5):642–8. doi: 10.1016/j.jand.2012.01.019.

125. Lu C., K. Toepel, R. Irish, R.A. Fenske, D.B. Barr, R. Bravo. 2006. Organic diets significantly lower children's dietary exposure to organophosphorus pesticides. *Environ Health Perspect.* 114(2):260–3.

126. Abdollahi M., A. Ranjbar, S. Shadnia, S. Nikfar, A. Rezaie. 2004. Pesticides and oxidative stress: a review. *Med Sci Monit.* 10(6):RA141–7.

127. Gordon C.J., B.K. Padnos. 2000. Prolonged elevation in blood pressure in the unrestrained rat exposed to chlorpyrifos. *Toxicology* 146(1):1–13.

128. Jansky L., D. Pospisilova, S. Honzova, B. Ulicny, P. Sramek, V. Zeman, J. Kaminkova. 1996. Immune system of cold-exposed and cold-adapted humans. *Eur J Appl Physiol Occup Physiol.* 72(5–6):445–50.

129. Brenner I.K., J.W. Castellani, C. Gabaree, A.J. Young, J. Zamecnik, R.J. Shephard, P.N. Shek. 1998. Immune changes in humans during cold exposure: effects of prior heating and exercise. *J Appl Physiol (1985).* 87(2):699–710.

130. Khurana V.G., L. Hardell, J. Everaet, A. Bortkiewicz, M. Carlberg, M. Ahonen. 2010. Epidemiological evidence for a health risk from mobile phone base stations. *Int J Occup Environ Health* 16(3):263–7.

131. Naviroglu M., B. Cig, S. Dogan, A.C. Uguz, S. Dilek, D. Faouzi. 2012. 2.45-Gz wireless devices induce oxidative stress and proliferation through cytosolic Ca^{2+} influx in human leukemia cancer cells. *Int J Radiat Biol.* 88(6):449–56. doi: 10.3109/09553002.2012.682192.

132. Avendano C., A. Mata, C.A. Sanchez Sarmiento, G.F. Doncel. 2012. Use of laptop computers connected to internet through Wi-Fi decreases human sperm motility and increases sperm DNA fragmentation. *Feril Steril.* 97(1):39–45. doi: 10.1016/j.fertnstert.2011.10.012.

133. Atasoy H.I., M.Y. Gunal, P. Atasoy, S. Elgun, G. Bugdayci. 2013. Immunohistopathologic demonstration of deleterious effects on growing rat testes of radiofrequency waves emitted from conventional Wi-Fi devices. *J Pediatr Urol.* 9(2):223–9. doi: 10.1016/j.jpurol.2012.02.015.

4 Marine-Derived Omega-3 Fatty Acids and Cardiovascular Disease

Thomas G. Guilliams

Jørn Dyerberg

CONTENTS

Omega-3 Fatty Acids 77
    Sources of Marine Omega-3 Ingredients 78
    Delivery Forms for Supplementation 79
The Epidemiology of Omega-3 Fatty Acids and CVD 79
    Omega-3 Index and CVD Risk 80
    CVD Intervention Studies Using Omega-3 Fatty Acids 80
        REDUCE-IT (2018) 82
        VITAL (2018) 82
        ASCEND (2018) 83
        STRENGTH (2020) 83
    Cardiometabolic Mechanisms and Biomarkers Related to EPA and/or DHA 84
LDL, HDL and Non-HDL Cholesterol 85
Inflammatory Biomarkers and Specialized Pro-Resolving Mediators 85
    Bioavailability of n-3 Supplements 86
Ethyl Esters vs Triglycerides 86
Krill Oil vs Fish Oil 87
Astaxanthin from Krill 88
Additional Considerations on Marine Omega-3 Sourcing 89
Allergies to Fish and Shellfish Related to Omega-3 Products 89
    Quality Control Issues of Fish Oil and Related Products 90
Conclusion and Recommendation 90
References 91

OMEGA-3 FATTY ACIDS

The relationship between dietary intake of marine-derived omega-3 fatty and cardiovascular risk challenged decades of assumptions about how fats contribute to human health.[1–6] Omega-3 (n-3) fatty acids are a class of polyunsaturated fatty acids (PUFA) derived from the 18-carbon essential fatty acid alpha-linolenic acid (ALA, 18:3 (n-3)). While ALA is only synthesized in plants, some plants (e.g., algae) and animals consuming ALA can elongate and desaturate this molecule to produce several different long-chain polyunsaturated fatty acids (LCPUFA) such as stearidonic acid

DOI: 10.1201/9781003137849-4

(SDA, 18:4 (n-3)), eicosatetraenoic acid (ETA, 20:4 (n-3)), eicosapentaenoic acid (EPA, 20:5 (n-3)), docosapentaenoic acid (DPA, 22:5 (n-3)) and docosahexaenoic acid (DHA, 22:6 (n-3)). While each of these fatty acids has been associated with health benefits in humans and garnered research attention, the two fatty acids that have gained the most attention and research focus are EPA and DHA. In fact, the vast majority of epidemiological studies connecting n-3 fatty acids and cardiovascular risk often only measure dietary intake of, or biomarkers for, EPA and DHA. Consequently, intervention trials using supplemental n-3 fatty acids are often described solely by their EPA and/or DHA content (even though they may contain other n-3 intermediates). Therefore, before diving into the epidemiological, intervention and mechanistic studies related to EPA and DHA, it is important to briefly describe the sources and molecular structures of these fatty acids delivered as foods, supplements and pharmaceuticals – since these factors can greatly influence their bioavailability, efficacy and cost.

SOURCES OF MARINE OMEGA-3 INGREDIENTS

For the most part, the marine n-3 fatty acid category is dominated by products best described as "fish oil"—that is, while there are products available that deliver n-3 fatty acids from other marine sources, nearly all the available research has been done with fish oil-derived fatty acids. These data using fish oil have become the benchmark for efficacy and safety, and are the standard to which we compare other sources. While pharmaceutical products often avoid the use of the term "fish oil," these products are currently all made from fish-derived fatty acids.

The following are the main sources of marine omega-3 fatty acids:

- **Fish Body Oil**: The largest biomass used to create marine-derived n-3 fatty acids are small oily fish caught in the cold waters off the coast of Chile and Peru. The fish species most commonly harvested are anchovies and sardines, with some mackerel. Various concentrations or fractions of these purified oils are the most common ingredient used in dietary supplements and pharmaceutical products throughout the world. Other species used to produce fish oil may include salmon, tuna, menhaden, herring and other minor species. The EPA and DHA (and other fatty acids) content, which is predominantly in the triglyceride form, is dependent on the species of fish, the water temperature and other variables on a seasonal basis.
- **Cod Liver**: As a byproduct of the cod meat market, cod livers are used to provide a blend of fatty acids similar to unconcentrated fish body oil.
- **Krill**: These small crustaceans feed on plankton and are subsequently eaten by many marine mammals, especially penguins and whales. Factory ships process krill immediately upon capture off the coast of Antarctica. Krill oil, in which the n-3 LCPUFAs are predominantly in a free fatty acid and phospholipid form, is relatively low in EPA and DHA, but contains small amount of the carotenoid astaxanthin.
- **Calamari**: A more recent, but small, player in the n-3 fatty acid industry is calamari or squid oil. This oil, which is predominantly in the triglyceride form, has a higher ratio of DHA over EPA than is typical of fish oil. This material is a byproduct of the calamari food industry.
- **Mussels**: Shellfish are only a minor source of commercially available n-3 fatty acids. Nonetheless, several products are currently available from the fatty acids derived from Green-Lipped Mussels (*Perna canaliculus*). These ingredients are not typically marketed for cardiovascular benefits.
- **Algae**: Various species of algae are commercial sources for n-3 fatty acids. Algae can be grown in large inland production sites where access to sunlight is plentiful. These products are very high in DHA, with only small amounts of EPA, predominantly in the triglyceride form. Most of the pure DHA raw materials, especially pure DHA used for the fortification

of infant formula, is sourced from algae. In addition, algae are currently the only vegan source of DHA available.

- **EPA and DHA from Genetically Modified Plants**: Various algae, plants and fungi have been genetically modified to produce various fatty acids, including both EPA and DHA. These ingredients are designed to help increase the global supply of these fatty acids, while limiting the harvesting burden on marine animals. As of 2020, these ingredients were only being produced for the supplementation of farm-raised fish (not directly used in dietary supplement ingredients).[7,8] It is likely these plant-derived EPA and DHA fatty acids may be approved for direct human consumption in the future.

DELIVERY FORMS FOR SUPPLEMENTATION

When fatty acids are harvested from their source, they are typically in the form of triglycerides (TG), phospholipids (PL) or free fatty acids (FFA) and are relatively low in total EPA and DHA (<30% of the total fatty acids). When consuming fish or unconcentrated fish oil (i.e., fish body oil or cod liver oil), these fatty acids are in the TG form, as they are in most plant and animal sources of fat. However, since the recommended doses of EPA and DHA are often difficult to consume using unconcentrated oils, several steps can be used to increase the EPA and DHA concentration of the product while increasing the purity of the fatty acids delivered. The EPA and DHA fatty acids can be removed from their glycerol backbone and separated from other fatty acids (via hydrolysis and distillation). The EPA and DHA can then be stabilized by esterification with ethanol to form ethyl esters (EEs) of EPA and then concentrated. These concentrated fatty acids can be re-attached to a glycerol backbone to form re-esterified TG (rTG) molecules which contain a much higher concentration of EPA and DHA compared to the original TG molecule. These two forms of concentrated fish oil (EE and rTG) are the most common sources used in clinical trials and are often recommended by physicians (as dietary supplements or pharmaceuticals). It is important to note the distinctions between the various delivery forms of these fatty acids, as this often impacts their bioavailability and efficacy. The use of FFA and phospholipids (PL, primarily from krill), as well as other factors affecting the quality, safety, and bioavailability of n-3 products (e.g., heavy metals, pesticides, oxidation), will be discussed further below.

THE EPIDEMIOLOGY OF OMEGA-3 FATTY ACIDS AND CVD

Epidemiological and cohort studies have repeatedly shown that higher dietary intake of fatty fish and/or a person's n-3 status (as measured by EPA and DHA in serum, plasma or red blood cell [RBC] membranes) is inversely associated with cardiovascular events and/or cardiovascular mortality.[9–12] For instance, in a cohort of 20,551 men from the Physician's Health Study, the multivariate relative risk for sudden cardiac death in those consuming one fish meal per week was 0.48 ($P=0.04$), compared with men who consumed fish less than once per month.[13] The adjusted relative risk in the highest quartile of RBC n-3 levels (compared to the lowest quartile) in this population was just 0.19 ($P=0.007$).[9] The Honolulu Heart Program followed Japanese-Americans living in Hawaii and found that the relative risk for coronary heart disease (CHD) mortality was cut in half for heavy smokers (>30 cig/day) if they consumed more than two fish meals per week.[14] Several recent meta-analyses of prospective cohort studies have confirmed these overall results. Chowdhury et al. (2014) analyzed 16 studies exploring the relationship between long-chain n-3 dietary intake (lowest vs highest tertile) and coronary outcomes, and reported a relative risk (RR) of 0.87 (95% confidence interval [CI], 0.78 to 0.97).[15] By comparison, ALA intake had no statistical relation to coronary outcomes (RR=0.99, N=7 studies), while total trans fatty acid intake contributed to a significant increase in coronary outcomes (RR=1.16, N=5). Furthermore, their analysis of studies comparing coronary outcomes based on circulating fatty acids (top vs lowest tertile, N=13) revealed statistically significant risk reduction for EPA (RR=0.78), DHA (RR=0.79) and EPA+DHA (RR=0.75).

In a more recent meta-analysis, Alexander et al. analyzed 17 prospective cohort studies and found a significant reduction in CHD events (RR=0.82), coronary deaths (RR=0.82) and sudden cardiac deaths (RR=0.53) comparing subjects consuming the highest vs lowest intake of n-3 fatty acids.[16] Notably, an analysis of data generated through the National Health and Nutrition Examination Survey (NHANES-2012) estimated that insufficient intake of marine n-3 fatty acids was the "cause" of over 54,000 cardiovascular disease-related deaths annually.[17]

OMEGA-3 INDEX AND CVD RISK

Since the dietary intake of omega-3 fatty acids from foods or supplements may not always correlate with biomarkers of omega-3 status, several investigators have focused on the incorporation of long-chain n-3 fatty acids (primarily EPA and DHA) within RBC membrane fatty acids as a way to measure the long-term absorption and tissue deposition of n-3 fatty acids.[18] In fact, the percentage of EPA and DHA within RBC membranes, known generally as the "omega-3 index" or O-3I, is inversely related to cardiovascular events and mortality, where the highest risk is associated with subjects with an omega-3 index less than 4%, and the lowest risk is in subjects with an omega-3 index greater than 8%.[19] A meta-analysis of 10 cohort studies measuring risk in subjects based on their estimated omega-3 index predicted that subjects with an omega-3 index of 8% had a 30% lower risk for fatal CHD compared to those with an omega-3 index of 4%.[20] A more recent (2021) pooled analysis of 17 prospective studies, including nearly 16,000 deaths among over 42,000 people, found a 15% reduction in CVD mortality between the highest and lowest quintiles of circulating long-chain omega-3 fatty acids.[21] This included risk reductions of 15% for EPA (*P* for Trend 0.006) and a 21% risk reduction for DHA (*P* for Trend 0.002) between the highest and lowest quintiles. These data, combined with data showing that the risk reduction potential of supplemental EPA and/or DHA is likely dependent on dose, absorption and tissue incorporation (see further below), determining a subject's baseline and post-supplemental omega-3 index, may be necessary to optimize risk reduction-related n-3 supplementation.

Testing a patient's omega-3 index may be especially important to ensure that they are being recommended the correct dose to optimize their CVD risk reduction. Flock et al. have convincingly shown that the treatment dose of EPA and DHA (TG from fish) has a predictable effect on the change in omega-3 index, but they also discovered that interindividual differences (especially based on a person's body weight) account for a high degree of variability in the omega-3 index changes seen after consuming EPA and DHA.[22] Therefore, it is essential for the clinician to understand that without testing a person's omega-3 index, it is difficult to predict the likely risk reduction they may experience upon n-3 supplementation based simply on the n-3 fatty acid dose given (an important factor in interpreting clinical trials where all subjects are given the same dose of n-3). The omega-3 index is readily available through numerous laboratories and can easily be incorporated into a clinician's CVD risk assessment.

CVD INTERVENTION STUDIES USING OMEGA-3 FATTY ACIDS

While epidemiological and cohort studies have consistently shown substantial risk reduction in subjects consuming higher amounts of long-chain n-3 fatty acids, primary and secondary prevention trials have resulted in much more heterogeneity. One of the first studies assessing the secondary prevention potential of n-3 fatty acids from fish was the Diet And Reinfarction Trial (DART).[23] Men (*N*=2033) recovering from a myocardial infarction (MI) were randomized to receive one of three different dietary recommendations: to increase fatty fish consumption, to increase fiber, or to reduce fat intake. Those advised to increase fatty fish consumption had a 29% reduction in 2-year all-cause mortality, while neither the low-fat nor fiber recommendation group had a meaningful risk reduction. Unfortunately, like many lifestyle changes, this advice was difficult to maintain over many years, and both compliance and benefits diminished after a decade.[24]

Until recently, the largest and most cited secondary prevention trial investigating the supplementation of EPA and DHA was the GISSI-prevention trial.[25] In this study, over 11,000 patients
(surviving a recent MI) were randomized to one of three supplement groups: those given one gelatin
capsule containing 850–882 mg of EPA and DHA (as EEs in the average ratio of EPA:DHA, 1:2),
those given 300 mg of vitamin E (as acetyl alpha tocopherol, synthetic *all racemic*) or those given
both n-3 fatty acids and vitamin E. Most of these patients were concomitantly on non-statin cardiovascular pharmaceuticals of various kinds, as well as advised about diet and lifestyle changes. Total
(RR = 0.59) and cardiovascular (RR = 0.66) mortalities were significantly reduced in the fish oil
groups as early as 3 and 4 months into the study, respectively. The most dramatic reduction was in
sudden deaths, for which relative risks of 0.37 (after 9 months) and 0.55 (42 months) were reported.[26]
Among the lipids measured, only triglyceride levels showed significant improvements. The results
of the GISSI-prevention trial initiated the wide-spread use of concentrated EPA and DHA products
around the world and justified numerous official recommendations for the use of EPA and DHA for
CVD prevention and management (e.g., American Heart Association's recommendation to consume
1 g/day of EPA and DHA from fatty fish or supplements).[27]

In the years between the publication of the DART and GISSI trials (1988–1999), there were
over 20 randomized clinical trials evaluating the role of n-3 supplementation or increased fatty fish
consumption on CVD, ten of which met the criteria for a meta-analytical study.[28] Though many of
these trials were of suboptimal quality, these data showed that the daily intake of long-chain n-3
fatty acids from fish for an average of 3 years resulted in a 16% decrease in all-cause mortality and
a 24% decrease in the incidence of death from MI. We should note that none of the subjects in these
ten trials were taking statin drugs and, with the exception of the GISSI-prevention trial, the n-3 fatty
acid doses given were all ≥ 1.5 g of EPA and DHA/day. Both are important factors in comparing
these data with more recent clinical trials, which are almost universally performed in statin-treated
individuals (for secondary prevention) and often use n-3 fatty acid doses below 1 g/day.

In the past two decades, hundreds of clinical trials have been performed using a variety of doses,
combinations and types of EPA and DHA, with respect to nearly every CVD-related endpoint.
While many of these were trials exploring the effects of n-3 fatty acids on a variety of biomarkers
(e.g., TG, C-reactive protein [CRP], LDL-cholesterol [LDL-C], lipoprotein number and size, blood
pressure), several of these studies were designed as primary and secondary prevention trials, measuring MACE (major adverse cardiac events; nonfatal MI/strokes, CVD deaths) and/or all-cause
mortality. In 2017 and 2018, several well-publicized meta-analyses examined and compared these
latter trials with some of the earlier trial mentioned before, determining that there was no significant
reduction in fatal or nonfatal CVD events in subjects randomized to n-3 fatty acids therapies in these
trials.[16,29,30] Of these, Aung et al.'s publication in *JAMA Cardiology* has had a significant negative
impact on cardiologists' view of n-3 supplementation.[29]

However, as with many large intervention trials evaluating nutrients for drug-like outcomes, this
meta-analysis, and the studies upon which it was based, has significant limitations. First, the analysis only included studies with greater than 500 participants treated for more than one year, which
restricted their analysis to only 10 trials. Further, 83.4% of the nearly 78,000 subjects included in the
analysis were concurrently using statin therapy, which reflects the changes in cardiovascular therapy
from the previously mentioned cohort of n-3 studies. Perhaps more problematic was the fact that the
omega-3 status was not used as an inclusion/exclusion criterion for any of these trials, nor reported as
a biomarker in these studies. This is important since, unlike drugs, participants would have started
each trial with varying levels of EPA and DHA, greatly influencing their ability to achieve risk reduction through n-3 supplementation. In addition, as pointed out by von Schacky, these trials used a fixed
dose of EPA and DHA, most often below 1 g (usually during a low-fat breakfast), which was likely to
result in poor bioavailability (overall) and a large interindividual dose-response on improved omega-3
index.[31] While some of the same limitations apply to the meta-analysis performed by Alexander
et al. published in *Mayo Clinic Proceedings*, a subgroup analysis of their 17 included trials revealed
statistically significant benefits in subjects with elevated baseline TG > 150 mg/dL (RR = 0.84; 95%

CI, 0.72–0.98) or baseline LDL-C > 130 mg/dL (RR = 0.86; 95% CI, 0.76–0.98). Importantly, in this study, the strongest benefit was seen in subjects with elevated baseline TG given an n-3 fatty acid dose greater than 1 g/day of EPA and DHA (RR = 0.75; 95% CI, 0.64–0.89).[16] This magnitude of risk reduction aligns with the prospective cohort data mentioned previously, suggesting that higher doses of n-3 fatty acids over a short-term period (i.e., less than 5 years) may be needed to realize benefits that are typically achieved by extended periods of low to moderate n-3 intake. Nonetheless, the recent publication of several large clinical trials using products that are approved as pharmaceuticals has dominated the narrative about omega-3 supplementation and cardiovascular risk; while this may not be completely warranted, we now turn our attention to these trials.

REDUCE-IT (2018)

One of these large clinical trials, the Reduction of Cardiovascular Events with Icosapent Ethyl-Intervention Trial (REDUCE-IT), has garnered much attention.[32] Like the successful Japan EPA Lipid Intervention Study (JELIS), the REDUCE-IT trial employed the use of the approved drug Vascepa®, which is an EPA-only, EE product.[33] In this secondary prevention study, 8,179 subjects with elevated fasting TG (between 150 and 499 mg/dL) and LDL-C of 41–100 mg/dL (all subjects were concurrently medicated with a stable dose of statin therapy) were randomized to receive placebo (mineral oil) or 4 g daily (2 g twice daily, with food) of EPA-EEs and followed for nearly 5 years. The major clinical endpoint was the cumulative incidence of cardiovascular events (CVD deaths, nonfatal MI, nonfatal stroke, coronary revascularization or unstable angina), which was 25% lower in the fish oil therapy group compared to placebo (hazard ratio 0.75, $P < 0.001$). As anticipated, TG levels in these subjects, which averaged 216.5 mg/dL at baseline, were significantly reduced (18.3%–21.7%) during the trial. Interestingly, while the company producing Vascepa (Amarin) often remarks that EPA therapy (as opposed to DHA therapy) does not raise LDL-C, these subjects realized a small but statistically significant increase in LDL-C from baseline (3.1%, $P < 0.001$). Since the LDL-C increase was coincident with an increase in high-density lipoprotein cholesterol (HDL-C) and a decrease in ApoB of similar magnitudes, these changes likely reflect a beneficial shift in LDL particle size and number (not reported). The lowest statistically significant hazard ratio following n-3 therapy was for subjects having baseline TG ≥ 200 mg/dL and HDL ≤ 35 mg/dL (HR = 0.62). There is significant debate (both scientifically and commercially) as to the applicability of these data to other (similar) available products (i.e., dietary supplements) that provide concentrated EPA or EPA/DHA in either the EE or rTG form. For a discussion of the potential differences between EPA and DHA and the bioavailability differences between EE and rTG, see further below.

VITAL (2018)

Published in the same November 2018 issue of the *New England Journal of Medicine* as the REDUCE-IT trial, the Vitamin D and Omega-3 Trial (VITAL) evaluated a more traditional n-3 dose and product in a large primary prevention study.[34] Participants (N = 25,871) were randomized to one of four groups: (1) n-3 fatty acids (1 g fish oil capsule/day [Omacor®/Lovaza®] providing EE forms of EPA [460 mg] and DHA [380 mg]), (2) vitamin D_3 (2000 IU/day), (3) both n-3 and vitamin D_3, or (4) both placebos (olive oil used for fish oil placebo). This dose and n-3 form was based on the recommendation of the American Heart Association (for cardio-protection) and the late-1990s GISSI-prevention trial. As a primary prevention trial in subjects over the age of 50 (mean 67.1 years), only 4.2% of the subjects in VITAL experienced a cardiovascular event (defined in the composite endpoints: MI, stroke, cardiovascular deaths, or coronary revascularization) during the 5 years of the trial, compared to greater than 19% of subjects in the REDUCE-IT trial. However, when subjects taking the n-3 supplements were compared to those taking olive oil, there was only a non-statistical trend in the reduction of major cardiovascular events (HR = 0.93; 95% CI, 0.80–1.04). Secondary endpoint analysis suggested some benefits with n-3 supplementation, such as total MI (HR = 0.72; 95% CI, 0.59–0.90), deaths from MI (HR = 0.50; 95% CI, 0.26–0.97) and events in subjects with fish consumption <1.5 servings per week (HR = 0.81; 95% CI, 0.67–0.98).

Overall, these data are not unexpected, based on the shortcomings of the trial design: primarily the low number of events in this populations, the comparatively low n-3 dose to achieve meaningful event reduction (evidenced by achieving an omega-3 index of only 4.1% [from 2.7% at baseline] after 1 year of n-3 supplementation), and the use of olive oil (known to reduce CVD events at higher doses) as a placebo.[35] These shortcomings should be considered when evaluating the (mostly) negative results of VITAL, one of the largest clinical trials performed using EPA and DHA for the primary prevention of CVD. Unfortunately, some of these same shortcomings exist in a similar trial published earlier in 2018, A Study of Cardiovascular Events in Diabetes (ASCEND).

ASCEND (2018)

ASCEND was also a primary prevention trial including only diabetic subjects ($N = 15,480$) with no evidence of CVD.[36] Subjects were randomized to receive a 1 g fish oil capsule/day (Omacor®/Lovaza®, providing EE forms of EPA [460 mg] and DHA [380 mg]) or placebo (olive oil) and followed for an average of 7.4 years. The primary outcome was a composite of nonfatal MI, stroke or vascular deaths, while secondary endpoints included other serious vascular events or any arterial revascularization. Over the length of the trial, the group randomized to fish oil had 689 events (8.9%), while the olive oil group had 712 events (9.2%); this difference was not statistically significant (RR = 0.97; 95% CI, 0.87–1.08). In fact, with the exception of vascular deaths (RR = 0.81; 95% CI, 0.67–0.99), there were no beneficial differences in events reported between the n-3 and olive oil groups.

Again, these data are not surprising for some of the same reasons discussed previously in the VITAL study (e.g., low n-3 dose, olive oil placebo), with two important differences. Since this group included only diabetic subjects (all types), these subjects had a higher CVD risk which was evidenced by the higher number of events recorded in ASCEND (9.0%) compared to VITAL (4.2%), though still much fewer than the secondary prevention REDUCE-IT trial (19%). However, unlike the American subjects recruited for VITAL who had a mean baseline omega-3 index of just 2.7% (high risk), the UK subjects recruited for ASCEND had a mean baseline omega-3 index of 7.1% (which increased to 9.1% after supplementation). This suggests that the ASCEND subjects were already at low risk based on their omega-3 index, limiting the ability of n-3 supplementation to alter that risk. On the other hand, since the VITAL group was only able to achieve an omega-3 index of 4.1% after supplementation, these subjects never achieved an omega-3 status associated with lower risk. Since neither trial reported TG levels of the participants, it is difficult to know whether either group included subjects with TG-associated risk and whether n-3 supplementation altered subjects' TG levels.

STRENGTH (2020)

The Long-Term Outcomes Study to Assess Statin Residual Risk with Epanova in High Cholesterol Risk Patients with Hypertriglyceridemia (STREGTH) trial randomized at-risk subjects already on statin drugs to either corn oil (placebo) or 4 g/day of n-3 fatty acids in the carboxylic acid form (i.e., FFA; providing 550 mg of EPA and 200 mg of DHA per gram).[37] This multinational study, involving 675 different academic and community hospitals, was intended to follow patients for 5 years but was stopped 6 months early when it was determined that the primary endpoint, the composite of CV deaths, nonfatal MIs, strokes, revascularizations and hospitalization for unstable angina, would be no different between groups.

The negative outcome of this study has left many confused about how to understand the role of omega-3 supplementation in the context of statin use and risk reduction, though adding the data from STRENGH to previous studies (pooled meta-analysis) does not change the benefits predicted for n-3 supplementation.[38] The use of corn oil placebo compared to mineral oil (used in REDUCE-IT) is often cited as a potential confounder, as is the inclusion of DHA with EPA in this trial. While we will discuss the potential differences between EPA and DHA supplementation further below, we should note here that a subset analysis of subjects with higher post-supplementation increases in RBC DHA had no statistical difference in outcomes compared to those with lower post-supplementation increases of DHA, suggesting that the inclusion of DHA had no impact on the negative outcome of this trial.

CARDIOMETABOLIC MECHANISMS AND BIOMARKERS RELATED TO EPA AND/OR DHA

While the use of large clinical trials using major cardiovascular events as primary endpoints is viewed as the standard for measuring effects in drug trials, there are many studies linking the intake of EPA and/or DHA to a range of well-established CVD risk biomarkers.[39] For the most part, EPA and DHA are considered to have similar health benefits; since they are most often delivered together, at various ratios, in fish meals and in most product used in clinical trials therefore, recommendations usually describe a combination of the two (EPA plus DHA), without differentiation. However, over the past decade, a number of studies have hinted at both mechanistic and clinically relevant differences between these two similar fatty acids, potentially leading to subtle therapeutic differences for each. In some cases, there are head-to-head comparisons between the two fatty acids in clinical trials; in other cases, there are epidemiological or basic science discoveries that are driving clinical focus on one fatty acid over the other for specific health outcomes (e.g., eye health, depression). Here, we will briefly overview some of these discoveries as they relate to CVD biomarkers and outcomes, outlining where these differences between EPA and DHA may be clinically relevant. These data are particularly helpful in balancing the discussion related to the results of REDUCE-IT, which used only EPA.

Interestingly, while it is generally assumed that EPA and DHA have identical benefits in preventing cardiovascular risk, and there is some limited evidence that the two molecules can be converted back and forth in humans,[40] there is accumulating evidence that DHA may be more favorable (overall) in changing cardiovascular-related biomarkers. Mori and Woodman concluded in a review published in 2006 that "The data in humans suggest that DHA may be more favorable in lowering blood pressure and improving vascular function, raising HDL-C and attenuating platelet function. Future studies will need to carefully assess the independent effects of EPA and DHA on other clinical and biochemical measures before decisions can be made with respect to dietary supplements and the fortification of foods with either EPA or DHA."[41] Others have published similar observations.[42,43] Since then, many advances, including the introduction and approval of an EPA-only EE pharmaceutical n-3 product, have been added to these early findings. Nonetheless, a systematic review published in 2018, came to a similar conclusion: "Both EPA and DHA lowered triglyceride concentration, with DHA having a greater triglyceride-lowering effect. While total cholesterol levels were largely unchanged by EPA and DHA, DHA increased HDL-C concentration, particularly HDL$_2$, and increased low-density lipoprotein (LDL) cholesterol concentration and LDL particle size. Both EPA and DHA inhibited platelet activity, while DHA improved vascular function and lowered heart rate and blood pressure to a greater extent than EPA."[44] Perhaps the ability of high-dose DHA to increase the omega-3 index to a greater extent than high-dose EPA helps explain some of these differences.[45] Below we will explore the data behind these statements further.

Triglyceride (TG) Reduction: One of the most consistent CVD-related biomarker changes resulting from supplementation with EPA and/or DHA preparations is the reduction in fasting and non-fasting serum TG.[46] These results have been consistently reported for decades, where the magnitude of reduction is often related to the dose of EPA and/or DHA, as well as the subject's baseline TG levels.[47–49] The TG-lowering effects of EPA and DHA are so well established that, currently, each of the omega-3 pharmaceutical products approved by the FDA is indicated specifically for severe hypertriglyceridemia (TG > 500 mg/dL).

In many cases, the magnitude of the TG-lowering effect following EPA and/or DHA supplementation influences changes in other lipoprotein biomarkers, such as VLDL number and size, LDL number and size, LDL-C and HDL-C. These effects are thought to be mostly driven by the effects of these fatty acids on lipid-modulating transcription factors in hepatocytes and adipocytes (e.g., PPAR family, RXR, SREBP1), and lipoprotein enzymes such as cholesterol ester transfer protein

(CETP) and apoCIII.[50] Ultimately, these effects result in reduced hepatic synthesis of VLDL-TG, an increased clearance of TG, reduced levels of ApoB100 and a shift in cholesterol from VLDL particles to HDL and LDL particles. When compared head to head, DHA is often reported to have a slightly greater ability to lower TG levels vs EPA.[44,51,52]

LDL, HDL AND NON-HDL CHOLESTEROL

There is much controversy surrounding the ability of fish oil supplementation to affect LDL-C and HDL-C levels, especially related to fish oil's ability to *raise* LDL-C. Research shows that long-chain n-3 fatty acid supplementation, and particularly DHA supplementation, raises both HDL-C and LDL-C, though it does not increase non-HDL-C. These increases in both HDL-C and LDL-C appear to be greater where TG-lowering is greatest.[53] As the triglyceride-rich lipoprotein VLDL is metabolized to LDL, a concomitant rise in LDL particles is, therefore, a natural consequence of triglyceride-lowering (i.e., VLDL-lowering). Since the increase in LDL-C does not translate to higher non-HDL-C, this effect is likely the result of shifting cholesterol from VLDL particles to LDL and HDL particles, which then shifts LDL particles toward a larger and less atherogenic phenotype (see the discussion below on particle size changes). The increase in LDL-C (and HDL-C) after DHA supplementation should therefore be viewed as metabolically favorable and indicative of shifting of lipids away from the triglyceride-rich VLDL particles, effects associated with reduced CVD risk.

Lipoprotein Particle Size: Combinations of EPA and DHA have been shown to favorably alter lipoprotein particle size: increasing both LDL and HDL particle sizes, as well as decreasing VLDL particle size. When EPA and DHA are compared with respect to their ability to improve HDL particle size, DHA-rich oils show more consistent improvements.[54,55] This may be due to the fact that DHA has a greater inhibition of CETP activity, one of the enzymes responsible for altering lipoprotein particle size.[56] DHA, but not EPA, was capable of increasing LDL particle size in treated hypertensive type 2 diabetic patients, as well as overweight hypercholesterolemic subjects.[54,57]

Blood Pressure: Omega-3 fatty acid therapy has shown modest improvements in both systolic and diastolic blood pressures and endothelial function, particularly in hypertensive patients.[58–60] In animal and human studies, DHA supplementation has a more significant impact on reducing both systolic and diastolic blood pressures than EPA supplementation.[61] DHA also showed greater improvement in endothelial function in these patients.[62] Both EPA and DHA improve arterial compliance.[63]

Heart Rate: An increased heart rate is an independent risk factor for CVD mortality. A meta-analysis of 30 studies investigating the role of fish oil supplements on heart rate showed a modest, statistically significant, improvement in subjects consuming fish oil, compared to placebo (1.6 bpm; $P=0.002$).[64] Heart rate was reduced by 2.6 bpm ($P<0.001$) in studies lasting longer than 12 weeks or in studies where the baseline median heartrate was above 69 bpm. In a study comparing DHA to EPA in their ability to affect heart rate, DHA was able to lower heart rate in overweight hyperlipidemic men, while EPA was not.[54] Other studies have shown similar superiority of heart rate lowering using DHA as compared to EPA.[52,65]

INFLAMMATORY BIOMARKERS AND SPECIALIZED PRO-RESOLVING MEDIATORS

Inflammation is a critical initiator and mediator of atherosclerosis and CVD events. Therefore, agents that reduce inflammatory biomarkers in at-risk subjects are considered to be helpful in risk reduction. CRP has been recognized as a universal biomarker of systemic and cardiovascular inflammation, and has been used as a biomarker of CVD risk for many years.[66] Numerous studies have investigated the ability of n-3 supplements (primarily EPA and DHA) to improve biomarkers of inflammation (e.g., CRP, TNF-α, IL-6, eicosanoids) in human clinical trials, animal studies and cell culture experiments, though many of these are in non-CVD-related experimental designs. A meta-analysis of 68 clinical trials evaluating the effects of marine-derived n-3 fatty acids on CRP,

IL-6 and TNF-α has been performed.[67] This included studies performed in healthy subjects, as well as in patients with chronic autoimmune and non-autoimmune diseases. Overall, subjects given n-3 supplements had clinically meaningful, statistically significant reduction in fasting blood CRP, IL-6 and TNF-α, when compared to subjects given placebo. The cohort of studies that included those with CVD (chronic non-autoimmune diseases) had reductions of −18% for CRP and −20% for IL-6, but the reduction in TNF-α was not statistically significant. Of the three biomarkers measured, only IL-6 lowering (−7.7%) reached statistical significance when these biomarkers were assessed based on n-3 from dietary intake (rather than supplementation). It is interesting to note that in subgroup analysis, significant lowering of CRP was only observed when n-3 supplementation was paired with a placebo that contained the n-6 fatty acid linolenic acid (primarily corn, sunflower or soybean-containing oils), whereas this difference was not statistically significant in trials where olive oil was used as the placebo. As noted earlier in our discussion of the VITAL and ASCEND clinical trials, olive oil has known benefits in CVD subjects, including documented anti-inflammatory activity.[68] In a meta-analysis of eight studies evaluating the effects of n-3 supplementation in type 2 diabetic subjects, there was a modest, but statistical mean reduction of CRP.[69]

There are numerous mechanisms that have been postulated to account for the anti-inflammatory activities of EPA and DHA including the downregulation of various eicosanoids (prostaglandins, thromboxanes and leukotrienes), PPAR-mediated modulation of NFκB pathways, and as precursors for specialized pro-resolving mediators (SPMs).[70,71] The latter mechanism has recently gained much attention, especially as it pertains to n-3 supplementation. SPMs are cell-signaling molecules derived from LCPUFA that function primarily to resolve (rather than inhibit) inflammatory processes.[72] Categories of SPMs include lipoxins (derived from arachidonic acid), resolvins (from EPA, DPA and DHA), protectins/neuroprotectins (from DPA and DHA) and maresins (from DPA and DHA).

Currently, there are several studies that associate biomarkers of SPMs with n-3 intake in human subjects.[73,74] For example, a secondary analysis of subjects with peripheral arterial disease given high doses of fish oil n-3 fatty acids (4.4 g of EPA and DHA/day) showed a significant 1-month increase in their omega-3 index (from 5% to 9%), which corresponded to significant increases in four different SPM precursors. Similarly, subjects with chronic kidney disease given 4 g/day of n-3 fatty acids (Omacor™) saw significant increases in E- and D-series resolvins after 8 weeks of supplementation. These studies, along with other similar findings, suggest that the intake of n-3 fatty acids (particularly EPA, DPA and DHA) may augment the fatty acid reserve needed for the local production of SPMs to allow for appropriate resolution of local inflammatory processes.[75–77]

BIOAVAILABILITY OF N-3 SUPPLEMENTS

The efficacy of omega-3 fatty acid therapy is significantly affected by tissue availability, particularly its ability to increase a person's omega-3 index, which is affected by its initial bioavailability.[78] Therefore, numerous studies have been performed to compare short- and long-term bioavailability in human subjects using omega-3 fatty acids from different sources and in different molecular forms. We will first discuss studies using fish oil preparations and subsequently address the question of krill vs fish oil.[79]

ETHYL ESTERS VS TRIGLYCERIDES

Since the initial production and use of EE forms of omega-3 fatty acids, many have questioned the potential difference between bioavailability of these forms compared to that of other natural fatty acid forms. The early studies were small, but these data revealed either a slightly reduced bioavailability of the EE forms (compared to TG forms) in the absence of additional dietary fat or a statistically similar bioavailability between EE and TG forms. More recently, several larger and better-designed studies have shown a superior bioavailability of rTG forms over EE forms.

One of the largest studies performed to date compared similar doses of EPA and DHA using five different forms: unconcentrated triglycerides (which the researchers called fish body oil [FBO]), cod liver oil (similar TG form as FBO), rTG, EE or FFA, along with a "placebo" of corn oil. In this study, 72 subjects were randomly assigned 3.3 g/day of an EPA+DHA blend as capsules for 2 weeks.[80] Serum fatty acids (combined serum TG, PL and cholesterol esters) were analyzed at baseline and after 2 weeks. In these subjects, the bioavailability of EPA+DHA from re-esterified tri-glycerides (rTG) was superior (+24%) when compared with natural fish oil (FBO or CLO), whereas the bioavailability from EEs was inferior (−27%) to natural TG and nearly 70% less bioavailable than rTG. The authors suggest that the increased bioavailability of rTG over the unconcentrated TG form may be due to diglycerides contained in the rTG products, along with a small amount of monoglycerides, which act as "partially digested forms" of the natural triglyceride, potentially enhancing bioavailability over the natural FBO. Concerning the EE form, studies have shown a decreased lipase enzymatic activity when ethyl ester substrates are used, perhaps accounting for their decreased absorption when consumed away from a meal containing fat.[81]

Ultimately, it is critical to know whether these differences in bioavailability over 2 weeks might translate into long-term differences in fatty acid incorporation into important tissues (e.g., RBC or cardiovascular tissues) and whether these differences can be measured in a clinically meaning-ful outcome (e.g., reductions in TG). These sorts of studies have been carried out by researchers in Germany, who looked at the incorporation of EPA and DHA into RBC membranes, commonly referred to as the omega-3 index, when individuals consumed either EE or rTG forms of fish oil.[82] One particular study included 150 hyperlipidemic subjects who were also taking statin drugs. Subjects were given soft gelatin capsules containing EPA (1,008 mg) and DHA (672 mg) daily as either rTG or EE form (corn oil used in placebo group) and were followed for 6 months. Subjects consuming the rTG form had, on average, a statistically higher omega-3 index than those consum-ing the EE form after 3 months, which was maintained after 6 months of daily intake. In a separate publication, the lipid-lowering effects of these two therapies were also reported.[83] While both the EE and rTG reduced serum TG levels in these patients compared to placebo, the change resulting from rTG was nearly double that of the EE form (−18.7% vs −9.4%). The only therapy to reach a statistically significant decrease from baseline was rTG therapy.

These differences between rTG and EE have become hotly debated, because pharmaceutical products are primarily delivered as EE, whereas dietary supplement forms are available as both EE and rTG. Therefore, in a more recent trial, researchers performed a head-to-head trial compar-ing the TG-lowering effects of one of the popular EE pharmaceutical products (Lovaza®) and a rTG fish oil product.[84] In this randomized, double-blind, placebo-controlled trial, 120 subjects with non-fasting plasma TG levels of 150–500 mg/dL were given 3 g/day EPA and DHA as either an EE or rTG (or placebo) for 8 weeks. After supplementation, non-fasting plasma TG decreased 28% in the rTG group and 22% in the EE group (both $P < 0.001$ vs placebo), with no statistically signifi-cant difference between the two groups. The TG-lowering effect was seen after 4 weeks and was inversely correlated with the omega-3 index, which increased 63.2% in the rTG group and 58.5% in the EE group. In addition, heart rate decreased by three beats per minute ($P = 0.045$) and HDL-C increased only in the rTG group ($P < 0.001$). These data confirm that rTG products delivering similar amounts of total EPA and DHA as pharmaceutical EE products are at least as effective for lowering TG and may provide other cardioprotective benefits beyond the EE forms.*

KRILL OIL VS FISH OIL

In the past decade, the market has been flooded with information about the use of, and purported superiority of, omega-3 fatty acids from krill.[85] These claims have primarily come from two proper-ties of krill oil: that it is composed mostly of phospholipids (as opposed to TG) and that it contains

---

* It may be important to note that the rTG fish oil product had a higher content of DHA than the pharmaceutical EE product (1,930 vs 1,382 mg), though the rTG product had a lower level of total EPA and DHA (2,885 vs 3,306 mg). Even though the rTG dose was lower, the higher level of DHA may have accounted for some of these differences.

trace levels of astaxanthin, a bioactive carotenoid. Additionally, some studies have suggested that these properties, particularly the PL nature of the fatty acids, account for superior bioavailability compared to fish oil. We will examine this claim first.

In general, only short-term and limited comparisons are available to ascertain the relative bioavailability of krill oil vs fish oil, a research question complicated by krill oil's very low concentration of EPA and DHA. One group studied the difference between the use of krill oil and menhaden oil (FBO, natural TG) or placebo (olive oil) in their ability to alter plasma fatty acids when consumed by overweight and obese subjects ($N=76$).[86] Each subject was to consume 2 g/day of each oil for 4 weeks before being tested for changes in plasma fatty acid levels. It is important to note that the 2 g of menhaden oil contained 212 mg of EPA and 178 mg of DHA (390 mg total), while the krill oil preparation contained 216 mg of EPA and 90 mg of DHA (306 mg total). Compared to olive oil, both the krill and menhaden oils significantly increased the EPA and DHA levels of the subjects: krill increased EPA by 89% and DHA by 23%, and menhaden increased EPA by 81% and DHA by 45%. These data suggest that the bioavailability of EPA and DHA from krill and unconcentrated menhaden oils are similar.

The second study often cited was a 7-week study comparing the change in plasma fatty acids in subjects with "normal or slightly elevated" lipids when given either krill or fish oil.[87] This study compared six capsules of krill oil, providing 543 mg of EPA+DHA, and three capsules of fish oil (unspecified form), providing 864 mg of EPA+DHA. Compared to control subjects (unsupplemented subjects), both krill and fish oils were able to statistically increase EPA and DHA in those consuming each. However, while the average increase in EPA and DHA was slightly higher in the fish oil group, the difference between the groups was not statistically significant.

Unfortunately, trials using equal amounts of EPA/DHA from fish and krill are limited or severely flawed. One recent study compared equivalent doses of EPA+DHA from krill, rTG and EE fish oils.[88] This was a single-dose, 72-hour study that measured changes in plasma phospholipids only, unlike the previous krill studies (measuring plasma fatty acids) or the long-term fish oil study (omega-3 index/RBC fatty acids). Here, 12 healthy males were recruited to consume each of the three omega-3 preparations (crossover design, 14 days apart) containing a total of 1,680 mg of EPA+DHA. The particular products used required 4 capsules of fish oil (rTG or EE) or 14 krill oil capsules to obtain the necessary EPA+DHA. Blood samples were taken before dosing (7 a.m.) and at 2, 4, 6, 8, 24, 48 and 72 hours after capsule intake. Like previous studies, there were no significant differences in the changes in plasma PL levels of EPA, DHA or the sum of EPA+DHA between the three treatments. The authors did note non-statistical "trends" of higher levels of plasma PL-EPA when subjects consumed krill. When one examines the data closely, it does appear that a higher plasma phospholipid level did indeed occur in individuals consuming equal levels of EPA+DHA from krill vs fish. However, since the authors measured plasma phospholipids only, and krill oil is enriched with the phospholipid form of the fatty acids, this trend may have been an artifact of fatty acid metabolism. Lastly, and perhaps most important for practical clinical consideration, it took 14 krill oil capsules to provide 1,680 mg of EPA+DHA, something now provided easily in two concentrated fish oil capsules (they used four in this study). We conclude, as others have, that the bioavailability of EPA and DHA from krill is not superior to that of fish oil TG or rTG forms, and the low concentration of EPA and DHA from krill makes it an especially uneconomical way to deliver these compounds.[89]

ASTAXANTHIN FROM KRILL

Astaxanthin is a reddish-colored xanthophyll (carotenoid, similar to the compound zeaxanthin) found in a variety of marine organisms, from algae to salmon. Krill biomass contains about 120 ppm astaxanthin, and most krill oil preparations claim a small amount of it on their label. To date, no human studies have been performed using krill oil-derived astaxanthin, making the various marketing claims difficult to evaluate. Microalgae sources, and some synthetic sources, are the commercially available forms used in the limited clinical studies that have evaluated astaxanthin. For context, the few studies available for astaxanthin supplementation in humans used doses ranging from 4 to 20 mg/day, and the average krill oil capsule claims to have 0.5–0.8 mg of astaxanthin per capsule.[90,91] Additional studies must be performed to understand the role and benefits of delivering astaxanthin from krill oil.

ADDITIONAL CONSIDERATIONS ON MARINE OMEGA-3 SOURCING

Kosher: Only products derived from fish or algae sources can be deemed truly "kosher;" however, additional manufacturing processes may influence the ability to officially label a finished product (e.g., soft gelatin capsules) with a particular kosher certificate.

Vegetarian/Vegan: While many vegetarians choose to consume fish oil products even if they avoid consuming fish, strict vegans will avoid all marine lipids with the exception of algae-sourced products. Since EPA can be formed by consuming either DHA from algae or ALA from flaxseed oil, these may be suitable options for strict vegan individuals. It should be noted that while these vegan omega-3 sources are likely to increase blood levels of EPA and DHA, there are limited data to suggest that these alternatives will have the same risk-lowering benefits as EPA and DHA from fish.

Gluten: Marine fatty acids are gluten-free, and softgel manufacturing typically does not introduce gluten to finished products.

Sustainability Issues: One of the concerns with using large quantities of marine omega-3 fatty acids for therapeutic use is the long-term sustainability of harvesting the needed biomass. The debate over which source(s) might be in danger of overharvesting or are being harvested in an ecologically sound manner is controversial and made more difficult by the fact that no single final authority defines "sustainability" for the global community. Fisheries that supply both fish meal and fish oil are managed by a number of regulatory bodies around the world, and harvest limits are set for certain fish species, fishing seasons and fishery zones. There is a seasonal variability in biomass, which is controlled by both local and global ocean conditions, affecting the year-to-year availability of EPA and DHA.[†]

Controversy over krill sustainability is especially keen. Most notably, in 2010 the retailer Whole Foods declared that they would not sell krill products because of data they believed linked krill harvesting with reduced levels of animals that depend on krill for food. Since that time, the Marine Stewardship Council and other organizations have approved several of the largest krill-harvesting companies as being "sustainable." The future of the sustainability of marine biomass is influenced by global ocean fluctuations and the growing need for EPA and DHA. Tension between marine-derived EPA and DHA sustainability and the development of more sustainable GMO-produced EPA and DHA from plants will no doubt heighten the controversy.

ALLERGIES TO FISH AND SHELLFISH RELATED TO OMEGA-3 PRODUCTS

Since the changes required for food allergen labeling went into effect in the United States in 2006, there is confusion as to how fish oil products should be labeled and whether individuals allergic to fish can safely consume fish oil. The eight allergens requiring mandatory labeling include both fish and shellfish (also soy, wheat, eggs, peanuts, tree nuts and milk). However, the labeling requirements exempt the need to label ingredients that are highly refined oils containing no allergenic proteins, specifically allergens. Therefore, highly refined fish oils, like certain soybean oils, do not need to be listed in a separate "contains the following allergens" statement on the label, though most companies using highly refined fish oils still choose to include "fish" in a list of allergens, primarily from a product liability standpoint. Nonetheless, the supplement facts box or front panel of a fish

---

[†] For detailed information about the status and environmental performance of fisheries worldwide (e.g., fish species, harvest statistics, regulations and sustainability), see www.fishsource.com.

oil product must still declare that the ingredient itself is concentrated fish oil, thereby notifying users that the content contains fish-derived oils, even if no official declaration is made pertaining to fish-derived allergens.

Labeling issues aside, what is the likelihood that individuals who have known allergies to finned fish might also have an allergic reaction to a fish oil product? The answer appears to be: *extremely unlikely*. First, allergic reactions to fish are well understood and linked to specific proteins. Highly refined fish oil products are virtually free from any detectable protein, and there are no known allergens in fish-derived fatty acids. This notion was actually tested in a small-scale study where individuals with known allergies to finned fish were given fish oil supplements to evaluate their reaction.[92] Two different fish oil supplements were tested in six subjects with known fish allergies by both skin and oral challenges. None of the subjects reacted in any way to either product.

These data, while limited, agree with the notion that highly refined fish oil products contain no reactive allergens and should be safe to consume by individuals with mild-to-moderate fish allergies, though published case reports suggest it may occur rarely.[93] Ironically, delivering fish oil using fish gelatin capsules (to avoid animal versions of gelatin) may inadvertently increase the likelihood of an allergic reaction in sensitive individuals.[94] Highly sensitive individuals and those with life-threatening fish allergies should probably avoid the use of fish oil products as a precaution and look to obtain omega-3 fatty acids from plant sources such as algae (DHA) or flax (ALA). Likewise, subjects with shellfish allergies should avoid krill- and mussel-derived oils.[95]

QUALITY CONTROL ISSUES OF FISH OIL AND RELATED PRODUCTS

Fish oil-derived omega-3 fatty acids have been used as dietary supplements and pharmaceutical products for several decades. The quality control issues that plagued the first few years of fish oil availability, such as heavy-metal contamination, pesticide residues, and oxidation, rarely occur in today's products. Several highly reputable organizations (e.g., Global Organization for EPA and DHA [GOED], The Council of Responsible Nutrition [CRN]) have developed quality and regulatory standards for fish oil and related omega-3 products, and set specific limits for heavy-metal contamination, a wide variety of organic pollutants, and oxidation.[96] Because of these standards, most global fish oil providers maintain their products to these high standards – this is especially true of the concentrated products (i.e., rTG and EE forms). Since heavy metals and pesticide residues are virtually impossible to be added during the manufacturing process, monitoring oxidation of the fatty acids is one of the critical steps in producing a high-quality product.

Fish oil oxidation is measured using two methods. The first measures oxidized fatty acids directly as a peroxide value (PV or POV). Since these peroxides are transient and can form secondary oxidized molecules, such as aldehydes, a second test is used to detect these oxidized compounds: the anisidine (or p-anisidine) test. By adding the anisidine value to twice the peroxide value (AV+2PV), we get the TOTOX value, which allows for evaluating an oil's rancidity.[97] To control the oxidation of the oil raw material and finished product, most manufacturers add a variety of antioxidants. The most popular are vitamin E, vitamin A, flavonoids, and rosemary or other spice extracts; synthetic antioxidants are rarely used. Most commercially available products contain one or more of these antioxidants, at very low doses, in the finished product. Manufacturers of liquid-filled bottles or softgel capsules also utilize nitrogen (to purge available oxygen), low light and cold temperatures in the manufacturing process to reduce oxidation and extend shelf life. Products that have passed their expiration date should be thrown away, as oxidized fish oil can act as a pro-oxidant and limit the benefits realized if consumed.[98,99]

CONCLUSION AND RECOMMENDATION

Based upon the current available evidence, there is a significant inverse relationship between a person's omega-3 status (as measured by their omega-3 index) and their risk for CVD. In addition, there is a strong correlation between their dietary intake and/or supplementation with EPA and DHA and their omega-3 index. Therefore, clinicians should routinely measure the n-3 status of their patients and make dietary and supplemental recommendations in accordance with those results. While many forms of n-3 supplements have been shown to improve a subject's n-3 status and reduce CVD risk, evidence suggests that rTG forms may increase a patient's omega-3 index greater than EE forms, though individual variability (and subject's BMI) can affect this relationship. Also, while most studies are performed on products providing both EPA and DHA (some with only EPA), head-to-head studies often favor DHA for CVD-related outcomes. Therefore, some subjects may benefit from rTG products providing more DHA than EPA for CVD-related outcomes. Subjects should be monitored to achieve an omega-3 index of greater than 8%, which will often require doses greater than 1.5 g of EPA/DHA per day. These doses are easy to achieve using rTG or EE forms of fish oil, though they are difficult to achieve using low-dose fish or krill oil products.

REFERENCES

1. Buja LM, Nikolai N. Anitschkow and the lipid hypothesis of atherosclerosis. *Cardiovasc. Pathol.* 2014; 23:183–4.
2. Mahmood SS, Levy D, Vasan RS, et al. The Framingham Heart Study and the epidemiology of cardiovascular disease: a historical perspective. *Lancet.* 2014; 383:999–1008.
3. Andrade J, Mohamed A, Frohlich J, et al. Ancel Keys and the lipid hypothesis: from early breakthroughs to current management of dyslipidemia. *B. C. Med. J.* 2009; 51:66–72.
4. Bang HO, Dyerberg J. Plasma lipids and lipoproteins in Greenlandic west coast Eskimos. *Acta Med. Scand.* 1972; 192:85–94.
5. Dyerberg J, Bang HO, Hjorne N. Fatty acid composition of the plasma lipids in Greenland Eskimos. *Am. J. Clin. Nutr.* 1975; 28:958–66.
6. Dyerberg J. Coronary heart disease in Greenland Inuit: a paradox. Implications for western diet patterns. *Arctic Med. Res.* 1989; 48:47–54.
7. Sprague M, Betancor MB, Tocher DR. Microbial and genetically engineered oils as replacements for fish oil in aquaculture feeds. *Biotechnol. Lett.* 2017; 39:1599–609.
8. Betancor MB, Li K, Sprague M, et al. An oil containing EPA and DHA from transgenic Camelina sativa to replace marine fish oil in feeds for Atlantic salmon (*Salmo salar* L.): effects on intestinal transcriptome, histology, tissue fatty acid profiles and plasma biochemistry. *PLoS One.* 2017; 12:e0175415.
9. Albert CM, Campos H, Stampfer MJ, et al. Blood levels of long-chain n-3 fatty acids and the risk of sudden death. *N. Engl. J. Med.* 2002; 346:1113–8.
10. Hu FB, Bronner L, Willett WC, et al. Fish and omega-3 fatty acid intake and risk of coronary heart disease in women. *JAMA.* 2002; 287:1815–21.
11. Gammelmark A, Nielsen MS, Bork CS, et al. Association of fish consumption and dietary intake of marine n-3 PUFA with myocardial infarction in a prospective Danish cohort study. *Br. J. Nutr.* 2016; 116:167–77.
12. Miyagawa N, Miura K, Okuda N, et al. Long-chain n-3 polyunsaturated fatty acids intake and cardiovascular disease mortality risk in Japanese: a 24-year follow-up of NIPPON DATA80. *Atherosclerosis.* 2014; 232:384–9.
13. Albert CM, Hennekens CH, O'Donnell CJ, et al. Fish consumption and risk of sudden cardiac death. *JAMA.* 1998; 279:23–8.
14. Rodriguez BL, Sharp DS, Abbott RD, et al. Fish intake may limit the increase in risk of coronary heart disease morbidity and mortality among heavy smokers. The Honolulu Heart Program. *Circulation.* 1996; 94:952–6.
15. Chowdhury R, Warnakula S, Kunutsor S, et al. Association of dietary, circulating, and supplement fatty acids with coronary risk: a systematic review and meta-analysis. *Ann. Intern. Med.* 2014; 160:398–406.
16. Alexander DD, Miller PE, Van Elswyk ME, et al. A meta-analysis of randomized controlled trials and prospective cohort studies of eicosapentaenoic and docosahexaenoic long-chain omega-3 fatty acids and coronary heart disease risk. *Mayo Clin. Proc.* 2017; 92:15–29.
17. Micha R, Penalvo JL, Cudhea F, et al. Association between dietary factors and mortality from heart disease, stroke, and type 2 diabetes in the United States. *JAMA.* 2017; 317:912–24.
18. Harris WS, Von Schacky C. The Omega-3 Index: a new risk factor for death from coronary heart disease? *Prev. Med.* 2004; 39:212–20.

19. Harris WS. The omega-3 index: clinical utility for therapeutic intervention. *Curr. Cardiol. Rep.* 2010; 12:503–8.

20. Harris WS, Del Gobbo L, Tintle NL. The Omega-3 Index and relative risk for coronary heart disease mortality: estimation from 10 cohort studies. *Atherosclerosis.* 2017; 262:51–4.

21. Harris WS, Tintle NL, Imamura F, et al. Blood n-3 fatty acid levels and total and cause-specific mortality from 17 prospective studies. *Nat. Commun.* 2021; 12(1):2329.

22. Flock MR, Skulas-Ray AC, Harris WS, et al. Determinants of erythrocyte omega-3 fatty acid content in response to fish oil supplementation: a dose-response randomized controlled trial. *J. Am. Heart Assoc.* 2013; 2:e000513.

23. Burr ML, Fehily AM, Gilbert JF, et al. Effects of changes in fat, fish, and fibre intakes on death and myocardial reinfarction: diet and reinfarction trial (DART). *Lancet.* 1989; 2:757–61.

24. Ness AR, Hughes J, Elwood PC, et al. The long-term effect of dietary advice in men with coronary disease: follow-up of the Diet and Reinfarction trial (DART). *Eur. J. Clin. Nutr.* 2002; 56:512–8.

25. Dietary supplementation with n-3 polyunsaturated fatty acids and vitamin E after myocardial infarction: results of the GISSI-Prevenzione trial. Gruppo Italiano per lo Studio della Sopravvivenza nell'Infarto miocardico. *Lancet.* 1999; 354:447–55.

26. Marchioli R, Barzi F, Bomba E, et al. Early protection against sudden death by n-3 polyunsaturated fatty acids after myocardial infarction: time-course analysis of the results of the Gruppo Italiano per lo Studio della Sopravvivenza nell'Infarto Miocardico (GISSI)-Prevenzione. *Circulation.* 2002; 105:1897–903.

27. Kris-Etherton PM, Harris WS, Appel LJ. Fish consumption, fish oil, omega-3 fatty acids, and cardiovascular disease. *Circulation.* 2002; 106:2747–57.

28. Yzebe D, Lievre M. Fish oils in the care of coronary heart disease patients: a meta-analysis of randomized controlled trials. *Fundam. Clin. Pharmacol.* 2004; 18:581–92.

29. Aung T, Halsey J, Kromhout D, et al. Associations of omega-3 fatty acid supplement use with cardiovascular disease risks: meta-analysis of 10 trials involving 77917 individuals. *JAMA Cardiol.* 2018; 3:225–34.

30. Abdelhamid AS, Brown TJ, Brainard JS, et al. Omega-3 fatty acids for the primary and secondary prevention of cardiovascular disease. *Cochrane Database Syst. Rev.* 2018; 11:Cd003177.

31. von Schacky C. Rebuttal to Aung et al, "Associations of omega-3 fatty acid supplement use with cardiovascular disease risks: meta-analysis of 10 trials involving 77 917 individuals". *Altern. Ther. Health Med.* 2018; 24:8–9.

32. Bhatt DL, Steg PG, Miller M, et al. Cardiovascular risk reduction with icosapent ethyl for hypertriglyceridemia. *N. Engl. J. Med.* 2019; 380:11–22.

33. Yokoyama M, Origasa H, Matsuzaki M, et al. Effects of eicosapentaenoic acid on major coronary events in hypercholesterolaemic patients (JELIS): a randomised open-label, blinded endpoint analysis. *Lancet.* 2007; 369:1090–8.

34. Manson JE, Cook NR, Lee IM, et al. Marine n-3 fatty acids and prevention of cardiovascular disease and cancer. *N. Engl. J. Med.* 2019; 380:23–32.

35. Guasch-Ferre M, Hu FB, Martinez-Gonzalez MA, et al. Olive oil intake and risk of cardiovascular disease and mortality in the PREDIMED Study. *BMC Med.* 2014; 12:78.

36. Bowman L, Mafham M, Wallendszus K, et al. Effects of n-3 fatty acid supplements in diabetes mellitus. *N. Engl. J. Med.* 2018; 379:1540–50.

37. Nicholls SJ, Lincoff AM, Garcia M, et al. Effect of high-dose omega-3 fatty acids vs corn oil on major adverse cardiovascular events in patients at high cardiovascular risk: the STRENGTH randomized clinical trial. *JAMA.* 2020; 324(22):2268–80.

38. Bernasconi AA, Lavie CJ, Milani RV, Laukkanen JA. Omega-3 benefits remain strong post-STRENGTH. *Mayo Clin. Proc.* 2021; 96(5):1371–2.

39. Thota RN, Ferguson JJA, Abbott KA, et al. Science behind the cardio-metabolic benefits of omega-3 polyunsaturated fatty acids: biochemical effects vs. clinical outcomes. *Food Funct.* 2018; 9:3576–96.

40. Arterburn LM, Hall EB, Oken H. Distribution, interconversion, and dose response of n-3 fatty acids in humans. *Am. J. Clin. Nutr.* 2006; 83:1467s–76s.

41. Mori TA, Woodman RJ. The independent effects of eicosapentaenoic acid and docosahexaenoic acid on cardiovascular risk factors in humans. *Curr. Opin. Clin. Nutr. Metab. Care.* 2006; 9:95–104.

42. Cottin SC, Sanders TA, Hall WL. The differential effects of EPA and DHA on cardiovascular risk factors. *Proc. Nutr. Soc.* 2011; 70:215–31.

43. Wei MY, Jacobson TA. Effects of eicosapentaenoic acid versus docosahexaenoic acid on serum lipids: a systematic review and meta-analysis. *Curr. Atheroscler. Rep.* 2011; 13:474–83.

44. Innes JK, Calder PC. The differential effects of eicosapentaenoic acid and docosahexaenoic acid on cardiometabolic risk factors: a systematic review. *Int. J. Mol. Sci.* 2018; 19:532.
45. Allaire J, Harris WS, Vors C, et al. Supplementation with high-dose docosahexaenoic acid increases the Omega-3 Index more than high-dose eicosapentaenoic acid. *Prostaglandins Leukot. Essent. Fatty Acids.* 2017; 120:8–14
46. Pirillo A, Catapano AL. Omega-3 polyunsaturated fatty acids in the treatment of atherogenic dyslipidemia. *Atheroscler. Suppl.* 2013; 14:237–42.
47. Skulas-Ray AC, Alaupovic P, Kris-Etherton PM, et al. Dose-response effects of marine omega-3 fatty acids on apolipoproteins, apolipoprotein-defined lipoprotein subclasses, and Lp-PLA2 in individuals with moderate hypertriglyceridemia. *J. Clin. Lipidol.* 2015; 9:360–7.
48. Balk EM, Lichtenstein AH, Chung M, et al. Effects of omega-3 fatty acids on serum markers of cardiovascular disease risk: a systematic review. *Atherosclerosis.* 2006; 189:19–30.
49. Backes J, Anzalone D, Hilleman D, et al. The clinical relevance of omega-3 fatty acids in the management of hypertriglyceridemia. *Lipids Health Dis.* 2016; 15:118.
50. Martinez-Fernandez L, Laiglesia LM, Huerta AE, et al. Omega-3 fatty acids and adipose tissue function in obesity and metabolic syndrome. *Prostaglandins Other Lipid Mediat.* 2015; 121:24–41.
51. Grimsgaard S, Bonaa KH, Hansen JB, et al. Effects of highly purified eicosapentaenoic acid and docosahexaenoic acid on hemodynamics in humans. *Am. J. Clin. Nutr.* 1998; 68:52–9.
52. Allaire J, Couture P, Leclerc M, et al. A randomized, crossover, head-to-head comparison of eicosapentaenoic acid and docosahexaenoic acid supplementation to reduce inflammation markers in men and women: the Comparing EPA to DHA (ComparED) Study. *Am. J. Clin. Nutr.* 2016; 104:280–7.
53. Mori TA, Burke V, Puddey IB, et al. Purified eicosapentaenoic and docosahexaenoic acids have differential effects on serum lipids and lipoproteins, LDL particle size, glucose, and insulin in mildly hyperlipidemic men. *Am. J. Clin. Nutr.* 2000; 71:1085–94.
54. Buckley R, Shewring B, Turner R, et al. Circulating triacylglycerol and apoE levels in response to EPA and docosahexaenoic acid supplementation in adult human subjects. *Br. J. Nutr.* 2004; 92:477–83.
55. Allaire J, Vors C, Tremblay AJ, et al. High-dose DHA has more profound effects on LDL-related features than high-dose EPA: the ComparED study. *J. Clin. Endocrinol. Metab.* 2018; 103:2909–17.
56. Hirano R, Igarashi O, Kondo K, et al. Regulation by long-chain fatty acids of the expression of cholesteryl ester transfer protein in HepG2 cells. *Lipids.* 2001; 36:401–6.
57. Woodman RJ, Mori TA, Burke V, et al. Docosahexaenoic acid but not eicosapentaenoic acid increases LDL particle size in treated hypertensive type 2 diabetic patients. *Diabetes Care.* 2003; 26:253.
58. Zehr KR, Walker MK. Omega-3 polyunsaturated fatty acids improve endothelial function in humans at risk for atherosclerosis: a review. *Prostaglandins Other Lipid Mediat.* 2018; 134:131–40.
59. Balakumar P, Taneja G. Fish oil and vascular endothelial protection: bench to bedside. *Free Radic. Biol. Med.* 2012; 53:271–9.
60. Cicero AF, Ertek S, Borghi C. Omega-3 polyunsaturated fatty acids: their potential role in blood pressure prevention and management. *Curr. Vasc. Pharmacol.* 2009; 7:330–7.
61. Mori TA, Bao DQ, Burke V, et al. Docosahexaenoic acid but not eicosapentaenoic acid lowers ambulatory blood pressure and heart rate in humans. *Hypertension.* 1999; 34:253–60.
62. Mori TA, Watts GF, Burke V, et al. Differential effects of eicosapentaenoic acid and docosahexaenoic acid on vascular reactivity of the forearm microcirculation in hyperlipidemic, overweight men. *Circulation.* 2000; 102:1264–9.
63. Nestel P, Shige H, Pomeroy S, et al. The n-3 fatty acids eicosapentaenoic acid and docosahexaenoic acid increase systemic arterial compliance in humans. *Am. J. Clin. Nutr.* 2002; 76:326–30.
64. Mozaffarian D, Geelen A, Brouwer IA, et al. Effect of fish oil on heart rate in humans: a meta-analysis of randomized controlled trials. *Circulation.* 2005; 112:1945–52.
65. Hidayat K, Yang J, Zhang Z, et al. Effect of omega-3 long-chain polyunsaturated fatty acid supplementation on heart rate: a meta-analysis of randomized controlled trials. *Eur. J. Clin. Nutr.* 2018; 72:805–17.
66. Avan A, Tavakoly Sany SB, Ghayour-Mobarhan M, et al. Serum C-reactive protein in the prediction of cardiovascular diseases: Overview of the latest clinical studies and public health practice. *J. Cell. Physiol.* 2018; 233:8508–25.
67. Li K, Huang T, Zheng J, et al. Effect of marine-derived n-3 polyunsaturated fatty acids on C-reactive protein, interleukin 6 and tumor necrosis factor alpha: a meta-analysis. *PLoS One.* 2014; 9:e88103.
68. Schwingshackl L, Christoph M, Hoffmann G. Effects of olive oil on markers of inflammation and endothelial function-a systematic review and meta-analysis. *Nutrients.* 2015; 7:7651–75.

69. Lin N, Shi JJ, Li YM, et al. What is the impact of n-3 PUFAs on inflammation markers in Type 2 diabetic mellitus populations?: a systematic review and meta-analysis of randomized controlled trials. *Lipids Health Dis.* 2016; 15:133.

70. Calder PC. Omega-3 fatty acids and inflammatory processes: from molecules to man. *Biochem. Soc. Trans.* 2017; 45:1105–15.

71. Conte MS, Desai TA, Wu B, et al. Pro-resolving lipid mediators in vascular disease. *J. Clin. Invest.* 2018; 128:3727–35.

72. Chiang N, Serhan CN. Specialized pro-resolving mediator network: an update on production and actions. *Essays Biochem.* 2020 Sep 23; 64(3):443–62.

73. Zaloga GP. Narrative review of n-3 polyunsaturated fatty acid supplementation upon immune functions, resolution molecules and lipid peroxidation. *Nutrients.* 2021; 13(2):662.

74. Calder PC. Eicosapentaenoic and docosahexaenoic acid derived specialised pro-resolving mediators: concentrations in humans and the effects of age, sex, disease and increased omega-3 fatty acid intake. *Biochimie.* 2020; 178:105–23.

75. Barden AE, Mas E, Mori TA. n-3 Fatty acid supplementation and proresolving mediators of inflammation. *Curr. Opin. Lipidol.* 2016; 27:26–32.

76. Barden AE, Mas E, Croft KD, et al. Specialized proresolving lipid mediators in humans with the metabolic syndrome after n-3 fatty acids and aspirin. *Am. J. Clin. Nutr.* 2015; 102:1357–64.

77. Mas E, Croft KD, Zahra P, et al. Resolvins D1, D2, and other mediators of self-limited resolution of inflammation in human blood following n-3 fatty acid supplementation. *Clin. Chem.* 2012; 58:1476–84.

78. von Schacky C. Omega-3 fatty acids in cardiovascular disease--an uphill battle. *Prostaglandins Leukot. Essent. Fatty Acids.* 2015; 92:41–7.

79. Schuchardt JP, Hahn A. Bioavailability of long-chain omega-3 fatty acids. *Prostaglandins Leukot. Essent. Fatty Acids.* 2013; 89:1–8.

80. Dyerberg J, Madsen P, Moller JM, et al. Bioavailability of marine n-3 fatty acid formulations. *Prostaglandins Leukot. Essent. Fatty Acids.* 2010; 83:137–41.

81. Krokan HE, Bjerve KS, Mork E. The enteral bioavailability of eicosapentaenoic acid and docosahexaenoic acid is as good from ethyl esters as from glyceryl esters in spite of lower hydrolytic rates by pancreatic lipase in vitro. *Biochim. Biophys. Acta.* 1993; 1168:59–67.

82. Neubronner J, Schuchardt JP, Kressel G, et al. Enhanced increase of omega-3 index in response to long-term n-3 fatty acid supplementation from triacylglycerides versus ethyl esters. *Eur. J. Clin. Nutr.* 2011; 65:247–54

83. Schuchardt JP, Neubronner J, Kressel G, et al. Moderate doses of EPA and DHA from re-esterified triacylglycerols but not from ethyl-esters lower fasting serum triacylglycerols in statin-treated dyslipidemic subjects: results from a six month randomized controlled trial. *Prostaglandins Leukot. Essent. Fatty Acids.* 2011; 85:381–6.

84. Hedengran A, Szecsi PB, Dyerberg J, et al. n-3 PUFA esterified to glycerol or as ethyl esters reduce non-fasting plasma triacylglycerol in subjects with hypertriglyceridemia: a randomized trial. *Lipids.* 2015; 50:165–75.

85. Kwantes JM, Grundmann O. A brief review of krill oil history, research, and the commercial market. *J. Diet. Suppl.* 2015; 12:23–35.

86. Maki KC, Reeves MS, Farmer M, et al. Krill oil supplementation increases plasma concentrations of eicosapentaenoic and docosahexaenoic acids in overweight and obese men and women. *Nutr. Res.* 2009; 29:609–15.

87. Ulven SM, Kirkhus B, Lamglait A, et al. Metabolic effects of krill oil are essentially similar to those of fish oil but at lower dose of EPA and DHA, in healthy volunteers. *Lipids.* 2011; 46:37–46.

88. Schuchardt JP, Schneider I, Meyer H, et al. Incorporation of EPA and DHA into plasma phospholipids in response to different omega-3 fatty acid formulations--a comparative bioavailability study of fish oil vs. krill oil. *Lipids Health Dis.* 2011; 10:145.

89. Salem N, Jr., Kuratko CN. A reexamination of krill oil bioavailability studies. *Lipids Health Dis.* 2014; 13:137.

90. Earnest CP, Lupo M, White KM, et al. Effect of astaxanthin on cycling time trial performance. *Int. J. Sports Med.* 2011; 32:882–8.

91. Choi HD, Kim JH, Chang MJ, et al. Effects of astaxanthin on oxidative stress in overweight and obese adults. *Phytother. Res.* 2011; 25:1813–8.

92. Mark BJ, Beaty AD, Slavin RG. Are fish oil supplements safe in finned fish-allergic patients? *Allergy Asthma Proc.* 2008; 29:528–9.

93. Howard-Thompson A, Dutton A, Hoover R, et al. Flushing and pruritus secondary to prescription fish oil ingestion in a patient with allergy to fish. *Int. J. Clin. Pharm.* 2014; 36:1126–9.
94. Sakaguchi M, Toda M, Ebihara T, et al. IgE antibody to fish gelatin (type I collagen) in patients with fish allergy. *J. Allergy Clin. Immunol.* 2000; 106:579–84.
95. Motoyama K, Suma Y, Ishizaki S, et al. Identification of tropomyosins as major allergens in antarctic krill and mantis shrimp and their amino acid sequence characteristics. *Mar. Biotechnol. (N. Y.).* 2008; 10:709–18.
96. Global Organization for EPA and DHA Omega-3. 2018. GOED Voluntary Monograph. http://goedomega3.com/index.php/goed-monograph.
97. Miller M. N/A. Oxidation of Food Grade Oils. https://www.oilsfats.org.nz/documents/Oxidation%20101.pdf.
98. Jackowski SA, Alvi AZ, Mirajkar A, et al. Oxidation levels of North American over-the-counter n-3 (omega-3) supplements and the influence of supplement formulation and delivery form on evaluating oxidative safety. *J Nutr Sci.* 2015; 4:e30.
99. Rundblad A, Holven KB, Ottestad I, et al. High-quality fish oil has a more favourable effect than oxidised fish oil on intermediate-density lipoprotein and LDL subclasses: a randomised controlled trial. *Br. J. Nutr.* 2017; 117:1291–8.

5 Nutrition and Nutritional Supplements in the Management of Dyslipidemia and Dyslipidemia-Induced Cardiovascular Disease

Mark C. Houston

CONTENTS

Introduction..98
Pathophysiology...98
Treatment 100
    Overview..100
Nutrition..102
    Framingham Heart Study and Seven Countries Study 102
    Pritikin Diet..102
    Ornish Diet..102
    Therapeutic Lifestyle Changes (TLC) Diet 103
    OmniHeart Trial..103
    Portfolio Diet 104
    Mediterranean Diets...104
    Lyon Diet Heart Study 104
    Indian Heart Study...104
    Nutrigenomics..105
The FUNGENUT Study 105
The GEMINAL Study...105
The PREDIMED Study..105
    Nutritional Conclusions and Recommendations 106
Specific Foods, Nutrients, and Dietary Supplements..106
    Omega-3 Fatty Acids 106
    Flax 114
    Monounsaturated Fats (MUFA)...114
    Garlic 114
    Green Tea...114
    Orange Juice 115
    Pomegranate Juice and Seeds 115

DOI: 10.1201/9781003137849-5

Sesame 115
Soy 115
Nutrients and Dietary Supplements 115
Citrus Bergamot 116
Curcumin 116
Guggulipids 116
Lycopene 116
Niacin (Vitamin B3) 116
Pantethine 119
Plant Sterols (Phytosterols) 119
Policosanol 120
Tocotrienols 120
Red Yeast Rice 121
Resveratrol 121
Vitamin C 121
Berberine 122
Combination Therapies 122
Future Perspectives 122
Summary and Conclusions 123
References 124

INTRODUCTION

The combination of a lipid-lowering diet with the judicious use of scientifically proven nutritional supplements and lipid-lowering drugs has the ability to significantly reduce total cholesterol (TC), low-density lipoprotein cholesterol (LDL-C), and LDL particle number (LDL-P); increase LDL particle size (LDL-P); lower triglycerides (TG), remnant particles, very-low-density lipoprotein (VLDL), and lipoprotein (a) levels; and increase high-density lipoprotein cholesterol (HDL-C) and HDL particle number (HDL-P), while providing a beneficial effect on HDL sub-fractions and HDL functionality. In addition, vascular inflammation, oxidative stress, and vascular immune responses are also decreased with aggressive lipid management. In several prospective clinical trials, coronary heart disease (CHD), myocardial infarction (MI), and cardiovascular disease (CVD) events have been reduced using nutraceutical supplements. Other trials show additional improvement in CHD events when lipid-lowering drugs such as statins are supplemented with nutraceuticals such as omega-3 fatty acids or niacin. This chapter will review the role of nutrition, nutritional supplements, and lipid-lowering drugs that favorably improve dyslipidemia and address the myriad steps and mechanisms involved in lipid-mediated atherosclerosis and clinical cardiovascular events such as MI and stroke.

PATHOPHYSIOLOGY

Dyslipidemia is a major risk factor for CHD, along with hypertension, diabetes mellitus (DM), smoking, and obesity [1]. The mechanisms by which certain plasma lipids induce vascular damage are complex, but from a pathophysiologic viewpoint, these include vascular inflammation, oxidative stress with reduced oxidative defense, and vascular immune dysfunction [2–4]. These pathophysiologic mechanisms lead to endothelial dysfunction (ED) and vascular smooth muscle dysfunction (VSMD) with loss of arterial elasticity and compliance. In addition, coronary artery obstruction, coronary artery ED, and coronary artery spasm cause cardiac myocyte dysfunction. The consequences are CHD, MI, and cerebrovascular accidents (CVAs) [4].

The causes of dyslipidemia include genetic inheritance and a number of acquired conditions such as poor nutrition, visceral obesity, numerous co-morbidities, and the use of pharmacological agents such as nonselective and non-vasodilating beta-blockers and diuretics (including hydrochlorothiazide and chlorthalidone), anti-retrovirals, retinoids and rexinoids, steroids, and sex hormones [5]. In addition, tobacco use, DM, hypothyroidism and other metabolic dysfunctions, an abnormal gut microbiome, acute and chronic infections, heavy metals, toxins, and lack of exercise may also induce dyslipidemia [5]. Often there are both genetic and acquired factors at play. For example, several genetic phenotypes, such as the common apolipoprotein E (apoE) polymorphism, regulate intestinal absorption of dietary fat and result in variable serum lipid responses to diet, thus controlling risk for CHD and MI [6,7]. In addition, variations in the HDL proteome, involving players such as paroxonase-1 (PON-1), scavenger receptor B-1 (SR-B1), SCARB-1, and apolipoprotein C 3 (APO C3), influence the risk for CHD and MI [8]. The Sortilin I allele variants on chromosome 1p13 increase LDL-C and CHD risk by 29% [9].

Recent studies suggest that dietary cholesterol intake has a minimal effect on serum cholesterol levels and rates of CHD and MI, and that only saturated fats (SFA) with a carbon length of C12 or greater have adverse effects on serum lipids and CHD risk [5,10–16]. However, consumption of monounsaturated (MUFA) and polyunsaturated fats (PUFA) has a favorable influence on serum lipids and CHD risk. Increased refined carbohydrate intake adversely affects serum lipoproteins and their subfractions more than do short-chain SFA with carbon length of C10 or less. Refined carbohydrates and sugars have significant effects on insulin resistance and adverse effects on LDL-C, LDL-P, LDL-P size, VLDL, TG, total HDL-C, HDL-P, HDL sub-fractions, HDL functionality, vascular inflammation, oxidative stress, and vascular immune function. All of these lipid changes from sugar intake contribute more to CHD risk than do short-chain SFA [5,10–16].

The validity of the long-standing "Diet Heart Hypothesis" which suggests that dietary SFA and dietary cholesterol increase the risk of CHD and MI has been questioned [11–13]. However, dietary trans fatty acids (TFA) do have definite adverse lipid effects, and increase the risk of sudden death due to MI, CVD, and CHD. TFA suppresses TGF-beta responsiveness, and this facilitates the deposition of cholesterol in vascular tissue [11,13–15]. In contrast, PUFA, omega-3 fatty acids (such as docosahexaenoic acid (DHA) and eicosapentaenoic acid (EPA)), and MUFA improve serum lipids and reduce CHD and MI risks [5,10–16].

Expanded lipid profiles (advanced lipid testing) that measure lipids, lipid sub-fractions, particle size, particle number, and apolipoproteins B and A are preferred over the standard lipid panel that measures only the TC, LDL-C, TG, and HDL-C (Figure 5.1).

Expanded lipid profiles are offered by numerous commercial laboratories, including Boston Labs, Berkeley Labs, Lab Corps, and Quest Diagnostics. These expanded lipid profiles have been shown to improve CHD risk profiling, better predict CHD and MI events, and allow a more accurate assessment of the lipid changes that occur with exercise, weight loss or weight gain, lifestyle changes, and use of nutritional supplements or pharmacotherapy [17,18]. Assessment of CHD risk, identification of the mechanisms of dyslipidemia-induced vascular disease, and evaluation of efficacy of natural or drug treatment are vastly improved using the new expanded lipid profiles [17,18]. In addition, new concepts in assessing dysfunctional or inflammatory HDL-C [19] directly or indirectly by measuring reverse cholesterol transport (RCT) [20], lipoprotein-associated phospholipase A2 (Lp-PLA2), platelet-activating factor acetylhydrolase (PAF-AH), high-sensitivity C-reactive protein (hsCRP), and myeloperoxidase (MPO) levels [21] will add to the intervention toolkit and allow improved assessment of CHD and MI risks.

An understanding of the pathophysiological steps and mechanisms in dyslipidemia-induced vascular damage and atheroma plaque formation that goes beyond measurement of lipid levels or even expanded lipid profiles, allows for the treatment of dyslipidemia and prevention of CHD and MI to be conducted in a more logical and efficacious manner (Figure 5.2).

The ability to interfere on most steps and mechanisms in this pathway will allow more specific approaches and treatments to reduce vascular injury, improve vascular repair systems, and maintain and restore vascular health. Native LDL, especially large type A LDL, is not usually atherogenic unless it accumulates in very high concentrations or it is oxidized or otherwise modified. However, effective pinocytosis mechanisms allow macrophage ingestion of native LDL-C in the setting of

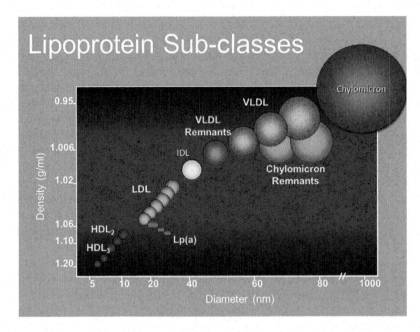

FIGURE 5.1   The various lipoprotein particles are shown below with NMR: HDL, LDL, IDL, VLDL, and chylomicrons.

chronic infection or inflammation, which could account for up to 30% of the foam cell formation in the subendothelium [22,23]. Identifying maneuvers to decrease modified LDL forms such as oxidized (oxLDL) and glycated (glyLDL) or glyco-oxidized LDL (gly-oxLDL) would represent a gigantic next step toward a revolution in management of this common condition. In addition, it would be important to have instruments to decrease the uptake of modified LDL-C into macrophages by the SR-A and CD 36 scavenger receptors (SR), inflammatory and oxidative stress, and abnormal vascular immune responses. All of these approaches would reduce vascular damage beyond just treating LDL-C levels [24–30]. There are at least 45 potential mechanisms that can be treated in the pathways involving dyslipidemia-induced vascular damage. We now know that lowering of serum hsCRP, an inflammatory marker and mediator, leads to fewer cardiovascular events independent of reductions in LDL-C cholesterol [29].

TREATMENT

OVERVIEW

Many patients cannot tolerate or will not in principle use pharmacologic treatments such as statins, fibrates, bile acid binders, ezetimibe, or PCSK9 inhibitors to treat dyslipidemia [5]. Other patients with definitive indications for use of statins and other anti-lipid therapies and prefer their use for many reasons such as cost, convenience, and proven efficacy. The most informed patients prefer to use an integrative approach to lipid management as clinical trials indicate an improved risk reduction in CHD and MI with combinations of nutraceuticals and drugs.

Drug-induced side effects (myopathy, myositis, rhabdomyolysis, abnormal liver function tests, neuropathy, memory loss, mental status changes, decreased focus and concentration, gastrointestinal disturbances, glucose intolerance or type 2 DM) are the largest reason why patients find lipid management notoriously disagreeable [31–34]. With prolonged or high-dose usage of statin medications, patients may experience other clinical symptoms such as chronic fatigue, exercise-induced fatigue with myalgias and muscle weakness, reduced exercise tolerance, and loss of lean muscle

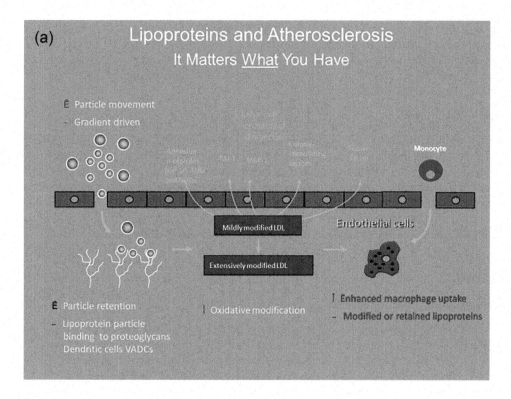

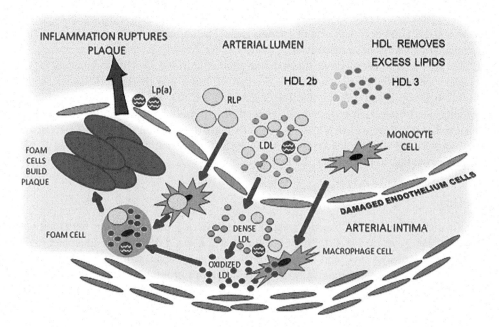

FIGURE 5.2 A and B lipoproteins and atherosclerosis and atherosclerotic plaque formation. Proposed mechanisms of actions of nutraceuticals and statins in the dyslipidemia-induced atherosclerotic vascular disease pathway to the development of an atherosclerotic plaque. Diagrammed here are the various steps in the uptake of LDL cholesterol, modification, macrophage ingestion with scavenger receptors, foam cell formation, oxidative stress, inflammation, autoimmune cytokines, and chemokine production.

mass. In addition, there may be reductions in both serum and tissue levels of coenzyme Q10, carnitine, copper, zinc, creatine, vitamin E (tocopherols and tocotrienols), vitamin D, vitamin A, vitamin K2, selenium, selenoproteins, heme A, steroid, and sex hormones. Statins also may reduce the level of conversion of thyroxine (T4) to free tri-iodothyronine (T3) by inhibiting the deiodinase enzyme resulting in hypothyroidism [5,31,35–42]

New treatment approaches that combine weight loss, reductions in visceral and total body fat with increases in lean muscle mass, optimal aerobic and resistance exercises, scientifically proven nutrition, and use of nutritional supplements and lipid-lowering drugs will improve serum lipids and reduce vascular inflammation, oxidative stress, abnormal vascular immune dysfunction, ED, and VSMD. In addition, both surrogate markers for vascular disease and rates of clinical endpoints such as CHD and MI are reduced in clinical trials [5]. This chapter will review nutrition, nutritional supplements, and lipid-lowering drugs in the treatment of dyslipidemia and dyslipidemia-induced vascular disease. The reader is referred to an extensive body of literature on the role of exercise, weight loss, and other lifestyle changes in the treatment of dyslipidemia.

NUTRITION

FRAMINGHAM HEART STUDY AND SEVEN COUNTRIES STUDY

Nutrition has long been recognized as an important modality for managing and preventing dyslipidemia and other risk factors for CVD, MI, and CHD [43]. The Framingham Heart Study (FHS) and Seven Countries Study (SCS) found associations between increased LDL-C and TC levels with increased risk of CVD, and between elevated levels of HDL-C and decreased risk of CVD. An association between CVD and dietary fat consumption was also identified at that time, and a general link was established between Western diet, lipid levels, CHD, and CVD [44–46]. The FHS initially included a cohort of 5,209 healthy, mostly Caucasian residents of Framingham, MA, aged 30–60 years and then added a second cohort of 5,124 offspring in 1971. The last FHS cohort included 500 minorities [47]. It should be noted that this is an epidemiologic, hypothesis-generating study with a small number of subjects of a single race. The ability to apply these conclusions to a broader population was to be verified later.

The SCS was a large prospective study that evaluated nutrition and lifestyle habits in 12,000 middle-aged men in Asia, Northern Europe, Southern Europe, and the United States. This study found a link between a high-fat diet and increased risk of CVD. The SCS has been criticized as to its validity due to selection bias and forced premises. It should also be noted that the high-fat diet consumed at that time was rich in TFA and long-chain SFA. Intake of omega-3 fatty acids and MUFA was associated with reduced risk of CHD. The SCS thus should not have bundled all dietary fats together in the link to increased risk of CVD.

PRITIKIN DIET

The Pritikin diet is a low-fat diet based primarily on vegetables, grains, and fruits with total fat supplying 10% of energy needs [48,49]. Studies of this diet suggested that dietary fat content reduced CVD, LDL-C, and triglycerides and increased HDL-C when coupled with a regular exercise program [50]. It cannot be concluded that any one modality in this program was the primary reason for the CVD and lipid outcomes. A plant-based diet with exercise could have been the primary reason for the positive outcomes, more than the dietary fat reduction per se.

ORNISH DIET

The Ornish diet [51] started from a randomized controlled trial that had as its 1- and 5-year endpoints LDL-C level, number of anginal episodes, and angiography-based regression of coronary stenosis [52–54]. It was based on a combined intensive therapeutic approach of diet, exercise, and other lifestyle changes, The diet consisted of a low-fat, whole foods vegetarian diet with 10% of total energy as fat, drastic reduction (10 mg/day) in dietary cholesterol, increased intake of complex carbohydrates (fiber- and plant-based nutrition), and minimal intake of simple sugars. Lifestyle modifications included moderate aerobic exercise, stress reduction, smoking cessation, and group psychosocial support. Compared with the control group, the experimental group had statistically significant reduction in LDL-C, a lower frequency of angina episodes, and regression of coronary artery stenosis at years 1 and 5. In contrast, the control group had minimal reduction in LDL-C, significant increase in frequency of angina episodes, and increase in coronary artery stenosis. The dietary fat reduction here was primarily in long-chain SFA and TFA, which are now known to increase CHD risk. There was a concomitant increase in intake of omega-3 fatty acids and MUFA. The effects due to reduced consumption of these types of fats in combination with a plant-based diet, more fiber, and lower simple sugars are consistent with those of other studies using the same nutritional components, also showing a reduction in CHD rates. The comprehensive approach of nutrition, exercise, stress reduction, and smoking cessation, while certainly efficacious, does not allow one to pinpoint any single treatment as the primary reason for the clinical findings.

THERAPEUTIC LIFESTYLE CHANGES (TLC) DIET

The National Heart, Lung, and Blood Institute (NHLBI) and the Adult Treatment Panel III of the National Cholesterol Education Program (ATP III) recommend Therapeutic Lifestyle Changes (TLC) nutritional program with dietary saturated fat (SFA) of <7% of total energy, dietary cholesterol of <200 mg/day, 10–25 g/day of viscous fiber, and 2 g/day of plant sterols/stanols [55,56]. A randomized crossover study of 36 moderately hypercholesterolemic subjects treated over a period of 1 month compared the TLC diet (28% total fat, <7% SFA, 66 mg cholesterol/1000 kcal) with a Western diet (38% total fat, 15% SFA, 164 mg cholesterol/1,000 kcal). Compared to the Western diet, the TLC diet significantly reduced plasma levels of both LDL-C (by 11%) and HDL-C (by 7%), with no significant effect on TG or TC/HDL-C ratio [57]. These net lipid changes are not impressive as the decrease in LDL was negated by the decrease in HDL. The lack of change in the TC/HDL ratio would predict no change in CHD risk over time. Moreover, in the 15-year Women's Health Initiative (WHI), a multi-center randomized clinical trial of 48,835 postmenopausal women with a diet low in fat (20% of total calories), high in fruits and vegetables (five or more servings/day), and high in grains (six or more servings/day) did not show an effect on CVD rates or improvement in lipid profile. The type of fat reduction and the relatively low intake of fruits and vegetables could account for the negative CV outcomes [58]. The addition of plant sterols in the TLC could also have biased the results in that study.

OMNIHEART TRIAL

The Optimal Macronutrient Intake for Heart Health Trial (OmniHeart Trial) investigated the effect of a Mediterranean-style diet on plasma lipids and blood pressure [47]. In this randomized controlled intervention crossover study of generally healthy adults, three diets (a carbohydrate-rich diet, a protein-rich diet, and a diet rich in MUFA) were compared for 6 weeks in each of the three groups (total 18 weeks). The MUFA diet did not change LDL-C levels but increased HDL-C levels, the protein-rich diet decreased LDL-C and HDL-C levels, and all three diets reduced serum TG. After adjustment for potential confounders, an OmniHeart score higher by 1 point was associated with systolic/diastolic BP differences of −1.0/−0.5 mmHg (both $P < 0.001$). Findings were comparable for men and women, for non-hypertensive participants, and with adjustment for antihypertensive treatment. The trial could not assess the effects on CHD as it was too short and underpowered with only 164 subjects.

PORTFOLIO DIET

The Portfolio diet [59–64] is a vegetarian version of the low-fat TLC diet, with the addition of soluble fiber, nuts, soy protein, and plant sterols. In a 1-month randomized control feeding trial, the Portfolio diet was compared to the TLC control diet [59]. The LDL-C fell an average of 35.0% compared with 12.1% on the control diet. A follow-up study found that the Portfolio diet reduced LDL-C equal to a statin medication [62]. In a subsequent study of hyperlipidemic adults who were followed for 1 year on the Portfolio diet, about 50% had reductions in LDL-C of >20% [60]. Increasing the MUFA content increased the HDL-C levels without changing LDL-C [63]. In the largest randomized controlled trial of the Portfolio diet to date, LDL-C levels in those following this diet were significantly lower than in those following a low-saturated fat diet [64]. Once again, the addition of plant sterols with fiber and more plant-based nutrition likely resulted in improved lipid profiles over the basic nutritional suggestions of just low-fat dieting in the TLC diet.

MEDITERRANEAN DIETS

The Mediterranean-style diet is characterized by a high intake of vegetables, fruits, bread and other cereal grains, potatoes, legumes, nuts, and seeds. MUFA with extra virgin olive oil (EVOO) and nuts are the primary fats consumed which is typically 15%–20% of total calories. Animal product intake such as meat, poultry, fish, dairy, and eggs are low to moderate, and wine consumption is regular but in moderation [65]. Several clinical trials on the Mediterranean-style diet and CVD are discussed below.

LYON DIET HEART STUDY

The Lyon Diet Heart Study (LDHS) was the first intervention trial to investigate the effect of a Mediterranean-style diet on cardiovascular disease (CVD) risk. This randomized single-blind secondary prevention trial was conducted in a single center in the Lyon region of France and included over 600 participants with prior MI [66–68]. The primary outcome measurement (fatal or nonfatal MI) was significantly reduced by the intervention over the four-year study period. CV outcomes including recurrent stable angina and restenosis of grafts were decreased by 47%, while the composite of MI, cardiovascular death, and major secondary events was decreased by 67%. These changes were independent of serum lipid changes, which were not significantly different between the groups. The design introduced changes to the usual Mediterranean diet consumed in southern Europe that the study is not generally considered an appropriate test of the efficacy of that diet on CVD risk. For example, the diet was 30.5% fat, with 12.5% as MUFA, which is much lower rather than the 15%–20% MUFA content in the diet of southern Europe. Further, the diet was enriched in alpha-linolenic acid (ALA), which is an omega-3 polyunsaturated fat, rather than the usual MUFA oleic acid.

INDIAN HEART STUDY

The Indian Heart Study was a case-control study of 350 Indian subjects with ischemic heart disease on the effect of a Mediterranean-style diet enriched in ALA [69]. The control group was advised on smoking cessation, stress management, regular exercise, and reduction of dietary fat and alcohol. Compared to the control group at the 1-year follow-up, the treatment group had a 38% reduction in nonfatal MI and a 32% reduction in fatal MI. There was a significant and dose-dependent inverse association between vegetable intake and CHD risk. The inverse association was stronger for green leafy vegetables; in a multivariate analysis, persons consuming a median of 3.5 servings/week had a 67% lower relative risk (risk ratio (RR): 0.33; 95% CI: 0.17, 0.64; P for trend=0.0001) than did those consuming 0.5 servings/week. Controlling for other dietary covariates did not alter the association.

Cereal intake was also associated with a lower risk. Use of mustard oil, which is rich in ALA, was associated with a lower risk than was use of sunflower oil (for use in cooking: RR: 0.49 (95% CI: 0.24, 0.99); for use in frying, RR: 0.29 (95% CI: 0.13, 0.64)). Diets that are rich in vegetables and using mustard oil could contribute to the lower risk of CHD among Indians. There are numerous other diets that have been recommended for weight management and blood sugar or lipid control. These include the Atkins diet, South Beach diet, ketogenic diet, Paleo diet, vegetarian, vegan, or plant-based diet, Esselstyn diet, and fasting mimicking diet. All of these will be discussed in other chapters. Of all these diets, the fasting mimicking diet (FMD) shows the best results for control of weight, glucose, lipids, and stem cell production and possibly slowing the aging process.

NUTRIGENOMICS

The importance of nutrigenomic effects on serum lipids, DM, CHD, MI, CVD, ASCVD, hypertension, inflammation, oxidative stress, immune function, and cancer has been demonstrated in numerous clinical trials such as the FUNGENUT Study, the Gene Expression Modulation by Intervention with Nutrition and Lifestyle (GEMINAL) Study, and the PREDIMED Study [73–80]. These are discussed in the section below.

THE FUNGENUT STUDY

Diet changes can influence both phenotypic outcomes and gene expression [73]. The Functional Genomics and Nutrition (FUNGENUT) Study of Finnish subjects with metabolic syndrome was conducted over 3 months, and the participants were randomly assigned to either a low-glycemic-load rye-pasta diet to curtail postprandial insulin response or a high-glycemic-load oat-wheat-potato diet promoting a high postprandial insulin response. Gene expression was determined on samples of subcutaneous adipose tissue [73].

In the low-glycemic-load rye-pasta group, the insulinogenic index improved and 71 genes were down-regulated, including genes involved in insulin signaling and apoptosis. In the high-glycemic-load oat-wheat-potato diet group, 62 genes were up-regulated such as those promoting oxidative stress and inflammation [73].

THE GEMINAL STUDY

The GEMINAL Study [74] reported changes in gene expression in 30 men with low-risk prostate cancer after a 3-month intensive diet-and-lifestyle intervention. The intervention consisted of a low-fat, plant-based diet, moderate exercise, stress management, and psychosocial group support. Microarray analysis of gene expression in prostate biopsies taken before and after the intervention detected 453 down-regulated genes, many of which associated with tumorigenesis, as a result of the intensive diet-lifestyle intervention.

THE PREDIMED STUDY

In the PREDIMED Study [75], three diets were evaluated for their effects on gene expression. The control diet was a low-fat TLC diet; the experimental diets were a Mediterranean-style diet enhanced with either EVOO or mixed nuts. The Mediterranean-style diets, particularly the EVOO, decreased expression of genes related to inflammation, foam cell formation, and thrombosis.

Another cohort of the PREDIMED Study [76] investigated the same three diets over a 3-year period to determine the effects on body weight parameters of a variant of the IL6 gene (IL6–174G>C, rs1800795) that overproduces this proinflammatory cytokine and is associated with increased body weight, waist circumference, and serum lipid levels. The change in weight was numerically greatest in the EVOO group, but was not statistically significant between groups. When the population was stratified by genotype (GG+GC vs. CC), the CC group experienced greater weight loss irrespective of diet type. Interestingly, these individuals had greater adiposity at baseline but lost significantly more weight than those with one or two copies of the G allele ($p=0.002$). Interestingly, in the CC group, the nut diet actually led to weight gain.

Analyses of intermediate markers of cardiovascular risk demonstrated beneficial effects of the Mediterranean diet on blood pressure, lipid profiles, lipoprotein particles, DM, inflammation, oxidative stress, and carotid atherosclerosis, as well as on the expression of proatherogenic genes [77–80]. Nutrigenomics studies also demonstrated favorable interactions of a Mediterranean diet with cyclooxygenase-2 (COX-2), interleukin-6 (IL-6), apolipoprotein A2 (APOA2), cholesteryl ester transfer protein plasma (CETP), transcription factor 7-like 2 (TCF7L2), beta adrenergic receptor gene (ADR B2), interleukin (IL7R), interferon (IFN gamma), monocyte chemotactic protein (MCP), and tumor necrosis factor alpha (TNF-α) gene polymorphisms [77–80].

NUTRITIONAL CONCLUSIONS AND RECOMMENDATIONS

Despite some apparent conflicts in these studies, due to variations in amount and types of fats, simple sugars, complex carbohydrates, fiber, and the use of plant sterols, one can draw fairly solid conclusions from these nutritional interventions:

1. TFA increases LDL-C, TG, reduces HDL-C, and increases CHD risk.
2. Fatty acids that are C12 and longer increase LDL-C and TG, and may increase or not change HDL-C. They are associated with increased risk of CHD. Shorter chain fatty acids of C10 and below instead lower LDL-C and TG increase HDL-C and are not associated with increased risk for CHD.
3. Increased dietary intake of simple sugars increase LDL-C and TG, lower HDL-C, and are associated with an increased risk of CHD.
4. Omega-3 fatty acids and MUFA lower LDL-C and TG, increase HDL-C, and reduce CHD risk. They also have effects that are independent of serum lipids that decrease CHD risk (Table 5.1).

SPECIFIC FOODS, NUTRIENTS, AND DIETARY SUPPLEMENTS

OMEGA-3 FATTY ACIDS

Observational, epidemiologic, and controlled clinical trials of dietary omega-3 fatty acids have shown significant reductions in serum TG, VLDL, and LDL-P and variable changes in LDL-C, along with an increase in HDL-C, HDL particle size, and HDL-P, all of which are associated with major reductions in all CVD events [5,81–88]. The Diet and Reinfarction Trial (DART) demonstrated a decrease in mortality of 29% in men post MI. In DART, 2033 men who had recovered from MI were allocated to receive advice on each of three dietary factors: a reduction in fat intake with increased ratio of polyunsaturated to saturated fat, an increase in fatty fish intake, and an increase in cereal fiber intake. The advice on fat was not associated with any difference in mortality. The subjects advised to eat fatty fish had a 29% reduction in 2-year all-cause mortality. This effect, which was significant, was not altered by adjusting for potential confounding factors. Subjects given fiber advice had slightly higher mortality (not significant). The 2-year incidence of reinfarction plus death from ischemic heart disease was not significantly affected by any of the dietary regimens. A modest intake of fatty fish (two or three portions per week) may reduce mortality in men who have recovered from MI.

The Gruppo Italiano per lo Studio della Sopravvivenza nell'Infarto Miocardico (GISSI) enrolled 11,324 patients surviving an MI (less than 3 months). The patients were randomly assigned supplements of n-3 PUFA (1 g daily, $n=2,836$), vitamin E (300 mg daily, $n=2,830$), both ($n=2,830$), or

TABLE 5.1

Nutrients for the Treatment of Dyslipidemia-Induced Vascular Disease [5]

Mechanism	Food or Nutrient Therapy (Alphabetically by Mechanism)
Inhibit LDL oxidation	Citrus bergamot
	Coenzyme Q10
	Curcumin
	Epigallocatechin gallate
	Flavonoids
	Garlic
	Glutathione
	Grape seed extract
	Lycopene
	Monounsaturated fatty acids
	Niacin
	Oleic acid
	Pantethine
	Polyphenols
	Pomegranate
	Pycnogenol
	Quercetin
	Red wine
	Resveratrol
	Sesame
	Tangerine extract
	Tocotrienols and tocopherols (gamma/delta)
Inhibit LDL glycation	Carnosine
	Histidine
	Kaempferol
	Morin
	Myricetin
	Organosulfur compounds Pomegranate
	Rutin
Reduce LDL	Astaxanthin
	Berberine
	Citrus bergamot
	Curcumin
	Epigallocatechin gallate
	Flax seed
	Garlic
	Gamma-linolenic acid
	Lycopene
	Monounsaturated fatty acids
	Niacin
	Omega-3 fatty acids
	Orange juice
	Pantethine
	Plant sterols
	Quercetin
	Red yeast rice
	Resveratrol
	Sesame
	Soluble fiber
	Tocotrienols (gamma/delta)

(Continued)

TABLE 5.1 (*Continued*)

Nutrients for the Treatment of Dyslipidemia-Induced Vascular Disease [5]

Mechanism	Food or Nutrient Therapy (Alphabetically by Mechanism)
Convert dense LDL B to large LDL A	Niacin
	Omega-3 fatty acids
	Plant sterols
Reduce intestinal cholesterol absorption	Berberine
	Epigallocatechin gallate
	Fiber
	Flax seeds
	Garlic
	Plant sterols
	Sesame
	Soy
Inhibit HMG-CoA reductase	Berberine
	Citrus bergamot
	Curcumin
	Epigallocatechin gallate
	Gamma-linolenic acid
	Garlic
	Lycopene
	Omega-3 fatty acids
	Pantethine
	Plant sterols
	Red yeast rice
	Sesame
	Tocotrienols (gamma/delta)
Reduce lipoprotein (a)	Berberine
	Coenzyme Q10
	Curcumin
	Flax seed
	L-Arginine
	L-Carnitine
	L-Lysine
	N-Acetylcysteine
	Niacin
	Omega-3 fatty acids
	Proline
	Quercetin
	Tocotrienols (gamma/delta)
	Vitamin C
Reduce triglycerides	Astaxanthin
	Berberine
	Citrus bergamot
	Coenzyme Q10
	Fiber
	Flax seed
	Krill oil
	Monounsaturated fatty acids
	Niacin
	Omega-3 fatty acids
	Orange juice
	Pantethine
	Red yeast rice
	Resveratrol

(Continued)

TABLE 5.1 (*Continued*)

Nutrients for the Treatment of Dyslipidemia-Induced Vascular Disease [5]

Mechanism	Food or Nutrient Therapy (Alphabetically by Mechanism)
Increase total HDL and HDL 2b levels and convert HDL 3 to HDL 2 and 2b	Astaxanthin
	Citrus bergamot
	Coenzyme Q10
	Curcumin
	Krill oil
	Lycopene
	Monounsaturated fatty acids
	Niacin
	Omega-3 fatty acids
	Orange juice
	Pantethine
	Pomegranate
	Red yeast rice
	Resveratrol
Alter scavenger receptor NADPH oxidase and oxLDL uptake into macrophages	N-Acetylcysteine
	Resveratrol
Increase reverse cholesterol transport	Anthocyanidins
	Coenzyme Q10
	Curcumin
	Flavonoids
	Glutathione
	Lycopene
	MUFA
	Niacin
	Plant sterols
	Phosphatidyl serine
	Quercetin
	Resveratrol
Decrease LDL particle number	Berberine
	Niacin
	Omega-3 fatty acids
	Red yeast rice
Reduce inflammation	Curcumin
	Flax seed
	Glutathione
	Monounsaturated fatty acids
	Niacin
	Omega-3 fatty acids
	Plant sterols
	Quercetin
	Resveratrol
Lower apolipoprotein B	Astaxanthin
	Berberine
	Epigallocatechin gallate
	Niacin
	Omega-3 fatty acids
	Plant sterols
	Red yeast rice
Increase apolipoprotein A-1	Niacin
	Coenzyme Q10

(*Continued*)

TABLE 5.1 (*Continued*)

Nutrients for the Treatment of Dyslipidemia-Induced Vascular Disease [5]

Mechanism	Food or Nutrient Therapy (Alphabetically by Mechanism)
Upregulate the LDL receptor	Berberine (PCSK9 inhibition)
	Curcumin (PCSK9 inhibition)
	Epigallocatechin gallate
	Fiber
	Niacin (PCSK9 inhibition)
	Plant sterols
	Quercetin (PCSK9 inhibition)
	Sesame
	Soy
	Tocotrienols (gamma/delta)
Increase PON 1 and PON 2	Epigallocatechin gallate
	Lycopene
	Quercetin
	Pomegranate
	Resveratrol
	Glutathione
Increase bile acid excretion	Berberine
	Citrus bergamot
	Fiber
	Resveratrol
	Probiotics
	Plant sterols
	Sesame
	RYR
	Plant sterols
Reduce fibrinogen	L Reuteri
	MUFA
	Omega-3 fatty acids
Reduce TNF-α	Plant sterols
	RYR
	Curcumin
	Luteolin
	Lycopene
Reduce CAMs	MUFA
	Niacin
	Resveratrol
	Berberine
	NAC
Reduce NADPH oxidase	Niacin
	Resveratrol
	RYR
Reduce Myeloperoxidase (MPO)	Curcumin
	Niacin
	Pomegranate
	Curcumin

(Continued)

TABLE 5.1 (*Continued*)
Nutrients for the Treatment of Dyslipidemia-Induced Vascular Disease [5]

Mechanism	Food or Nutrient Therapy (Alphabetically by Mechanism)
	Niacin
	Omega-3 fatty acids (PPAR)
	RYR
Increase adiponectin and lower leptin	
	Berberine
	Curcumin
	EGCG
	Lycopene (PPAR)
	Omega-3 fatty acids (PPAR)
	Quercetin (PPAR)
	RYR
Improve insulin sensitivity	
	RYR
Reduce MMP	Luteolin

HDL, high-density lipoprotein; LDL, low-density lipoprotein; NADPH, nicotinamide adenine dinucleotide phosphate, PON, ParaxONase.

none (control, $n=2,828$) for 3.5 years. The primary combined efficacy endpoint was death, nonfatal MI, and stroke. Treatment with n-3 PUFA, but not vitamin E, significantly lowered the risk of the primary endpoint (relative-risk decrease 10%). There was a decrease in total mortality of 20%. CV deaths decreased by 30%, and sudden death was reduced by 45%. The Kuopio Ischemic Heart Disease Risk Factor Study [5,81,82] was a prospective population study of 871 men aged 42–60 years who had no clinical CHD at baseline examination. A total of 194 men had a fatal or nonfatal acute coronary event during follow-up. In a Cox proportional hazards' model adjusting for other risk factors, men in the highest quintile of serum DHA in all fatty acids had a 44% reduced risk ($P=0.014$) of acute coronary events compared with men in the lowest quintile. Men in the highest quintile who had a low hair content of mercury had a 67% reduced risk ($P = 0.016$) of acute coronary events compared with men in the lowest quintile and with a high hair content of mercury. There was no association between eicosapentaenoic acid (EPA) levels and the risk of acute coronary events. Fish oil-derived fatty acids reduce the risk of acute coronary events. However, a high mercury content in fish could attenuate this protective effect [5,81,82].

The range of omega-3 fatty acids was from 500 to 1,000 mg/day in these studies and included both food and supplemental sources. Omega-3 fatty acids reduce CHD progression, stabilize plaque, reduce coronary artery stent restenosis, and reduce graft restenosis [5,83]. In the Japan EPA Lipid Intervention Study (JELIS), the addition of 1.8 g of EPA to a statin resulted in an additional 19% relative-risk reduction (RRR) in major coronary events and nonfatal MI, and a 20% decrease in CVA [5,84]. A recent very large meta-analysis of 825,000 subjects [81] included 18 randomized controlled trials and 16 prospective cohort studies examining the combination of EPA+DHA from foods or supplements and CHD, including MI, sudden cardiac death, coronary death, and angina. In the randomized controlled trials, there was a non-statistically significant reduction in CHD risk of 6% with EPA+DHA (summary relative-risk elements (SRRE)=0.94; 95% CI: 0.85–1.05).

However, subgroup analyses of data from these randomized controlled trials indicate a statistically significant CHD risk reduction with the combination of EPA+DHA (dose range of 340–5,000 mg/day) among higher-risk populations with TG levels over 150 mg/dL (16% reduction in CHD) and/or LDL-C over 130 mg/dL (14% reduction in CHD). A meta-analysis of data from these 16 prospective cohort studies resulted in an 18% statistically significant reduction in risk of any CHD event for higher intakes of EPA+DHA from diet and supplement. Although not statistically significant, a 6% reduced risk of any CHD event was observed among randomized controlled trials, a finding supported by a statistically significant 18% reduced risk of CHD among the prospective cohort studies. From a clinical perspective, these results indicate that EPA+DHA are associated with reducing CHD risk to a greater extent in populations with elevated triglyceride levels or LDL cholesterol, which affect a significant portion of the general adult population in the United States [81]. In addition, a significant reduction in CHD rates in patients with known CHD was reported for a dietary intake over 1,000 mg daily of combined DHA and EPA with longer duration of treatment.

EPA and DHA in combination demonstrate a dose-related reduction in VLDL and TG of up to 50%, with a decrease in total TC and ApoB, slight increase in LDL size, and increase in HDL-C, HDL-P, and HDL size at the very high dose of 5 g/day. Lower doses, used by most, have less favorable effects on lipids [5,85–88]. Despite a small increase in LDL-C in some subjects, the other lipid changes were beneficial and reduced the risk of CHD and MI. Patients with LDL-C over 100 mg/dL usually have reductions in total LDL-C, and those that are below 80 mg/dL have mild increases [87]. The rate of entry of VLDL particles into the circulation is decreased by omega-3 fatty acids, and the lowering of APOCIII allows lipoprotein lipase to be more active. There was also a decrease in remnant chylomicrons and remnant lipoproteins [5,86]. Omega-3 fats are also anti-inflammatory and antithrombotic, lower blood pressure and heart rate, and improve heart rate variability (HRV) [5,81].

Long-term supplementation with omega-3 fatty acids at doses up to 5,000 mg/day improves insulin resistance and slightly decreases or makes no significant changes in fasting glucose or hemoglobin A1c [5,89]. Interestingly, the combination of plant sterols and omega-3 fatty acids appears to be synergistic in improving lipids and inflammation [88].

A recent meta-analysis of omega-3 fatty acids and CVD has suggested no beneficial effect on CHD (*JAMA Cardiol.* doi:10.1001/jamacardio.2017.5205, Published online January 31, 2018). This is at variance with the Mayo Clinic meta-analysis as well as large body of published literature showing improved CHD risk with omega-3 fatty acids. The more recent meta-analysis in included only ten trials involving 77,917 individuals compared with 34 trials and 825,000 subjects in the Mayo Clinic meta-analysis. Its limitations include:

- **Exclusion of Data with Arbitrary Selection of Studies**: 500 individuals for at least 1 year (1–6.2 years) and no minimum dose of omega-3 fatty acids are required. It included both randomized controlled trials [8] and open-label studies [2]. Only ten studies included with a total of 77,917 individuals.
- Many studies used nontherapeutic, low doses of DHA and EPA. The EPA dose ranged from 226 to 800 mg/day and the DHA dose from 0 to 1,700 mg/day. Most studies used <1,800 mg EPA/DHA in high-risk CV population. Only three studies used >1,800 mg EPA/DHA per day.
- There was no monitoring of blood or tissue levels of omega-3 fatty acids, no compliance evaluations, and no omega-3 index data showing achievement of the minimal therapeutic level of 8%.
- The studies with the best results used higher doses of DHA and EPA.
- The larger studies with over 10,000 subjects and those consuming 1,000 mg or more of omega-3 fatty acids all had reductions in CV events (JELIS R and P, GISSI–P).
- There were insufficient numbers of subjects in many studies to show any CV effect.
- The quality of DHA/EPA may not have been good, or it was not mentioned. Omega-3 fatty acids were from the ester form in 9/10 trials.
- CV morbidity and mortality were nominally lower in most of the studies, which suggest that benefits favor treatment.

In another recent Cochrane analysis of 79 randomized controlled trials with 112,059 subjects, the authors concluded that increasing consumption of EPA and DHA has little to no effect on mortality or CV health (http://cochranelibrary-wiley.com/wol1/doi/10.1002/14651858.CD012345.pub2/full). Randomized controlled trials that lasted at least 12 months were evaluated and compared supplementation and/or advice to increase LCn3 or ALA intake versus usual or lower intake. It included 79 randomized controlled trials with 12–72 months' duration and included adults at varying cardiovascular risks, mainly in high-income countries. Most studies assessed LCn3 supplementation with capsules, but some used LCn3- or ALA-rich or enriched foods or dietary advice compared to placebo or usual diet. Meta-analysis and sensitivity analyses suggested little or no effect of increasing LCn3 on all-cause mortality (RR: 0.98; 95% CI: 0.90–1.03; 92,653 participants; 8,189 deaths in 39 trials), cardiovascular mortality (RR: 0.95; 95% CI: 0.87–1.03, 67,772 participants; 4,544 CVD deaths in 25 randomized controlled trials), cardiovascular events (RR: 0.99; 95% CI: 0.94–1.04; 90,378 participants; 14,737 events in 38 trials), CHD mortality (RR: 0.93; 95% CI: 0.79–1.09; 73,491 participants; 1,596 CHD deaths in 21 randomized controlled trials), stroke (RR: 1.06; 95% CI: 0.96–1.16; 89,358 participants; 1,822 strokes in 28 trials), or arrhythmia (RR: 0.97; 95% CI: 0.90–1.05; 53,796 participants; 3,788 events in 28 randomized controlled trials). There was a suggestion that LCn3 reduced CHD events (RR: 0.93; 95% CI: 0.88–0.97; 84,301 participants; 5,469 events in 28 randomized controlled trials); however, this was not maintained in sensitivity analyses.

Increasing ALA intake does not impact all-cause mortality (RR: 1.01; 95% CI: 0.84–1.20; 19,327 participants; 459 deaths; 5 randomized controlled trials) and cardiovascular mortality (RR: 0.96; 95% CI: 0.74–1.25; 18,619 participants; 219 cardiovascular deaths; 4 randomized controlled trials), though it may slightly benefit CHD events (RR: 1.00; 95% CI: 0.80–1.22; 19,061 participants; 397 CHD events; 4 randomized controlled trials).

There was no evidence that increasing LCn3 or ALA produced serious adverse events, adiposity or lipids, although LCn3 slightly reduced triglycerides and increased HDL. Interestingly, the authors actually show a 5%–7% reduction in CHD mortality with omega-3 fatty acids despite their negative conclusion. There are potential limitations, and sources of variability should be noted in all meta-analyses. The individual randomized controlled trials differed in terms of CHD prevalence at baseline, the EPA+DHA dosage provided, follow-up duration, and the methods of patient selection and randomization. The benefit of $n-3$ LCPUFA (you should standardize the name and not mix omega-3, LC3, and $n-3$ LCPUFA) intake is likely to accrue over time, but randomized controlled trials of longer duration may suffer from poorer compliance with dietary supplementation. The variable use of terminology specific to CHD outcomes, or a lack of specificity required to discern CHD from broader cardiovascular disease outcomes is problematic. Many randomized controlled trials lacked statistical power to detect an effect because of relatively small sample sizes and/or few observed events due to the increased survival rate associated with current standards of care. Finally, most randomized controlled trials did not measure baseline intake of EPA+DHA from the diet nor did they track EPA+DHA intake from sources other than that supplemented during the course of study, thus making it impossible to determine whether background dietary EPA+DHA intake affected the relationship between supplemental EPA+DHA and CHD.

Neither the JAMA nor the Cochrane analysis has the validity of the Mayo Clinic meta-analysis which included more appropriate types of studies, more than 825,000 subjects, better analysis, and less bias. Based on all published clinical trials, randomized controlled trials, cohort studies, and meta-analysis, these are the most valid conclusions regarding omega-3 fatty acid dietary intake and CHD:

1. CHD is reduced by 16% in patients with TG over 150 mg/dL.
2. CHD is reduced by 14% in patients with LDL-C over 130 mg/dL.
3. DHA and EPA over 1,000 mg/day significantly reduce CHD in both primary and secondary prevention settings.
4. A longer duration of treatment results in a greater reduction in CHD.
5. Secondary prevention trials with known CHD have shown more robust reductions of CHD event rates.

FLAX

Flax seeds and flax lignan complexed with SDG (secoisolariciresinol diglucoside) have been shown in several meta-analyses to reduce TC and LDL-C by 5%–15%, Lp(a) by 14%, and TG by up to 36%, with either no change or a slight reduction in HDL [5,90–92]. These properties do not apply to flax seed oil. Flax seeds contain fiber and lignans that reduce the levels of 7 alpha hydrolase and acyl CoA cholesterol transferase to decrease LDL-C, TG, and Lp(a) [5,90–92]. Flax seeds and ALA are anti-inflammatory, increase endothelial nitric oxide synthase (eNOS), improve ED, decrease vascular smooth muscle hypertrophy, reduce oxidative stress, and reduce the risk of CHD [5,90–92]. The dose required for these effects is from 14 to 40 g of flax seed per day [5,90–92].

MONOUNSATURATED FATS (MUFA)

Monounsaturated fats such as those in olive oil, especially in EVOO, and nuts reduce LDL-C by 5%–10%, lower TG by 10%–15%, increase HDL by 5%, improve HDL function, increase cholesterol efflux capacity (CEC), and decrease oxLDL. In addition, MUFA reduce vascular inflammation and oxidation; decrease IL-23, IL-8, intracellular adhesion molecule (ICAM), and vascular cell adhesion molecule (VCAM); decrease TNF-α; improve ED; lower blood pressure; and decrease thrombosis. The net effect is to reduce the incidence of CHD by 30% (PREDIMED diet) [5,75,76,93–95]. In a study of 195 subjects [94], replacing SFAs with MUFAs or n-6 PUFAs did not affect the percentage change in flow-mediated dilatation (primary endpoint) or other measures of vascular reactivity, but the substitution of SFAs with MUFAs attenuated the increase in night systolic blood pressure (-4.9 mmHg, $P=0.019$) and reduced E-selectin (-7.8%, $P=0.012$). Replacement of SFAs with MUFAs or n-6 PUFAs lowered fasting serum TC (-8.4% and -9.2%, respectively), LDL-C (-11.3% and -13.6%, respectively), and the TC/HDL ratio (-5.6% and -8.5%, respectively) ($P \leq 0.001$). These changes in LDL-C equate to an estimated 17%–20% reduction in CVD mortality. MUFA are one of the most potent agents to reduce oxLDL [5]. The equivalent of 3–4 tablespoons (30–40 g) per day of EVOO in MUFA content is recommended for the maximum effect in conjunction with omega-3 fatty acids. The best ratio of EVOO to combined DHA and EPA is about 5:1 [5]. The polyphenol content of EVOO is important for its overall lipid and CV effects. However, the caloric intake of this amount of MUFA must be balanced with the other beneficial effects.

GARLIC

Numerous placebo-controlled clinical trials in humans indicate reductions in TC and LDL-C of about 9%–12% with a standardized extract of allicin and ajoene [5,96] at doses of 600–900 mg/day. However, many studies have been poorly controlled and used different types and doses of garlic, which have given inconsistent results [5,96]. The best form of garlic is the CV formulation of aged garlic. Garlic reduces intestinal cholesterol absorption and inhibits enzymes involved in cholesterol synthesis [5,96]. In addition, garlic lowers blood pressure, has fibrinolytic and anti-platelet activities, reduces oxLDL, and may decrease coronary artery calcification [5,96,97].

GREEN TEA

Catechins, especially epigallocatechin gallate (EGCG), as green tea or in supplement form, may improve the lipid profile by interfering with micellar solubilization of cholesterol in the GI tract and reduce its absorption [5]. In addition, EGCG reduces fatty acid gene expression, inhibits HMG-CoA reductase, increases mitochondrial energy expenditure, reduces oxLDL, increases paroxonase (PON-1), upregulates the LDL receptor, decreases ApoB secretion, mimics the action of insulin, improves ED, and decreases body fat [5,98–101]. A meta-analysis of 14 clinical trials shows that EGCG at 224–674 mg/day or 60 oz of green tea per day minimally reduced TC (7 mg/dL) and

LDL-C (2 mg/dL) ($p<0.001$ for both) [101]. Recent studies have confirmed similar reductions in TC and LDL-C in postmenopausal women [98]. There is no significant change in HDL or TG levels [101]. The recommended dose is a standardized EGCG extract 500–700 mg/day or green tea 12–60 oz/day.

ORANGE JUICE

In one human study, 750 mL of concentrated orange juice per day over 2 months decreased LDL-C by 11% and had positive effects on ApoB, TG, and HDL (up by 21%) [102]. The effects are due to polymethoxylated flavones, hesperidin naringin, pectin, and essential oils [102]. Additional studies are needed to verify these data.

POMEGRANATE JUICE AND SEEDS

Pomegranate seeds and juice increase PON 1 binding to HDL-C, increase PON 2 and HDL-C, lower the TG/HDL ratio, and decrease TG [103–108]. As a potent antioxidant, it increases total anti-oxidant status, lowers oxLDL, decreases antibodies to oxLDL, inhibits platelet function, reduces glycosylated LDL, decreases macrophage LDL uptake, and reduces lipid deposition in the arterial wall [103–108]. Pomegranate juice at 6 oz/day and seeds at ¼ cup twice a day decrease progression of carotid artery IMT and stabilize or reduce carotid artery plaque, especially in those with the higher levels of serum TG and HDL-C [103–108]. In addition, it may reduce blood pressure at the doses above within 2 months especially in subjects with the highest levels of oxidative stress. Consuming about 6–8 oz of pomegranate juice or ¼ to ½ cup of seeds per day is recommended.

SESAME

Sesame seeds and oil at 40 g/day reduce LDL-C by 9% through inhibition of intestinal absorption and increased biliary secretion of cholesterol [109,110]. Sesame also decreases HMG-CoA reductase activity and upregulates the LDL receptor gene, 7-alpha hydroxylase gene expression, and sterol regulatory element-binding proteins (SREBP) 2 genes [109,110]. A randomized placebo-controlled crossover study of 26 postmenopausal women who consumed 50 g of sesame powder daily for 5 weeks had a 5% decrease in TC and a 10% decrease in LDL-C (109).

SOY

Numerous studies have shown mild improvements in serum lipids with consumption of soy-containing foods at doses of about 30–50 g/day [5,111,112]. In most studies, the average reduction in TC is 9.3%, LDL-C decreased by 4%–12.9%, TG fell 10.5%, and HDL increased 2.4% [5,111,112]. However, the studies are conflicting due to differences in the type and dose of soy used (fermented, powders, foods, etc.) in many of the clinical trials, as well as non-standardized methodologies [5,111,112]. Soy decreases the micellar content and absorption of lipids through a combination of fiber, isoflavones (genistein, glycitein, daidzein), and phytoestrogens [5,111,112]. The greatest reduction is seen with soy-enriched isoflavones with soy protein.

NUTRIENTS AND DIETARY SUPPLEMENTS

New important scientific information and clinical studies are required to understand the present role of these natural agents in the management of dyslipidemia [5,80]. Several clinical trials that show excellent reductions in both serum lipids and risk of CHD with niacin, omega-3 fatty acids, red yeast rice, fiber, and ALA [5,80,97,113]. Smaller studies show reductions in surrogate vascular markers such as carotid intimal medial thickness and obstruction, plaque progression, stabilization and regression, coronary artery calcium (CAC) score, generalized atherosclerosis, and endothelial function with numerous other nutritional supplements [5,80,97,113]. The mechanisms by which nutritional supplements exert their effects are variable and will be discussed in detail with each of the supplements below.

CITRUS BERGAMOT

Citrus bergamot has been evaluated in several clinical prospective trials in humans. In doses of 1,000 mg/day, citrus bergamot lowers LDL-C up to 36% and TG by 39%, while it increases HDL-C by 40% [114,115]. Citrus bergamot inhibits HMG-CoA reductase, increases cholesterol and bile acid excretion, and reduces radical oxygen species (ROS) and oxLDL [114,115]. The active ingredients include naringin, neroeriocitrin, neohesperidin, poncerin, rutin, neodesmin, rhoifolin, melitidine, and brutelidine [114,115].

CURCUMIN

Curcumin is one of the phenolic compounds in turmeric and curry [5,116]. It induces changes in the expression of genes involved in cholesterol synthesis such as LDL receptor mRNA, HMG-CoA reductase, SREBP, cholesterol 7 alpha hydroxylase, peroxisome proliferator-activated receptors (PPARs), liver X receptor (LXR), activated protein kinase (AMPK), ATP-binding cassette transporters (ABCA1 and ABCG1), receptors for RCT, and CEC [5,116]. In one human study of ten patients consuming 500 mg/day of curcumin, the HDL increased 29% and TC fell 12% [5,116]. This needs confirmation in larger randomized clinical trials.

GUGGULIPIDS

Guggulipids are resins from the mukul myrrh tree (*Commiphora Mukul*) that contain active lipid-lowering compounds called guggulsterones [5,117,118]. These increase hepatic LDL receptors and bile acid secretion, and decrease cholesterol synthesis in animal experiments [5,117]. However, controlled human clinical trials have not shown these agents to be effective in improving serum lipids [117,118]. One study of 103 subjects on 50–75 mg of guggulsterones per day for 8 weeks actually had a 5% increase in LDL-C; no change in TC, TG, or HDL-C; and insignificant reductions in Lp(a) and hsCRP [117]. Guggulipids are not recommended at this time pending more studies in humans.

LYCOPENE

Lycopene has been shown in tissue culture to inhibit HMG-CoA reductase, increase PON 1 and HDL-C, improve HDL functionality, decrease oxLDL, induce Rho inactivation, increase PPAR gamma and LXR receptor activities, and increase RCT and CEC with ATP-binding cassette (ABCA1) and caveolin 1 expression [119,120]. There are no prospective clinical trials with lycopene, tomatoes, or tomato extract on CHD risk reduction to date.

NIACIN (VITAMIN B3)

Niacin has a dose-related effect (1–4 g/day) on serum lipids and CVD [5,121–127]. Niacin reduces TC, LDL-C, Apo-B, LDL-P, TG, and VLDL. Niacin increases LDL size from small type B to large type A, increases HDL by 15%–35%, increases HDL-P, especially the protective and larger HDL 2b particle, and increases APO A1 by 15%–35% [5,121–127]. The average changes in lipids in the dose range of 1–4 g/day are TC 20%–25% decrease, LDL-C and ApoB 10%–25% decrease, and LDL-P 10%–25% reduction, with an increase in LDL size. Niacin reduces Lp(a) by 25%–35%, lowers TG by 20%–25% with a decrease in VLDL size, improves HDL functionality, inhibits proprotein convertase subtilisin/kexin type 9 (PCSK9), and lowers oxLDL. The inhibition of PCSK9 and increases in RCT and CEC all may contribute to its anti-atherogenic effects [124,125].

These dose-related changes range from approximately 10% to 30% for each lipid level as noted above [5,121,122]. Many of the anti-atherosclerotic effects of niacin may be independent of the favorable effects on serum lipids [5,122,126]. Niacin increases TG lipolysis in adipose tissue, increases Apo-B degradation, reduces the fractional catabolic rate of HDL-ApoA-1, inhibits platelet function, induces fibrinolysis, decreases cytokines, inhibits inflammation, decreases cell adhesion molecules (CAMs), increases adiponectin, and has potent antioxidant activities [5,121,122].

Randomized controlled clinical trials such as the Coronary Drug Project (CDP), HDL-Atherosclerosis Treatment Study (HATS), Arterial Biology for the Investigation of the Treatment Effects of Reducing Cholesterol (ARBITER 2 and 6), Oxford Niaspan Study, Familial Atherosclerosis Treatment (FATS), Cholesterol Lowering Atherosclerosis Studies (CLAS I and II), and Air Force Regression Study (AFRS) have shown reduction in coronary events and decreases in coronary atheroma, carotid necrotic core and atheroma, and carotid IMT as monotherapy or in combination with other anti-lipid therapies and superiority to some anti-lipid agents [5,121–126]. Eleven trials of 9,959 subjects found that niacin use was associated with significant reductions in the composite endpoints of any CVD event (odds ratio (OR): 0.66; 95% confidence interval (CI): 0.49–0.89; $p=0.007$) and major CHD even (OR: 0.75; 95% CI: 0.59 to 0.96; $p=0.02$). No significant association was observed between niacin therapy and stroke incidence (OR: 0.88; 95% CI: 0.5–1.54; $p=0.65$) [124]. The magnitude of on-treatment HDL-C difference between treatment arms was not significantly associated with the magnitude of the effect of niacin on outcomes [124].

In a meta-analysis of 13 trials ($N=35,206$), niacin led to significant increases in serum HDL-C levels by 21.4% (95% CI: 5.11–13.51) from baseline trial enrollment [123]. Niacin treatment was associated with a trend toward lower risk of cardiovascular mortality (RR: 0.91; 95% CI: 0.81–1.02), coronary death (RR: 0.93; 95% CI: 0.78–1.10), nonfatal MI (RR: 0.85; 95% CI: 0.73–1.0), revascularization (coronary and noncoronary) (RR: 0.83; 95% CI: 0.65–1.06), and stroke (RR: 0.89; 95% CI: 0.72–1.10), compared with control. The recent negative findings in the AIM HIGH and HPS 2 THRIVE studies [126,127] do not detract from positive results in previous trials.

The AIM-HIGH study was designed to test whether extended-release niacin added to intensive statin therapy, as compared to statin therapy alone, would reduce the risk of CV events in patients with established atherosclerotic CV disease (defined as stable coronary, cerebrovascular, or peripheral arterial disease) and atherogenic dyslipidemia (low baseline levels of HDL-C < 40 mg/dL for men; <50 mg/dL for women; and elevated triglyceride levels 150–400 mg/dL). A total of 3,414 patients, aged 45 years or older, were randomly assigned to receive high-dose (1,500–2,000 mg) extended-release niacin or placebo. Both groups received simvastatin adjusted to maintain LDL-C level below 80 mg/dL. The primary endpoint was the composite of death from CHD, nonfatal MI, ischemic stroke, hospitalization (>23 hours) for an acute coronary syndrome (ACS), or symptom-driven coronary or cerebral revascularization. Secondary endpoints included the composite of death from CHD, nonfatal MI, ischemic stroke, and hospitalization for a "high-risk" ACS (characterized by accelerating ischemic symptoms or prolonged chest pain with electrocardiographic evidence of ischemia or biomarker values greater than, but less than, two times the upper limit of the normal range); death from CHD; nonfatal MI, ischemic stroke, or death from CV causes. The study was terminated after a mean follow-up period of 3 years due to lack of clinically meaningful efficacy. Over 3 years, HDL-C levels increased by 9.6 mg/dL (35%) in the niacin group compared to 4.2 mg/dL (9.8%) in the placebo group ($p<0.001$), whereas triglycerides levels decreased by 28.6% in the niacin group compared to 8.1% in the placebo group. The use of aspirin, beta-blockers, and inhibitors of renin angiotensin system was similar in both groups. Niacin was discontinued after randomization in 25.4% compared to 20.1% in the placebo. The primary endpoint occurred in 16.4% of the niacin group and in 16.2% of the placebo group (hazard ratio with niacin = 1.02; 95% CI: 0.87–1.21; $p=0.8$). There was no statistically significant difference in the composite secondary endpoint between patients assigned to niacin and those assigned to placebo (hazard ratio: 1.08;

95% CI: 0.87–1.34; $p=0.49$). Among the components of primary endpoint, unexpected increase in the rate of ischemic stroke was noticed in the niacin group (1.6%) compared to the placebo group (0.9%). The primary problem with the AIM-HIGH study was the patient selection bias. All patients were on statins with very low LDL levels of about 60 mg/dL or less. At this level of LDL-C, the ability of any additional anti-lipid agent is not likely to show any additional significant reduction in CHD. HPS2-THRIVE was a study of an investigational drug (Tredaptive, Merck) containing both extended-release niacin (Niaspan) (ERN) and the drug laropiprant, a selective antagonist of the prostaglandin D2 receptor subtype 1((DP1R), which partially blocks the dermal flushing response to niacin. HPS2-THRIVE randomized 25,673 high-risk patients who could tolerate niacin to either placebo or ERN plus laropiprant (ERNL). The study subjects were all on simvastatin 40 mg/day. The primary endpoint was the time to the first major vascular event, defined as the composite of nonfatal MI or coronary death, any stroke or any arterial revascularization.

The primary composite endpoint of major vascular events (MVE) was not significantly reduced (RR: 0.96; 95% CI: 0.90–1.03; $p=0.3$) in the active arm. "Serious adverse events" were found in 3% more subjects in the active arm, although most were "minor hyperglycemic problems." Myopathy generally was uncommon (0.34% per year), but was four-fold higher overall in the active arm, and ten-fold higher among Chinese subjects. The study subjects had excellent baseline control of serum lipids on statin therapy (simvastatin 40 mg/day) with an average LDL-C of 63mg/dL, HDL of 44 mg/dL, and triglycerides of 125 mg/dL. The National Lipid Association (NLA) in the March 2013 position paper stated that in HPS2-THRIVE, "niacin was clinically irrelevant in the average study subject, and there was substantial subgroup heterogeneity. However, the investigators "tested a drug in patients who, on average, had no indication to take it." MVE reduction with ERNL was strongly predicted by baseline LDL-C (heterogeneity $p=0.02$), with apparent net benefit if LDL-C was above 58 mg/dL at study entry. Thus, this study population was not likely to have any significant CVD reduction. In addition to the early data from the Coronary Drug Project (CDP) [5,6], which showed significant reductions in cardiovascular events when niacin was used *alone* in individuals with documented heart disease as well as many other niacin trials, there are documented benefits of additive therapy on top of statins when LDL-C or triglyceride remains elevated and HDL remains low.

Nevertheless, there were several positive effects of treated patients on ERNL, including reductions in weight, blood pressure, and lipoprotein (a); a significant reduction in arterial vascularization procedures ($p=0.03$); and a significant reduction in CV risk in the subgroup with the higher baseline LDL cholesterol level ($p=0.02$). The adherence rate was poor at one year and at completion of the study which may have altered hard CV outcomes. The average age was 64.9 years, and the patients studied were mostly men. The data cannot be totally extrapolated to a younger population or perhaps to women.

The claim that in HPS2-THRIVE, niacin induced more harm than statin alone is baseless. However, the study did show increases in serious adverse events (3.7% absolute excess adverse events) including myalgia (0.7%; $p<0.001$), new onset diabetes (NOD) (1.3%; $p<0.001$), gastrointestinal problems (1.0%; $p<0.001$), skin problems (0.3%; $p<0.003$), infections (1.4%; $p<0.001$), and bleeding (0.7%; $p<0.001$). The dose of niacin was high and fixed resulting in dose-related adverse effects. About 43% of the study subjects were Chinese. This influenced many of the adverse effects, especially myopathy and skin eruptions. As noted in the paper, "the absolute risk of myopathy in the placebo group was higher in China than in Europe and the relative risk with ERNL versus placebo was 5.2 in China, as compared to 1.5 in Europe. This is 10× greater in China participants, with 50 cases per 10,000, compared to 3 cases per 10,000 in Europe."

The investigational drug laropiprant has documented mechanisms of harm similar to the Cox-2 inhibitors and non-steroidal anti-inflammatory drugs to which it is related, as well as many other potential adverse effects). Laropiprant with aspirin or clopidogrel induces a prolongation of bleeding time and an inhibitory effect on platelet aggregation ex vivo in healthy subjects and in patients with dyslipidemia.

These studies are too far from reality. It is very unlikely that niacin (or any other HDL-C raising medications) would be prescribed in practice to patients with lipoprotein profile as in these studies before randomization. In the HPS2-THRIVE study, average baseline LDL-C was 63 mg/dL, HDL-C was 44 mg/dL, and triglycerides was 125 mg/dL before study drug treatment. Of further concern, major vascular event reduction in the niacin-laropiprant group was strongly predicted by baseline LDL-C ($p=0.02$), with apparent clinical benefit if baseline LDL-C level was above 58 mg/dL. Indeed, it might not be expected to get clinical benefit if patients were on the flat part of the event curve. Patients in the placebo group in the AIM-HIGH study had received 50 mg immediate-release niacin in each placebo tablet in order to mask the identity of treatment to patients or study personnel. Per protocol, the placebo group in all studies received also high dose of statin with or without ezetimibe. The early termination of the AIM-HIGH might not allow detection of positive results.

The effective dosing range of niacin is from 500 to 4,000 mg/day. The niacin dose should be gradually increased, starting at 100 mg/day and administered at meal time. Niacin-induced flushing can be reduced by giving a daily dose of 81 mg aspirin and taken with a quercetin supplement at 500–1,000 mg/day. Niacin should not be taken within 6 hours of alcohol [5]. Only vitamin B3 niacin is effective for dyslipidemia. The no-flush (inositol hexanicotinate (IHN)) does not improve lipid profiles and is not recommended [5]. The potential side effects of niacin include hyperglycemia, hyperuricemia, gout, hepatitis, flushing, rash, pruritus, hyperpigmentation, hyper-homocysteinemia, gastritis, ulcers, bruising, tachycardia, and palpitations [5,121,122]. At lower doses of niacin, these side effects are not common.

PANTETHINE

Pantethine is the disulfide derivative of pantothenic acid and is metabolized to cystamine-SH which is the active form for treating dyslipidemia [5]. Over 28 clinical trials have shown consistent and significant improvement in serum lipids. TC is decreased by 15%, LDL-C falls by 20%, ApoB is decreased by 27.6%, and TG are reduced by 36.5% over 4–9 months. HDL-C and APO A1 are increased by 8% [5,128–132]. The effects on lipids are slow to occur and have a peak effect at 4 months but may take up to 6–9 months. Pantethine reduces lipid peroxidation of LDL-C and decreases lipid deposition, intimal thickening, and fatty streak formation in the aorta and coronary arteries [5,128–132]. Pantethine inhibits cholesterol synthesis, accelerates fatty acid metabolism in the mitochondria by inhibiting hepatic acetyl-CoA carboxylase, increases CoA in the cytoplasm which stimulates the oxidation of acetate at the expense of fatty acid and cholesterol synthesis, and increases the Krebs cycle activity [5,128–132]. In addition, cholesterol esterase activity increases and HMG-CoA reductase activity is decreased. There is 50% inhibition of fatty acid synthesis and 80% inhibition of cholesterol synthesis [5]. It has an additive effect when used with RYR, statins, niacin, and fibrates [5,128–132]. The recommended effective dose is 450 mg twice per day with or without food [5,128–132].

PLANT STEROLS (PHYTOSTEROLS)

The plant sterols are naturally occurring cholesterol-like compounds with different side chain substitutions that give them unique properties. These include B-sitosterol (the most abundant), campesterol, and stigmasterol (4-desmethyl sterols of the cholestane series), and the stanols which are saturated sterols [5,133–135]. The plant sterols are much better absorbed than the plant stanols. The daily intake of plant sterols in the United States is about 150–400 mg/day, mostly from soybean oil and various nuts [5,133–135]. Consumption of these compounds results in a dose-dependent reduction in serum lipids [134]. TC is decreased by 8%, and LDL-C is decreased by 10% (range 6%–15%) with no change in TG and HDL-C, from doses of 2 to 3 g/day in divided doses with meals [5,133,134]. A recent meta-analysis of 84 trials showed that an average intake of 2.15 g/day reduced LDL-C by 8.8% with no improvement with higher doses [134]. They are additive with other anti-lipid therapies such as statins, niacin, fibrates, and curcumin. The mechanism of action is primarily to decrease the incorporation of dietary and biliary cholesterol into micelles due to lowered micellar solubility of cholesterol, which reduces cholesterol absorption and increases bile acid secretion. In addition, there is an interaction with enterocyte ATP-binding cassette transport proteins (ABCG8 and ABCG 5) that directs cholesterol back into the intestinal lumen [5,133]. The only difference between cholesterol and sitosterol consists of an additional ethyl group at position C24 in sitosterol, which is responsible for its poor absorption. The plant sterols have a higher affinity than cholesterol for micelles.

The plant sterols are also anti-inflammatory and decrease the levels of proinflammatory cytokines such as interleukins (IL-6, IL1b) and TNF-α, as well as hsCRP, LpPLA 2, and fibrinogen; however, these effects vary among the various phytosterols [135]. Other potential mechanisms include modulation of signaling pathways, activation of cellular stress responses, cellular growth arrest, reduction of Apo-B48 secretion from intestinal and hepatic cells, reduction of cholesterol synthesis with suppression of HMG-CoA reductase and cytochrome P 450 (CYP7A1), interference with SREBP, and promotion of RCT via ABCA1 and ABCG1 [135]. The biological activity of phytosterols is both cell-type and sterol-specific [133].

The plant sterols can interfere with absorption of lipid-soluble compounds such as the fat-soluble vitamins and carotenoids (vitamins A D, E, K, and alpha carotene) [5]. Some studies have shown reduction in atherosclerosis progression, reduced carotid IMT, and decreased plaque progression, but the results have been conflicting [5]. There are no studies on CHD or other CVD outcomes. The recommended dose is about 2–2.5 g/day (average 2.15 g/day). Patients that have the rare homozygote mutations of sitosterolemia and abnormal ATP-binding cassette are hyper-absorbers of sitosterol (absorbing 15%–60% instead of the normal 5%) and will develop premature atherosclerosis. The patients can be identified with genetic testing and should avoid plant sterols.

POLICOSANOL

Policosanol is a sugar cane extract of eight aliphatic alcohols that has undergone extensive clinical studies with variable results [5,136–139]. Most of the earlier studies that showed positive results were performed in Cuba, and these have been questioned as to their validity [5,137]. More recent double-blind placebo-controlled clinical trials have not shown any significant improvement in any measured lipids including TC, LDL-C, TG, or HDL-C. A recent small study (14 subjects, underpowered) suggested that policosanol may improve HDL-C functionality, increase paraoxonase (PON), lower glucose, reduce uric acid, decrease blood pressure and the oxidative stress marker malondialdehyde (MDA), and improve the lipid profile [136]. Other studies have found that policosanol may enhance the effects of statins and improve hepatic function [139]. Policosanol is not recommended at this time for the treatment of any form of dyslipidemia pending more definitive studies with a larger study population [5,137,138].

TOCOTRIENOLS

Tocotrienols are a family of unsaturated forms of vitamin E termed alpha, beta, gamma, and delta tocotrienols [5,140,141]. The gamma and delta tocotrienols lower TC up to 17%, LDL-C by 24%, ApoB by 15%, and Lp(a) by 17% with minimal changes or slightly increase HDL-C and Apo-A1 in 50% of subjects at doses of 200 mg/day given at night with food [5,140,141]. In addition, the LDL-C receptor is augmented, and the tocotrienols exhibit antioxidant activity [5,140,141]. The gamma/delta from of tocotrienols inhibits cholesterol synthesis by suppression of HMG-CoA reductase activity by two post-transcriptional actions [5,140,141]. These include increased controlled degradation of the reductase protein and decreased efficiency of translation of HMG-CoA reductase mRNA. These effects are mediated by sterol binding of the reductase enzyme to the endoplasmic reticulum membrane proteins called INSIGS. The tocotrienols have natural farnesylated analog of tocopherols which give them their effects on HMG-CoA reductase [140].

The tocotrienol dose is very important due to the fact that increased dosing will induce its own metabolism and reduce effectiveness, whereas lower doses are not as effective [5]. Also, concomitant intake within 12 hours of alpha tocopherol reduces tocotrienol absorption. Increased intake of alpha tocopherol over 20% of the total tocopherol intake may interfere with the lipid-lowering effect [5,140]. Tocotrienols are metabolized by successive beta-oxidation, and then catalyzed by the CYP 450 enzymes 3A4 and CYP 4F2 [5]. The combination of a statin with gamma/delta tocotrienols further reduces LDL-C cholesterol by 10% [140]. The tocotrienols block the adaptive response of upregulation of HMG-CoA reductase secondary to competitive inhibition by the statins [5,140]. Tocotrienols lower hsCRP, advanced glycation endproducts, CAMs, and thrombotic risk and suppress matrix metalloproteinases [141]. In addition, they suppress, regress, and slow down the progression of atherosclerosis, stabilize atherosclerotic plaques, and reduce the risk of cardiac events in established CHD [141]. Carotid artery stenosis regression has been reported in about 30% of subjects given tocotrienols over 18 months. They also slow down the progression of generalized atherosclerosis [5,141]. The recommended dose is 200 mg of gamma delta tocotrienol at night with food.

RED YEAST RICE

Red yeast rice (RYR) (*Monascus purpureus*) is a fermented product of rice that contains monocolins which inhibit cholesterol synthesis via HMG-CoA reductase and thus has "statin-like" properties [5,142,143]. RYR also contains sterols, isoflavones, and MUFA. At 2,400 mg/day, LDL-C is reduced by 22% ($p < 0.001$) and TG falls by 12% with little change in HDL-C [5,142,143]. A meta-analysis by Xiong showed that RYR reduced LDL by 17.6% ($p < 0.001$) and increased HDL by 4.2% ($p < 0.001$) at doses of up to 1,600 mg/day dose [143]. In addition, the CV mortality was decreased by 30% ($p < 0.005$) and total mortality by 33% ($p < 0.0003$) in the treated subjects. The overall primary endpoints for MI and death are decreased by 45% ($p < 0.001$) [5,143]. Numerous previous controlled clinical trials of RYR showed similar effects [5]. RYR lowers metalloproteinases 2 and 3, leptin, insulin resistance, hsCRP, tissue factor, NADPH oxidase, thrombosis, caveolin-1, TNF-α, pulse wave velocity, and angiotensin II and decreases the risk of abdominal aortic aneurysms [5,142,143]. RYR increases nitric oxide and eNOS [5,142,143]. A highly purified and certified RYR must be used to avoid potential renal damage induced by a mycotoxin, citrinin [5,143]. The recommended dose is 2,400–4,800 mg of a standardized RYR at night with food. No adverse clinical effects have been reported with long-term use. Reductions in coenzyme Q10 may occur in predisposed patients and those on prolonged high-dose RYR due to its weaker "statin-like" effect. RYR provides an alternative to patients with statin-induced myopathy or other statin-induced adverse effects [5,142,143].

RESVERATROL

Resveratrol reduces oxLDL-C; inhibits ACAT activity and cholesterol ester formation; increases bile acid excretion; reduces TC, TG, and LDL-C; and increases PON-1 activity and HDL-C. In vitro studies showed that resveratrol inhibits NADPH oxidase in macrophages, and blocks the uptake of modified LDL-C by CD36 SR (scavenger receptors [5]). N-acetylcysteine (NAC) has the same effect on CD 36 SR and should be used in conjunction with resveratrol [5]. The dose of *trans* resveratrol is 250 mg/day and NAC is 1,000 mg once or twice per day [5].

VITAMIN C

Vitamin C supplementation lowers serum LDL-C and TG [144]. A meta-analysis of 13 randomized controlled trials in subjects given at least 500 mg of vitamin C daily for 3–24 weeks found a reduction in LDL-C cholesterol of 7.9 mg/dL ($p < 0.0001$) and a decrease of TG by 20.1 mg/dL ($P < 0.003$). HDL-C did not change. The reductions in LDL-C and TG were greatest in those with the highest initial lipid levels and the lowest serum vitamin C levels [145]. High-dose vitamin C is part of a therapeutic regimen to neutralize the negative effects of elevated Lp(a) levels.

BERBERINE

Berberine, an alkaloid present in plant roots, rhizomes, and stem barks, is effective as either monotherapy or in combination with other nutritional supplements to improve serum lipids [146–149]. In one study, at 3 months, berberine at 500 mg bid decreased TC by 29%, LDL-C fell by 25%, and TG reduced by 35% [147]. A meta-analysis of 11 trials in 874 subjects demonstrated significant reductions in TC (23 mg/dL), LDL-C (25 mg/dL), and TG (44 mg/dL) and an increase in HDL-C (2mg/dL) [148]. Berberine suppresses PCSK9 expression and increases hepatic LDL R (mRNA/protein) 2.6–3.5-fold, reduces cholesterol absorption, increases biliary excretion of LDL, inhibits HMG-CoA reductase, decreases fatty acid synthesis, and increases fatty acid oxidation [146–148]. Berberine is additive for the reduction of LDL-C, TC, and TG with ezetimibe, RYR, and phytosterols [146–149]. Berberine may inhibit CYP enzymes in increased serum levels of statins. The recommended dose of berberine HCL is 500–1,000 mg/day.

COMBINATION THERAPIES

A prospective open-label human clinical trial of 30 patients for 2 months showed significant improvement in serum lipids using a proprietary product (LS) with a combination of pantethine, plant sterols, EGCG, and gamma/delta tocotrienols [150]. The TC fell by 14%, LDL-C decreased by 14%, VLDL dropped by 20% and small dense LDL-C particles fell by 25% (types III and IV) [146]. In another study using the same proprietary product with RYR 2,400–4,800 mg/day and niacin 500 mg/day, the TC fell by 34%, LDL-C decreased by 34%, LDL-C particle number fell by 35%, VLDL dropped by 27%, and HDL-C increased by 10% [151–156].

The most recent study of a proprietary lipid-lowering product (LC) found significant improvement in the expanded lipid profile particle numbers, size and total lipid levels, and inflammatory markers [152]. Forty participants were recruited for a single-center, double-blind randomized, placebo-controlled trial. The 40 participants were randomly assigned to receive either the proprietary multi-ingredient lipid-lowering supplement (LC) $n=20$ or placebo $n=20$. The trial consisted of a screening visit, a 2-week run-in, and a 4-month treatment period. Results from the trial showed that the LC significantly reduced TC, LDL-C, VLDL-C, oxLDL, Apo B, TG, LDL-P heart rate, and diastolic blood pressure compared to placebo at 1 and 4 months. The LC significantly increased HDL-P and LDL particle size from dense type III and IV to larger type I and II LDL particle compared to placebo at 1 and 4 months. In addition, LC significantly lowered hsCRP, TNF-α, and IL-6 within the treatment group from baseline. There were no adverse effects noted in the treatment group after 4 months of supplementation.

Clinical studies indicate a RRR of CVD mortality with omega-3 fatty acids of 0.68, with resins of 0.70 and statins of 0.78 [153]. Combining statins with omega-3 fatty acids further decreases CHD by 19% [84]. The combination of gamma/delta tocotrienols with a statin reduces LDL-C an additional 10% [139]. Plant sterols with omega-3 fatty acids have synergistic lipid-lowering and anti-inflammatory effects [88]. Future studies are needed to evaluate various other combinations on serum lipids, surrogate vascular endpoints, CHD, and CVD morbidity and mortality [154–156].

FUTURE PERSPECTIVES

Advances in the understanding of pathophysiology and causes of dyslipidemia and dyslipidemia-induced CVD coupled with new diagnostic CV biomarkers, genetics, microbiome analysis and non-invasive testing will allow for more personalized treatment in the future. The most common secondary causes for dyslipidemia are:

1. Chronic inflammatory macro- and micro-nutrient intakes (metabolic endotoxemia).
2. Chronic infections (all types including bacteria, virus, fungi, TB, and parasites).
3. Heavy metals (mercury, cadmium, lead, arsenic) and other toxins.

It is estimated that approximately 70% of secondary dyslipidemia is due to one of these three etiologies. All dyslipidemia patients should be evaluated and treated for these causes as well as the traditional metabolic causes such as hypothyroidism, renal and liver diseases, and autoimmunity, and secondary causes such as dietary factors and drugs affecting lipids. Proper therapy of the underlying cause can often correct the dyslipidemia over time. Such therapies would include optimal diets, probiotics, prebiotics, anti-infectives, improvement in the natural immune function, and chelation therapy in addition to the drugs discussed above, if ever needed.

SUMMARY AND CONCLUSIONS

The combination of a lipid-lowering diet, select foods, and nutraceutical supplements have the ability to reduce TC and LDL-C by 65% or more, decrease LDL-C particle number, increase LDL-C particle size, lower TG and VLDL, increase total HDL-C and HDL-P, and improve HDL functionality. In addition, vascular inflammation, oxidative stress, and immune responses are decreased, and vascular target organ damage, atherosclerosis, CHD, and CVD are reduced by many of the dietary interventions, by RYR, omega-3 fatty acids niacin, statins, or a combination of these (Table 5.2).

The LDL-P is the primary lipid component that drives the risk for CHD and MI. RYR, omega-3 fatty acids, niacin, and berberine are very effective in reducing LDL-P and increasing

---

TABLE 5.2

Summary of Nutraceutical Supplements at Recommended Doses for the Treatment of Dyslipidemia

- Red yeast rice: 2,400–4,800 mg at night with food
- Plant sterols: 2.5 g/day
- Berberine: 500 mg/day to twice per day
- Niacin (nicotinic acid B3: 500–3,000 mg/day as tolerated pretreated with quercetin, apples, ASA. Take with food and avoid alcohol. Never interrupt therapy)
- Omega-3 fatty acids with EPA/DHA at 3/2 ratio: 4 g per day with GLA at 50% of total EPA and GLA and gamma/delta tocopherol
- Gamma delta tocotrienols: 200 mg hs
- Aged garlic-Kyolic standardized 600 mg twice per day
- Sesame 40 g/day
- Phosphatidyl serine: 300 mg bid
- Pantethine: 450 mg bid
- MUFA: 20–40 g/day (EVOO 4 tablespoons per day)
- Lycopene: 20 mg/day
- Luteolin: 10 per day
- Astaxanthin: 15 mg/day
- Trans resveratrol: 250 mg/day
- NAC: 500 mg twice per day
- Carnosine: 500 mg twice per day
- Citrus bergamot: 1,000 mg/day
- Quercetin: 500 mg twice per day
- Probiotics standardized: 15–50 billion organisms bid
- Curcumin: 500–1,000 mg twice per day
- EGCG: 500–1,000 mg bid or 60–100 oz of green tea per day
- Pomegranate: 1/4–1/2 cup of seeds per day or 6 oz of juice per day

small dense LDL size. Statins will decrease LDL-P approximately 30%–50% of the time, and the new PCSK9 inhibitors are very effective on both LDL-C and LDL-P but limited in scope to the patients at the highest risk of CVD. Recent new proprietary nutritional supplements have combined many of these supplements to favorably affect all the components of the advanced lipid profile as well as interrupt many of the 45 mechanisms involved in dyslipidemia and dyslipidemia-induced vascular disease. This approach broadens treatment options by leveraging the effects of diet, food, and nutritional supplements, and complex pathophysiology of lipid-induced vascular damage.

REFERENCES

1. Kannel WB, Castelli WD, Gordon T. et al. Serum cholesterol, lipoproteins and risk of coronary artery disease. The Framingham study. *Ann Intern Med* 1971;74:1–12.
2. Houston MC. Nutrition and nutraceutical supplements in the treatment of hypertension. *Exp Rev Cardiovasc Ther* 2010;8:821–33.
3. Tian N, Penman AD, Mawson AR, Manning RD Jr and Flessner MF. Association between circulating specific leukocyte types and blood pressure: the atherosclerosis risk in communities (ARIC) study. *J Am Soc Hypertens* 2010;4(6):272–83.
4. Ungvari Z, Kaley G, de Cabo R, Sonntag WE and Csiszar A. Mechanisms of vascular aging: new perspectives. *J Gerontol A Biol Sci Med Sci* 2010;65(10):1028–41.
5. Houston, M. The role of nutrition and nutritional supplements in the treatment of dyslipidemia. *Clin Lipidol* 2014;9(3):333–3.
6. Plourde M, Vohl MC, Vandal M, Couture P, Lemieux S and Cunnane SC. Plasma n-3 fatty acid supplement is modulated by apoE epsilon 4 but not by the common PPAR-alpha L162 polymorphism in men. *Br J Nutr* 2009;102:1121–4.
7. Neiminen T, Kahonen M, Viiri LE, Gronroos P and Lehtimaki T. Pharmacogenetics of apolipoprotein E gene during lipid-lowering therapy: lipid levels and prevention of coronary heart disease. *Pharmacogenomics* 2008;9(10):1475–86.
8. Shih DM and Lusis AJ. The roles of PON 1 and PON 2 in cardiovascular disease and innate immunity. *Curr Opin Lipidol* 2009;20(4):288–92.
9. Calkin AC and Tontonoz P. Genome-wide association studies identify new targets in cardiovascular disease. *Sci Transl Med* 2010;2(48):48.
10. Djousse L and Caziano JM. Dietary cholesterol and coronary artery disease: a systematic review. *Curr Atheroscler Rep* 2009;11(6):418–22.
11. Houston M. The role of noninvasive cardiovascular testing, applied clinical nutrition and nutritional supplements in the prevention and treatment of coronary heart disease. *Ther Adv Cardiovasc Dis* 2018;12(3):85–108.
12. Erkkila A, de Mello VD, Riserus U and Laaksonen DE. Dietary fatty acids and cardiovascular disease: an epidemiological approach. *Prog Lipid Res* 2008;47(3):172–87.
13. Houston M, Minich D, Sinatra ST, Kahn JK and Guarneri M. Recent science and clinical application of nutrition to coronary heart disease. *J Am Coll Nutr* 2018;37(3):169–87.
14. Mozaffarian D and Willet WC. Trans fatty acids and cardiovascular risk: a unique cardiometabolic imprint. *Curr Atheroscler Rep* 2007;9(6):486–93.
15. Chen CL, Tetri LH, Neuschwander-Tetri BA, Huang SS and Huang JS. A mechanism by which dietary trans fats cause atherosclerosis. *J Nutr Biochem* 2011;22:649–55.
16. Siri-Tarino PW, Sun Q, Hu FB and Krauss RM. Saturated fat, carbohydrate and cardiovascular disease. *Am J Clin Nutr* 2010;91(3):502–9.
17. Otvos JD, Mora S, Shalaurova I, Greenland P, Mackey RH and Goff DC Jr. Clinical implications of discordance between low-density lipoprotein cholesterol and particle number. *J Clin Lipidol* 2011;5(2):105–13.
18. Hodge AM, Jenkins AJ, English DR, O'Dea K and Giles GG. NMR determined lipoprotein subclass profile is associated with dietary composition and body size. *Nutr Metab Cardiovasc Dis* 2011;21(8):603–609.
19. Asztalos BF, Tani M and Schaefer E. Metabolic and functional of HDL subspecies. *Curr Opin Lipidol* 2011;22:176–185.

20. Khera AV, Cuchel M, de la Llera-Moya M, Rodriguez A, Burke MF Jafri K, French BC, Phillips JA, Mucksavage ML, Wilensky RL, Mohler ER, Rothblat GH and Rader DJ. Cholesterol efflux capacity, high-density lipoprotein function, and atherosclerosis. *N Engl J Med* 2011;64:127–35.

21. Karakas M, Koenig W, Zierer A, Herder C, Rottbauer W, Meisinger C and Thorand B. Myeloperoxidase is associated with incident coronary heart disease independently of traditional risk factors: results from the MONICA/KORA Augsburg study. *J Intern Med* 2011;66:132–145; May 2 E PUB.

22. Lamarche B, Tchernof A, Mooriani S, Cantin B, Dagenais GR, Lupien PJ and Despres JP. Small, dense low-density lipoprotein particles as a predictor of the risk of ischemic heart disease in men. Prospective results from the Quebec cardiovascular study. *Circulation* 1997;95(1);69–75.

23. Kruth HS. Receptor-independent fluid-phase pinocytosis mechanisms for induction of foam cell formation with native low density lipoprotein particles. *Curr Opin Lipidol* 2011;22(5):386–93.

24. Zhao ZW, Zhu XL, Luo YK, Lin CG and Chen LL. Circulating Soluble lectin-like oxidized low-density lipoprotein redeptor-1 levels are associated with angiographic coronary lesion complexity in patients with coronary artery disease. *Clin Cardiol* 2011;34(3):172–77.

25. Ehara S, Ueda M, Naruko T, Haze K, Itoh A, Otsuka M, Komatsu R, Matsuo T, Itabe H, Takano T, Tsukamoto Y, Yoshiyama M, Takeuchi K, Yoshikawa J and Becker AE. Elevated levels of oxidized low density lipoprotein show a positive relationship with the severity of acute coronary syndromes. *Circulation* 2001;103(15):1955–60.

26. Hansson GK. Inflammation, atherosclerosis, and coronary artery disease. *N Engl J Med* 2005;352(16):1685–95.

27. Harper CR and Jacobson TA. Using apolipoprotein B to manage dyslipidemic patients: time for a change? *Mayo Clin Proc* 2010;85(5):440–5.

28. Curtiss LK. Reversing atherosclerosis? *N Engl J Med* 2009;360(11):1144–6.

29. Ridker PM, Danielson E, Fonseca FA, Genest J, Gotto AM Jr, Kastelein JJ, Koenig W, Libby P, Lorenzatti AJ, MacFadyen JG, Nordestgaard BG, Shepherd J, Willerson JT, Glynn RJ, Jupiter Study Group. Rosuvastatin to prevent vascular events in men and women with elevated C-eactive protein. *N Engl J Med* 2008;359(21):2195–207.

30. Shen GX. Impact and mechanism for oxidized and glycated lipoproteins on generation of fibrinolytic regulators from vascular endothelial cells. *Mol Cell Biochem* 2003;246(1–2):69–74.

31. Krishnan GM and Thompson PD. The effects of statins on skeletal muscle strength and exercise performance. *Curr Opin Lipidol* 2010;21(4):324–8.

32. Mills EJ, Wu P, Chong G, Ghement K, Singh S, Aki EA, Eyawo O, Guyatt G, Berwanger O and Briel M. Efficacy and safety of statin treatment for cardiovascular disease: a network meta-analysis of 170,255 patients from 76 randomized trials. *QJM* 2011;104(2):109–24.

33. Mammen AL and Amato AA. Statin myopathy: a review of recent progress. *Curr Opin Rheumatol* 2010;22(6):544–50.

34. Russo MW, Scobev M and Bonkovsky HL. Drug-induced liver injury associated with statins. *Semin Liver Dis* 2009;29(4):412–22.

35. Moosmann B and Behl C. Selenoproteins, cholesterol-lowering durgs, and the consequences: revisiting of the mevalonate pathway. *Trends Cardiovasc Med* 2004;14(7):273–81.

36. Liu CS, Lii CK, Chang LL, Kuo CL, Cheng WL, Su SL, Tsai CW and Chen HW. Atorvastatin increases blood ratios of vitamin E/low-density lipoprotein cholesterol and coenzyme Q10/low-density lipoprotein cholesterol in hypercholesterolemic patients. *Nutr Res* 2010;30(2):118–24.

37. Wyman M, Leonard M and Morledge T. Coenzyme Q 10: a therapy for hypertension and statin-induced myalgia? *Clev Clin J Med* 2010;77(7):435–42.

38. Mortensen SA. Low coenzyme Q levels and the outcome of statin treatment in heart failure. *J Am Coll Cardiol* 2011;57(14):1569.

39. Shojaei M, Djalali M, Khatami M, Siassi F and Eshraghian M. Effects of carnitine and coenzyme Q 10 on lipid profile and serum levels of lipoprotein (a) in maintenance hemodialysis patients on statin therapy. *Iran J Kidney Dis* 2011;5(20):114–8.

40. Gupta A and Thompson PD. The relationship of vitamin D deficiency to statin myopathy. *Atherosclerosis* 2011;215(1):23–9.

41. Avis HJ, Hargreaves IP, Ruiter JP, Land JM, Wanders RJ and Wijburg FA. Rosuvastatin lowers coenzyme Q 10 levels, but not mitochondrial adenosine triphosphate synthesis, in children with familial hypercholesterolemia. *J Pediatr* 2011;158(3):458–62.

42. Kiernan TJ, Rochford M and McDermott JH. Simvastatin induced Rhapdomyloysis and an important clinical link with hypothyroidism. *Int J Cardiol* 2007;119(3):374–6.

43. Van Horn L, McCoin M, Kris-Etherton PM, et al. The evidence for dietary prevention and treatment of cardiovascular disease. *J Am Diet Assoc* 2008;108:287–331.
44. Dawber TR, Meadors GF and Moore FE. Epidemiological approaches to heart disease: the Framingham Study. *Am J Public Health* 1951;41:279–86.
45. Keys A. 1970. Coronary heart disease in seven countries. *Circulation* 41(Suppl 1):1–21.
46. Keys A, Menotti A, Karvonen MJ, et al. The diet and 15-year death rate in the seven countries study. *Am J Epidemiol* 1986;124:903–15.
47. Appel LJ, Sacks FM, Carey VJ, et al. Effects of protein, monounsaturated fat, and carbohydrate intake on blood pressure and serum lipids: results of the OmniHeart randomized trial. *JAMA* 2005;294:2455–64.
48. Pritikin N. Dietary factors and hyperlipidemia. *Diabetes Care* 1982;5:647–8.
49. Pritikin N. The Pritikin diet. *JAMA* 1984;251:1160–1.
50. Barnard RJ, Lattimore L, Holly RG, et al. Response of non-insulin-dependent diabetic patients to an intensive program of diet and exercise. *Diabetes Care* 1982;5:370–4.
51. Ornish D, Scherwitz LW, Doody RS, et al. Effects of stress management training and dietary changes in treating ischemic heart disease. *JAMA* 1983;249:54–9.
52. Ornish D, Brown SE, Scherwitz LW, et al. Can lifestyle changes reverse coronary heart disease? The lifestyle heart trial. *Lancet* 1990;336:129–33.
53. Ornish D, Scherwitz LW, Billings JH, et al. Intensive lifestyle changes for reversal of coronary heart disease. *JAMA* 1998;280:2001–7. Erratum in: *JAMA* 1999;281:1380.
54. Chainani-Wu N, Weidner G, Purnell DM, et al. Changes in emerging cardiac biomarkers after an intensive lifestyle intervention. *Am J Cardiol* 2011;108:498–507.
55. Expert Panel on Detection, Evaluation, and Treatment of High Blood Cholesterol in Adults. Executive summary of the third report of the National Cholesterol Education Program (NCEP) expert panel on detection, evaluation, and treatment of high blood cholesterol in adults (Adult Treatment Panel III). *JAMA* 2001;16(285):2486–97. 2004 update available at http://www.nhlbi.nih.gov/guidelines/cholesterol/atp3upd04.htm. Accessed 27 November 2011.
56. Lichtenstein AH, Appel LJ, Brands M, et al. Summary of American Heart Association Diet and lifestyle recommendations revision 2006. *Arterioscler Thromb Vasc Biol* 2006;26:2186–91.
57. Lichtenstein AH, Ausman LM, Jalbert SM, et al. Efficacy of a therapeutic lifestyle change/step 2 diet in moderately hypercholesterolemic middle-aged and elderly female and male subjects. *J Lipid Res* 2002;43:264–73.
58. Howard BV, Van Horn L and Hsia J. Low-fat dietary pattern and risk of cardiovascular disease: the Women's health initiative randomized controlled dietary modification trial. *JAMA* 2006;8(295):655–66.
59. Jenkins DJ, Kendall CW, Marchie A, et al. The effect of combining plant sterols, soy protein, viscous fibers, and almonds in treating hypercholesterolemia. *Metabolism* 2003;52:1478–83.
60. Jenkins DJ, Kendall CW, Faulkner DA, et al. Assessment of the longer-term effects of a dietary portfolio of cholesterol-lowering foods in hypercholesterolemia. *Am J Clin Nutr* 2006;83:582–91.
61. Jenkins DJ, Kendall CW, Faulkner D, et al. A dietary portfolio approach to cholesterol reduction: combined effects of plant sterols, vegetable proteins, and viscous fibers in hypercholesterolemia. *Metabolism* 2002;51:1596–604.
62. Jenkins DJ, Kendall CW, Marchie A, et al. Effects of a dietary portfolio of cholesterol-lowering foods vs lovastatin on serum lipids and C-reactive protein. *JAMA* 2003;290:502–10.
63. Jenkins DJ, Chiavaroli L, Wong JM, et al. Adding monounsaturated fatty acids to a dietary portfolio of cholesterol-lowering foods in hypercholesterolemia. *CMAJ* 2010;182:1961–7.
64. Jenkins DJ, Jones PJ, Lamarche B, et al. Effect of a dietary portfolio of cholesterol-lowering foods given at 2 levels of intensity of dietary advice on serum lipids in hyperlipidemia: a randomized controlled trial. *JAMA* 2011;306:831–9.
65. Kris-Etherton P, Eckel RH, Howard BV, et al. AHA Science Advisory: Lyon Diet Heart Study. Benefits of a Mediterranean-style, National Cholesterol Education Program/American Heart Association step I dietary pattern on cardiovascular disease. *Circulation* 2001;103:1823–5.
66 de Lorgeril M, Renaud S, Mamelle N, et al. Mediterranean alpha-linolenic acid-rich diet in secondary prevention of coronary heart disease. *Lancet* 1994;343:1454–9. Erratum in: *Lancet* 1994;345:738.
67. de Lorgeril M, Salen P, Martin JL, et al. Mediterranean diet, traditional risk factors, and the rate of cardiovascular complications after myocardial infarction: final report of the Lyon Diet Heart Study. *Circulation* 1999;99:779–85.
68. de Lorgeril M and Salen P. The Mediterranean diet: rationale and evidence for its benefit. *Curr Atheroscler Rep* 2008;10:518–22.

69. Rastogi T, Reddy KS, Vaz M. et al. Diet and risk of ischemic heart disease in India. *Am J Clin Nutr* 2004;79:582–92.

70. PREDIMED Investigators. PREDIMED Study (protocol), 2011, available at: http://predimed.onmedic. net/LinkClick.aspx?fileticket=PPjQkaJqs20%3D&tabid=574. Accessed 26 November 2011.

71. Estruch R, Martínez-González MA, Corella D, et al. Effects of a Mediterranean-style diet on cardiovascular risk factors: a randomized trial. *Ann Intern Med* 2006;145:1–11.

72. Salas-Salvadó J, Garcia-Arellano A, Estruch R, et al. Components of the Mediterranean-type food pattern and serum inflammatory markers among patients at high risk for cardiovascular disease. *Eur J Clin Nutr* 2008;62:651–9.

73. Kallio P, Kolehmainen M, Laaksonen DE, et al. Dietary carbohydrate modification induces alterations in gene expression in abdominal subcutaneous adipose tissue in persons with the metabolic syndrome: the FUNGENUT study. *Am J Clin Nutr* 2007;85:1417–27.

74. Ornish D, Magbanua MJ, Weidner G, et al. Changes in prostate gene expression in men undergoing an intensive nutrition and lifestyle intervention. *Proc Natl Acad Sci U S A* 2008;105:8369–74.

75. Llorente-Cortés V, Estruch R, Mena MP, et al. Effect of Mediterranean diet on the expression of proatherogenic genes in a population at high cardiovascular risk. *Atherosclerosis* 2010;208:442–50.

76. Razquin C, Martinez JA, Martinez-Gonzalez MA, et al. A Mediterranean diet rich in virgin olive oil may reverse the effects of the -174G/C IL6 gene variant on 3-year body weight change. *Mol Nutr Food Res* 2010;54(Suppl 1):S75–82.

77. Ros E, Martínez-González MA, Estruch R, Salas-Salvadó J, Fitó M, Martínez JA. Mediterranean diet and cardiovascular health: teachings of the PREDIMED study. *Adv Nutr* 2014;5(3):330S–6S.

78. Castañer O, Corella D, Covas MI, Sorlí JV, Subirana I, Flores-Mateo G, Nonell L, Bulló M, de la Torre R, Portolés O, Fitó M and PREDIMED Study Investigators. In vivo transcriptomic profile after a Mediterranean diet in high-cardiovascular risk patients: a randomized controlled trial. *Am J Clin Nutr* 2013;98(3):845–53.

79. Konstantinidou V, Covas MI, Sola R. and Fitó M. Up-to date knowledge on the in vivo transcriptomic effect of the Mediterranean diet in humans. *Mol Nutr Food Res* 2013;57(5):772–83.

80. Estruch R, Ros E, Salas-Salvadó J, Covas MI, Corella D, Arós F, Gómez-Gracia E, Ruiz-Gutiérrez V, Fiol M, Lapetra J, Lamuela-Raventos R.M, Serra-Majem L, Pintó X, Basora J, Muñoz MA, Sorlí JV, Martínez JA, Martínez-González MA and PREDIMED Study Investigators. Primary prevention of cardiovascular disease with a Mediterranean diet. *N Engl J Med* 2013;368(14):1279–90.

81. Alexander DD, Miller PE, Van Elswyk ME, Kuratko CN and Bylsma LC. A meta-analysis of randomized controlled trials and prospective cohort studies of eicosapentaenoic and docosahexaenoic long-chain omega-3 fatty acids and coronary heart disease risk. *Mayo Clin Proc* 2017;92(1):15–29.

82. Rissanen T, Voutilainen S, NyyssonenK, Lakka TA and Salonen JT Fish oil-derived fatty acids, docosahexaenoic acid and docosapentaenoic acid and the risk of acute coronary events: the Kuopio ischaemic heart disease risk factor study. *Circulation* 2000;102(22):2677–79.

83. Davis W, Rockway S and Kwasny M. Effect of a combined therapeutic approach of intensive lipid management, omega 3 fatty acid supplementation, and increased serum 25(OH) D on coronary calcium scores in asymptomatic adults. *Am J Ther* 2009;16(4):326–332.

84. Yokoyama M, Origasa H, Matsuzaki M, Matsuzawa Y, Saito Y, Ishikawa Y, Oikawa S, Sasaki J, Hishida H, Itakura H, Kita I, Kitabatake A, Nakaya N, Sakata T, Shimada K, Shirato K. Japan EPA lipid intervention study (JELIS) Investigators. *Lancet* 2007;369(9567):1090–8.

85. Ryan AS, Keske MA, Hoffman JP and Nelson EB. Clinical overview of algal-docosahexaenoic acid: effects on triglyceride levels and other cardiovascular risk factors. *Am J Ther* 2009;16(2):183–92.

86. Kelley DS, Siegal D, Vemuri M, Chung GH and Mackey BE. Docosahexaenoic acid supplementation decreases remnant-like particle cholesterol and increases the (n-3) index in hypertriglyceridemic men. *J Nutr* 2008;138(1):30–35.

87. Maki KC, Dicklin MR, Davidson MH, Doyle RT, Ballantyne CM. Combination of prescription omega-3 with Simvastatin (COMBOS) investigators. *Am J Cardiol* 2010;105(10):1409–12.

88. Micallef MA and Garg ML. The lipid-lowering effects of phytosterols and (n-3) polyunsaturated fatty acids are synergistic and complementary in hyperlipidemic men and women. *J Nutr* 2008;138 (6):1085–90.

89. Mori TA, Burke V, Puddey IB, Watts GF, O'Neal DN, Best JD and Beilin LJ. Purified eicosapentaenoic and docosahexaenoic acids have differential effects on serum lipids and lipoproteins, LDL particle size, glucose and insulin in mildly hyperlipidemic men. *Am J Clin Nutr* 2000;71(5):1085–94.

90. Prasad K. Flaxseed and cardiovascular health. *J Cardiovasc Pharmacol* 2009;54(5):369–77.

91. Bioedon LT, Balkai S, Chittams J, Cunnane SC, Berlin JA, Rader DJ and Szapary PO. Flaxseed and cardiovascular risk factors: results from a double-blind, randomized controlled clinical trial. *J Am Coll Nutr* 2008;27(1):65–74.

92. Mandasescu S, Mocanu V, Dascalita AM, Haliga R, Nestian I, Stitt PA and Luca V. Flaxseed supplementation in hyperlipidemic patients. *Rev Med Chir Soc Med Nat Iasi* 2005;109(3):502–6.

93. Bester D, Esterhuyse AJ, Truter EJ, van Rooven J. Cardiovascular effects of edible oils: a comparison between four popular edible oils. *Nutr Res Rev* 2010;23(2):334–48.

94. Vafeiadou K, Weech M, Altowaijri H, Todd S, Yaqoob P, Jackson KG, Lovegrove JA. Replacement of saturated with unsaturated fats had no impact on vascular function but beneficial effects on lipid biomarkers, E-selectin, and blood pressure: results from the randomized, controlled Dietary Intervention and VAScular function (DIVAS) study. *Am J Clin Nutr* 2015;102(1):40–8.

95. Bogani P, Gali C, Villa M and Visioli F. Postprandial anti-inflammatory and antioxidant effects of extra virgin olive oil. *Atherosclerosis* 2007;190(1):181–6.

96. Reid K. Garlic lowers blood pressure in hypertensive individuals, regulates serum cholesterol, and stimulates immunity: an updated meta-analysis and review. *J Nutr* 2016;146(2):389S–96S.

97. Ried K, Toben C and Fakler P. Effect of garlic on serum lipids: an updated meta-analysis. *Nutr Rev* 2013;71(5):282–99.

98. Samavat H, Newman AR, Wang R, Yuan JM, Wu AH and Kurzer MS. Effects of green tea catechin extract on serum lipids in postmenopausal women: a randomized, placebo-controlled clinical trial. *Am J Clin Nutr* 2016;104(6):1671–1682.

99. Tinahones FJ, Rubio MA, Garrido-Sanchez L, Ruiz C, Cordillo E, Cabrerizo L and Cardona F. Green tea reduces LDL oxidizability and improves vascular function. *J Am Coll Nutr* 2008;27(2):209–13.

100. Brown AL, Lane J, Holyoak C, Nicol B, Mayes AE and Dadd T. Health effects of green tea catechins in overweight and obese men: a randomized controlled cross-over trial. *Br J Nut* 2011;7:1–10.

101. Zheng XX, Xu YL, Li SH, Liu XX, Hui R and Huang XH. Green tea intake lowers fasting serum total and LDL cholesterol in adults: a meta-analysis of 14 randomized controlled trials. *Am J Clin Nutr* 2011;94:601–10.

102. Cesar TB, Aptekman NP, Araujo MP, Vinagre CC and Maranhao RC. Orange juice decreases low-density lipoprotein cholesterol in hypercholesterolemic subjects and improves lipid transfer to high-density lipoprotein in normal and hypercholesterolemic subjects. *Nutr Res* 2010;30(10):689–94.

103. Mirmiran P, Fazeli MR, Asghari G, Shafiee A, Azizi F. Effect of pomegranate seed oil on hyperlipidaemic subjects: a double-blind placebo-controlled clinical trial. *Br J Nutr* 2010;104(3):402–6.

104. Fuhrman B, Volkova N and Aviram M. Pomegranate juice polyphenols increase recombinant paroxonase-1 binding to high density lipoprotein: studies in vitro and in diabetic patients. *Nutrition* 2010;26(4):359–366.

105. Avairam M, Rosenblat M, Gaitine D, Nitecki S, Hoffman A, Dornfeld L, Bolkova N, Presser D, Attias J, Liker H and Hayek T Pomegranate juice consumption for 3 years by patients with carotid artery stenosis reduces common carotid intima-media thickness, blood pressure and LDL oxidation. *Clin Nutr* 2004;23(3):423–33.

106. Mattiello T, Trifiro E, Jotti GS and Pulcinelli FM. Effects of pomegranate juice and extract polypyenols on platelet function. *J Med Food* 2009;12(2):334–9.

107. Aviram M, Dornfeld L, Rosenblat M, Volkova N, Kaplan M, Coleman R, Hayek T, Presser D and Fuhrman B. Pomegranate juice consumption reduces oxidative stress, atherogenic modifications to LDL, and platelet aggregation: studies in humans and in atherosclerotic apolipoprotein E-deficient mice. *Am J Clin Nutr* 2000;71(5):1062–76.

108. Davidson MH, Maki KC, Dicklin MR, Feinstein SB, Witcher M. Bell M, McGuire DK, Provost JC, Liker H and Aviram M. Effects of consumption of pomegranate juice on carotid intima-media thickness in men and women at moderate risk for coronary heart disease. *Am J Cardiol* 2009;104(7):936–42.

109. Devarajan S, Singh R, Chatterjee B, Zhang B and Ali A. A blend of sesame oil and rice bran oil lowers blood pressure and improves the lipid profile in mild-to-moderate hypertensive patients. *J Clin Lipidol* 2016;10(2):339–49.

110. Namiki M. Nutraceutical functions of sesame: a review. *Crit Rev food Sci Nutr* 2007;47(7):651–73.

111. Sacks FM, Lichtenstein A, Van Horn L, Harris W, Kris-Etherton P, Winston M and American Heart Association Nutrition Committee. Soy protein, isoflavones, and cardiovascular health: an American Heart Association Science Advisory for professionals from the Nutrition Committee. *Circulation* 2006;113(7):1034–44.

112. Harland JI and Haffner TA. Systemic review, meta-analysis and regression of randomized controlled trials reporting an association between an intake of circa 25 g soya protein per day and blood cholesterol. *Atherosclerosis* 2008;200(1):13–27.

113. Houston MC. Juice Powder concentrate and systemic blood pressure, progression of coronary artery cal-cium and antioxidant status in hypertensive subjects: a pilot study Evid based complementary. *Alternat Med* 2007;4(4):455–62.

114. Toth PP, Patti AM, Nikolic D, Giglio RV, Castellino G, Biancucci T, Geraci F, David S, Montalto G, Rizvi A and Rizzo M. Bergamot reduces plasma lipids, atherogenic small dense LDL, and subclinical atherosclerosis in subjects with moderate hypercholesterolemia: a 6 months prospective study. *Front Pharmacol* 2016;6:299.

115. Mollace V, Sacco I, Janda E, Malara C, Ventrice D, Colica C, Visalli C, Muscoli S, Ragusa S, Muscoli C, Rotiroti D and Romeo F. Hypolipidemic and hypoglycaemic activity of bergamot polyphenols: from animal models to human studies. *Fitotherapia* 2011;82(3): 309–16.

116. Soni KB and Kuttan R. Effect of oral curcumin administration on serum peroxides and cholesterol levels in human volunteers. *Indian J Physiol Pharmacol* 1992;36(4):273–5.

117. Ulbricht C, Basch E, Szapary P, Hammerness, P, Axentsev S, Boon H, Kroll D, Garraway L, Vora M, Woods J and Natural Standard Research Collaboration. Guggul for hyperlipidemia: a review by the Natural Standard Research Collaboration. *Complement Ther Med* 2005;13(4):279–90.

118. Nohr LA, Rasmussen LB and Straand J. Resin from the Mukul Myrrh tree, guggul, can it be used for treating hypercholesterolemia: a randomized, controlled study. *Complement Ther Med* 2009;17 (1):16–22.

119. McEneny J, Wade L, Young IS, Masson L, Duthie G, McGinty A, McMaster C and Thies F. Lycopene intervention reduces inflammation and improves HDL functionality in moderately overweight middle-aged individuals. *J Nutr Biochem* 2013;24(1):163–8.

120. Palozza P, Simone R, Gatalano A, Parrone N, Monego G and Ranelletti F. Lycopene regulation of cho-lesterol synthesis and efflux in human macrophages. *J Nutr Biochem* 2011;22: 971–978.

121. Ruparelia N, Digby JE, Choudhury RP. Effects of niacin on atherosclerosis and vascular function. *Curr Opin Cardiol* 2011;26(1):66–70.

122. Al-Mohissen MA, Pun SC and Frohlich JJ. Niacin: from mechanisms of action to therapeutic uses. *Mini Rev Med Chem* 2010;10(3):204–17.

123. Garg A, Sharma A, Krishnamoorthy P, Garg J, Virmani D, Sharma T, Stefanini G, Kostis JB, Mukherjee D and Sikorskaya E. Role of niacin in current clinical practice: a systematic review. *Am J Med* 2017;130(2):173–87.

124. Lavigne PM and Karas RH. The current state of niacin in cardiovascular disease prevention: a system-atic review and meta-regression. *J Am Coll Cardiol* 2013;61(4):440–6.

125. Khera AV, Qamar A, Reilly MP, Dunbar RL and Rader DJ. Effects of niacin, statin, and fenofibrate on circulating proprotein convertase subtilisin/kexin type 9 levels in patients with dyslipidemia. *Am J Cardiol* 2015;115(2):178–82.

126. Houston M and Pizzorno J. "Niacin doesn't work and is harmful/" proclaim the headlines. Yet another highly publicized questionable study to discredit integrative medicine. *Integr Med* 2014; 13(5):8–11.

127. AIM HIGH Investigators. The role of niacin in raising high density lipoprotein cholesterols to reduce cardiovascular events in patients with atherosclerotic cardiovascular disease and optimally treated low density lipoprotein cholesterol: baseline characteristics of study participants. The atherothrombosis intervention in metabolic syndrome with low HDL/high triglycerides: impact on Global Health out-comes (AIM-HIGH) trial. *Am Heart J* 2011;161(3):538–43.

128. McRae MP. Treatment of hyperlipoproteinemia with pantethine: a review and analysis of efficacy and tolerability. *Nutr Res* 2005;25:319–333.

129. Kelly G. Pantethine: a review of its biochemistry and therapeutic applications. *Altern Med Rev* 1997;2:365–377.

130. Rumberger JA, Napolitano J, Azumano I, Kamiya T and Evans M. Pantethine, a derivative of vitamin B(5) used as a nutritional supplement, favorably alters low-density lipoprotein cholesterol metabolism in low- to moderate-cardiovascular risk North American subjects: a triple-blinded placebo and diet-controlled investigation. *Nutr Res* 2011;31(8):608–15.

131. Evans M, Rumberger JA, Azumano I, Napolitano JJ, Citrolo D and Kamiya T. Pantethine, a derivative of vitamin B5, favorably alters total, LDL and non-HDL cholesterol in low to moderate cardiovascular risk subjects eligible for statin therapy: a triple-blinded placebo and diet-controlled investigation. *Vasc Health Risk Manag* 2014;10:89–100.

132. No Authors listed. Pantethine monograph. *Altern Med Rev* 2010;15(3):279–82.

133. Plat J, Baumgartner S and Mensink RP. Mechanisms underlying the health benefits of plant sterol and stanol ester consumption. *J AOAC Int* 2015;98(3):697–700.

134. Demonty I, Ras RT, van der Knaap HC, Duchateau GS, Meijer L, Zock PL, Geleijnse JM and Trautwein EA. Continuous dose response relationship of the LDL cholesterol lowering effect of phytosterol intake. *J Nutr* 2009;139(2):271–84.
135. Sabeva NS, McPhaul CM, Li X, Cory TJ, Feola DJ and Graf GA. Phytosterols differently influence ABC transporter expression, cholesterol efflux and inflammatory cytokine Secretion in macrophage foam cells. *J Nutr Biochem* 2011;22:777–783.
136. Kim JY, Kim SM, Kim SJ, Lee EY, Kim JR and Cho KH. Consumption of policosanol enhances HDL functionality via CETP inhibition and reduces blood pressure and visceral fat in young and middle-aged subjects. *Int J Mol Med* 2017;39(4):889–99.
137. Berthold HK, Unverdorben S, Degenhardt R, Bulitta M and Gourni-Berthold I. Effect of policosanol on lipid levels among patients with hypercholesterolemia or combined hyperlipidemia: a randomized controlled trial. *JAMA* 2006;295(19):2262–9.
138. Greyling A, De Witt C, Oosthuizen W and Jerling JC. Effects of a policosanol supplement on serum lipid concentrations in hypercholesterolemic and heterozygous familial hypercholesterolaemic subjects. *Br J Nutr* 2006;95(5):968–75.
139. Solomenchuk TM, Vosukh V, Bedzay A, Koval VG, Chepka IM and Trotsko VV. Efficiency of concomitant use of policosanol and rosuvastatin in patients with stable coronary artery disease and moderate hepatic dysfunction. *Lik Sprava.* 2015;7–8:29–37.
140. Qureshi AA, Sami SA, Salser WA and Khan FA. Synergistic effect of tocotrienol-rich fraction (TRF 25) of rice bran and lovastatin on lipid parameters in hypercholesterolemic humans. *J Nutr Biochem* 2001;12(6):318–29.
141. Prasad K. Tocotrienols and cardiovascular health. *Curr Pharm Des* 2011;17(21):2147–54.
142. Cicero AFG. Red yeast rice, monacolin K, and pleiotropic effects. *Recent Prog Med* 2018;109(2):154e–7e.
143. Xiong X, Wang P, Li X, Zhang Y and Li S. The effects of red yeast rice dietary supplement on blood pressure, lipid profile, and C-reactive protein in hypertension: a systematic review. *Crit Rev Food Sci Nutr* 2017;57(9):1831–51.
144. McRae MP. Vitamin C supplementation lowers serum low-density cholesterol and triglycerides: a meta-analysis of 13 randomized controlled trials. *J Chiropr Med* 2008;7(2):48–58.
145. McRae MP. The efficacy of vitamin C supplementation on reducing total serum cholesterol in human subjects: a review of 51 experimental trials. *J Chiropr Med* 2006;5(1):2–12.
146. Sahebkar A and Watts GF. Mode of action of berberine on lipid metabolism: a new-old phytochemical with clinical applications? *Curr Opin Lipidol* 2017;28(3):282–283.
147. Kong W, Wei J, Abidi P, Lin M, Inaba S, Li C, Wang Y, Wang Z, Si S, Pan H, Wang S, Wu J, Wang Y, Li Z, Liu J, Jiang JD. Berberine is a novel cholesterol-lowering drug working through a unique mechanism distinct from statins. *Nat Med* 2004;10(12):1344–51.
148. Dong H, Zhao Y, Zhao L, Lu F. The effects of berberine on blood lipids: a systemic review and meta-analysis of randomized controlled trials. *Planta Med* 2013;79(6):437–46.
149. McCarty MF, O'Keefe JH, DiNicolantonio JJ. Red yeast rice plus berberine: practical strategy for promoting vascular and metabolic health. *Altern Ther Health Med* 2015;21(Suppl 2):40–5.
150. Houston M and Sparks W. Effect of combination pantethine, plant sterols, green tea extract, delta-tocotrienol and phytolens on lipid profiles in patients with hyperlipidemia. *JANA* 2010;13(1):15–20.
151. Houston MC. Unpublished data. Personal Communication, 2017.
152. Houston M, Rountree R, Lamb J, Phipps S, Meng S and Zhang R. A placebo-controlled trial of a proprietary lipid-lowering nutraceutical supplement in the management of dyslipidemia. *J Biol Regul Homeost Agents* 2016;30(4):1115–23.
153. Studer M, Briel M, Leimenstoll B, Glass TR and Bucher HC. Effect of different anti-lipidemic agents and diets on mortality: a systemic review. *Arch Int Med* 2005; 165(7): 725–30.
154. Nijjar PS, Burke FM, Bioesch A and Rader DJ. Role of dietary supplements in lowering low-density lipoprotein cholesterol: a review. *J Clin Lipidol* 2010;4:248–58.
155. Cicero AFG, Colletti A, Bajraktari G, Descamps O, Djuric DM, Ezhov M, Fras Z, Katsiki N, Langlois M, Latkovskis G, Panagiotakos DB, Paragh G, Mikhailidis DP, Mitchenko O, Paulweber B, Pella D, Pitsavos C, Reiner Ž, Ray KK, Rizzo M, Sahebkar A, Serban MC, Sperling LS, Toth PP, Vinereanu D, Vrablík M, Wong ND and Banach M. Lipid lowering nutraceuticals in clinical practice: position paper from an International Lipid Expert Panel. *Arch Med Sci* 2017;13(5):965–1005.
156. Mannarino MR, Ministrini S and Pirro M. Nutraceuticals for the treatment of hypercholesterolemia. *Eur J Intern Med* 2014;25(7):592–9.

6 The Role of Nitric Oxide Supplements and Foods in Cardiovascular Disease

Nathan S. Bryan

Ernst R. von Schwarz

CONTENTS

Introduction..131
Loss of Nitric Oxide Production Is Responsible for CVD 132
Diet and Lifestyle Habits That Disrupt NO Production...133
     Standard American Diet..133
Use of Mouthwash and Antibiotics..134
Antacids Inhibit NO Production 135
Certain Food Patterns Increase NO Production 135
Resveratrol 136
Curcumin..136
Nitric Oxide Supplements...137
Conclusions..137
References..138

KEY POINTS

- Nitric oxide is essential for normal blood pressure and delivery of oxygen and nutrients to every cell in the body.
- Loss of nitric oxide production is recognized as the earliest event in the onset and progression of cardiovascular disease (CVD).
- Use of mouthwash, antacids and antibiotics inhibits nitric oxide production.
- Certain foods, dietary patterns and supplements have been clinically shown to improve nitric oxide production.
- Restoration of nitric oxide is the most important consideration in the prevention and treatment of CVD.

INTRODUCTION

Cardiovascular disease (CVD) has been and remains the number one killer of men and women worldwide accounting for nearly 18 million deaths every year representing 31% of all deaths. CVD is a class of disorders of the heart and all blood vessels throughout the body. Four out of five CVD-related deaths are due to heart attacks and strokes, and one-third of these deaths occur prematurely in people

DOI: 10.1201/9781003137849-6

under 70 years of age.[1] There are recognized risk factors for the development of CVD which include high blood pressure, obesity, diabetes, smoking and lack of physical exercise. Probably not coincidental, all of the above are either caused by lack of NO production or lead to the loss of NO production.[2] Each minute of every day someone dies from an event due to CVD. These statistics are unacceptable, especially since science has revealed the cause of CVD, loss of NO production, and that it can be mitigated by diet and lifestyle. Moderate physical exercise and a diet rich in vegetables is proven to prevent or even reverse heart disease.[3–5] The mechanism of action of both physical exercise and a vegetarian diet is activation and promotion of nitric oxide.[6–8] Hypertension, the number one risk factor for development of CVD, is poorly managed. In the United States, about 78 million (one out of every three) people have high blood pressure or hypertension. Another one out of three have pre-hypertension (CDC fact sheet). That puts over 200 million Americans at an increased risk for developing CVD. Despite major advances in understanding the pathophysiology of hypertension and availability of antihypertensive drugs, management of blood pressure is still not achieved, even with multiple drugs. According to the AHA 2015 Statistics Fact Sheet, 75% of Americans are aware of their hypertension and take medication to treat it. However, only about half of those are adequately managed. Since blood pressure remains elevated in approximately half of all treated hypertensive patients,[9,10] better and more effective strategies are needed. Better management of blood pressure reduces all-cause mortality.[11] Adding additional drug therapy is not the solution. Loss of nitric oxide production and signaling is the cause of hypertension.[12,13] Implementing food, supplements and lifestyle changes may prove to be the missing link in the eradication of CVD. This approach is supported by biochemical, physiological and epidemiological evidence. Identifying risk factors and ensuring those patients receive appropriate treatment can prevent premature deaths. Any treating physician should recognize NO as a primary cause of CVD, and implement strategies and drug therapy to positively restore NO production.

LOSS OF NITRIC OXIDE PRODUCTION IS RESPONSIBLE FOR CVD

Loss of endothelial NO production, termed endothelial dysfunction, precedes all other structural and biochemical changes that lead to CVD.[14] Getting older and hypertension are well-known risk factors.[15,16] The vascular changes that are hallmark of CVD, oxidative stress, immune dysfunction and inflammation, are similar in older patients that have aged normally without hypertension to those younger adults that have aged with high blood pressure.[17] Furthermore, the vascular dysfunction seen in essential hypertension is an accelerated form of vascular dysfunction seen with normal aging.[18] Young healthy individuals have normal and sufficient endothelial production of NO through L-arginine. However, as we age, we lose our ability to synthesize NO from L-arginine; this is termed endothelial dysfunction. This leads to oxidative stress through production of superoxide,[19] immune dysfunction and inflammation. Aging also causes a decrease in expression of the NO-producing enzyme.[20,21] There is also an upregulation of arginase (an enzyme that degrades the natural substrate for nitric oxide synthase (NOS), L-arginine) in the blood vessels as we age that causes a reduction in NO production[22] due to a shuttling of L-arginine away from the NOS enzyme. Aging leads to a gradual decline in NO production.[23] Some studies show a more than 75% loss of NO in the coronary circulation in patients in their 70s and 80s compared to younger patients.[24] Others have shown[25] that age is a strong predictor of NO production. These data clearly demonstrate that NO production from L-arginine declines as we get older. This is due to uncoupling of the NOS enzyme which is then unable to convert L-arginine into NO. This process can be accelerated or decelerated depending on diet and lifestyle. The majority of studies reveal that loss of NO production was clearly evident by 40 years of age. However, the vasodilation to exogenous NO (endothelium-independent vasodilation) does not change over time with aging, illustrating that the body does not lose its ability to respond to NO, but it only loses its ability to generate it with age. These observations allow scientists and physicians to conclude that reduced production of NO occurs as we age, and this creates the environment that is conducive to the onset and progression of CVD. This is illustrated in Figure 6.1.

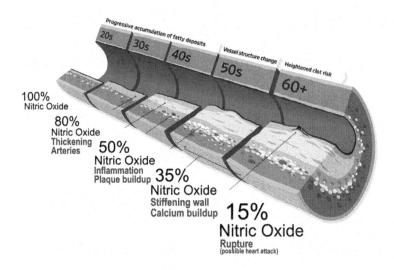

FIGURE 6.1 Fat deposition and increased thickness of the media along with plaque formation occurs as we age. Loss of endothelial nitric oxide production precedes structural changes that occur during progression of CVD.

DIET AND LIFESTYLE HABITS THAT DISRUPT NO PRODUCTION

STANDARD AMERICAN DIET

In addition to the oxidation of L-arginine by the NOS enzyme, nitric oxide can be produced through the serial reduction of inorganic nitrate from out diet (Figure 6.2).

Diet is the most important consideration for prevention and management of chronic disease. The Mediterranean diet, Japanese diet, plant-based diet and even the Dietary Approaches to Stop Hypertension (DASH) diet are scientifically and clinically proven to prevent and even reverse heart disease. There are many studies now revealing that the mechanism of action of all of these diets is from inorganic nitrate and nitrite found in these dietary patterns and foods.[8] These studies establish that 300–400 mg of nitrate per meal is required to see any changes in blood pressure or improvements in exercise performance.[8] This can be achieved through the consumption of specific nitrate-rich foods, such as spinach, beets, kale and other green leafy vegetables. However, there is more than tenfold difference in nitrate content of the same vegetable across different geographical regions in the United States and also more than tenfold difference between nitrate contents of different vegetables.[26] Interestingly, organically grown vegetables have much less nitrate than conventionally grown, in some cases up to ten times less. Based on existing databases, the estimated intake for nitrate and nitrite in the United States for a Western-type diet is about 40–100 mg/day.[27,28] We know from above that 300–400 mg as a bolus is required to see any improvement in NO production. Americans are only consuming about a third of what is required. Therefore, the US diet is depleted in nitrate, and as a result, Americans are a nitrate-deficient society. The research suggests that this deficiency may be partly responsible for the increased incidence of all CVDs in the US population.[29] This deficiency may be due to insufficient vegetable consumption, lack of nitrate in organically grown vegetables or cooking techniques such as boiling vegetables that remove any water-soluble minerals such as nitrate.

The standard American diet (SAD) is also enriched in simple carbohydrates and high sugar. Excess carbohydrate or sugar consumption leads to advanced glycosylation end-products (AGEs).

Two **Nitric Oxide** Production Pathways

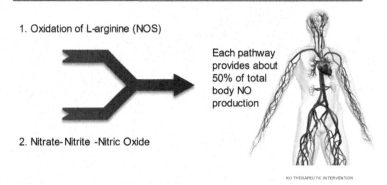

1. Oxidation of L-arginine (NOS)

Each pathway provides about 50% of total body NO production

2. Nitrate- Nitrite -Nitric Oxide

NO THERAPEUTIC INTERVENTION

FIGURE 6.2 There are two primary production pathways in the human body. The first pathway is through the enzymatic oxidation of L-arginine by the NOS enzyme. The second pathway is through the serial reduction of inorganic nitrate (found primarily in green leafy vegetables) to nitrite and nitric oxide from commensal bacteria. One can compensate for the other. When both systems fail, disease ensues.

AGEs reduce the production and activity of NO. NO inhibits many of the mechanisms that lead to CVD, such as leukocyte adhesion to the vessel wall, vascular smooth muscle growth, and platelet adhesion and aggregation. The NO inhibitory effect of AGEs on NO will accelerate CVD.[30] In fact, studies reveal that AGEs inhibit the antiproliferative effects of NO.[31] Moreover, impaired vasodilation in diabetes may be a result of AGEs' reduction of NO activity.[30] Mechanistically, it is clear that AGEs reduce the half-life of endothelial NO synthase (eNOS) mRNA through an increased rate of mRNA degradation and reduced eNOS activity.[32] Another mechanism proposes that AGEs impair NO production by causing a reduction in phosphorylation of serine residues in eNOS, resulting in deactivation of the enzyme.[33] AGEs may also quench and inactivate endothelium-derived NO.[30] AGE formation from high sugar and carbohydrate intake also results in the production of reactive oxygen species through the activation of nicotinamide adenine dinucleotide phosphate (NADPH) oxidase.[34]

The lack of consumption of plants and vegetables that contain inorganic nitrate combined with the high sugar and carbohydrate intake of the Western diet leads to a complete disruption of NO production, and the consequences are obvious.

USE OF MOUTHWASH AND ANTIBIOTICS

We now know an American diet is devoid of nitrate and replete with glycosylating sugars, both of which disrupt NO production. However, it gets worse. Even if you do consume a plant-based diet and get regular physical exercise, if you use mouthwash, you abolish the benefits of both. The NO effects of dietary nitrate are completely abolished if mouthwash is used which disrupts the oral microbiome.[35–38] Kapil demonstrated that use of antiseptic mouthwash for 7 days caused a decrease in salivary and plasma nitrite with a concomitant increase in systolic and diastolic blood pressures.[36] Increases in salivary and plasma levels of nitrite are completely abolished in subjects that use an antiseptic mouthwash,[35] which demonstrates that the removal of these bacteria with an antibacterial mouthwash will very likely attenuate the NO-dependent biological effects of dietary nitrate. Over 180 million Americans use mouthwash on a daily basis, and between 2000 and 2015, antibiotic consumption, expressed in defined daily doses (DDD), increased 65% (21.1–34.8 billion DDDs), and the antibiotic consumption rate increased 39% (11.3–15.7 DDDs per 1,000 inhabitants per day). CDC estimates that about 47 million antibiotic courses are prescribed each year for infections that don't need antibiotics, which represents that about 30% of these antibiotic prescriptions were unnecessary.[39] In 2015 alone, approximately 269 million antibiotic prescriptions were dispensed from outpatient pharmacies in the United States, enough for five out of every six people to receive one antibiotic prescription each year. Use of both antiseptic mouthwash and antibiotics disrupts the oral microbiome and leads to a complete lack of nitrate reduction or at least a decreased efficiency of nitrate reduction. Also given the diversity and variability of the oral microbiome between certain individuals and cultures, it is uncertain how many people have the correct nitrate-reducing bacteria.[40] With the prevalence of antibiotic and antiseptic mouthwash use in the United States along with periodontal disease due to poor oral hygiene, it would not be surprising if over half of the population is unable to reduce dietary nitrate. This means that although they may be consuming what is considered a healthy diet even with sufficient nitrate, they are unable to get a nitric oxide benefit due to lack of nitrate reduction by bacteria. This should be a new consideration in patient assessment.

ANTACIDS INHIBIT NO PRODUCTION

Even if you have the right oral nitrate-reducing bacteria, this does not always mean you will get a benefit from the nitrate consumed in your diet that is then reduced to nitrite. Stomach acid is required for optimal effects of salivary nitrite that results from consuming dietary nitrate. Nitrite concentration in the saliva from reduction of dietary nitrite when swallowed becomes protonated (nitrite pKa ~ 3.4) to form nitrous acid. Nitrous acid can spontaneously release NO.[41] Proton pump inhibitors (PPIs), by inhibiting stomach acid production and increasing gastric pH, may prevent formation of nitrous acid from inorganic nitrite, and, accordingly, NO release. Indeed, giving PPIs to rodents blocks the blood pressure-lowering effects of orally administered sodium nitrite.[42] Furthermore, PPIs blunt the favorable effects of antioxidants on nitrite-to-NO conversion in the stomach[43] and disrupts the formation of S-nitrosothiols. S-nitrosothiols are an important circulating reservoir of NO that also contributes to the blood pressure-lowering effects of orally administrated nitrates/nitrites.[44] PPIs also specifically lead to the accumulation of asymmetric dimethyl L-arginine (ADMA).[45] ADMA is generated during metabolism of cellular proteins containing methyl-arginine residues. ADMA is broken down by the enzyme dimethylarginine dimethylaminohydrolase,[46] an intracellular enzyme ubiquitously expressed in many cells. The inhibition of the dimethylarginine dimethylaminohydrolase (DDAH) enzyme is known to be the major contributor to increases in ADMA in animal models and patients with cardiovascular risk factors.[47,48] Evidence now reveals that PPI drugs directly inhibit DDAH activity.[49] In addition to inhibiting DDAH, PPIs affect NOS expression. Both phosphorylated (active) and unphosphorylated endothelial NOS proteins are downregulated by omeprazole.[49] Altogether, these findings provide a proof-of-concept that PPIs are able to impair nitric oxide pathway in the endothelium as well as NO production from the nitrate-nitrite-NO pathway. There are approximately 64.6 million prescriptions written for gastroesophageal reflux disease (GERD) medications in the United States on an annual basis,[68] accounting for over $11 billion in total healthcare expenditures in the United States, and this does not even include the over the counter (OTC) market. Any therapy that increases stomach pH will interrupt NO generation from salivary nitrite. Clear evidence is emerging that PPIs have adverse cardiovascular effects. These effects may be mediated primarily or at least in part through a disruption in NO production/signaling and should be considered when PPIs are prescribed, especially, in patients at increased cardiovascular risk.

CERTAIN FOOD PATTERNS INCREASE NO PRODUCTION

Epidemiological evidence reveal that diets such as the Mediterranean diet, Japanese diet and plant-based diet are healthy and prevent CVD and even cancer. It is clear that the mechanism of these dietary patterns is promoted to produce NO by inorganic nitrate content combined with antioxidants. Consistent with this notion, certain diets provide much more nitrate. For example, the DASH diet can provide as much as 1,200 mg nitrate per day from selection of certain foods.[50] The Japanese diet also provides sufficient nitrate that has been shown to reduced blood pressure and improve athletic performance.[51] Similarly, the Mediterranean diet provides sufficient nitrate along with antioxidants to support reduction of nitrate to nitrite and nitric oxide.[52] There is strong evidence that it is the inorganic nitrate in these foods and diets that confers the protective and health-promoting activities.[29] Although many clinical trials have been performed to try to identify the mechanism of action of these diets, looking primarily at antioxidants, vitamins and minerals, most if not all have failed to recapitulate the effects of the whole food diets. Evidence strongly suggests that it is the nitrate/nitrite content along with the antioxidants that accounts for the effects.

Although it is difficult, if not impossible, to ensure you are getting sufficient nitrate from you diet, you can supplement with standardized nitrate and/or nitrite dietary supplements or nutritional products. One should look for products with a known and standardized amount of nitrate or products backed by published clinical trials. Such products are Superbeets Original, BeetElite, Beet It, Berkeley Life and Resync.

RESVERATROL

Resveratrol (*trans*-3, 4′, 5-trihydroxystilbene) is a non-flavonoid polyphenol mainly found in grapes, berries, peanuts and medicinal plants.[53] Red wine is an important and common source of resveratrol due to the high concentrations found in grape skin.[54] It became popular as a result of epidemiological studies linking red wine consumption to reduced mortality of the French population from CVDs. Resveratrol was identified as the source of beneficial properties of red wine.[55] Resveratrol protects the cardiovascular system in several ways but primarily through an increase in the production and bioavailability of NO. Resveratrol acts to stimulate and activate endothelial production of NO, reduce oxidative stress, inhibit vascular inflammation and prevent platelet aggregation.[56] Several in vitro studies demonstrate that resveratrol inhibits oxygen free radical formation by inhibiting NADPH oxidases and subsequent reactive oxygen species production.[57] Similarly, resveratrol induces the expression of antioxidative enzymes and their substrates, thereby contributing to the overall reduction in oxidative stress. Resveratrol upregulates endothelial NOS (eNOS) expression and subsequent NO production from endothelial cells.[58] Additionally, resveratrol exerts beneficial cardiovascular effects by inhibiting platelet aggregation.[55] By decreasing oxidative stress, disrupting proinflammatory pathways, minimizing endothelial dysfunction and inhibiting platelet aggregation, resveratrol promotes NO production and confers cardioprotective characteristics. To support this, in a study assessing the effect of resveratrol on endothelial function,[59] patients with metabolic syndrome and associated cardiovascular risk factors were followed for 6 months where treatment with 100 mg resveratrol was given for 3 months and then discontinued for 3 months. Endothelial function was measured using flow mediated dilatation (FMD). Patients receiving treatment showed marked improvement of endothelial function, with an FMD increasing from 4% to 9%, a more than doubling of endothelial function. The treatment showed no significant changes on blood pressure, insulin resistance, lipid profile or inflammatory markers. The study demonstrated improved endothelial function with standard resveratrol treatment.

CURCUMIN

Curcumin is a naturally occurring phenolic compound that is the active ingredient of the spice turmeric. Turmeric has been used for centuries in traditional medicine to treat various human ailments. Modern science has attributed the anti-inflammatory properties of turmeric to curcumin, a diferuloylmethane. The health benefits seen with curcumin can be attributed to anti-inflammation, antioxidation, cardiovascular protection, immunomodulation, enhancement of the apoptotic process and antiangiogenic properties. Oxidative stress is present in all forms of CVD, particularly in the development of atherosclerosis. The phenolic group on the structural component of curcumin is critical to the antioxidant and reactive oxygen species scavenging properties of curcumin.[60] Curcumin's effect on oxidative stress may also be due to the fact that oxidative antioxidant enzymes are augmented by curcumin and effectively inhibit the oxidation and modification of LDL which is shown to significantly reduce atherosclerotic lesions.[60] In another human clinical trial, 39 healthy men and postmenopausal women between ages 45 and 74 years were given either 2,000 mg/day of Longvida curcumin ($n=20$) or placebo ($n=19$) for 12 weeks. Resistant artery endothelium-dependent dilation (EDD) and independent dilation were tested by measuring forearm blood flow after acetylcholine infusions using strain gauge venous occlusion plethysmography. Although curcumin did not seem to have an effect on large elastic artery stiffness ($P>0.1$), subjects treated with curcumin demonstrated improvement in resistance artery endothelial function with a 36% increase of endothelial function versus no change in the placebo group. Subjects using curcumin presented with greater NO bioavailability, and reduced vascular oxidative stress.[61]

NITRIC OXIDE SUPPLEMENTS

Collectively, the evidence suggests that the US diet is deficient in nitrate. Products that contain a standardized amount of nitrate to replace what is missing in our diet is a great first approach. Berkeley Life nitrate capsule provides a safe and effective dose of nitrate shown to normalize blood pressure and improve athletic performance. Common drug therapy and lifestyle decisions disrupt metabolism of nitrate into nitrite and nitric oxide. So, how does one overcome deficiencies in dietary nitrate, variability between individual microbiome, mouthwash use, PPI use or achlorhydria? In addition to the Berkeley Life nitrate capsule, consider a product that actually delivers NO gas. Although there are many products sold on the market as nitric oxide products, there are only a handful that are patented and clinically proven to restore and/or generate nitric oxide. Neo40 and Superbeets are examples. Neo40™ and HumanN, Inc.™ are 15 mg of supplemental sodium nitrite to account for missing nitrite due to differences in endogenous production or use of mouthwash or antibiotics. Neo40 also has an active nitrite reductase that helps facilitate nitrite reduction to NO along the physiological oxygen gradient. Neo40 has also been shown to improve cardiovascular risk factors in patients over the age of 40, significantly reduce triglycerides, and normalize blood pressure.[61] In pediatric patients with argininosuccinic aciduria (ASA), the Neo40 lozenge shows a statistically significant reduction in blood pressure when prescription medications were ineffective. Results also demonstrated an improvement in renal function, cognition and even reversed cardiac hypertrophy.[62] In a study in unmedicated hypertensive patients, Neo40 significantly reduced blood pressure, dilated blood vessels by as much as 13% within 10 minutes and significantly improved endothelial function and arterial compliance.[63] Furthermore, in pre-hypertensive patients (BP >120/80< 139/89), administration of one lozenge twice daily for 30 days showed a significant reduction in blood pressure (12 mmHg systolic and 6 mmHg diastolic)[64] as well as improvements in functional capacity of the heart as measured by a 6-minute walk test. In an exercise study of well-trained athletes, Neo40 significantly improved performance.[65] Neo40 has also been shown to cause a 11% reduction in carotid plaque after 6 months.[66] To put this in perspective, a meta-analysis of trials using treatment with statins (mean treatment duration of 25.6 months) reveals that a total of seven trials showed regression and four trials showed slowdown of the progression of carotid intima media thickness (CIMT) of approximately 2.7% (−0.04) after over 2 years.[67] Using Neo40, the data show an average of 0.073 mm or 10.9% after 6 months.[66] Similarly, the same patented technology in the form of a concentrated beet root powder (Superbeets™, HumanN, Inc.™) attenuates peripheral chemoreflex sensitivity without concomitant change in spontaneous cardiovagal baroreflex sensitivity while also reducing systemic blood pressure and mean arterial blood pressure in older adults.[68] These studies clearly demonstrate the safety and efficacy of specific nitric oxide supplements in humans that can correct for any insufficiencies from dietary exposure, pharmacological inhibition by antiseptics or PPIs.

CONCLUSIONS

We have made very little progress on combating CVD and early deaths from CVD over the past few decades, despite enormous innovations in imaging, diagnostic biomarkers and recognition of

TABLE 6.1

Clinical Benefits of Nitric Oxide

Benefits of Nitric Oxide

Maintains normal blood pressure

Inhibits platelet aggregation

Prevents oxidative stress

Inhibits immune dysfunction

Mitigates inflammation

Facilitates oxygen delivery from hemoglobin

Anti-microbial

the cause of CVD. It may be due to the fact that no prescription therapeutic used in the treatment of CVD is directed toward restoration of NO. Furthermore, it appears that the everyday lifestyle of most Americans is directed toward disrupting NO production from our poor diet to use of mouthwash, antacids and antibiotics. If we are to effectively combat CVD, we must first stop doing the things that disrupt NO production and start implementing safe and effective strategies that are clinically shown to improve NO production. There are clinically and scientifically proven benefits of nitric oxide. These benefits are summarized in Table 6.1. There are simple steps one can take that can have a profound impact on public health. Physicians should recommend all patients stop using mouthwash, wean patients off antacids and only use antibiotics when necessary. Changes in diet, including cost-effective supplementation of resveratrol, curcumin and nitric oxide products, can and will have a positive impact on our global war on CVD. Science favors this approach.

REFERENCES

1. Mensah GA, Roth GA, Fuster V. The global burden of cardiovascular diseases and risk factors: 2020 and beyond. *J Am Coll Cardiol* 2019;74:2529–32.
2. Torregrossa AC, Aranke M, Bryan NS. Nitric oxide and geriatrics: implications in diagnostics and treatment of the elderly. *J Geriatr Cardiol* 2011;8:230–42.
3. Tuso P, Stoll SR, Li WW. A plant-based diet, atherogenesis, and coronary artery disease prevention. *Perm J* 2015;19:62–7.
4. Cooper KH, Pollock ML, Martin RP, White SR, Linnerud AC, Jackson A. Physical fitness levels vs selected coronary risk factors. A cross-sectional study. *JAMA* 1976;236:166–9.
5. Blair SN, Kohl HW, 3rd, Paffenbarger RS, Jr., Clark DG, Cooper KH, Gibbons LW. Physical fitness and all-cause mortality. A prospective study of healthy men and women. *JAMA* 1989;262:2395–401.
6. Rassaf T, Lauer T, Heiss C, et al. Nitric oxide synthase-derived plasma nitrite predicts exercise capacity. *Br J Sports Med* 2007;41:669–73; discussion 73.
7. Green DJ, O'Driscoll G, Blanksby BA, Taylor RR. Control of skeletal muscle blood flow during dynamic exercise: contribution of endothelium-derived nitric oxide. *Sports Med* 1996;21:119–46.
8. Bryan NS, Ivy JL. Inorganic nitrite and nitrate: evidence to support consideration as dietary nutrients. *Nutr Res* 2015;35:643–54.
9. Wang YR, Alexander GC, Stafford RS. Outpatient hypertension treatment, treatment intensification, and control in Western Europe and the United States. *Arch Intern Med* 2007;167:141–7.
10. Cutler JA, Sorlie PD, Wolz M, Thom T, Fields LE, Roccella EJ. Trends in hypertension prevalence, awareness, treatment, and control rates in United States adults between 1988–1994 and 1999–2004. *Hypertension* 2008;52:818–27.
11. Wright JT, Jr., Williamson JD, Whelton PK, et al. A randomized trial of intensive versus standard blood-pressure control. *N Engl J Med* 2015;373:2103–16.
12. Arnold WP, Mittal CK, Katsuki S, Murad F. Nitric oxide activates guanylate cyclase and increases guanosine 3':5'-cyclic monophosphate levels in various tissue preparations. *Proc Natl Acad Sci U S A* 1977;74:3203–7.

13. Bryan NS, Bian K, Murad F. Discovery of the nitric oxide signaling pathway and targets for drug development. *Front Biosci* 2009;14:1–18.
14. Vita JA, Treasure CB, Nabel EG, et al. Coronary vasomotor response to acetylcholine relates to risk factors for coronary artery disease. *Circulation* 1990;81:491–7.
15. Lakatta EG, Yin FC. Myocardial aging: functional alterations and related cellular mechanisms. *Am J Physiol* 1982;242:H927–41.
16. Kannel WB, Gordon T, Schwartz MJ. Systolic versus diastolic blood pressure and risk of coronary heart disease. The Framingham study. *Am J Cardiol* 1971;27:335–46.
17. Ross R. Atherosclerosis—an inflammatory disease. *N Engl J Med* 1999;340:115–26.
18. Soltis EE. Effect of age on blood pressure and membrane-dependent vascular responses in the rat. *Circ Res* 1987;61:889–97.
19. van der Loo B, Labugger R, Skepper JN, et al. Enhanced peroxynitrite formation is associated with vascular aging. *J Exp Med* 2000;192:1731–44.
20. Pie JE, Baek SY, Kim HP, et al. Age-related decline of inducible nitric oxide synthase gene expression in primary cultured rat hepatocytes. *Mol cells* 2002;13:399–406.
21. Zhou XJ, Vaziri ND, Zhang J, Wang HW, Wang XQ. Association of renal injury with nitric oxide deficiency in aged SHR: prevention by hypertension control with AT1 blockade. *Kidney Int* 2002;62:914–21.
22. Berkowitz DE, White R, Li D, et al. Arginase reciprocally regulates nitric oxide synthase activity and contributes to endothelial dysfunction in aging blood vessels. *Circulation* 2003;108:2000–6.
23. Taddei S, Virdis A, Ghiadoni L, et al. Age-related reduction of NO availability and oxidative stress in humans. *Hypertension* 2001;38:274–9.
24. Egashira K, Inou T, Hirooka Y, et al. Effects of age on endothelium-dependent vasodilation of resistance coronary artery by acetylcholine in humans. *Circulation* 1993;88:77–81.
25. Gerhard M, Roddy MA, Creager SJ, Creager MA. Aging progressively impairs endothelium-dependent vasodilation in forearm resistance vessels of humans. *Hypertension* 1996;27:849–53.
26. Nunez de Gonzalez MT, Osburn WN, Hardin MD, et al. A survey of nitrate and nitrite concentrations in conventional and organic-labeled raw vegetables at retail. *J Food Sci* 2015;80:C942–9.
27. Mensinga TT, Speijers GJ, Meulenbelt J. Health implications of exposure to environmental nitrogenous compounds. *Toxicol Rev* 2003;22:41–51.
28. Gangolli SD, van den Brandt PA, Feron VJ, et al. Nitrate, nitrite and N-nitroso compounds. *Eur J Pharmacol* 1994;292:1–38.
29. Lundberg JO, Feelisch M, Bjorne H, Jansson EA, Weitzberg E. Cardioprotective effects of vegetables: is nitrate the answer? *Nitric Oxide* 2006;15:359–62.
30. Bucala R, Tracey KJ, Cerami A. Advanced glycosylation products quench nitric oxide and mediate defective endothelium-dependent vasodilatation in experimental diabetes. *J Clin Invest* 1991;87:432–8.
31. Hogan M, Cerami A, Bucala R. Advanced glycosylation endproducts block the antiproliferative effect of nitric oxide. Role in the vascular and renal complications of diabetes mellitus. *J Clin Invest* 1992;90:1110–5.
32. Rojas A, Romay S, Gonzalez D, Herrera B, Delgado R, Otero K. Regulation of endothelial nitric oxide synthase expression by albumin-derived advanced glycosylation end products. *Circ Res* 2000;86:E50–4.
33. Xu B, Chibber R, Ruggiero D, Kohner E, Ritter J, Ferro A. Impairment of vascular endothelial nitric oxide synthase activity by advanced glycation end products. *FASEB J* 2003;17:1289–91.
34. Yan SD, Schmidt AM, Anderson GM, et al. Enhanced cellular oxidant stress by the interaction of advanced glycation end products with their receptors/binding proteins. *J Biol Chem* 1994;269:9889–97.
35. Govoni M, Jansson EA, Weitzberg E, Lundberg JO. The increase in plasma nitrite after a dietary nitrate load is markedly attenuated by an antibacterial mouthwash. *Nitric Oxide* 2008;19:333–7.
36. Kapil V, Haydar SM, Pearl V, Lundberg JO, Weitzberg E, Ahluwalia A. Physiological role for nitrate-reducing oral bacteria in blood pressure control. *Free Radic Biol Med* 2013;55:93–100.
37. Petersson J, Carlstrom M, Schreiber O, et al. Gastroprotective and blood pressure lowering effects of dietary nitrate are abolished by an antiseptic mouthwash. *Free Radic Biol Med* 2009;46:1068–75.
38. Webb AJ, Patel N, Loukogeorgakis S, et al. Acute blood pressure lowering, vasoprotective, and antiplatelet properties of dietary nitrate via bioconversion to nitrite. *Hypertension* 2008;51:784–90.
39. Fleming-Dutra KE, Hersh AL, Shapiro DJ, et al. Prevalence of inappropriate antibiotic prescriptions among US Ambulatory Care Visits, 2010–2011. *JAMA* 2016;315:1864–73.
40. Hyde ER, Andrade F, Vaksman Z, et al. Metagenomic analysis of nitrate-reducing bacteria in the oral cavity: implications for nitric oxide homeostasis. *PLoS One* 2014;9:e88645.
41. Lundberg JO, Weitzberg E, Lundberg JM, Alving K. Intragastric nitric oxide production in humans: measurements in expelled air. *Gut* 1994;35:1543–6.

42. Pinheiro LC, Montenegro MF, Amaral JH, Ferreira GC, Oliveira AM, Tanus-Santos JE. Increase in gastric pH reduces hypotensive effect of oral sodium nitrite in rats. *Free Radic Biol Med* 2012; 53:701–9.

43. Amaral JH, Montenegro MF, Pinheiro LC, et al. TEMPOL enhances the antihypertensive effects of sodium nitrite by mechanisms facilitating nitrite-derived gastric nitric oxide formation. *Free Radic Biol Med* 2013;65:446–55.

44. Pinheiro LC, Amaral JH, Ferreira GC, et al. Gastric S-nitrosothiol formation drives the antihypertensive effects of oral sodium nitrite and nitrate in a rat model of renovascular hypertension. *Free Radic Biol Med* 2015;87:252–62.

45. Porst H, Padma-Nathan H, Giuliano F, Anglin G, Varanese L, Rosen R. Efficacy of tadalafil for the treatment of erectile dysfunction at 24 and 36 hours after dosing: a randomized controlled trial. *Urology* 2003;62:121–5; discussion 5–6.

46. Perros F, Ranchoux B, Izikki M, et al. Nebivolol for improving endothelial dysfunction, pulmonary vascular remodeling, and right heart function in pulmonary hypertension. *J Am Coll Cardiol* 2015;65:668–80.

47. Cooke JP, Ghebremariam YT. DDAH says NO to ADMA. *Arterioscler Thromb Vasc Biol* 2011;31:1462–4.

48. Dayoub H, Achan V, Adimoolam S, et al. Dimethylarginine dimethylaminohydrolase regulates nitric oxide synthesis: genetic and physiological evidence. *Circulation* 2003;108:3042–7.

49. Ghebremariam YT, LePendu P, Lee JC, et al. Unexpected effect of proton pump inhibitors: elevation of the cardiovascular risk factor asymmetric dimethylarginine. *Circulation* 2013;128:845–53.

50. Hord NG, Tang Y, Bryan NS. Food sources of nitrates and nitrites: the physiologic context for potential health benefits. *Am J Clin Nutr* 2009;90:1–10.

51. Sobko T, Marcus C, Govoni M, Kamiya S. Dietary nitrate in Japanese traditional foods lowers diastolic blood pressure in healthy volunteers. *Nitric Oxide* 2010;22:136–40.

52. Nadtochiy SM, Redman EK. Mediterranean diet and cardioprotection: the role of nitrite, polyunsaturated fatty acids, and polyphenols. *Nutrition* 2011;27:733–44.

53. Baur JA, Sinclair DA. Therapeutic potential of resveratrol: the in vivo evidence. *Nat Rev Drug Discov* 2006;5:493–506.

54. Smoliga JM, Baur JA, Hausenblas HA. Resveratrol and health—a comprehensive review of human clinical trials. *Mol Nutr Food Res* 2011;55:1129–41.

55. Tome-Carneiro J, Larrosa M, Gonzalez-Sarrias A, Tomas-Barberan FA, Garcia-Conesa MT, Espin JC. Resveratrol and clinical trials: the crossroad from in vitro studies to human evidence. *Curr Pharm Des* 2013;19:6064–93.

56. Li H, Xia N, Forstermann U. Cardiovascular effects and molecular targets of resveratrol. *Nitric Oxide* 2012;26:102–10.

57. Yousefian M, Shakour N, Hosseinzadeh H, Hayes AW, Hadizadeh F, Karimi G. The natural phenolic compounds as modulators of NADPH oxidases in hypertension. *Phytomedicine* 2019;55:200–13.

58. Wallerath T, Deckert G, Ternes T, et al. Resveratrol, a polyphenolic phytoalexin present in red wine, enhances expression and activity of endothelial nitric oxide synthase. *Circulation* 2002;106:1652–8.

59. Fujitaka K, Otani H, Jo F, et al. Modified resveratrol Longevinex improves endothelial function in adults with metabolic syndrome receiving standard treatment. *Nutr Res* 2011;31:842–7.

60. Motterlini R, Foresti R, Bassi R, Green CJ. Curcumin, an antioxidant and anti-inflammatory agent, induces heme oxygenase-1 and protects endothelial cells against oxidative stress. *Free Radic Biol Med* 2000;28:1303–12.

61. Zand J, Lanza F, Garg HK, Bryan NS. All-natural nitrite and nitrate containing dietary supplement promotes nitric oxide production and reduces triglycerides in humans. *Nutr Res* 2011;31:262–9.

62. Nagamani SC, Campeau PM, Shchelochkov OA, et al. Nitric-oxide supplementation for treatment of long-term complications in argininosuccinic aciduria. *Am J Hum Genet* 2012;90:836–46.

63. Houston M, Hays L. Acute effects of an oral nitric oxide supplement on blood pressure, endothelial function, and vascular compliance in hypertensive patients. *J Clin Hypertens (Greenwich)* 2014; 16:524–9.

64. Biswas OS, Gonzalez VR, Schwarz ER. Effects of an oral nitric oxide supplement on functional capacity and blood pressure in adults with prehypertension. *J Cardiovasc Pharmacol Ther* 2015;20:52–58.

65. Lee J, Kim HT, Solares GJ, Kim K, Ding Z, Ivy JL. Caffeinated nitric oxide-releasing lozenge improves cycling time trial performance. *Int J Sports Med* 2015;36:107–12.

66. Lee E. Effects of nitric oxide on carotid intima media thickness: a pilot study. *Altern Ther Health Med* 2016;22:32–4.

67. Bedi US, Singh M, Singh PP, et al. Effects of statins on progression of carotid atherosclerosis as measured by carotid intimal–medial thickness: a meta-analysis of randomized controlled trials. *J Cardiovasc Pharmacol Ther* 2010;15:268–73.

68. Bock JM, Ueda K, Schneider AC, et al. Inorganic nitrate supplementation attenuates peripheral chemoreflex sensitivity but does not improve cardiovagal baroreflex sensitivity in older adults. *Am J Physiol Heart Circ Physiol* 2018;314:H45–51. doi:10.1152/ajpheart.00389.2017.

7 The Treatment of Hypertension with Nutrition, Nutritional Supplements, Lifestyle and Pharmacologic Therapies

Mark C. Houston

CONTENTS

Introduction 144
Epidemiology and Pathophysiology 145
The Three Finite Vascular Responses and Cardiovascular Disease (Figures 7.1 and 7.2) 145
    Oxidative Stress, Inflammation and Vascular Immune Dysfunction 145
The Balance of Hypertension 147
Treatment of Hypertension with Nutrition and Nutritional Supplements 148
Sodium (Na⁺) — $Sodium (Na^+)$ 150
Potassium 150
Magnesium (Mg^{++}) 151
Calcium (Ca^{++}) 151
Zinc (Zn^{++}) 151
Protein 151
L-Arginine 152
Taurine 153
Omega-3 Fats and Selected Omega-6 Fats 153
Monounsaturated Fatty Acids (MUFA): Olive Oil, Mediterranean Diet, Omega-9 Fats,
    Oleic Acid and Olive Leaf Extract 154
Vitamin C 154
Vitamin E 155
Vitamin D 155
Vitamin B6 (Pyridoxine) 156
Flavonoids: Resveratrol and Pomegranate 156
    Lycopene 157
    Coenzyme Q10 (Ubiquinone) 157
    Alpha Lipoic Acid 158
    Pycnogenol 158
    Garlic 158
    Seaweed 159
Cocoa: Dark Chocolate 159
Melatonin 159

DOI: 10.1201/9781003137849-7

Grape Seed Extract 160
Dietary Nitrates and Nitrites: Beetroot Juice and Extract... 160
Teas 161
L-Carnitine and Acetyl–L-Carnitine 161
    Fiber.. 162
    Sesame 162
Hesperidin.. 162
N-Acetylcysteine (NAC)... 162
Hawthorn.. 163
Quercetin.. 163
Probiotics 163
Drug Therapy for Hypertension... 164
Clinical Considerations... 166
Summary 166
References... 171

INTRODUCTION

Cardiovascular disease (CVD) remains the leading cause of death in the United States and is the most common reason for visits to primary care physicians [1–19]. The annual expenditure in the United States is over 20 billion USD for antihypertensive drugs [1–19]. Hypertension is one of the top five coronary heart disease (CHD) risk factors [1–19]. At this time, there are over 100 million people in the United States with hypertension based on recent hypertension guidelines [19]. In numerous clinical trials, pharmacotherapy will control blood pressure (BP) and reduce stroke, CHD, myocardial infarction (MI), congestive heart failure (CHF) and renal disease (CKD) [16–17]. However, some hypertensive patients either refuse to take drugs or prefer to be treated with nutrition, nutritional supplements or other lifestyle changes, if appropriate, as recognized by national and international guidelines [1–20].

Hypertension is a consequence of micro- and macronutrient insufficiencies, abnormal vascular biology, reduced bioavailability of nitric oxide (NO), and the three finite vascular responses to injury that include inflammation, oxidative stress and vascular immune dysfunction [2–5,11–14].

These abnormalities coexist and interact with genetics, epigenetics, nutrient-gene expression and other environmental and lifestyle factors [2–5,11–14]. Hypertension is the "correct" but chronic dysregulated response to numerous infinite insults to the endothelium with gene expression patterns in which the vascular system becomes an innocent bystander [2–5,11–14]. Hypertension is one of several responses of the blood vessel that include endothelial dysfunction (ED) and cardiac and vascular smooth muscle dysfunctions with abnormalities of both microvascular function and structure which may precede the development of hypertension by decades. These changes lead to vascular and cardiac hypertrophy, remodeling, functional and structural network rarefaction, decreased vasodilatory reserve, altered vascular media to lumen ratio (MLR), stiffness, loss of arterial elasticity, fibrosis, increased pulse pressure, elevated pulse-wave velocity (PWV) and increased augmentation index (AI) [2–5,11–14].

Significant functional and then structural microvascular impairment begins before elevations in BP in normotensive offspring of hypertensive parents [2–5,11–14].

As the BP increases, a bidirectional feedback occurs that exacerbates and perpetuates the cardiovascular functional and structural abnormalities. Macro- and micronutrients are crucial in the regulation of BP and subsequent cardiovascular target organ damage and these are more common in patients with hypertension than in the general population [2–5,11–14]. The appropriate measurement, interpretation and treatment of these nutrient deficiencies may effectively lower BP and improve ED, vascular and cardiac functional and structural abnormalities, and cardiovascular events [2–5,11–14].

TABLE 7.1

Contrasting the Intake of Nutrients Involved in Vascular Biology: Evolutionary Nutritional Impositions

Nutrient	Paleolithic Intake	Modern Intake
Potassium	>10,000 meq/day (256 g)	150 meq/day (6 g)
Sodium	<50 mmol/day (1.2 g)	175 mmol/day (4 g)
Sodium/potassium ratio	<0.13 per day	>0.67 per day
Fiber	>100 g/day	9 g/day
Protein	37%	20%
Carbohydrate	41%	40%–50%
Fat	22%	30%–40%
Polyunsaturated/saturated fat ratio	1.4	0.4

This chapter will primarily review the role of nutrition, selected nutraceutical supplements, minerals, vitamins, antiinflammatory agents, natural immune modulators and antioxidants in the treatment of hypertension.

EPIDEMIOLOGY AND PATHOPHYSIOLOGY

The human genome is 99.9% identical to our Paleolithic ancestors; however, the pattern of modern nutritional (macro- and micronutrients) intake has altered our gene expression resulting in an epidemic of hypertension and CVD [21] (Table 7.1).

Vascular biology assumes a pivotal role in the initiation and progression of hypertension [2–5,11–14]. Radical oxygen species (ROS) and radical nitrogen species (RNS), coupled with impaired oxidative defense, inflammatory mediators, vascular immune dysfunction and loss of nitric oxide bioavailability, contribute to hypertension through complex nutrigenomic interactions [2–5,11–14,22–32]. The high Na^+/K^+ ratio of modern diets and the reduced intake of magnesium, fiber, protein and omega-3 fatty acids coupled with increased consumption of omega-6 FA, saturated fat (SFA) and trans fatty acids (TFA) contribute to hypertension [2–5,11–14,21].

THE THREE FINITE VASCULAR RESPONSES AND CARDIOVASCULAR DISEASE (FIGURES 7.1 AND 7.2)

OXIDATIVE STRESS, INFLAMMATION AND VASCULAR IMMUNE DYSFUNCTION

Oxidative stress is an imbalance of ROS and RNS with a decrease in antioxidant defenses that contribute to hypertension [2–5,11–14,23–37]. The predominant ROS produced is superoxide anion, which is generated by numerous cellular sources, will uncouple endothelium-derived NO synthase (eNOS), reduce nitric oxide bioavailability, cause ED and elevate BP [24,27]. Antioxidant deficiency and excess free radical production have been implicated in human hypertension in epidemiologic, observational and interventional studies [29–31]. These ROS and RNS degrade NO, influence eicosanoid metabolism and increase catecholamine levels in serum and urine [2–5,11–14,24,26–27]. The inter-relation of neurohormonal systems, oxidative stress and CVD is shown in Figure 7.3.

Acute and chronic inflammations with abnormal vascular immune responses with involvement of pattern recognition receptors (PRR) such as toll-like receptors (TLR) are involved in hypertension [2–5,11–14,33–50]. Low levels of IL-10 (interleukin 10) and increased levels of high-sensitivity C-reactive protein (hsCRP), numerous inflammatory cytokines such as interleukins (IL-6, IL-b, IL-2 and IL-8), and tumor necrosis alpha (TNF-alpha) are excellent markers for hypertension and hypertension-related CVDs such as CHD, CHF and increased carotid IMT [2–5,11–14,33–50].

Mechanism of Model

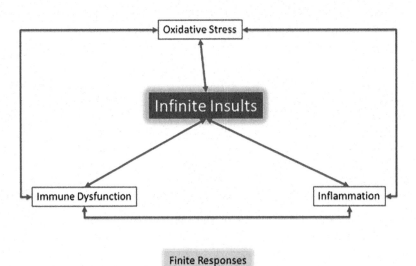

FIGURE 7.1 Infinite insults to the blood vessel result in only three finite responses of inflammation, oxidative stress and vascular immune dysfunction.

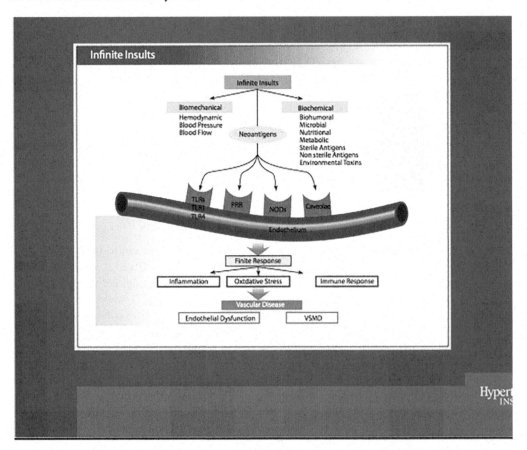

FIGURE 7.2 Infinite insults and the three finite vascular responses of inflammation, oxidative stress and vascular immune dysfunction lead to endothelial dysfunction and cardiac and vascular dysfunction.

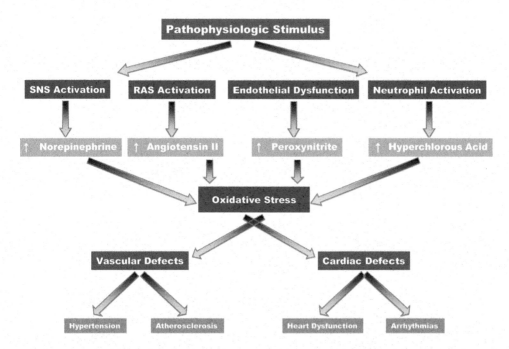

FIGURE 7.3   The neurohormonal and oxidative stress systems with interactions on cardiac and vascular muscles.

Elevated hsCRP is both a risk marker and a risk factor for hypertension and CVD [2,38–39]. Increase in hsCRP of over 3 ug/mL proportionately and positively increases BP rapidly [38–39]. Nitric oxide and eNOS are inhibited by hsCRP [38,39]. The angiotensin 2 receptor (AT2R), which increases NO when stimulated, normally counterbalances AT1R, but it is down-regulated or blocked by hsCRP [2,38–39]. Angiotensin II (A-II) is inflammatory, atherogenic, increases oxidative stress and vascular immune dysfunction, and upregulates many of the cytokines and increases BP [2,44,49].

Innate and adaptive immune responses induce hypertension by numerous mechanisms that include angiotensin II, antibodies to the AT1R, cytokine and chemokine production, PRR and TLR activation, central nervous system (CNS) stimulation and renal damage [2–4,35–36,40–50]. Monocytes cross the endothelial lining, invade the subintimal layer, transform into macrophages and various T-cell subtypes which regulate BP, cause vascular damage and promote vascular immune dysfunction [41]. Angiotensin II activates immune cells directly. In the CNS, angiotensin II activates T cells, macrophages and dendritic cells, and promotes cell infiltration into target organs [41,44,49]. The activation of the AT1R and PPAR gamma receptors, expressed on CD4+T lymphocytes, leads to the release of TNF-alpha, interferon and interleukins within the vascular wall [41,50]. Interleukin 17 (IL-17) produced by T-17 cells may play a pivotal role in the genesis and chronic progression of hypertension caused by angiotensin II [41].

THE BALANCE OF HYPERTENSION

Hypertension is a balance of vascular damage and repair that is mediated through the three finite vascular responses: angiotensin II, endothelin and aldosterone [2–5,11–14] (Figures 7.4 and 7.5).

The vascular protection and repair is mediated by bone marrow-derived endothelial progenitor cells (EPCs) which produce nitric oxide and superoxide dismutase (SOD) [2–5,11–14]. The endothelium maintains communication and homeostasis between the circulating blood cells and the vascular media by modulation of the permeability, contractile state, proliferation, migratory response and the redox balance in the vascular media. In addition, the endothelium modulates

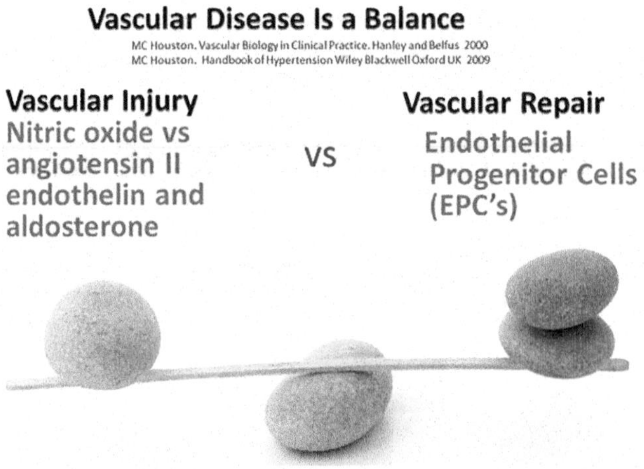

Vascular Disease Is a Balance

MC Houston. Vascular Biology in Clinical Practice. Hanley and Belfus 2000
MC Houston. Handbook of Hypertension Wiley Blackwell Oxford UK 2009

Vascular Injury   **Vascular Repair**
Nitric oxide vs   Endothelial
angiotensin II   VS   Progenitor Cells
endothelin and   (EPC's)
aldosterone

FIGURE 7.4   Cardiovascular disease is a balance between vascular injury and vascular repair.

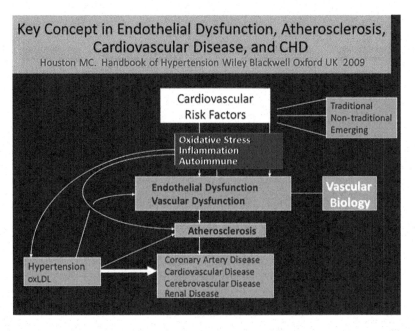

FIGURE 7.5   The three finite responses and vascular biology play a key role between CHD risk factors, endothelial and cardiovascular dysfunction, and CVD.

platelet function, coagulation, monocyte and leukocyte adhesion, inflammation, oxidative stress and immune responses in the blood [2–5,11–14] (Figures 7.6 and 7.7).

TREATMENT OF HYPERTENSION WITH NUTRITION AND NUTRITIONAL SUPPLEMENTS

Nutrition, nutraceutical supplements, antioxidants, vitamins, minerals and natural compounds in food produce physiologic effects that mimic specific classes of antihypertensive medications, improve vascular biology and lower BP [2–14]. These natural compounds can be classified into the major antihypertensive drug groups such as diuretics, serum aldosterone receptor antagonists (SARAs), beta-blockers, central alpha agonists, calcium channel blockers (CCB), angiotensin-converting

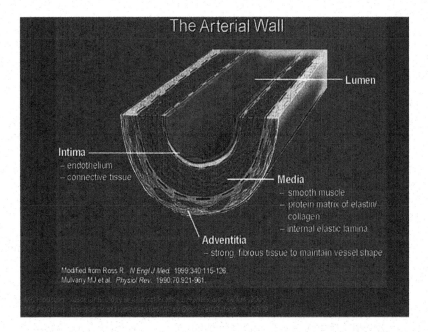

FIGURE 7.6 The blood vessel structure: endothelium, smooth muscle and adventitia.

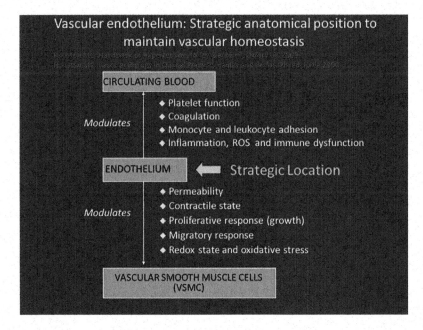

FIGURE 7.7 The endothelium has a strategic location and function to maintain communication and homeostasis between the circulating blood elements and the vascular smooth muscle.

enzyme inhibitors (ACEI) and angiotensin receptor blockers (ARBs), and direct renin inhibitors (DRI) [2–14].

Numerous clinical nutrition studies have demonstrated the efficacy of dietary interventions for the prevention and treatment of hypertension. These include Dietary Approaches to Stop Hypertension (DASH 1 and DASH 2), the Mediterranean diet, PREDIMED, Trials of Hypertension Prevention (TOHP 1 and TOHP 2), Trial of Nonpharmacologic Intervention in the Elderly (TONE),

Treatment of Mild Hypertension (TOMHS), INTERMAP, INTERSALT, Premier and Vanguard [2–5,10–14,51–52].

SODIUM (Na⁺)

Increased dietary sodium intake is associated with hypertension, cerebrovascular accident (CVA), left ventricular hypertrophy (LVH), diastolic dysfunction (DD), CHD, MI, renal insufficiency, proteinuria, arterial stiffness, platelet dysfunction and increased sympathetic nervous system (SNS) activation. A reduction in dietary sodium intake lowers BP and the risk of all of these diseases [2–5,10–15,18,19,53–61]. Decreasing dietary sodium intake in hypertensive patients, especially in the salt-sensitive patients and those with an overactive renal epithelial sodium channel, lowers BP by 4–6/2–3 mmHg proportional to the amount of sodium restriction, reduces the intravascular volume, and may prevent or delay hypertension in high-risk patients [54].

Salt sensitivity, defined as ≥10% increase in mean arterial pressure (MAP) with salt loading, increases the BP response to dietary salt intake in 51% of hypertensive patients [57,58]. Cardiovascular events may be more common in salt-sensitive patients compared to salt-resistant patients, independent of their BP level due to increased sodium content in both cardiac and vascular smooth muscles with loss of elasticity, DD and arterial stiffness with increases in PWV and augmentation index (AI) [57–64]. Decreasing sodium intake to below 1,500–2,300 mg/day was associated with lower BP and a decrease in all-cause mortality, whereas increasing the intake to >2,300 mg/day was associated with an increase in all-cause mortality and CVD [56].

Sodium promotes hypertension by increasing endothelial cell and arterial stiffness, reducing the size and pliability of endothelial cells, promoting DD and LVH, decreasing eNOS and NO production, elevating asymmetric dimethyl arginine (ADMA), increasing oxidative stress and TGF-b, and abolishing the AT 2 receptor-mediated vasodilation [59–64]. All of these effects are increased in the presence of aldosterone, which mimics these same pathophysiologic changes [59–60,63]. Endothelial cells act as **vascular salt sensors** [59–60].

A balance of sodium with potassium and magnesium improves BP control and lowers cardiovascular and cerebrovascular events [2,63,65–68]. Increasing the sodium to potassium ratio increases BP and the risk of CVD, but increasing the potassium to sodium ratio lowers BP and CVD risk [65–68]. A potassium/sodium ratio of 4:1 is recommended with a daily dietary sodium intake of 1,500 mg and a dietary potassium intake of 6,000 mg [2,66–69].

POTASSIUM

Increased dietary potassium intake reduces BP, CVA and CVD [66–73]. The minimal recommended intake of K⁺ is 4,700 mg day (120 mmol) with a K⁺/Na⁺ ratio of 4–5:1 [65–72]. Potassium supplementation at 60 mmol of KCl per day for 12 weeks significantly reduced systolic BP (SBP) by 5.0 mmHg in 150 Chinese subjects [69]. Prospective studies reviewed in a meta-analysis found that 1.64 g or more per day of potassium intake resulted in a 21% lower risk of stroke ($p = 0.0007$) and a lower risk of CHD and total CVD. In another meta-analysis, potassium supplementation resulted in modest but significant reductions in both SBP by 4.25 mmHg and diastolic BP (DBP) by 2.53 mmHg [71]. Studies indicate a dose-related reduction in BP of 4.4/2.5 mmHg to 8/4.1 mmHg with potassium supplementation with doses ranging between 60 and 120 mmol/day [2–14,65–72]. Increased dietary potassium reduces CHD, MI, CHF, LVH, diabetes mellitus (DM) and cardiac arrhythmias independent of BP reduction [69]. The incidence of CVA is reduced proportional to BP reduction but also is independent of the BP reduction [2–14,65–72]. Chronic serum levels of potassium below 4.0 meq/dL increase CVD mortality, ventricular tachycardia, ventricular fibrillation and CHF [2–14,-65–72]. Red blood cell potassium is a better indication of total body stores than serum potassium [2–14]. Potassium also lowers NADPH oxidase, which reduces oxidative stress by decreasing superoxide anion, indirectly increases NO and reduces inflammation [2–14,65–72].

For each 1,000 mg increase of daily dietary potassium, the all-cause mortality is reduced by 20%, and for each 1,000 mg decrease of daily dietary sodium intake, all-cause mortality is decreased by 20% [65]. The recommended daily dietary intake of potassium is 6 grams in hypertensive patients with normal renal function, in those not taking potassium-retaining medications or in those with some other contraindication [2–14,65–72]. Potassium sources include dark green leafy vegetables and fruits, nutritional supplements such as "No Salt" (KCL) substitutes, pure potassium powders or capsules or combined potassium/magnesium powders or capsules and prescription KCL [2–4].

MAGNESIUM (Mg^{++})

There is an inverse relationship between dietary magnesium intake and BP [66,73–77]. In clinical trials, an increased dietary magnesium of 500–1,000 mg/day lowers BP, but compared to dietary potassium intake, the BP results are less prominent [66,73–77]. Significant reductions in BP of 5.6/2.8 mmHg, as documented by 24-hour ambulatory BP monitoring and home and office blood BP readings, usually take about 2 months [73]. A meta-analysis of trials found that Mg^{++} supplementation of over 370 mg daily reduced BP by 3–4±2 mmHg/2.5±1 mmHg [76]. A more recent meta-analysis (34 trials and 2,028 participants) showed that Mg^{++} supplementation dosed at 368 mg/day for 3 months reduced BP by 2.0/1.78 mm Hg [75]. The combination of high potassium and magnesium combined with a low sodium intake potentiates the antihypertensive effects in both treated and untreated hypertensive subjects [66,73–77]. Magnesium also competes with Na$^+$ and calcium on vascular smooth muscle binding sites, simulates the effects of CCB, increases nitric oxide levels and improves endothelial function [2,73–77].

Intracellular erythrocyte levels of magnesium are a more accurate assessment of total body stores compared to serum levels [2,66,77]. Magnesium formulations chelated to an amino acid, especially magnesium with taurine, provides additional BP reduction [2,66,77]. Transdermal preparations of magnesium and magnesium salt baths are also effective in lowering BP [2,66,77]. A high-magnesium diet or magnesium supplements must be used with caution in patients taking medications that promote magnesium retention, in those with known renal insufficiency or in those with other contraindications to high doses of magnesium intake [2,66,77].

CALCIUM (Ca^{++})

Calcium supplementation is not recommended as an effective means to reduce BP until more studies are done on specific populations, both genders and age groups, and the proper formulation and dose is identified [78–81]. The only exception is that calcium may reduce the risk of pre-eclampsia and its comorbidities for both mother and fetus [81].

ZINC (Zn^{++})

Low serum zinc levels correlate with hypertension and other cardiovascular problems [2,82,83]. There is an inverse correlation between BP, serum Zn^{++} and the Zn^{++}-dependent enzyme-lysyl oxidase activity in hypertensive subjects [2,83]. Zinc is transported into cardiac and vascular muscles and other tissues by metallothionein [82]. Genetic deficiencies of metallothionein lead to vascular and cardiac muscle zinc deficiencies, CHF and hypertension [82]. Zinc reduces oxidative stress, inflammation and immune dysfunction, and balances the renin angiotensin aldosterone system (RAAS) and SNS [1,2,57,58,82,83]. Dietary zinc intake should be approximately 50 mg/day, and its levels should be monitored [1].

PROTEIN

Lower BP is associated with an increased intake of animal protein and plant-based protein depending on the type of fat present in animal protein [2,6,84–114]. Lean or wild animal protein with a higher content of essential omega-3 fatty acids and reduced saturated fat improves hypertension [85–88,114]. Dietary protein intake 30% above the mean had a 3.0/2.5 mmHg lower BP compared to those that were 30% below the mean (81 g versus 44 g/day) [2,84].

In a meta-analysis of 40 RCTs compared with carbohydrate, dietary animal and vegetable protein intake was associated with significant changes in mean BP 1.2/0.6 mmHg [6,87].

In a randomized crossover study of 352 prehypertension and stage I hypertension subjects, soy protein and milk protein significantly reduced SBP 2.0 and 2.3 mmHg, respectively, with no change in DBP compared to a high-glycemic-index diet [88]. Soy protein intake of 25 g/day over 3 years was associated with lower BP by 1.9/0.9 mmHg in 45,694 Chinese women [100]. Randomized clinical trials and meta-analysis of soy protein in hypertensive subjects indicate an average reduction in BP by 5.9/3.3 mmHg [100–102,104,105,107]. The recommended daily intake of fermented soy protein is 25 g [2].

Whey protein, milk peptides, fermented milk and casein significantly lower BP in humans [2,6,89–94,103,109–114]. Administration of 20 g/day of hydrolyzed whey protein lowered BP within 6 weeks by 8.0/5.5 mmHg [90]. Milk peptides are rich in ACEI peptides, which lower BP by approximately 4.8/2.2 mmHg with doses of 5–60 mg/day [2,6,89–94,103]. Powdered fermented milk containing *Lactobacillus helveticus and active ACEI peptides*, dosed at 12 g daily significantly reduced BP by 11.2/6.5 mmHg in 1 month [91]. Administration of 20 g of hydrolyzed whey protein to hypertensive subjects lowered BP by 11/7 mmHg compared to controls within 1 week [94]. The WHEY2Go trial [109] was a double-blinded, randomized, three-way-crossover, controlled intervention study of 42 participants who were randomly assigned to consume 56 g of whey protein, 56 g of calcium caseinate or 54 g of maltodextrin (control)/day for 8 weeks separated by a 4-week washout.

The 24-hour ambulatory blood pressure monitor (ABM) reductions in BP were 3.9/2.5 mmHg ($p=0.05$), and the peripheral and central SBP fell by 5.7 mmHg ($p=0.007$) and 5.4 mmHg ($p=0.012$), respectively, after whey-protein consumption compared with the control group [109].

Whey protein improves endothelial function, stimulates opioid receptors and improves PWV. Marine collagen peptides (MCPs) derived from deep sea fish have antihypertensive activity [96–98]. Protein from bonito (*Sarda orientalis*, from the tuna and mackerel family) has natural ACEI inhibitory peptides and lowers BP by 10.2/7 mmHg with a dose of 1.5 g daily [96]. Administration of MCPs in a double-blind, placebo-controlled trial of 100 hypertensive diabetic subjects for 3 months significantly reduced DBP and MAP [95].

Sardine muscle protein lowered BP by 9.7/5.3 mmHg ($p<0.05$) over 4 weeks in 29 hypertensive subjects at a dose of 3 mg of VAL-TYR (a sardine muscle-concentrated extract) [98]. A vegetable drink with sardine protein hydrolysates also reduced BP by 8/5 mmHg over 13 weeks [99].

The daily recommended intake of protein from all sources is 1.0–1.5 g/kg body weight, depending on exercise level, gender, age, hepatic and renal function, medications such as proton pump inhibitors and H2 blockers, and concomitant medical diseases [2].

L-ARGININE

L-arginine lowers BP in humans with a low-side-effect profile, and reductions in BP are similar to the DASH diet [115–127]. L-arginine and endogenous methylarginines are the primary precursors for the eNOS to produce nitric oxide (NO) [115–121].

Intracellular arginine levels far exceed the K(m) of eNOS under normal physiological conditions, but endogenous NO formation depends on extracellular arginine concentration. Endothelial cell NO production is closely coupled to cellular arginine transport mechanisms to regulate NO-dependent functions such as increasing renal vascular flow, renal perfusion, renal tubular NO bioavailability and BP [121].

Parenteral and oral L-arginine administration in hypertensive and normotensive subjects lowers BP significantly at doses of 10–12 g/day in food or as a supplement by about 6.2/6.8 mmHg in both office and 24-hour ABM readings [115,116,122,124,125]. Arginine administered at 4 g daily significantly lowered BP in gestational hypertension, reduced concomitant antihypertensive therapy, and improved maternal and neonatal outcomes with normal delivery time [122,123]. The combination of arginine (1,200 mg/day) and N-acetyl cysteine (600 mg bid) administered over 6 months to hypertensive patients with type 2 diabetes lowered SBP and DBP ($p < 0.05$) [124]. Arginine may have a pro-oxidative effect and increase mortality in patients with advanced atherosclerosis, CHD, acute coronary syndrome (ACS) and MI [126]. Pending more studies, arginine is best avoided in these situations.

TAURINE

Taurine is a conditionally essential sulfur-based amino acid that is efficacious for the treatment of hypertension and a variety of cardiovascular diseases. Taurine reduces SNS activity, plasma norepinephrine, and plasma and urinary epinephrine [2–5,14,128–133]. In addition, taurine increases urinary sodium and water excretion, atrial natriuretic factor (ANF), NO bioavailability and EPCs and improves ED, while it decreases plasma renin activity (PRA), angiotensin II (A-II) and aldosterone [2–5,128–130]. Nineteen hypertensive subjects administered 6 g of taurine lowered BP by 9/4.1 mmHg ($p < 0.05$) in 7 days [129]. In a randomized, double-blind, placebo-controlled study over 12 weeks in 120 prehypertensive individuals, taurine supplementation (1.6 g/day) significantly improved endothelial function and decreased the clinic and 24-hour ambulatory BP reading by 7.2/2.6 and 4.7/1.3 mmHg, respectively [133]. In another 4-month study of 97 prehypertensive individuals, 1.6 g/day of taurine significantly decreased the clinic and 24-hour ambulatory BPs, improved endothelium-vasodilation and reduced the carotid IMT [133].

In a double blind randomized placebo controlled trial (DBRPC) study of 42 hypertensive subjects evaluated over 1 month, a combination powder dietary supplement was given once daily [134]. The supplement included 6 g of taurine, vitamin C (as magnesium ascorbate) at 1,000 mg, grape seed extract at 150 mg, magnesium ascorbate at 87 mg, vitamin B6 (pyridoxine HCl) at 100 mg, vitamin D3 at 2,000 IU and biotin at 2 mg. The active group had a reduction in BP of 16/11.35 mmHg ($p < 0.001$) at week 4. The recommended dose of taurine is 1.5–6 g/day in as a single dose or as divided doses [2,128–133].

OMEGA-3 FATS AND SELECTED OMEGA-6 FATS

Omega-3 fatty acids derived from food or nutritional supplements produce a dose-related reduction in BP and CVD in published human studies [2–14,114,135–150].

A meta-analysis of 70 RCTs found that, compared with placebo, the consumption of omega-3 PUFAs (0.3–15 g/day) for 4–26 weeks significantly reduced BP by 1.5/1.0 mmHg [144]. The largest BP reductions were in untreated hypertensive subjects (SBP = −4.5 [95% confidence interval (CI): −6.1, −2.8] mmHg; DBP = −3.0 [95% CI: −4.3, −1.7] mmHg) [144]. A second meta-analysis of RCTs found that omega-3 fatty acid supplementation for 6–105 weeks at 900–3,000 mg/day improved the PWV ($P < 0.01$) and arterial compliance ($P < 0.001$) [145]. Dexohexanoic acid (DHA) is more effective than eicsopentanoic acid (EPA) in reducing the BP by an average of 8/5 mmHg and also lowering the resting heart rate by 6 beats per minute and improving heart rate variability (HRV) [2–14,135–137,140–142].

Administration of EPA and DHA is preferred to alpha lipoic acid (ALA) due to minimal conversion to these longer-chain omega-3 fatty acids [2–14,136,138]. The consumption of cold-water fish three times per week reduces BP due to the combination of protein and omega-3 fatty acids [2–14,108,136]. In patients with chronic kidney disease, 4 g of omega-3 fatty acids significantly lowered 24-hour BP (ABM) by 3.3/2.9 mmHg compared to placebo ($p < 0.0001$) [137]. The omega-6 fatty acids, gamma linolenic acid (GLA) and dihomo-gamma linolenic acid (DGLA) reduce BP and prevent elevations in BP induced by saturated fats [141]. GLA blocks stress-induced hypertension, lowers aldosterone levels, decreases the adrenal AT1R density and affinity, and increases the vasodilating prostaglandins E 1 (PGE1) and PGI 2 [2–14,141].

Omega-3 fatty acids reduce CHD and MI [150]; increase eNOS and NO; improve endothelial function; reduce arterial stiffness; decrease PWV, insulin resistance and plasma norepinephrine; suppress angiogenin converting enzyme (ACE) activity; and increase parasympathetic tone at doses of 900–3,000 mg daily [2–14,135,143,146]. The recommended daily dose is 3,000–5,000 mg/day of combined DHA and EPA in a ratio of three parts EPA to two parts DHA with 50% of this dose as GLA combined with gamma/delta tocopherol at 100 mg/g of DHA and EPA to get the RBC membrane and omega-3 index at 8% [2–5]. There are no adverse effects or safety concerns at these recommended doses [2–14].

MONOUNSATURATED FATTY ACIDS (MUFA): OLIVE OIL, MEDITERRANEAN DIET, OMEGA-9 FATS, OLEIC ACID AND OLIVE LEAF EXTRACT

The Mediterranean diet (MedDiet), which is rich in olive oil and the supplement olive leaf extract (OLE), reduces BP and CVD in most clinical trials [2–14,151–173]. In an open study over 2 months, 40 borderline hypertensive monozygotic twins given either 500 or 1,000 mg/day of olive leaf extract had significant reductions in BP of 6/5 mmHg (500 mg of OLE) and 13/5 mmHg reduction (1,000 of OLE) compared to controls [171]. In another randomized doublle blind placebo control and control (RDBPC) trial, the BP decreased 8/6 mmHg ($p \leq 0.01$) in office and 24-hour ABM, and the need for antihypertensive medications was reduced by 48% in the MUFA group ($p < 0.005$) [151]. Extra virgin olive oil (EVOO) lowered the SBP by 14 mmHg in elderly hypertensive patients ($p < 0.01$) [152,153]. EVOO contains lipid-soluble phytonutrients such as nitrates and polyphenols which lower BP by reducing oxidative stress and oxLDL, blocking the AT1R, altering RAAS and endothelin gene expression, increasing nitric oxide levels and endothelial-induced vasodilation, and blocking calcium channels similar to a CCB [148,151,155,162–164]. EVOO with a total phenol content of at least 161 mg/kg at 20–40 g (2–4 tablespoons) per day will significantly lower SBP in about 3 weeks. EVOO with 300 mg/kg of total phenols may also decrease DBP [2–5,168].

A total of 166 elderly subjects were prescribed a MedDiet or their habitual diet (HabDiet; control) for 6 months [172]. The MedDiet, compared with the HabDiet, lowered SBP by 1.1 mmHg and improved flow-mediated vasodilation at 6 months ($p = 0.01$). The INTERMAP trial found that dietary MUFA intake, especially oleic acid from vegetable sources, may prevent adverse BP levels in general populations [173].

In the European Prospective Investigation into Cancer and Nutrition (EPIC) study (20, 343 subjects), the intake of EVOO and polyphenols documented an inverse relationship with SBP and DBP [169]. In the Prevention with Mediterranean Diet (PREDIMED) trial, that included 7,447 patients at high risk for CVD, the participants on the Mediterranean diet supplemented with EVOO had a significantly lower DBP than those in the control group (1.5 mmHg) [170].

OLE has a dose-dependent reduction in both office BP measurements and 24-hour ABM with a range of 4/3–11/5 mmHg with [165–167,171]. A total of 60 prehypertensive male subjects in a 6-week study with OLE demonstrated a reduction in BP about 4/3 mmHg [165]. Leaf extract of olive (*Olea europaea*), at the dosage regimen of 500 mg twice daily, was similarly effective in lowering SBP and DBP in subjects with stage 1 hypertension compared to captopril, given at its effective dose of 12.5–25 mg twice daily (reduction of about 11/5 mmHg) [167].

VITAMIN C

Dietary intake of vitamin C and plasma ascorbate concentration in humans are inversely correlated to BP [2–14,174–195]. The administration of vitamin C orally and intravenously reduces BP in clinical trials [2–14,174–195]. Thirty-one patients were randomized to 500, 1,000 or 2,000 mg of oral vitamin C daily with a mean reduction in BP by 4.5/2.8 mmHg ($p < 0.05$) [192]. There was no difference between the three vitamin C groups indicating that 500 mg daily or 250 mg twice per day is sufficient to reduce BP [191]. In a meta-analysis of 29 trials, with a median dose of vitamin C of 500 mg/day and a median duration of 2 months, there was a significant reduction in BP of 3.84/ 1.48 mmHg ($p=0.04$) [199]. Published clinical trials show that vitamin C at a dose of 250 mg twice daily reduces BP by an average of 7/4 mmHg [2–14,174–195]. Vitamin C is a potent water-soluble antioxidant and electron donor that recycles vitamin E and other antioxidants and enhances total antioxidant capacity [174]. In elderly patients with refractory hypertension already on maximum pharmacologic therapy, 600 mg of vitamin C daily lowered the BP by an additional 20/16 mmHg [183]. Plasma ascorbate is inversely correlated with BP in healthy, normotensive individuals, and those with the lowest initial ascorbate serum levels have the best BP reduction [2–5,184,190]. The SBP and 24 ABM show the most significant reductions with chronic oral administration of vitamin C [2,178–183]. Block et al. [184], in a depletion-repletion study of vitamin C, demonstrated an inverse correlation of plasma ascorbate levels, SBP and DBP. In a meta-analysis of 13 clinical trials with 284 patients, vitamin C at 500 mg/day over 6 weeks reduced BP by 3.9/2.1 mmHg [185]. Hypertensive subjects have significantly lower plasma ascorbate levels compared to normotensive subjects (40 umol/L versus 57 umol/L, respectively) [187,195]. A serum level of 100 micromol/L is recommended for optimal BP lowering [2–5].

VITAMIN E

Very few clinical studies demonstrated improved BP with the various types of tocopherols or tocotrienols [2,196–200]. Patients with type 2 DM on prescription medications with controlled BP (average BP of 136/76 mmHg) were administered mixed tocopherols containing 60% gamma, 25% delta and 15% alpha tocopherols [196]. The BP increased by 6.8/3.6 mmHg in the study patients on the mixed tocopherols ($p<0.0001$) and increased even more in those subjects taking alpha tocopherol (BP increased 7/5.3 mmHg $-p<0.0001$) [196]. The BP increase was likely due to drug interactions with tocopherols via cytochrome P 450-3A 4 and 4F2 that decreased the effective serum levels of the antihypertensive medications [196]. Gamma tocopherol has an antihypertensive and natriuretic effect through the inhibition of the 70pS potassium channel in the thick ascending limb of the loop of Henle [197]. Both alpha and gamma tocopherols improve insulin sensitivity and enhance adiponectin expression via a PPAR gamma-dependent process which has the potential to lower BP and serum glucose [198].

In a retrospective analysis and data from NHNS, the medium and high tertiles of vitamin E intake were associated with a significantly lower odds ratio for hypertension, 0.73 and 0.81, respectively [199]. Fifty-eight individuals with type 2 DM given 500 mg/day of RRR-α-tocopherol, 500 mg/day of mixed tocopherols or placebo for 6 weeks did not significantly alter the rate of daytime or nighttime SBP, DBP or pulse pressure variation compared to placebo ($P>0.05$) [200]. If vitamin E has an antihypertensive effect, it is probably small and may be limited to untreated hypertensive patients, those with vitamin E deficiency, known vascular disease, mild volume overload or other concomitant problems such as diabetes or hyperlipidemia [2–5,196–200].

VITAMIN D

Vitamin D3 has variable BP-lowering effects [2–5,201–218]. Vitamin D may have an independent and direct role in the regulation of BP, insulin metabolism and dysglycemia [201–213], but the results have not been consistent in prospective studies or in meta-analysis in which there has been little or no significant BP reduction [214,215,217]. If the vitamin D level is below 30 ng/mL, the circulating PRA levels are higher, which increases angiotensin II and elevates BP [211]. Patients in the lowest quartile of serum vitamin D have a 52% incidence of hypertension versus the highest quartile which have a 20% incidence [211]. Compared with a 25-hydroxyvitamin D > 30 ng/mL, a 25-hydroxyvitamin D < 20 ng/mL was associated with a greater hypertension risk (OR: $1.225-p=0.04$) [211]. In another study during a median follow-up of 2 years, 42.6% of the cohort developed hypertension [213]. Compared with the 25-hydroxyvitamin D > 30 ng/mL, 25-hydroxyvitamin D < 20 ng/mL was associated with a greater hypertension risk (OR: 1.225 [95% CI: 1.010–1.485]; $p=0.04$) [213]. This meta-analysis, including seven prospective studies of 53,375 participants, showed a significant association between vitamin D deficiencies and incident hypertension (HRs $= 1.23 - p = 0.002$) [213]. A recent meta-analysis from eight randomized controlled trials (RCTs), who received treatment with vitamin D for more than 3 months, showed that vitamin D supplementation slightly decreased SBP by 1.964 mmHg ($p=0.016$), but DBP did not change [215]. Compared to placebo, there was also no statistical difference in SBP lowering by vitamin D supplementation [215]. Vitamin D3 markedly suppresses renin transcription by a VDR-mediated mechanism via the juxtaglomerular apparatus (JGA) apparatus which alters electrolyte balance, volume and BP [2,203]. Vitamin D reduces ADMA, suppresses pro-inflammatory cytokines, increases nitric oxide, improves endothelial function and arterial elasticity, and decreases vascular smooth muscle hypertrophy [204–211].

The hypotensive effect of vitamin D was inversely related to the pretreatment serum levels of $1,25$ $(OH)_2$ D_3 and has additive BP reduction when used concurrently with antihypertensive medications [212].

Blacks have significantly higher rates of hypertension than whites and lower circulating levels of 25-hydroxyvitamin D [218]. In a 3-month study of placebo, 1,000, 2,000 or 4,000 international units of cholecalciferol per day, the difference in SBP between baseline and 3 months was +1.7 mmHg for those receiving placebo, −0.66 mmHg for 1,000 U/day, −3.4 mmHg for 2,000 U/day and −4.0 mmHg for 4,000 IU/day of cholecalciferol (−1.4 mmHg for each additional 1,000 IU/day of cholecalciferol; $p=0.04$). For each 1-ng/mL increase in plasma 25-hydroxyvitamin D, there was a significant 0.2 mmHg reduction in SBP ($p=0.02$) [218]. There was no effect of cholecalciferol supplementation on DBP ($p=0.37$). Vitamin D levels are lower in patients with non-dipping hypertension [216]. A vitamin D level of 80 ng/mL is recommended for optimal BP reduction and cardiovascular risk reduction [2–5].

VITAMIN B6 (PYRIDOXINE)

Low serum vitamin B6 (pyridoxine) levels are associated with hypertension in humans [2–5,219–223]. High dose of vitamin B6 significantly lowered BP by 14/10 mmHg ($p<0.005$) and serum catecholamine levels ($p<0.05$) in a placebo-controlled study of 20 hypertensive subjects who were administered vitamin B6 at 5 mg/kg/day for 4 weeks [220].

In a placebo-controlled trial over 12 weeks, 800 mg lipoic acid and 80 mg pyridoxine lipoic acid and pyridoxine, urinary albumin, serum malondialdehyde (MDA) and SBP decreased significantly in the supplement group compared to the placebo group ($p<0.05$) [223]. Serum NO increased in the supplement group compared to the placebo group ($p<0.05$). No statistically significant differences were observed between the two groups in mean changes of serum endothelin-1, glucose and DBP [223].

Vitamin B6 thus has similar action to central alpha agonists, diuretics and CCB [2–5]. The recommended dose is 200 mg/day orally [2–5].

FLAVONOIDS: RESVERATROL AND POMEGRANATE

Flavonoids (flavonols, flavones and isoflavones) are potent free radical scavengers that prevent atherosclerosis, promote vascular relaxation and have antihypertensive properties [224–234].

Resveratrol administration to humans reduces augmentation index, improves arterial compliance and lowers central arterial pressure when administered as 250 mL of either regular or dealcoholized red wine [226–230]. Aortic augmentation index fell by 6.1% with the dealcoholized red wine and by 10.5% with regular red wine, central arterial pressure was reduced with dealcoholized red wine by 7.4 and with regular red wine by 5.4 mmHg. Resveratrol increases flow-mediated vasodilation in a dose-related manner, improves ED, prevents uncoupling of eNOS, and blocks the effects of angiotensin II [226–230]. The recommended dose is 250 mg/day of trans-resveratrol [2–5,228].

Pomegranate (*Punica granatum* L.) reduces serum ACE activity by 36%, improves endothelial function, lowers BP and reduces carotid IMT [2–4,231–234]. A meta-analysis from 8 RCTs showed significant reductions in both SBP (4.96 mmHg − $p < 0.001$) and DBP ($p = 0.021$) after 6 oz of pomegranate juice consumption [231].

LYCOPENE

Lycopene produces a significant reduction in BP, serum lipids and oxidative stress markers [2–14,235–241]. Its dietary sources include grapefruit, watermelon, tomatoes, guava, pink apricots and papaya [2–14,235–241]. In patients with grade I hypertension, tomato lycopene extract (10 mg lycopene/day) given for 2 months lowered BP by 9/7 mmHg ($p < 0.01$) [235,237]. Tomato extract administered to 31 hypertensive subjects over 3 months lowered BP by 10/4 mmHg [236]. Patients on antihypertensive agents including ACEI, CCB and diuretics had an additional significant BP reduction of 5.4/3 mmHg over 6 weeks when administered a standardized tomato extract [237]. A meta-analysis of the effect of lycopene on SBP showed a significant BP-reducing effect (mean SBP change ± SE: −5.60 ± 5.26 mmHg, $p = 0.04$) [240]. The doses ranged from 10 to 25 mg/day of lycopene in these trials [240]. Other studies have not shown changes in BP with lycopene [238]. The recommended daily intake of lycopene is 10–25 mg in food or in a supplement form, but it is not clear which has the best effect on BP and CVD risk [241]. However, present data suggest that supplemental forms of lycopene are superior for BP reduction [241].

COENZYME Q10 (UBIQUINONE)

Coenzyme Q10 (CoQ-10, ubiquinone) has shown consistent and significant antihypertensive effects in hypertensive subjects [2–14,242–258]. CoQ-10 increases eNOS and NO, and improves endothelial function and vascular elasticity [2–14,250,251]. Serum levels of COQ-10 decrease with age, chronic diseases, oxidative stress, dyslipidemia, CHD, hypertension, DM, statin and beta-blocker use, exercise and atherosclerosis [2–14,250,251,256]. Compared to normotensive patients, essential hypertensive patients have a higher incidence of CoQ-10 serum deficiency (39% vs 6% of controls) [2–5,245,253,256]. In a 12-week RDBPCT of subjects with isolated systolic hypertension (ISH) (165/81–82 mmHg), CoQ-10 administered orally at 60 mg twice daily reduced SBP by 18 mmHg ($p < 0.01$) and DBP by 2.6 mmHg (NS) [244]. The serum level increased by 2.2 ug/dL ($p < 0.01$). There was a 55% response rate defined as a reduction in SBP of over 4 mmHg. The responders had an average reduction in SBP of 26 mmHg [244]. The therapeutic serum level of CoQ-10 should be 3 ug/mL [2,210,242,245,252,253]. This dose is usually 3–5 mg/kg/day of CoQ-10 [1–5,242,246,252,253]. Combination of a targeted intracellular cardiac CoQ-10 (MitoQ10) and low-dose losartan provides additive therapeutic benefit, significantly attenuating development of hypertension, increasing NO levels and reducing LVH in the spontaneously hypertensive rat (SHRSP) [257]. In addition, MitoQ10 mediates a direct antihypertrophic effect on rat cardiomyocytes in vitro.

Patients with the lowest CoQ-10 serum levels may have the best antihypertensive response to supplementation [2–5,244]. The average reduction in BP is about 15/10 mmHg with office readings (range of 11–17/8–10 mmHg) [2–5,242–258] and 18/10 mmHg with 24-hour ABM ($p < 0.0001$) [245,258]. The antihypertensive effect peaks at 4 weeks, and then the BP remains stable during long-term treatment [2–5,244], but within 2 weeks after discontinuation of Co-Q-10, the antihypertensive effect dissipates [2–5,244]. The reductions in BP and systemic vascular resistance (SVR) are correlated with the pre- and post-treatment levels of CoQ-10 and the percent increase in serum levels [2–5,244,245]. About 50% of patients respond to oral supplemental CoQ-10 [2–5,244]. Patients administered CoQ-10 with enalapril have better 24-hour ABM control compared to enalapril monotherapy and better endothelial function [249]. Approximately

50% of patients on antihypertensive drugs may be able to stop between one and three agents. A recent meta-analysis that suggested that CoQ-10 did not reduce BP is seriously flawed and biased in its data selection [247]. The literature is supportive of significant reductions in BP in human clinical trials [2–5,242–246,248–256,258]. Adverse effects have not been seen in patients in the literature [2–5,242–246,248–256,258].

ALPHA LIPOIC ACID

ALA is effective in the treatment of hypertension, especially as part of the metabolic syndrome [2–5,259–263]. Lipoic acid reduces oxidative stress, inflammation and serum aldehydes, closing calcium channels which leads to vasodilation, improved endothelial function and lower BP [2–5,259–263]. Urinary albumin excretion is stabilized in DM subjects given 600 mg of ALA compared to placebo for 18 months ($p < 0.05$) [263]. In a double-blind crossover study of 36 patients with CHD given 200 mg of lipoic acid with 500 mg of acetyl-L-carnitine twice daily for 8 weeks [262], there was a 2% increase in brachial artery diameter and a decrease in SBP from 151 ± 20 to 142 ± 18 mmHg ($p < 0.03$) with no change in DBP [262]. However, patients with metabolic syndrome had a reduction in SBP from 139 ± 21 to 132 ± 15 mmHg ($p < 0.03$) and DBP from 76 ± 8 to 73 ± 8 mmHg ($p < 0.06$) [262]. In a 2-month double-blind crossover study of 40 patients with DM and stage I hypertension, quinapril 40 mg daily vs quinapril 40 mg with lipoic acid 600 mg daily reduced urinary albumin excretion by 30% with quinapril and 53% quinapril with lipoic acid ($p < 0.005$), the BP was reduced significantly by 10% in both groups, and the flow medicated dilation (FMD) increased 58% with quinapril and 116% with the combination ($p < 0.005$) [261]. The HOMA-IR decreased 19% with quinapril and 40% with quinapril with lipoic acid ($p < 0.005$). The combined administration of lipoic acid and pyridoxine improves albuminuria in patients with diabetic nephropathy [223]. The recommended dose is 100–200 mg/day of R-lipoic acid with biotin 2–4 mg/day to prevent biotin depletion with long-term use of lipoic acid. R-lipoic acid is recommended instead of the L isomer because of its preferred use by the mitochondria [2–5].

PYCNOGENOL

Pycnogenol is a bark extract from the French maritime pine that significantly reduces BP in human trials [2–14,264–272]. Pycnogenol administered at 200 mg/day lowered SBP 2.7 mmHg ($p < 0.05$) and DBP fell by 1.8 mmHg (NS) [223]. The antihypertensive effect is mediated by an ACEI effect, reductions in ET–1, increases in NO and prostaglandins, reduction in inflammation, oxidative stress and improvement in endothelial function [2–14,264–272]. Other studies have shown reductions in BP and a decreased need for ACEI and CCB [2–5,264,265,267,269].

GARLIC

Meta-analysis and clinical trials of garlic administration have shown consistent reductions in BP in hypertensive patients both on antihypertensive medications and not on antihypertensive medications with an average reduction in BP of 7–16/5–9 mmHg [273–283]. Garlic is a vasodilator with ACEI activity, calcium channel blocking activity and ability to increase nitric oxide [2–14,278]. In a DBRPCT over 3 months, subjects given 900 mg of aged garlic extract with 2.4 mg of S-allylcysteine reduced SBP by 10.2 mmHg ($p = 0.03$) [275]. In another DBRPC trial of 81 prehypertensive and mild hypertensive patients given 300 mg of garlic homogenate for 12 weeks, the BP reduction was 6.6–7.5/4.6–5.2 mmHg [276]. Aged garlic extract at 480 mg/day had the best BP reduction of 11.8 ± 5.4 mmHg ($p = 0.006$) [277]. Garlic improves central BP, central pulse pressure, MAP, augmentation pressure, PWV and arterial stiffness [281].

SEAWEED

Wakame seaweed (*Undaria pinnatifida*) is the most popular, edible seaweed in Japan [284]. A daily dose of 3.3 g of dried wakame for 4 weeks significantly reduced BP by $14\pm3/5\pm2$ mmHg ($p<0.01$) [285]. In a study of 62 middle-aged, male subjects with mild hypertension given a potassium-loaded, ion-exchanging sodium-adsorbing, potassium-releasing seaweed preparation, significant BP reductions occurred at 4 weeks on 12 and 24 g/day ($p<0.01$) [286]. The MAP fell by 11.2 mmHg ($p<0.001$) in the sodium-sensitive subjects and 5.7 mmHg ($p<0.05$) in the sodium-insensitive subjects, correlating with PRA.

Seaweed and sea vegetables contain 771 minerals and rare earth elements, fiber and alginate in a colloidal form [284–286]. Wakame has ACEI activity from at least four parent tetrapeptides and possibly their dipeptide and tripeptide metabolites, especially those containing the amino acid sequence Val-Tyr, Ile-Tyr, Phe-Tyr and Ile-Try in some combination [284,287,288]. Its long-term use in Japan has demonstrated its safety.

COCOA: DARK CHOCOLATE

Dark chocolate (100 g) and cocoa with a high content of polyphenols (30 mg or more) significantly reduce BP in various meta-analysis and clinical prospective trials [2–14,289–300]. A meta-analysis of 173 hypertensive subjects given cocoa for 2 weeks lowered BP by 4.7/2.8 mmHg ($p=0.002–0.006$) [289]. Fifteen subjects given 100 g of dark chocolate with 500 mg of polyphenols for 15 days had a 6.4 mmHg reduction in SBP ($p<0.05$) [290]. Cocoa at a dose of 30 mg of polyphenols lowered BP in prehypertensive and stage I hypertensive patients by 2.9/1.9 mmHg at 18 weeks ($p<0.001$) [291]. Two meta-analyses of 23 trials with a total of 297 patients found a significant reduction in BP of 3.2/2.0–4.5/3.2 mmHg [293,296]. The BP reduction is the greatest in those with the highest baseline BP and those with a least 50%–70% cocoa at doses of 6–100 g/day [2–5,289–293,296].

A meta-analysis in 2012 included 20 DBRPC clinical trials involving 856 healthy participants found a statistically significant BP-reducing effect of flavanol-rich cocoa products, compared with control, in short-term trials of 2–18 weeks' duration (mean difference in SBP – 2.8 mmHg; $p = 0.005$; mean difference in DBP – 2.2 mmHg, $p=0.006$) [300]. The participants were given 30–1,080 mg of flavanols (mean 545.5 mg) in 3.6–105.0 g of cocoa products per day in the active intervention group [300]. Cocoa improves insulin resistance, nitric oxide production and endothelial function in patients with or without hyperglycemia [290,296–299].

MELATONIN

Melatonin demonstrates significant antihypertensive effects in humans in numerous double-blind, randomized, placebo-controlled clinical trials as single therapy or in conjunction with antihypertensive medications [301–327].

Melatonin inhibits plasma A-II levels both centrally and in peripheral tissues to reduce BP [6,314–316,319].

Melatonin levels are reduced by shortened sleep cycle of less than 6 hours, shift work, age, brief light exposure after darkness, trespass light, and specific medications such as beta-blockers and benzodiazepines [319]. Melatonin lowers nocturnal BP in diabetic and non-diabetic hypertensive patients and in those with CHD, and improves the dipping pattern in patients with nocturnal non-dipping status [302–308,310,312].

In a DBRPCXO study, chronic administration (3 weeks) of melatonin at 2.5 mg before bedtime in hypertensive men, not taking any antihypertensive medications, reduced nocturnal BP by 6/4 mmHg. In addition, melatonin reduced day-night amplitudes of SBP by 15% and DBP by 25%, improved sleep and reduced cortisol levels [301]. In a meta-analysis of DBPC RCTs of 221 participants treated with controlled-release melatonin 2–5 mg/night for 7–90 days, there was a significant decrease in night BP of 6.1/3.5 mmHg ($p = 0.009$) [324].

GRAPE SEED EXTRACT

Grape seed extract (GSE) produces a significant reduction in BP in clinical trials and in meta-analyses [2–5,328–332]. A meta-analysis of 9 randomized trials with 390 subjects administered GSE in variable doses and variable amounts of resveratrol demonstrated a significant reduction in SBP of 1.54 mmHg ($p < 0.02$), but no reduction in DBP [328]. Significant reduction in BP of 11/8 mmHg ($P < 0.05$) occurs with a dose of 300 mg/day in 1 month [329]. In a meta-analysis of 16 clinical trials in 2016 with 810 subjects [331], there were significant reductions in BP with GSE 6/3 mmHg ($p = 0.001$) especially in young patients and those with obesity or metabolic syndrome [331]. A single-center, randomized, two-arm, double-blinded, placebo-controlled, 12-week parallel study was conducted in 36 middle-aged adults with prehypertension [332]. Subjects consumed a juice containing placebo or 300 mg/day GSE, 150 mg twice daily, for 6 weeks preceded by a 2-week placebo run-in and followed by 4-week no-beverage follow-up [332]. GSE significantly reduced SBP by 5.6% ($P = 0.012$) and DBP by 4.7% ($P = 0.049$) [332]. BP returned to baseline after the 4-week discontinuation period of GSE beverage. The higher the initial BP, the greater the response.

DIETARY NITRATES AND NITRITES: BEETROOT JUICE AND EXTRACT

The Mediterranean and DASH diets and the ingestion of fruits and vegetables rich in inorganic nitrate (NO3(–)) are effective methods for elevating vascular nitric oxide (NO) levels through formation of an NO2(–) intermediate that reduces BP, and improves arterial compliance and endothelial function [6,333–343].

The pathway for NO generation involves the activity of facultative oral microflora and the gastric/entero-salivary cycle to facilitate the reduction of inorganic NO3(–), ingested in the diet, to inorganic NO2(–). This NO2(–) eventually enters the circulation where, through the activity of numerous and distinct NO2(–) reductases, it is chemically reduced to NO [6,333–334]. Raw or cooked beets, beet juice and extract of dark green leafy vegetables (kale and spinach) are concentrated dietary sources of inorganic nitrates. This is the alternate pathway to the arginine NO/eNOS pathway mediated though eNOS. Beet juice at a dose of 250 mL/day reduces BP in 30–60 minutes in normotensive, prehypertensive or mild hypertensive subjects [335,336]. A meta-analysis of DBRPCTs shows that daily beetroot juice consumption of 5.1–45 mmol (321–2,790 mg) over a period from 2 hours to 15 days is associated with dose-dependent changes in SBP (mean reduction −4.4 mmHg; $p < 0.001$) [337]. In a blinded, placebo-controlled, crossover study, the acute effects of an orally disintegrating lozenge that generates nitric oxide (NO) in the oral cavity evaluated the effects on BP response, endothelial function and vascular compliance in 30 unmedicated hypertensive patients with an average baseline BP of $144 \pm 3/91 \pm 1$ mmHg [338].

Nitrate supplementation vs placebo resulted in a significant decrease of 4/5 mmHg ($P < 0.002$) from baseline after 20 minutes. In addition, there was a further significant reduction of 6 mmHg in both SBP and DBP after 60 minutes ($P < 0.0001$ vs baseline). After a half hour of a single dose, there was a significant improvement in vascular compliance as measured by augmentation index and, after 4 hours, a statistically significant improvement in endothelial function as measured by the EndoPAT (Itamar Medical, Franklin, MA) [338]. In another DBRPC study of 68 drug-naïve and treated patients with hypertension, a daily dietary supplementation was given for 4 weeks with either dietary nitrate (250 mL daily, as beetroot juice) or a placebo (250 mL daily, as nitrate-free beetroot juice) after a 2-week run-in period and followed by a 2-week washout [335]. Daily supplementation with dietary nitrate was associated with reduction in BP measured by three different methods. The mean reduction in clinic BP was 7.7/2.4 mmHg (3.6–11.8/0.0–4.9, $p < 0.001$ and $p = 0.050$).

Twenty-four-hour ambulatory BP was reduced by 7.7/5.2 mmHg (4.1–11.2/2.7–7.7, $p < 0.001$ for both). Home BP was reduced by 8.1/3.8 mmHg (3.8–12.4/0.7–6.9, $p < 0.001$ and $p < 0.01$) [335]. There was no evidence of tachyphylaxis, and the study supplement was well tolerated. Endothelial function improved by ≈20% ($P < 0.001$) and arterial stiffness reduced by 0.59 m/s (0.24–0.93; $p < 0.01$) after dietary nitrate consumption with no change after placebo [335].

In a randomized, crossover study of 24 hypertensive subjects, raw beet juice was administered for 2 weeks followed by cooked beets [341]. After 2 weeks, both groups had a washout for 2 weeks and then switched to the alternative treatment. Each participant consumed 250 mL/day of beet juice or 250 g/day of cooked beets. FMD was significantly ($p < 0.05$) increased and SBP and DBP were significantly ($p < 0.05$) decreased with beet juice and cooked beet [341].

Based on these studies, there is a dose-related response to SBP, DBP, endothelial function and other vascular parameters with beet juice, beet extract, and raw and cooked beets [333–343]. The consumption of dietary nitrate at 0.1 mmol/kg of body weight per day (high intake of F and V at 4–6 servings a day) reduces SBP and DBP about 3.5–4.0 mmHg, and this effect is potentiated by vitamin C and polyphenols [333–343].

Vegetables are the primary source of nitrates (80%–85%) [342,343]. About 500 mg of beetroot juice with 45 mmol/L or 2.79 g/L of inorganic nitrate lowers BP by 10.4/8.1 mmHg and increases FMD by 30% [342,343]. Beetroot tends to be dosed based on the *nitrate* content, with around 0.1–0.2 mmol/kg (6.4–12.8 mg/kg) being the target for nitrate consumption. This is about 436 mg for a 150 lb person, which is comparable to half a kilogram (500 g) of the beetroots themselves (wet weight) [342,343].

TEAS

Green tea, black tea and their respective extracts of active components have demonstrated reductions in BP in human clinical trials and meta-analysis [344–354]. In a DBRPCT of 379 hypertensive subjects given green tea extract 370 mg/day for 3 months, BP was reduced significantly at 4/4 mmHg [348].

A meta-analysis of regular consumption of either green or black tea for 4–24 weeks (2–6 cups per day) reduced BP significantly. Green tea lowered SBP by 2.1 mmHg and DBP by 2.0 mmHg, while black tea reduced SBP by 1.4 mmHg and DBP by 1.1 mmHg [344]. A small 4-week crossover RDBPCT of 21 women administered 1,500 mg of green tea extract (GTE, containing 780 mg of polyphenols) or a matching placebo for 4 weeks, with a washout period of 2 weeks between treatments, had significant reductions in SBP [352]. The 24-hour ABM showed an overall decrease in SBP of 3.6 mmHg, daytime reduction of 3.61 mmHg and nighttime reduction of 3.9 mmHg [352]. There was no reduction in DBP. A meta-analysis of 10 trials with 834 subjects noted a reduction in BP of 2.36/1.77 mmHg with green and black teas in 3 months. The best results were with non-caffeinated tea. The required amount is about 500 mg flavonoid content (2 cups of tea/day) [354]. Green tea lowers systemic vascular resistance and induces microvascular vasodilation [348,353].

L-CARNITINE AND ACETYL–L-CARNITINE

Carnitine has mild systemic antihypertensive effects by upregulation of eNOS and inhibition of RAAS [2–5,355–365]. Endothelial function, NO and oxidative defense are improved, while oxidative stress and BP are reduced [355–359].

Human studies on the effects of L-carnitine and acetyl-L-carnitine are limited, with minimal to no change in BP [2–5,360–365]. In patients with metabolic syndrome, acetyl-L-carnitine at 1 g bid over 8 weeks improved dysglycemia and reduced SBP by 7–9 mmHg, but DBP was significantly decreased only in those with higher glucose levels [366]. Low carnitine levels are associated with a non-dipping BP pattern in type 2 DM [365]. The clinical role of carnitine in hypertension and CVD must be carefully evaluated as carnitine may increase trimethylamine oxidase (TMAO) via the gut microbiome which is associated with atherosclerosis and CHD [366]. Doses of 2–3 g twice per day are recommended if carnitine is used [2–5].

FIBER

The clinical trials with various types of fiber to reduce BP have been inconsistent [2–5,367–372].

Soluble fiber, guar gum, guava, psyllium, flax seed and oat bran may reduce BP and decrease the need for antihypertensive medications in hypertensive subjects, diabetic subjects and hypertensive diabetic subjects especially when incorporated into the Mediterranean diet [2–5,367–372]. In a meta-analysis, dietary fiber intake was associated with a significant 1.65 mmHg reduction in DBP but a non-significant 1.15 mmHg reduction in SBP [367]. However, a significant reduction in both SBP and DBP was observed in trials conducted among patients with hypertension (5.95/4.20 mmHg) and in trials with a duration of ≥8 weeks (BP 3.12/2.57 mmHg) [367]. A recent meta-analysis of 14 RCTs with flaxseed, which is a rich dietary source of α-linolenic acid, lignans and fiber, lowered BP by 1.8/1.6 mmHg ($p = 0.003$) [372].

SESAME

Sesame has been shown to reduce BP in a several small randomized, placebo-controlled human studies over 30–60 days [373–381]. Sesame lowers BP alone [182–186] or in combination with nifedipine [181,185], diuretics or beta-blockers [182,186]. In a group of 13 mild hypertensive subjects, consumption of 60 mg of sesamin for 4 weeks lowered SBP by 3.5 mmHg ($p < 0.044$) and DBP by 1.9 mmHg ($p < 0.045$) [183]. Black sesame meal at 2.52 g/day over 4 weeks in 15 subjects reduced SBP by 8.3 mmHg ($p < 0.05$), but there was a non-significant reduction in DBP of 4.2 mmHg [184]. Sesame oil at 35 g/day significantly lowered central BP within 1 hour and also maintained BP reduction chronically in 30 hypertensive subjects, and reduced heart rate, arterial stiffness, augmentation index, PWV and hsCRP [381]. Also, sesame oil improved NO and antioxidant capacity, while it decreased endothelin-I [381]. In addition, sesame lowers serum glucose, HgbA1C and LDL-C; increases HDL; reduces oxidative stress markers; and increases glutathione, SOD, GPx, CAT and vitamins C, E and A [181,182,184–186]. The active ingredients are natural ACEIs such as sesamin, sesamolin, sesaminol glucosides and furofuran lignans which also suppress NF-kappa B and inflammatory cytokine production [187,188]. All of these effects lower inflammation, decrease oxidative stress, improve oxidative defense, improve endothelial function, vasodilate and reduce BP [187,188].

HESPERIDIN

Hesperidin significantly lowered DBP by 3–4 mmHg ($p < 0.02$) and improved microvascular endothelial reactivity in 24 obese hypertensive male subjects in a randomized, controlled, crossover study over 4 weeks for each of three treatment groups consuming 500 mL of orange juice, hesperidin or placebo [382].

N-ACETYLCYSTEINE (NAC)

Combination of N-acetylcysteine (NAC) and L-arginine (ARG) reduces endothelial activation and BP in hypertensive patients with and without type 2 DM [124,383–385]. In 24 subjects with type 2 DM and hypertension treated for 6 months with placebo or NAC with ARG, both SBP and DBP were significantly reduced ($p = 0.05$) [124]. Nitric oxide and endothelial post-ischemic vasodilation increased [124]. NAC increases NO via IL-1b and increases iNOS mRNA, increases glutathione by increasing cysteine levels, reduces the affinity for the AT1 receptor by disrupting disulfide groups, blocks the L-type calcium channel, lowers homocysteine and improves carotid IMT [124,383–385]. The recommended dose is 500–1,000 mg twice a day.

HAWTHORN

Hawthorn extract has been used for centuries for the treatment of hypertension, CHF and other cardiovascular diseases, but the studies are limited and are not convincing of any significant clinical responses [386–390]. A recent four-period crossover design, dose response study of 21 subjects with prehypertension or mild hypertension over 3½ days did not show changes in FMD or BP on standardized extract with 50 mg of oligomeric procyanidin per 250 mg extract with 1,000, 1,500 or 2,500 mg of the extract [386]. Hawthorn showed non-inferiority of ACEI and diuretics in the treatment of 102 patients with NYHC II CHF over 8 weeks [388]. Patients with hypertension and type 2 DM on medications for BP and DM that were randomized to 1,200 mg of hawthorn extract for 16 weeks showed significant reductions in DBP of 2.6 mmHg ($p=0.035$) [389]. Thirty-six mildly hypertensive patients administered 500 mg of hawthorn extract for 10 weeks showed a non-significant trend in DBP reduction ($p=0.081$) compared to placebo [390]. Hawthorn acts like an ACEI, beta-blockers (BB), CCB and diuretic. More studies are needed to determine the efficacy, long-term effects and dose of hawthorn for the treatment of hypertension.

QUERCETIN

Quercetin is an antioxidant flavonol found in apples, berries and onions that reduces BP in hypertensive individuals [391–393], but the hypotensive effects do not appear to be mediated by changes in HSCRP, TNF-alpha, ACE activity, ET-1, NO, vascular reactivity or FMD [391]. Quercetin is metabolized by CYP 3A4 and should be used with caution in patients on drugs metabolized by this cytochrome system [391–393]. Quercetin was administered to 12 hypertensive men at an oral dose of 1,095 mg with reduction in mean BP by 5 mmHg, SBP by 7 mmHg and DBP by 3 mmHg [391]. Forty-one prehypertensive and stage I hypertensive subjects were enrolled in a randomized, double-blind, placebo-controlled, crossover study with 500 mg of quercetin per day vs placebo [392]. In the stage I hypertensive patients, the BP was reduced by 7/5 mmHg ($p<0.05$) [392]. Quercetin administered to 93 overweight or obese subjects at 150 mg/day (plasma levels of 269 nmol/L) over 6 weeks lowered SBP by 2.9 mmHg in the hypertensive group and up to 3.7 mmHg in SBP in the patients 25–50 years of age [393]. The recommended dose of quercetin is 500 mg twice daily.

PROBIOTICS

Gut dysbiosis in hypertension is characterized by a gut microbiome that are less diverse with an increased Firmicutes/Bacteroidetes ratio, a decrease in acetate- and butyrate-producing bacteria and an increase in lactate-producing bacterial populations. There are several meta-analysis in humans that support the role of probiotic supplementation to reduce BP [111,394–396].

A meta-analysis of RCTs suggested that consuming probiotics results in a modest lowering of BP with a potentially greater effect with an elevated baseline BP, when multiple species of probiotics are consumed, the duration of the intervention is ≥8 weeks and the daily dose is ≥10^{11} colony-forming units [394].

Another meta-analysis of 14 RCTs involving 702 participants showed that compared with placebo, probiotic-fermented milk produced a slight but significant reduction of 3.1/1.1 mmHg in BP. Subgroup analyses suggested a slightly greater effect on SBP in hypertensive than in normotensive participants [110]. In a meta-analysis of 11 eligible randomized controlled trial ($n=641$), probiotic consumption significantly decreased SBP (WMD, −3.28 mmHg; 95% CI: −5.38 to −1.18) and DBP (WMD, −2.13 mmHg; 95% CI: −4.5–0.24) in type 2 diabetic patients compared with placebo [395].

Hypertension may be caused by many factors including hypercholesterolemia, chronic inflammation and inconsistent modulation of the RAAS that are modified by probiotics [396–398].

DRUG THERAPY FOR HYPERTENSION

The 2017 ACC/AHA Guidelines for the Prevention, Detection, Evaluation, and
Management of Hypertension in Adults provides the following summary [2–5,11–15,399,400]:

1. **Classification of BP**: Four new BP categories based on the average of two or more in-office BP readings.
   Normal: <120 mmHg SBP and <80 mmHg DBP
   Elevated: 120–129 mmHg SBP and <80 mmHg DBP
   Stage 1 Hypertension: 130–139 mmHg SBP or 80–89 mmHg DBP
   Stage 2 Hypertension: ≥140 mmHg SBP or ≥90 mmHg DBP
2. **Prevalence of High BP**: Substantially higher prevalence of under the new guideline, 46% of U.S. adults versus 32%, based on the JNC 7 definition. However, for most U.S. adults meeting the new definition of hypertension that would not meet the JNC 7 definition, nonpharmacological treatment is recommended. Because most people between 130–139 mmHg SBP or 80–89 mmHg DBP will not require medication to treat their hypertension, there will only be a small increase in the percentage of U.S. adults for whom antihypertensive medication is recommended in conjunction with lifestyle modification. Commit to helping your patients by implementing a BP improvement program.
3. **Treatment of High BP**: All patients with BPs above normal should be treated with nonpharmacological interventions. For most adults, these include consuming a heart-healthy diet such as DASH, reducing sodium intake, increasing physical activity, limiting alcohol consumption and losing weight for those who are overweight. Pharmacological Interventions: Use of BP-lowering medications is recommended based on the stage of hypertension, an individual's medical history or estimated 10-year CVD risk ≥ 10% using the ACC/AHA Risk Estimator.
4. **BP Goal for People with High BP**: For adults with confirmed hypertension and known CVD, or 10-year atherosclerotice cardiovascular disease (ASCVD) event risk of 10% or higher, a BP goal of less than 130/80 mmHg is recommended. For adults without additional markers of increased CVD risk, a BP goal of less than 130/80 mmHg may also be reasonable. The totality of the available information provides evidence that a lower BP target is generally better than a higher BP target. The SBP target recommended in the new guideline (<130 mmHg) is higher than that which was used in the SPRINT trial (<120 mmHg). Learn how to improve BP control rates.
5. **Use Self-Measured Blood Pressure Monitoring (SMBP) to Diagnose, Reassess and Activate Patients with High BP**: SMBP refers to the regular measurement of BP by an individual, at their home or elsewhere outside the clinic setting. SMBP can be used for confirmation of hypertension diagnosis based on elevated office readings and for titration of BP-lowering medication, in conjunction with telehealth counseling or clinical interventions. SMBP can help differentiate between sustained, white coat, and masked hypertension. SMBP can also be used for reassessment of patients (at 1-, 3-, 6- or 12-month intervals) per new guideline recommendations.

The selection of antihypertensive drug therapy should be based on all of the following considerations [2–5,11–15]:

- Level of BP.
- Presence of other CHD risk factors.

- Calculation of CHD risk with COSHEC, ACC/AHA or Rasmussen risk calculator that indicates high risk.
- Presence of clinical CVD target organ damage (TOD).
- Presence of other preclinical tests for vascular damage such as EndoPAT.
   CAPWA, CAC, CORUS, Carotid Duplex, CPET, ECHO and autonomic function testing.
- Presence of clinical symptoms related to BP such as headache, chest pain at rest or with exercise and dyspnea, etc.
- PRA, aldosterone and ARR (aldosterone renin ratio). Low renin hypertension (LRH) has an increased intravascular volume (volume dependent) with a PRA < 0.65 ng/mL/hour. This represents about 30% of hypertensive patients. High renin hypertension (HRH) has a decreased intravascular volume with a PRA > 0.65 ng/mL/hour. This is about 70% of hypertensive patients. The ARR (pg/mL/ng/mL/hour) helps to further establish if the patient has LRH or HRH as follows:
   ARR over 80 is LRH or primary hyperaldosteronism
   ARR over 40 is probably LRH with a sensitivity and specificity of
   100% and 92% for primary aldosteronism.
   ARR less than 10 is HRH
   ARR between 10 and 40: not sure
   The measurement of PRA and aldosterone plasma levels may be done in a random ambulatory setting, is most accurate in drug-naïve patients, does not require alterations in patient position, time of day, sodium intake, etc. However, the levels of PRA will be altered by concomitant antihypertensive medications which requires more sophisticated interpretation.
- Nutritional depletion evaluation.
- Demographics.
- Subsets of Hypertension: Individualized Treatment.
- Genetic phenotype (SNP)
   1. Those that predispose an individual to hypertension in some or all conditions
   2. Those that predict response to a drug or nutrient.

Aggressive, early BP reduction results in the best CVD reduction. The recommended new BP goal is 120/80 mmHg [2–5,11–15]. The 24-hour ABM and brachial and central BPs are recommended over office or home brachial BP to assess dipping status, nocturnal BP, lability, BP load, BP surges and mean BP. Non-invasive vascular testing for functional and structural abnormalities of the vasculature should be done such as pulse-wave analysis, augmentation index central BP, ED and arterial compliance. Nocturnal BP drives the risk for CVD. If a patient is a non-dipper, then medications should be administered at night. This approach will reduce cardiovascular events to a greater extent compared to giving the medications in the morning.

Initial therapy in most hypertensive patients should be amlodipine/ACEI or amlodipine/ARB combinations, as these have the best reductions in BP and cardiovascular TOD [2–5,11–15]. However, this selection will depend on the PRA:

- LRH is best treated with CCB, diuretics and SARAs like spironolactone and epleronone.
- HRH is best treated with renal artery stenosis (RAS) or renin drugs such as ACEI, ARBs, DRI, certain BB or central alpha agonists (CAA).

Long-acting ACEIs with tissue selectivity are preferred. This would include all of the ACEIs except captopril, enalapril and lisinopril. An ARB with high affinity for the AT 1 receptor and longer effect on both BP and vascular protection is preferred. These would include most of the ARBs except losartan. The DHP CCBs such as amlodipine and nifedipine are preferred over verapamil and diltiazem. Indapamide is diuretic of choice for a third drug, and then chlorthalidone. However, hydrochlorothiazide (HCTZ) alone or in combination with other agents should be avoided due to its lack of efficacy in reducing CVD and CHD, increase in glucose and risk of type 2 DM, inducing an abnormal lipid profile, increasing homocysteine and causing numerous nutritional deficiencies and other metabolic problems such as hypokalemia, hypomagnesemia and hyponatremia [2–5,11–15].

Nebivolol (vasodilating and increases nitric oxide) and carvedilol (an alpha-/beta-blocker with antioxidant activity) are the BB of choice. One should avoid other older BB for hypertension as they do not reduce CVD or CHD compared to the other antihypertensive agents. Renin inhibitors (DRI) are appropriate for add-on treatment but should not be given with an ACEI or an ARB. An ACEI should not be administered with an ARB. Spironolactone 12.5–25 mg QD is very effective in resistant hypertension or in patients with LRH or those with the genetic SNP CYP11 B2. Amiloride 5–20 mg/day is very effective in patients with hyperactive epithelial sodium channel with a genetic SNP CYP4A11 or LRH.

If the patient develops edema on a CCB, then the best treatment to reduce the edema is with and ACEI or ARB not a diuretic. Also giving the CCB at night may reduce edema during the day. Drugs that may increase serum potassium should be monitored carefully if administered simultaneously (ACEI, ARB, spironolactone, epleronone, amiloride) and also used carefully in those with renal impairment. Rationale combinations are preferred that have different mechanisms of action such as ACEI or ARB with CCB, diuretic and a vasodilating beta-blocker. The addition of spironolactone or amiloride will depend on the BP and clinical setting as well as PRA and ARR levels, and genetics.

CLINICAL CONSIDERATIONS

A comprehensive clinical approach to the categories and clinical use of nutraceutical supplements is detailed in Tables 7.2 and 7.3.

Several of the strategic combinations of nutraceutical supplements with antihypertensive drugs have been shown to lower BP more than the medication alone [2–5]. These are:

- Pycnogenol with ACEI
- Lycopene with various antihypertensive medications
- R-Lipoic acid with ACEI
- Vitamin C with CCB
- N-Acetylcysteine with arginine
- Garlic with ACEI, diuretics and BB
- Coenzyme Q-10 with ACEI and CCB.

Many antihypertensive drugs may cause nutrient depletions that can actually interfere with their antihypertensive action or cause other metabolic adverse effects manifest through the laboratory results with clinical symptoms [401,402]. Diuretics decrease potassium, magnesium, phosphorous, sodium, chloride, folate, vitamin B6, zinc, iodine and coenzyme Q-10; increase homocysteine, calcium and creatinine; and elevate serum glucose by inducing insulin resistance. BB reduce coenzyme Q-10, and ACEI and ARBs reduce zinc [401,402].

Clinical monitoring of BP is required as well as patient awareness that dietary and supplemental interventions need to be taken as consistently as medications. Additional laboratory tests can inform clinical decision-making such as the measurement of intracellular micronutrients in lymphocytes, antioxidant capacity, oxidative stress, inflammation biomarkers such as hsCRP, PRA and serum aldosterone followed by repletion of all micronutrient depletions with selected higher doses of nutritional supplements based on the clinical studies that have been reviewed [403].

SUMMARY

- Vascular biology such as endothelial, vascular and cardiac smooth muscle dysfunction plays a primary and pivotal role in the initiation and perpetuation of hypertension.

TABLE 7.2

Natural Antihypertensive Compounds Categorized by Antihypertensive Class

Antihypertensive Therapeutic Class (Alphabetical Listing)	Foods and Ingredients Listed by Therapeutic Class	Nutrients and Other Supplements Listed by Therapeutic Class
Angiotensin-converting enzyme inhibitors	Egg yolk	Melatonin
	Fish (specific):	Omega-3 fatty acids
	Bonito	Pomegranate
	Dried salted fish	Probiotics
	Fish sauce	Pycnogenol
	Sardine muscle/protein	Quercetin (?)
	Tuna	Zinc
	Garlic	
	Gelatin	
	Hawthorn berry	
	Isoflavones/flavonoids	
	Milk products (specific):	
	Casein	
	Sour milk	
	Whey (hydrolyzed)	
	Protein	
	Sake	
	Sea vegetables (kelp)	
	Seaweed (wakame)	
	Sesame (also ET1)	
	Wheat germ (hydrolyzed)	
	Zein (corn protein)	
Angiotensin receptor blockers	Celery	Coenzyme Q-10
	Fiber	Gamma linolenic acid
	Garlic	NAC
	MUFA	Oleic acid
		Resveratrol
		Potassium
		Taurine
		Vitamin C
		Vitamin B6 (pyridoxine)
Beta-blockers	Hawthorn berry	
Calcium channel blockers	Celery	Alpha lipoic acid
	Garlic	Calcium
	Hawthorn berry	Magnesium (PGE,NO)
	MUFA	N-Acetyl cysteine
		Oleic acid
		Omega-3 fatty acids:
		Eicosapentaenoic acid
		Docosahexaenoic acid
		Taurine
		Vitamin B6
		Vitamin C
		Vitamin E

(Continued)

TABLE 7.2 (*Continued*)
Natural Antihypertensive Compounds Categorized by Antihypertensive Class

Antihypertensive Therapeutic Class (Alphabetical Listing)	Foods and Ingredients Listed by Therapeutic Class	Nutrients and Other Supplements Listed by Therapeutic Class
Central alpha agonists (reduce sympathetic nervous system activity)	Celery Fiber Garlic Protein	Coenzyme Q-10 Gamma linolenic acid Potassium Probiotics Restriction of sodium Taurine Vitamin C Vitamin B6 Zinc
Direct renin inhibitors		Vitamin D
Direct vasodilators	Beets (NO, ED) Celery Cocoa (NO, ED) Cooking oils with monounsaturated fats Fiber Garlic Hesperidin and OJ Lycopene food (NO, ED) MUFA Soy Teas: green and black	Alpha linolenic acid Arginine Calcium Carnitines (eNOS, NO) Flavonoids Grape seed extract Lycopene (NO, ED) Magnesium Melatonin (NO, ED) Omega-3 fatty acids (NO, ED) Potassium (NO, ED) Taurine Vitamin C Vitamin E
Diuretics	Celery Fiber Hawthorn berry Protein	Calcium Coenzyme Q-10 Fiber Gamma linolenic acid L-carnitine Magnesium Potassium Taurine Vitamin B6 Vitamin C Vitamin E : high gamma/delta tocopherols and tocotrienols

- Nutrient-gene interactions and epigenetics are predominant factors in promoting beneficial or detrimental effects in cardiovascular health and hypertension.
- Oxidative stress, inflammation and vascular immune dysfunction initiate and propagate hypertension and cardiovascular disease.
- Nutrition, natural whole food, nutraceutical supplements, antioxidants, antiinflammatory agents, vitamins and minerals can prevent, control and treat hypertension through numerous vascular biology mechanisms and may mimic the effects of the various antihypertensive drug classes.

TABLE 7.3

An Integrative Approach to the Treatment of Hypertension

Intervention Category	Therapeutic Intervention	Daily Intake
Diet characteristics	DASH I, DASH II-Na$^+$ or PREMIER diet	Diet type
	Sodium restriction	1,500 mg
	Potassium	5,000–10,000 mg
	Potassium/sodium ratio	>4:1
	Magnesium	1,000 mg
	Zinc	50 mg
Macronutrients	*Protein*: Total intake from non-animal sources, organic lean or wild animal protein, or cold-water fish	30% of total calories, which 1.5–1.8 g/kg body weight
	Whey protein	30 g
	Soy protein (fermented sources are preferred)	30 g
	Sardine muscle concentrate extract	3 g
	Milk peptides (VPP and IPP)	30–60 mg
	Fat	30% of total calories
	Omega-3 fatty acids	2–3 g
	Omega-6 fatty acids	1 g
	Omega-9 fatty acids (MUFA)	4 Tablespoons (40 g) of EVOO or nuts
	Saturated fatty acids from wild game, bison, or other lean meat	<10% Total calories
	Polyunsaturated to saturated fat ratio	>2.0
	Omega-3 to omega-6 ratio	1.1–1.2
	Synthetic *trans* fatty acids	None (completely remove from diet)
	Nuts in variety	4 Servings
	Carbohydrates as primarily complex carbohydrates and fiber	40% of total calories
	Oatmeal or	60 g
	Oatbran or	40 g
	Beta-glucan or	3 g
	Psyllium	7 g
Specific foods	Garlic as fresh cloves or aged Kyolic garlic	4 Fresh cloves (4 g) or 600 mg aged garlic taken twice daily
	Sea vegetables, specifically dried wakame	3.0–3.5 g
	Lycopene as tomato products, guava, watermelon, apricots, pink grapefruit, papaya or supplements	10–20 mg
	Dark chocolate	100 g
	Pomegranate juice or seeds	8 ounces or one cup
	Sesame	60 mg sesamin or 2.5 g <u>sesame meal</u> <u>500 g</u>
	Beet juice	<u>60 oz of 500 mg bid</u> 2–6 g per day
	Green tea or EGCG extract	
	Carnitine	
Exercise	Aerobic	20 minutes daily at 4,200 KJ/week
	Resistance	40 minutes per day

(Continued)

TABLE 7.3 (*Continued*)
An Integrative Approach to the Treatment of Hypertension

Intervention Category	Therapeutic Intervention	Daily Intake
Weight reduction	Body mass index < 25 Waist circumference: <35 in. for women <40 in. for men Total body fat: <22% for women <16% for men	Lose 1–2 pounds per week and increasing the proportion of lean muscle
Other lifestyle recommendations	Alcohol restriction: Among the choice of alcohol red wine is preferred due to its vasoactive phytonutrients	<20 grams/day Wine <10 ounces Beer <24 ounces Liquor <2 ounces
	Caffeine restriction or elimination depending on CYP 1A2 450 SNP	<100 mg/day
	Tobacco and smoking	Stop
Medical considerations	Medications which may increase BP	Minimize use when possible, such as by using disease-specific nutritional interventions
Supplemental foods and nutrients	Alpha lipoic acid with biotin	100–200 mg twice daily
	Amino acids: Arginine	2 g twice daily
	Carnitine	1–2 g twice daily
	Taurine	1–3 g twice daily
	Chlorogenic acids	150–200 mg
	Coenzyme Q-10	100 mg once to twice daily
	Grape seed extract	300 mg
	Hawthorn extract	500 mg twice a day
	Melatonin (long acting)	3 mg
	N-Acetyl cysteine (NAC)	500 mg twice a day
	Olive leaf extract (oleuropein)	500 mg twice a day
	Pycnogenol	200 mg
	Quercetin	500 mg twice a day
	Probiotics	10^{11} CFU
	Resveratrol (*trans*)	250 mg
	Vitamin B6	100 mg once to twice daily
	Vitamin C	250–500 mg twice daily
	Vitamin D3	Dose to raise 25-hydroxyvitamin D serum level to 60 ng/ml
	Vitamin E as mixed tocopherols	400 IU

- There is a role for the selected use of single and combined nutraceutical supplements, vitamins, antioxidants and minerals in the treatment of hypertension based on prospective randomized placebo-controlled studies and meta-analysis as a complement to optimal nutrition and other lifestyle modifications.
- A clinical approach that incorporates optimal nutrition with scientifically proven nutraceutical supplements, exercise, weight reduction, smoking cessation, alcohol and caffeine restriction, and other lifestyle strategies can be systematically and successfully incorporated into clinical practice for the prevention and treatment of hypertension (Tables 7.2 and 7.3).
- BP should be lowered aggressively and early with a combination of nutrition, supplements, lifestyle changes and drugs.
- Antihypertensive drugs should be directed at both BP and CVD reduction with improvement in vascular function and structure.
- ACEI, ARB, indapamide and DHP-CCB, nebivolol, carvedilol and spironolactone are preferred drugs comparted to HCTZ and the older beta-blocker. Logical combinations are recommended.

REFERENCES

1. Wesa KM, Grimm RH Jr. Recommendations and guidelines regarding the preferred research protocol for investigating the impact of an optimal healing environment on patients with hypertension. *J Altern Complement Med* 2004;10(Suppl 1):S245–50.
2. Houston MC. The role of nutrition and nutraceutical supplements in the treatment of hypertension. *World J Cardiol* 2014;6(2):38–66.
3. Houston MC. Nutrition and nutraceutical supplements for the treatment of hypertension: part 1. *J Clin Hypertens* 2013;15:752–7.
4. Houston MC. Nutrition and nutraceutical supplements for the treatment of hypertension: part II. *J Clin Hypertens* 2013;15:845–51.
5. Houston MC. Nutrition and nutraceutical supplements for the treatment of hypertension: part III. *J Clin Hypertens* 2013;15:931–7.
6. Borghi C, Cicero AF. Nutraceuticals with a clinically detectable blood pressure-lowering effect: a review of available randomized clinical trials and their meta-analyses. *Br J Clin Pharmacol* 2017;83(1):163–71.
7. Sirtori CR, Arnoldi A, Cicero AF. Nutraceuticals for blood pressure control. *Rev Ann Med* 2015;47(6):447–56.
8. Cicero AF, Colletti A. Nutraceuticals and blood pressure control: results from clinical trials and meta-analyses. *High Blood Press Cardiovasc Prev* 2015;22(3):203–13.
9. Turner JM, Spatz ES. Nutritional supplements for the treatment of hypertension: a practical guide for clinicians. *Curr Cardiol Rep* 2016;18(12):126. Review.
10. Caligiuri SP, Pierce GN. A review of the relative efficacy of dietary, nutritional supplements, lifestyle and drug therapies in the management of hypertension. *Crit Rev Food Sci Nutr* 2016 Aug 5:0 [Epub ahead of print].
11. Houston MC, Fox B, Taylor N. *What Your Doctor May Not Tell You About Hypertension. The Revolutionary Nutrition and Lifestyle Program to Help Fight High Blood Pressure.* AOL Time Warner, Warner Books, New York. 2003.
12. Houston MC. *Handbook of Hypertension.* Wiley-Blackwell, Oxford. 2009.
13. Houston MC. *What Your Doctor May Not Tell You About Heart Disease.* Grand Central Press, New York. 2012.
14. Sinatra S and Houston M, Editors. *Nutrition and Integrative Strategies in Cardiovascular Medicine.* CRC Press, Boca Raton, FL. 2015.
15. Joint National Committee on Prevention, Detection, Evaluation, and Treatment of High Blood Pressure. The seventh report of the joint national committee on prevention, detection, evaluation, and treatment of high blood pressure (JNC-7). *JAMA* 2003;289:2560–72.
16. Thomopoulos C, Parati G, Zanchetti A. Effects of blood pressure lowering on outcome incidence in hypertension: 7. Effects of more vs. less intensive blood pressure lowering and different achieved blood pressure levels – updated overview and meta-analyses of randomized trials. *J Hypertens* 2016;34(4):613–22.

17. Ettehad D, Emdin CA, Kiran A, Anderson SG, Callender T, Emberson J, Chalmers J, Rodgers A, Rahimi K. Blood pressure lowering for prevention of cardiovascular disease and death: a systematic review and meta-analysis. *Lancet* 2016;387(10022):957–67.
18. ESH/ESC Task Force for the Management of Arterial Hypertension. 2013 Practice guidelines for the management of arterial hypertension of the European Society of Hypertension (ESH) and the European Society of Cardiology (ESC): ESH/ESC Task Force for the management of arterial hypertension. *J Hypertens* 2013;31:1925–38.
19. Flack JM, Calhoun D, Schiffrin EL. The new ACC/AHA hypertension guidelines for the prevention, detection, evaluation, and management of high blood pressure in adults. *Am J Hypertens* 2018;31(2):133–5.
20. Appel LJ. American society of hypertension writing group. ASH position paper: dietary approaches to lower blood pressure. *J Am Soc Hypertens* 2009;3:321–31.
21. Eaton SB, Eaton SB III, Konner MJ. Paleolithic nutrition revisited: a twelve-year retrospective on its nature and implications. *Eur J Clin Nutr* 1997;51:207–16.
22. Layne J, Majkova Z, Smart EJ, Toborek M, Hennig B. Caveolae: a regulatory platform for nutritional modulation of inflammatory diseases. *J Nutr Biochem* 2011;22:807–11.
23. Dandona P, Ghanim H, Chaudhuri A, Dhindsa S, Kim SS. Macronutrient intake induces oxidative and inflammatory stress: potential relevance to atherosclerosis and insulin resistance. *Exp Mol Med* 2010;42(4):245–53.
24. Kizhakekuttu TJ, Widlansky ME. Natural antioxidants and hypertension: promise and challenges. *Cardiovasc Ther* 2010;28(4): e20–32.
25. Houston MC. New insights and approaches to reduce end organ damage in the treatment of hypertension: subsets of hypertension approach. *Am Heart J* 1992;123:1337–67.
26. Nayak DU, Karmen C, Frishman WH, Vakili BA. Antioxidant vitamins and enzymatic and synthetic oxygen-derived free radical scavengers in the prevention and treatment of cardiovascular disease. *Heart Dis* 2001;3:28–45.
27. Ritchie RH, Drummond GR Sobey CG, De Silva TM, Kemp-Harper BK. The opposing roles of NO and oxidative stress in cardiovascular disease. *Pharmacol Res* 2017;116:57–69.
28. Russo C, Olivieri O, Girelli D, Faccini G, Zenari ML, Lombardi S, Corrocher R. Antioxidant status and lipid peroxidation in patients with essential hypertension. *J Hypertens* 1998;16:1267–71.
29. Tse WY, Maxwell SR, Thomason H, Blann A, Thorpe GH, Waite M, Holder R. Antioxidant status in controlled and uncontrolled hypertension and its relationship to endothelial damage. *J Hum Hypertens* 1994;8:843–9.
30. Galley HF, Thornton J, Howdle PD, Walker BE, Webster NR. Combination oral antioxidant supplementation reduces blood pressure. *Clin Sci* 1997;92:361–5.
31. Dhalla NS, Temsah RM, Netticadam T. The role of oxidative stress in cardiovascular diseases. *J Hypertens* 2000;18:655–673.
32. Loperena R, Harrison DG. Oxidative stress and hypertensive diseases. *Med Clin North Am* 2017;101(1):169–93.
33. Pietri P, Vlachopoulos C, Tousoulis D. Inflammation and Arterial hypertension: from pathophysiological links to risk prediction. See comment in PubMed Commons below *Curr Med Chem* 2015; 22(23):2754–61.
34. Amer MS, Elawam AE, Khater MS, Omar OH, Mabrouk RA, Taha HM. Association of high-sensitivity C reactive protein with carotid artery intimamedia thickness in hypertensive older adults. *J Am Soc Hypertens* 2011 April 23;5:395–400 [Epub].
35. Kvakan H, Luft FC, Muller DN. Role of the immune system in hypertensive target organ damage. *Trends Cardiovasc Med* 2009;19(7):242–6.
36. Rodriquez-Iturbe B, Franco M, Tapia E, Quiroz Y, Johnson RJ. Renal inflammation, autoimmunity and salt-sensitive hypertension. *Clin Exp Pharmacol Physiol* 2011; 32,:24–32 [Epub].
37. Mansego ML, Solar Gde M, Alonso MP, Martinez F, Saez GT, Escudero JC, Redon J, Chaves FJ. Polymorphisms of antioxidant enzymes, blood pressure and risk of hypertension. *J Hypertens* 2011;29(3):492–500.
38. Vongpatanasin W, Thomas GD, Schwartz R, Cassis LA, Osborne-Lawrence S, Hahner L, Gibson LL, Black S, Samois D, Shaul PW. C-reactive protein causes downregulation of vascular angiotensin subtype 2 receptors and systolic hypertension in mice. *Circulation* 2007;115(8) 1020–8.
39. Razzouk L, Munter P, Bansilal S, Kini AS, Aneja A, Mozes J, Ivan O, Jakkula M, Sharma S, Farkouh ME. C reactive protein predicts long-term mortality independently of low-density lipoprotein cholesterol in patients undergoing percutaneous coronary intervention. *Am Heart J* 2009;158(2):277–83.

40. Tian N, Penman AD, Mawson AR, Manning RD Jr, Flessner MF. Association between circulating specific leukocyte types and blood pressure. The atherosclerosis risk in communities (ARIC) study. *J Am Soc Hypertens* 2010;4(6):272–83.

41. Muller DN, Kvakan H, Luft FC. Immune-related effects in hypertension and target-organ damage. *Curr Opin Nephrol Hypertens* 2011;20(2):113–7.

42. Leibowitz A, Schiffin, EL. Immune mechanisms in hypertension. *Curr Hypertens Rep* 2011;13(6):465–72.

43. Xiong S, Li Q, Liu D, Zhu Z. Gastrointestinal tract: a promising target for the management of hypertension. *Curr Hypertens Rep* 2017;19(4):31.

44. Caillon A, Mian MO, Fraulob-Aquino JC, Huo KG, Barhoumi T, Ouerd S, Sinnaeve PR, Paradis P, Schiffrin EL. Gamma delta T cells mediate angiotensin II-induced hypertension and vascular injury. *Circulation* 2017 Mar 22. pii: CIRCULATIONAHA.116.027058. doi:10.1161/CIRCULATIONAHA.116.027058 [Epub ahead of print].

45. Rudemiller NP, Crowley SD. The role of chemokines in hypertension and consequent target organ damage. *Pharmacol Res* 2017;119:404–11.

46. De Ciuceis C, Agabiti-Rosei C, Rossini C, Airò P, Scarsi M, Tincani A, Tiberio GA, Piantoni S, Porteri E, Solaini L, Duse S, Semeraro F, Petroboni B, Mori L, Castellano M, Gavazzi A, Agabiti-Rosei E, Rizzoni D. Relationship between different subpopulations of circulating CD4+ T lymphocytes and microvascular or systemic oxidative stress in humans. *Blood Press* 2017 Feb 15;30:1–9.

47. Caillon A, Schiffrin EL. Role of inflammation and immunity in hypertension: recent epidemiological, laboratory, and clinical evidence. *Curr Hypertens Rep* 2016 Mar;18(3):21.

48. Abais-Battad JM, Dasinger JH, Fehrenbach DJ, Mattson DL. Novel adaptive and innate immunity targets in hypertension. *Pharmacol Res* 2017 Mar 20. pii: S1043-6618(16)30860-X. doi:10.1016/j.phrs.2017.03.015 [Epub ahead of print].

49. Biancardi VC, Bomfim GF, Reis WL, Al-Gassimi S, Nunes KP. The interplay between angiotensin II, TLR4 and hypertension. *Pharmacol Res* 2017 Mar 19. pii: S1043-6618(16)30910-0. doi:10.1016/j.phrs.2017.03.017 [Epub ahead of print].

50. Justin Rucker A, Crowley SD. The role of macrophages in hypertension and its complications. *Pflugers Arch* 2017;469(3–4):419–30.

51. Miller ER 3rd, Erlinger TP, Appel LJ. The effects of macronutrients on blood pressure and lipids: an overview of the DASH and OmniHeart trials. *Curr Atheroscler Rep* 2006;8:460–5.

52. Pérez-López FR, Chedraui P, Quadro JL. Effects of the Mediterranean diet on longevity and age-related morbid conditions. *Maturitas* 2009;64:67–79.

53. Cutler JA, Follmann D, Allender PS. Randomized trials of sodium reduction: an overview. *Am J Clin Nutr* 1997;65:643S–51S.

54. Sacks FM, Svetkey LP, Vollmer WM, Appel LJ, Bray GA, Harsha D, Obarzanek E, Conlin PR, Miller ER 3rd, Simons-Morton DG, Karanja N, Lin PH, DASH-Sodium Collaborative Research Group. Effects on blood pressure of reduced dietary sodium and the dietary approaches to stop hypertension (DASH) diet. DASH-Sodium Collaborative Research Group. *N Engl J Med* 2001;344(1):3–10.

55. Messerli FH, Schmieder RE, Weir MR. Salt: a perpetrator of hypertensive target organ disease? *Arch Intern Med* 1997;157:2449–52.

56. Merino J, Guasch-Ferré M, Martínez-González MA, Corella D, Estruch R, Fitó M, Ros E, Arós F, Bulló M, Gómez-Gracia E, Moñino M, Lapetra J, Serra-Majem L, Razquin C, Buil-Cosiales P, Sorlí JV, Muñoz MA, Pintó X, Masana L, Salas-Salvadó J. Is complying with the recommendations of sodium intake beneficial for health in individuals at high cardiovascular risk? Findings from the PREDIMED study. *Am J Clin Nutr* 2015;101(3):440–8.

57. Weinberger MH. Salt sensitivity of blood pressure in humans. *Hypertension* 1996;27:481–90.

58. Morimoto A, Usu T, Fujii T, et al. Sodium sensitivity and cardiovascular events in patients with essential hypertension. *Lancet* 1997;350:1734–737.

59. Kanbay M, Chen Y, Solak Y, Sanders PW. Mechanisms and consequences of salt sensitivity and dietary salt intake. *Curr Opin Nephrol Hypertens* 2011;20(1):37–43.

60. Toda N, Arakawa K. Salt-induced hemodynamic regulation mediated by nitric oxide. *J Hypertens* 2011;29(3):415–24.

61. Rust P, Ekmekcioglu C. Impact of salt intake on the pathogenesis and treatment of hypertension. *Adv Exp Med Biol* 2016;L22:15–25 Oct 19 [Epub ahead of print].

62. Oberleithner H, Callies C, Kusche-Vihrog K, Schillers H, Shahin V, Riethmuller C, Macgregor GA, deWardener HE. Potassium softens vascular endothelium and increases nitric oxide release. *Proc Natl Acad Sci USA* 2009;106(8):2829–34.

63. Feis J, Oberleithner H, Kusche-Vihrog K. Menage a trios: aldosterone, sodium and nitric oxide in vascular endothelium. *Biochim Biophys Acta* 2010;1802(12):1193–202.
64. Foulquier S, Dupuis F, Perrin-Sarrado C, Maquin Gate K, Merhi-Soussi F, Liminana P, Kwan YW, Capdeville-Atkinson C, Lartaud I, Atkinson J. High salt intake abolishes AT (2) – mediated vasodilation of pial arterioes in rats. *J Hypertension* 2011;29(7):1392–9.
65. Yang Q, Liu T, Kuklina EV, Glanders WD, Hong Y, Gillespie C, Chang MH, Gwinn M, Dowling N, Khoury MJ, Hu FB. Sodium and potassium intake and mortality among US adults: prospective data from the third national health and nutrition examination survey. *Arch Int Med* 2011;171(13):1183–91.
66. Houston MC, Harper KJ. Potassium, magnesium, and calcium: their role in both the cause and treatment of hypertension. *J Clin Hypertens* 2008;10(7Suppl 2):3–11.
67. Perez V, Chang ET. Sodium-to-potassium ratio and blood pressure, hypertension, and related factors. *Adv Nutr* 2014;5:712–41.
68. Filippini T, Violi F, D'Amico R, Vinceti M. The effect of potassium supplementation on blood pressure in hypertensive subjects: a systematic review and metaanalysis. *Int J Cardiol* 2017;230:127–35.
69. Gu D, He J, Xigui W, Duan X, Whelton PK. Effect of potassium supplementation on blood pressure in Chinese: a randomized, placebo-controlled trial. *J Hypertens* 2001;19:1325–31.
70. D'Elia L, Barba G, Cappuccio FP, Strazzullo P. Potassium intake, stroke, and cardiovascular disease a meta-analysis of prospective studies. *J Am Coll Cardiol* 2011;57:1210–9.
71. Poorolajal J, Zeraati F, Soltanian AR, Sheikh V, Hooshmand E, Maleki A. Oral potassium supplementation for management of essential hypertension: a meta-analysis of randomized controlled trials. *PLoS One* 2017;12(4):e0174967. doi:10.1371/journal.pone.0174967.
72. Houston MC. The importance of potassium in managing hypertension. *Curr Hypertens Rep* 2011;13(4):309–17.
73. Widman L, Wester PO, Stegmayr BG, Wirell MP. The dose dependent reduction in blood pressure through administration of magnesium: a double-blind placebo controlled cross-over trial. *Am J Hypertens* 1993;6:41–5.
74. Laurant P, Touyz RM. Physiological and pathophysiological role of magnesium in the cardiovascular system: implications in hypertension. *J Hypertens* 2000;18:1177–1191.
75. Zhang X, Li Y, Del Gobbo LC, Rosanoff A, Wang J, Zhang W, Song Y. Effects of magnesium supplementation on blood pressure: a meta-analysis of randomized double-blind placebo-controlled trials. *Hypertension* 2016 Aug;68(2):324–33.
76. Kass L, Weekes J, Carpenter L. Effect of magnesium supplementation on blood pressure: a meta-analysis. *Eur J Clin Nutr* 2012;66:411–18.
77. Houston MC. The role of magnesium in hypertension and cardiovascular disease. *J Clin Hypertens* 2011;13:843–7.
78. Cormick G, Ciapponi A, Cafferata ML, Belizán JM. Calcium supplementation for prevention of primary hypertension. *Cochrane Database Syst Rev* 2015 Jun 30;6:CD010037. doi:10.1002/14651858.CD010037.
79. Resnick LM. Calcium metabolism in hypertension and allied metabolic disorders. *Diabetes Care* 1991;14:505–520.
80. Garcia Zozaya JL, Padilla Viloria M. Alterations of calcium, magnesium, and zinc in essential hypertension: their relation to the renin-angiotensin-aldosterone system. *Invest Clin* 1997;38:27–40.
81. Hofmeyr GJ, Lawrie TA, Atallah AN, Duley L. Calcium supplementation during pregnancy for preventing hypertensive disorders and related problems. *Cochrane Database Syst Rev* 2010;8:CD001059.
82. Shahbaz AU, Sun Y, Bhattacharya SK, Ahokas RA, Gerling IC, McGee JE, Weber KT. Fibrosis in hypertensive heart disease: molecular pathways and cardioprotective stratgies. *J Hypetens* 2010;28:S25–32.
83. Bergomi M, Rovesti S, Vinceti M, Vivoli R, Caselgrandi E, Vivoli G. Zinc and copper status and blood pressure. *J Trace Elem Med Biol* 1997;11:166–9.
84. Stamler J, Elliott P, Kesteloot H, Nichols R, Claeys G, Dyer AR, Stamler R. Inverse relation of dietary protein markers with blood pressure. Findings for 10,020 men and women in the intersalt study. Intersalt Cooperative Research Group. International study of salt and blood pressure. *Circulation* 1996;94:1629–34.
85. Altorf-van der Kuil W, Engberink MF, Brink EJ, van Baak MA, Bakker SJ, Navis G, van t'Veer P, Geleijnse JM. Dietary protein and blood pressure: a systematic review. *PLoS One* 2010;5(8);e12102–17.
86. Jenkins, DJ, Kendall CW, Faulkner DA, Kemp T, Marchie A, Nquyen TH, Wong JM, de Souza R. Emam A, Vidgen E, Trautwein EA, Lapsley KG, Josse RG, Leiter LA, Singer W. Long-term effects of a plant-based dietary portfolio of cholesterol-lowering foods on blood pressure. *Eur J Clin Nutr* 2008;62(6):781–8.
87. Rebholz CM, Friedman EE, Powers LJ, Arroyave WD, He J, Kelly TN. Dietary protein intake and blood pressure: a meta-analysis of randomized controlled trials. *Am J Epidemiol* 2012;176(S7):S27–43.

88. He J, Wofford MR, Reynolds K, Chen J, Chen CS, Myers L, Minor DL, ElmerPJ, Jones DW, Whelton PK. Effect of dietary protein supplementation on blood pressure: a randomized controlled trial. *Circulation* 2011;124(5);589–95.

89. FitzGerald RJ, Murray BA, Walsh DJ. Hypotensive peptides from milk proteins. *J Nutr* 2004:134(4):980S–8S.

90. Pins JJ, Keenan JM. Effects of whey peptides on cardiovascular disease risk factors. *J Clin Hypertens* 2006;8(11):775–82.

91. Aihara K, Kajimoto O, Takahashi R, Nakamura Y. Effect of powdered fermented milk with lactobacillus helveticus on subjects with high-normal blood pressure or mild hypertension. *J Am Coll Nutr* 2005;24(4):257–65.

92. Gemino FW, Neutel J, Nonaka M, Hendler SS. The impact of lactotripeptides on blood pressure response in stage 1 and stage 2 hypertensives. *J Clin Hypertens* 2010;12(3):153–9.

93. Geleijnse JM, Engberink MF. Lactopeptides and human blood pressure. *Curr Opin Lipidol* 2010;21(1):58–63.

94. Pins J, Keenan J. The antihypertensive effects of a hydrolyzed whey protein supplement. *Cardiovasc Drugs Ther* 2002;16:68.

95. Zhu CF, Li GZ, Peng HB, Zhang F, Chen Y, Li Y. Therapeutic effects of marine collagen peptides on Chinese patients with type 2 diabetes mellitus and primary hypertension. *Am J Med Sci* 2010;340(5):360–6.

96. De Leo F, Panarese S, Gallerani R, Ceci LR. Angiotensin converting enzyme (ACE) inhibitoroy peptides: production and implementation of functional food. *Curr Pharm Des* 2009;15(31):3622–43.

97. Lordan S, Ross P, Stanton C. Marine bioactives as functional food ingredients: potential to reduce the incidence of chronic disease. *Mar Drugs* 2011;9(6):1056–1100.

98. Kawasaki T, Seki E, Osajima K, Yoshida M, Asada K, Matsui T, Osajima Y. Antihypertensive effect of valyl-tyrosine, a short chain peptide derived from sardine muscle hydrolyzate, on mild hypertensive subjects. *J Hum Hypertens* 2000;14:519–23.

99. Kawasaki T, Jun CJ, Fukushima Y, Seki E. Antihypertensive effect and safety evaluation of vegetable drink with peptides derived from sardine protein hydrolysates on mild hypertensive, high-normal and normal blood pressure subjects. *Fukuoka Igaku Zasshi* 2002:93(10):208–18.

100. Yang G, Shu XO, Jin F, Zhang X, Li HL, Li Q, Gao YT, Zheng W. Longitudinal study of soy food intake and blood pressure among middle-aged and elderly Chinese women. *Am J Clin Nutr* 2005;81(5):1012–7.

101. Teede HJ, Giannopoulos D, Dalais FS, Hodgson J, McGrath BP. Randomised, controlled, cross-over trial of soy protein with isoflavones on blood pressure and arterial function in hypertensive patients. *J Am Coll Nutr* 2006;25(6):533–40.

102. Welty FK, Lee KS, Lew NS, Zhou JR. Effect of soy nuts on blood pressure and lipid levels in hypertensive, prehypertensive and normotensive postmenopausal women. *Arch Inter Med* 2007;167(10):1060–7.

103. Mohanty DP, Mohapatra S, Misra S, Sahu P, Saudi S. Milk derived bioactive peptides and their impact on human health. A review.*J Biol Sci* 2016;23(5):577–83.

104. Nasca MM, Zhou JR, Welty FK. Effect of soy nuts on adhesion molecules and markers of inflammation in hypertensive and normotensive postmenopausal women. *Am J Cardiol* 2008;102(1):84–6.

105. He J, Gu D, Wu X, Chen J, Duan X, Chen J, Whelton PK. Effect of soybean protein on blood pressue: a randomized, controlled trial. *Ann Intern Med* 2005:143(1):1–9.

106. Hasler CM, Kundrat S, Wool D. Functional foods and cardiovascular disease. *Curr Atheroscler Rep* 2000;2(6):467–75.

107. Liu XX, Li SH, Chen JZ, Sun K, Wang XJ, Wang XG, Hui RT. Effect of soy isoflavones on blood pressure: a meta-analysis of randomized controlled trials. *Nutr Metab Cardiovasc Dis* 2012;22:463–70.

108. Begg DP, Sinclari AJ, Stahl LA, Garg ML, Jois M, Weisinger RS. Dietary proteins level interacts with omega-3 polyunsaturated fatty acid deficiency to induce hypertension. *Am J Hypertens* 2009; Nov 5;12:-55–67 [Epub ahead of print].

109. Fekete ÁA, Giromini C, Chatzidiakou Y, Givens DI, Lovegrove JA. Whey protein lowers blood pressure and improves endothelial function and lipid biomarkers in adults with prehypertension and mild hypertension: results from the chronic Whey2Go randomized controlled trial. *Am J Clin Nutr* 2016;104(6):1534–44.

110. Dong JY, Szeto IM, Makinen K, Gao Q, Wang J, Qin LQ, Zhao Y. Effect of probiotic fermented milk on blood pressure: a meta-analysis of randomised controlled trials. *Br J Nutr* 2013;110:1188–94.

111. Cicero AF, Gerocarni B, Laghi L, Borghi C. Blood pressure lowering effect of lactotripeptides assumed as functional foods: a meta-analysis of current available clinical trials. *J Hum Hypertens* 2011;25:425–36.

112. Cicero AF, Aubin F, Azais-Braesco V, Borghi C. Do the lactotripeptides isoleucine-proline-proline and valine-proline-proline reduce systolic blood pressure in European subjects? A meta-analysis of randomized controlled trials. *Am J Hypertens* 2013;26:442–9.
113. Cicero AF, Rosticci M, Gerocarni B, Bacchelli S, Veronesi M, Strocchi E, Borghi C. Lactotripeptides effect on office and 24-h ambulatory blood pressure, blood pressure stress response, pulse wave velocity and cardiac output in patients with high-normal blood pressure or first-degree hypertension: a randomized double-blind clinical trial. *Hypertens Res* 2011;34:1035–40.
114. Morris MC. Dietary fats and blood pressure. *J Cardiovasc Risk* 1994;1:21–30.
115. Siani A, Pagano E, Iacone R, Iacoviell L, Scopacasa F, Strazzullo P. Blood pressure and metabolic changes during dietary L-arginine supplementation in humans. *Am J Hypertens* 2000;13:547–51.
116. Vallance P, Leone A, Calver A, Collier J, Moncada S. Endogenous dimethyl-arginine as an inhibitor of nitric oxide synthesis. *J Cardiovasc Pharmacol* 1992;20:S60–2.
117. Ruiz-Hurtado G, Delgado C. Nitric oxide pathway in hypertrophied heart: new therapeutic uses of nitric oxide donors. *J Hypertens* 2010;28(Suppl 1):56–61.
118. Sonmez A, Celebi G, Erdem G, Tapan S, Genc H, Tasci K, Ercin CN, Dogru T, Kilic S, Uckaya G, Yilmaz MI, Erbil MK, Kutlu M. Plasma apelin and ADMA levels in patients with essential hypertension. *Clin Exp Hypertens* 2010;32(3):179–83.
119. Michell DL, Andrews KL, Chin-Dusting JP. Endothelial dysfunction in hypertension: the role of arginase. *Front Biosci (Schol Ed)* 2011;3:946–60.
120. Rajapakse NW, Mattson DL. Role of L-arginine in nitric oxide production in health and hypertension. *Clin Exp Pharmacol Physiol* 2009;36(3):249–55.
121. Tsioufis C, Dimitriadis K, Andrikou E, Thomopoulos C, Tsiachris D, Stefanadi E, Mihas C, Miliou A, Papademetriou V and Stefanadis C. ADMA, C-reactive protein and albuminuria in untreated essential hypertension: a cross-sectional study. *Am J Kidney Dis* 2010;55(6):1050–9.
122. Facchinetti F, Saade GR, Neri I, Pizzi C, Longo M, Volpe A. L-arginine supplementation in patients with gestational hypertension: a pilot study. *Hypertens Pregnancy* 2007;26(1):121–30.
123. Neri I, Monari F, Sqarbi L, Berardi A, Masellis G, Facchinetti F. L-arginine supplementation in women with chronic hypertension: impact on blood pressure and maternal and neonatal complications. *J Matern Fetal Neonatal Med* 2010;23(12):1456–60.
124. Martina V, Masha A, Gigliardi VR, Brocato L, Manzato E, Berchio A, Massarenti P, Settanni F, Della Casa L, Bergamini S, Iannone A. Long-term N-acetylcysteine and L-arginine administration reduces endothelial activation and systolic blood pressure in hypertensive patients with type 2 diabetes. *Diabetes Care* 2008;31(5):940–4.
125. Ast J, Jablecka A, Bogdanski I, Krauss H, Chmara E. Evaluation of the antihypertensive effect of L-arginine supplementation in patients with mild hypertension assessed with ambulatory blood pressure monitoring. *Med Sci Monit* 2010;16(5):266–71.
126. Schulman SP, Becker LC, Kass DA, Champion HC, Terrin ML, Forman S. Ernst KV, Kelemen MD, Townsend SN, Capriotti A, Hare JM, Gerstenblith G. L arginine therapy in acute myocardial infraction: the vascular interaction with age in myocardial infarction (VINTAGE MI) randomized clinical trial. *JAMA* 2006;295(1):58–64.
127. Dong JY, Qin JQ, Zhang ZL, Zhao Y, Wang J, Arigoni F, Zhang W. Effect of oral L-arginine supplementation on blood pressure: a meta-analysis of randomized, double-blind, placebo-controlled trials. *Am Heart J* 2011;162:959–65.
128. Huxtable RJ. Physiologic actions of taurine. *Physiol Rev* 1992;72:101–63.
129. Fujita T, Ando K, Noda H, Ito Y, Sato Y. Effects of increased adrenomedullary activity and taurine in young patients with borderline hypertension. *Circulation* 1987;75:525–32.
130. Huxtable RJ, Sebring LA. Cardiovascular actions of taurine. *Prog Clin Biol Res* 1983;125:5–37.
131. Tanabe Y, Urata H, Kiyonaga A, Ikede M, Tanake H, Shindo M, Arakawa K. Changes in serum concentrations of taurine and other amino acids in clinical antihypertensive exercise therapy. *Clin Exp Hypertens* 1989;11:149–65.
132. Yamori Y, Taguchi T, Mori H, Mori M. Low cardiovascular risks in the middle age males and females excreting greater 24-hour urinary taurine and magnesium in 41 WHO-CARDIAC study populations in the world. *J Biomed Sci* 2010;17(Suppl 1): s21–6.
133. Sun Q, Wang B, Li Y, Sun F, Li P, Xia W, Zhou X, Li Q, Wang X, Chen J, Zeng X, Zhao Z, He H, Liu D, Zhu Z. Taurine supplementation lowers blood pressure and improves vascular function in prehypertension: randomized, double-blind, placebo-controlled study. *Hypertension* 2016;67(3):541–9.
134. Houston MC. Combination nutraceutical supplement lowers blood pressure in hypertensive individuals. *Integr Med* 2013;12(3):22–8.

135. Mori TA, Bao DQ, Burke V, Puddey IB, Beilin LJ. Docosahexaenoic acid but not eicosapentaenoic acid lowers ambulatory blood pressure and heart rate in humans. *Hypertension* 1999;34:253–60.
136. Bønaa KH, Bjerve KS, Straume B, Gram IT, Thelle D. Effect of eicosapentaenoic and docosahexanoic acids on blood pressure in hypertension: a population-based intervention trial from the Tromso study. *N Engl J Med* 1990;322:795–801.
137. Mori TA, Burke V, Puddey I, Irish A. The effects of omega 3 fatty acids and coenzyme Q 10 on blood pressure and heart rate in chronic kidney disease: a randomized controlled trial. *J Hypertens* 2009;27(9):1863–72.
138. Ueshima H, Stamler J, Elliot B, Brown, CQ. Food omega 3 fatty acid intake of individuals (total, linolenic acid, long chain) and their blood pressure: INTERMAP study. *Hypertension* 2007; 50(20):313–9.
139. Mon TA. Omega 3 fatty acids and hypertension in humans. *Clin Exp Pharmacol Physiol* 2006; 33(9):842–6.
140. Liu JC, Conkin SM, Manuch SB, Yao JK, Muldoon MF. Long-chain omega-3 fatty acids and blood pressure. *Am J Hypertens* 2011 July 14;24:1121–6 (Epub).
141. Engler MM, Schambelan M, Engler MB, Goodfriend TL. Effects of dietary gamma-linolenic acid on blood pressure and adrenal angiotensin receptors in hypertensive rats. *Proc Soc Exp Biol Med* 1998;218(3):234–7.
142. Sagara M, Njelekela M, Teramoto T, Taquchi T, Mori M, Armitage L, Birt N, Birt C, Yamori Y. Effects of docoahexaenoic acid supplementation on blood pressure, heart rate, and serum lipid in Scottish men with hypertension and hypercholesterolemia. *Int J Hypertens* 2011;8:8091–8.
143. Colussi G, Catena C, Novello M, Bertin N, Sechi LA. Impact of omega-3 polyunsaturated fatty acids on vascular function and blood pressure: relevance for cardiovascular outcomes. *Nutr Metab Cardiovasc Dis* 2017;27(3):191–200.
144. Miller PE, Van Elswyk M, Alexander DD. Long-chain omega-3 fatty acids eicosapentaenoic acid and docosahexaenoic acid and blood pressure: a meta-analysis of randomized controlled trials. *Am J Hypertens* 2014;27:885–96.
145. Pase MP, Grima NA, Sarris J. Do long-chain n-3 fatty acids reduce arterial stiffness? A meta-analysis of randomised controlled trials. *Br J Nutr* 2011;106:974–80.
146. Cicero AF, Ertek S, Borghi C. Omega-3 polyunsaturated fatty acids: their potential role in blood pressure prevention and management. *Curr Vasc Pharmacol* 2009;7:330–7.
147. Minihane AM, Armah CK, Miles EA, Madden JM, Clark AB, Caslake MJ, Packard CJ, Kofler BM, Lietz G, Curtis PJ, Mathers JC, Williams CM, Calder PC. Consumption of fish oil providing amounts of eicosapentaenoic acid and docosahexaenoic acid that can be obtained from the diet reduces blood pressure in adults with systolic hypertension: a retrospective analysis. *J Nutr* 2016;146(3):516–23.
148. Rodriguez-Leyva D, Weighell W, Edel AL, LaVallee R, Dibrov E, Pinneker R, Maddaford TG, Ramjiawan B, Aliani M, Guzman R, Pierce GN. Potent antihypertensive action of dietary flaxseed in hypertensive patients. *Hypertension* 2013 Dec;62(6):1081–9.
149. Saravanan P, Davidson NC, Schmidt EB and Calder PC. Cardiovascular effects of marine omega-3 fatty acids. *Lancet* 2010;376(9740):540–50.
150. Alexander DD, Miller PE, Van Elswyk ME, Kuratko CN, Bylsma LC. A meta-analysis of randomized controlled trials and prospective cohort studies of eicosapentaenoic and docosahexaenoic long-chain omega-3 fatty acids and coronary heart disease risk. *Mayo Clin Proc* 2017 Jan;92(1):15–29.
151. Ferrara LA, Raimondi S, d'Episcopa I. Olive oil and reduced need for antihypertensive medications. *Arch Intern Med* 2000;160:837–42.
152. Perona JS, Canizares J, Montero E, Sanchez-Dominquez JM, Catala A, Ruiz Gutierrez V. Virgin olive oil reduces blood pressure in hypertensive elderly patients. *Clin Nutr* 2004;23(5):1113–21.
153. Perona JS, Montero E, Sanchez-Dominquez JM, Canizares J, Garcia M, Ruiz- Gutierrez V. Evaluation of the effect of dietary virgin olive oil on blood pressure and lipid composition of serum and low-density lipoprotein in elderly type 2 subjects. *J Agric Food Chem* 2009;57(23):11427–33.
154. Lopez-Miranda J, Perez-Jimenez F, Ros E, De Caterina F, Badimon L, Cocas MI, Escrich E, Ordovas JM et al. Olive oil and health: summary of the II international conference on olive oil and health consensus report, Jaen and Cordoba (Spain) 2008. *Nutr Metab Cardiovasc Dis* 2010;20(4):284–94.
155. Thomsen C, Rasmussen OW, Hansen KW, Vesterlund M, Hermansen K. Comparison of the effects on the diurnal blood pressure, glucose, and lipid levels of a diet rich in monounsaturated fatty acids with a diet rich in polyunsaturated fatty acids in type 2 diabetic subjects. *Diabet Med* 1995;12:600–6.
156. Sofi F, Abbate R, Gensini GF, Casini A. Accruing evidence on benefits of adherence to the Mediterranean diet on health: an updated systematic review and meta-analysis. *Am J Clin Nutr* 2010;92(5):1189–96.

157. Estruch R, Ros E, Salas-Salvadó J, Covas MI, Corella D, Arós F, Gómez-Gracia E, Ruiz-Gutiérrez V, Fiol M, Lapetra J, Lamuela-Raventos RM, Serra-Majem L, Pintó X, Basora J, Muñoz MA, Sorlí JV, Martínez JA, Martínez-González MA, PREDIMED Study Investigators. Primary prevention of cardiovascular disease with a Mediterranean diet. *N Engl J Med* 2013;368(14):1279–90.

158. Nadtochiy SM, Redman EK. Mediterranean diet and cardioprotection: the role of nitrite, polyunsaturated fatty acids, and polyphenols. *Nutrition* 2011;27(7–8):733–44.

159. Salas-Salvadó J, Bulló M, Estruch R, Ros E, Covas MI, Ibarrola-Jurado N, Corella D, Arós F, Gómez-Gracia E, Ruiz-Gutiérrez V, Romaguera D, Lapetra J, Lamuela-Raventós RM, Serra-Majem L, Pintó X, Basora J, Muñoz MA, Sorlí JV, Martínez-González MA. Prevention of diabetes with Mediterranean diets: a subgroup analysis of a randomized trial. *Ann Intern Med* 2014;160(1):1–10.

160. Lopez S, Bermudez B, Montserrat-de la Paz S, Jaramillo S, Abia R, Muriana FJ. Virgin olive oil and hypertension. *Curr Vasc Pharmacol* 2016;14(4):323–9.

161. Martín-Peláez S, Castañer O, Konstantinidou V, Subirana I, Muñoz-Aguayo D, Blanchart G Gaixas S, de la Torre R, Farré M, Sáez GT, Nyyssönen K, Zunft HJ, Covas MI, Fitó M. Effect of olive oil phenolic compounds on the expression of blood pressure-related genes in healthy individuals. *Eur J Nutr* 2017;56(2):663–70.

162. Storniolo CE, Casillas R, Bulló M, Castañer O, Ros E, Sáez GT, Toledo E, Estruch R, Ruiz-Gutiérrez V, Fitó M, Martínez-González MA Salas-Salvadó J, Mitjavila MT, Moreno JJ. A Mediterranean diet supplemented with extra virgin olive oil or nuts improves endothelial markers involved in blood pressure control in hypertensive women. *Eur J Nutr* 2017;56(1):89–97.

163. Hohmann CD, Cramer H, Michalsen A, Kessler C, Steckhan N, Choi K, Dobos G. Effects of high phenolic olive oil on cardiovascular risk factors: a systematic review and meta-analysis. *Phytomedicine* 2015;22(6):631–40.

164. Doménech M, Roman P, Lapetra J, García de la Corte FJ, Sala-Vila A, de la Torre R, Corella D, Salas-Salvadó J, Ruiz-Gutiérrez V, Lamuela-Raventós RM, Toledo E, Estruch R, Coca A, Ros E. Mediterranean diet reduces 24-hour ambulatory blood pressure, blood glucose, and lipids: one-year randomized, clinical trial. *Hypertension* 2014;64(1):69–76.

165. Lockyer S, Rowland I, Spencer JP, Yaqoob P, Stonehouse W. Impact of phenolic-rich olive leaf extract on blood pressure, plasma lipids and inflammatory markers: a randomized controlled trial. *Eur J Nutr* 2016; 14:2–18 Mar 7 [Epub ahead of print].

166. Cabrera-Vique C, Navarro-Alarcón M, Rodríguez Martínez C, Fonollá-Joya J. Hypertensive effect of an extract of bioactive compounds olive leaves preliminary clinical study. *Nutr Hosp* 2015;32(1):242–9.

167. Susalit E, Agus N, Effendi I, Tjandrawinata RR, Nofiarny D, Perrinjaquet-Moccetti T, Verbruggen M. Olive (Olea europaea) leaf extract effective in patients with stage-1 hypertension: comparison with Captopril. *Phytomedicine* 2011;18(4):251–8.

168. Flynn M, Wang S. Olive oil as medicine: the effect on blood pressure. The Report of UCD Olive Center. 2015.

169. Psaltopoulou T, Naska A, Orfanos P, Trichopoulos D, Mountokalakis T, Trichopoulou A. Olive oil, the Mediterranean diet, and arterial blood pressure: the Greek European prospective investigation into cancer and nutrition (EPIC) study. *Am J Clin Nutr* 2004;80:1012–8.

170. Toledo E, Hu FB, Estruch R, Buil-Cosiales P, Corella D, Salas-Salvadó J, Covas MI, Arós F, Gómez-Gracia E, Fiol M, Lapetra J, Serra-Majem L, Pinto X, Lamuela-Raventós RM, Saez G, Bulló M, Ruiz-Gutiérrez V, Ros E, Sorli JV, Martinez-Gonzalez MA. Effect of the Mediterranean diet on blood pressure in the PREDIMED trial: results from a randomized controlled trial. *BMC Med* 2013;11:207.

171. Perrinjaquet-Moccetti T, Busjahn A, Schmidlin C, Schmidt A, Bradl B, Aydogan C. Food supplementation with an olive (Olea uropaea L.) leaf extract reduces blood pressure in borderline hypertensive monozygotic twins. *Phytother Res* 2008;22(9):1239–42.

172. Hodgson JM, Woodman R, Bryan J, Wilson C, Murphy KJ. A Mediterranean diet lowers blood pressure and improves endothelial function: results from the MedLey randomized intervention trial. *Am J Clin Nutr* 2017 Apr 19. pii: ajcn146803.

173. Miura K, Stamler J, Brown IJ, Ueshima H, Nakagawa H, Sakurai M, Chan Q, Appel LJ, Okayama A, Okuda N, Curb JD, Rodriguez BL, Robertson C, Zhao L, Elliott P, INTERMAP Research Group. Relationship of dietary monounsaturated fatty acids to blood pressure: the international study of macro/micronutrients and blood pressure. *J Hypertens* 2013 Jun;31(6):1144–50.

174. Sherman DL, Keaney JF, Biegelsen ES, et al. Pharmacological concentrations of ascorbic acid are required for the beneficial effect on endothelial vasomotor function in hypertension. *Hypertension* 2000;35:936–941.

175. Ness AR, Khaw K-T, Bingham S, Day NE. Vitamin C status and blood pressure. *J Hypertens* 1996;14:503–8.
176. Duffy SJ, Bokce N, Holbrook M. Treatment of hypertension with ascorbic acid. *Lancet* 1999;354:2048–9.
177. Enstrom JE, Kanim LE, Klein M. Vitamin C intake and mortality among a sample of the United States population. *Epidemiology* 1992;3:194–202.
178. Block G, Jensen, CD, Norkus EP, Hudes M, Crawford PB. Vitamin C in plasma is inversely related to blood pressure and change in blood pressure during the previous year in young black and white women. *Nutr J* 2008;17(7):35–46.
179. Hatzitolios A, Iliadis F, Katsiki N, Baltatzi M. Is the antihypertensive effect of dietary supplements via aldehydes reduction evidence based: a systemic review. *Clin Exp Hypertens* 2008:30(7) 628–39.
180. Mahajan AS, Babbar R, Kansai N, Agarwai SK, Ray PC. Antihypertensive and antioxidant action of amlodipine and Vitamin C in patients of essential hypertension. *J Clin Biochem Nutr* 2007;402:141–7.
181. Ledlerc PC, Proulx, CD, Arquin G, Belanger S. Ascorbic acid decreases the binding affinity of the AT! Receptor for angiotensin II. *Am J Hypertens* 2008;21(1):67–71.
182. Plantinga Y, Ghiadone L, Magagna A, Biannarelli C. Supplementation with vitamins C and E improves arterial stiffness and endothelial function in essential hypertensive patients. *Am J Hypertens* 2007;20(4):392–7.
183. Sato K, Dohi Y, Kojima M, Miyagawa K. Effects of ascorbic acid on ambulatory blood pressure in elderly patients with refractory hypertension. *Arzneimittelforschung* 2006;56(7):535–40.
184. Block G, Mangels AR, Norkus EP, Patterson BH, Levander OA, Taylor PR. Ascorbic acid status and subsequent diastolic and systolic blood pressure. *Hypertension* 2001;37:261–7.
185. McRae MP. Is vitamin C an effective antihypertensive supplement? A review and analysis of the literature. *J Chiropr Med* 2006;5(2):60–4.
186. Simon JA. Vitamin C and cardiovascular disease: a review. *J Am Coll Nutr* 1992;11(2):107–25.
187. Ness AR, Chee D, Elliott P. Vitamin C and blood pressure—an overview. *J Hum Hypertens* 1997;11(6):343–50.
188. Trout DL. Vitamin C and cardiovascular risk factors. *Am J Clin Nutr* 1991;53(1 Suppl):322S–5S.
189. Ried K, Travica N, Sali A The acute effect of high-dose intravenous vitamin C and other nutrients on blood pressure: a cohort study. *Blood Press Monit* 2016 Jun;21(3):160–7.
190. Buijsse B, Jacobs DR Jr, Steffen LM, Kromhout D Gross MD. Plasma ascorbic acid, a priori diet quality score, and incident hypertension: a prospective cohort study. *PLoS One* 2015;10(12):e0144920.
191. Hajjar IM, George V, Sasse EA, Kochar MS. A randomized, double-blind, controlled trial of vitamin C in the management of hypertension and lipids. *Am J Ther* 2002 Jul–Aug;9(4):289–93.
192. National Center for Health Statistics, Fulwood R, Johnson CL, Bryner JD. *Hematological and Nutritional Biochemistry Reference Data for Persons 6 Months-74 Years of Age: United States, 1976–80.* US Public Health Service, Washington, DC. 1982. Vital and Health Statistics Series 11, No. 232, DHHS Publication No. (PHS) 83-1682.
193. McCartney DM, Byrne DG, Turner MJ. Dietary contributors to hypertension in adults reviewed. *Ir J Med Sci* 2015;184:81–90.
194. Enstrom JE, Kanim LE, Klein M. Vitamin C intake and mortality among a sample of the United States population. *Epidemiology* 1992;3:194–202.
195. Juraschek SP, Guallar E, Appel LJ, Miller ER 3rd. Effects of vitamin C supplementation on blood pressure: a meta-analysis of randomized controlled trials. *Am J Clin Nutr* 2012;95:1079–88.
196. Ward NC, Wu JH, Clarke MW and Buddy IB. Vitamin E effects on the treatment of hypertension in type 2 diabetics. *J Hypertens* 2007;227:227–34.
197. Murray ED, Wechter WJ, Kantoci D, Wang WH, Pham T, Quiggle DD, Gibson KM, Leipold D, Anner BM. Endogenous natriuretic factors 7: biospecificity of a natriuetic gamma-tocopherol metabolite LLU alpha. *J Pharmacol Exp Ther* 1997;282(2):657–62.
198. Gray B, Swick J, Ronnenberg AG. Vitamin E and adiponectin: proposed mechanism for vitamin E-induced improvement in insulin sensitivity. *Nutr Rev* 2011;69(3):155–61.
199. Kuwabara A, Nakade M, Tamai H, Tsuboyama-Kasaoka N, Tanaka K. The association between vitamin E intake and hypertension: results from the re-analysis of the National Health and Nutrition Survey. *J Nutr Sci Vitaminol (Tokyo)* 2014;60(4):239–45.
200. Hodgson JM, Croft KD, Woodman RJ, Puddey IB, Bondonno CP, Wu JH, Bilin LJ, Lukoshkova EV, Head GA, Ward NC. Effects of vitamin E, vitamin C and polyphenols on the rate of blood pressure variation: results of two randomised controlled trials. *Br J Nutr* 2014;112(9):1551–61.
201. Hanni LL, Huarfner LH, Sorensen OH, Ljunghall S. Vitamin D is related to blood pressure and other cardiovascular risk factors in middle-aged men. *Am J Hypertens* 1995;8:894–901.

202. Bednarski R, Donderski R, Manitius L. Role of vitamin D in arterial blood pressure control. *Pol Merkur Lekarski* 2007;136:307–10.

203. Li YC, Kong H, Wei M, Chen ZF. 1, 25 Dihydroxyvitamin D 3 is a negative endocrine regulator of the renin angiotensin system. *J Clin Invest* 2002;110(2):229–38.

204. Ngo DT, Sverdlov AL, McNeil JJ, Horowitz JD. Does vitamin D modulate asymmetric dimethylargine and C-reactive protein concentrations? *Am J Med* 2010;123(4):335–41.

205. Rosen CJ. Clinical practice. Vitamin D insufficiency. *N Engl J. Med* 2011;364(3):248–54.

206. Boldo A, Campbell P, Luthra P, White WB. Should the concentration of vitamin D be measured in all patients with hypertension? *J Clin Hypertens* 2010;12(3):149–52.

207. Pittas AG, Chung M, Trikalinos T, Mitri J, Brendel M, Patel K, Lichtenstein HA, Lau J, Balk EM. Systematic review: vitamin D and cardiometabolic outcomes. *Ann Intern Med* 2010;152(5):307–14.

208. Movano Peregrin C, Lopez Rodriguez R, Castilla Castellano MD. Vitamin D and hypertension. *Med Clin (Barc)* 2011 June 22;138:397–401 (Epub).

209. Motiwala SR, Want TJ. Vitamin D and cardiovascular disease. *Curr Opin Nephrol Hypertens* 2011;20(4):345–53.

210. Cosenso-Martin LN, Vitela-Martin JF. Is there an association between vitamin D and hypertension. *Recent Pat Cardiovasc Drug Discov* 2011;6(2):140–7.

211. Bhandari SK, Pashayan S, Liu IL, Rasgon SA, Kujubu DA, Tom TY, SimJJ. 25-Hydroxyvitamin D levels and hypertension rates. *J Clin Hypertens* 2011;13(3):170–7.

212. Pfeifer M, Begerow B, Minne HW, Nachtigall D, Hansen C. Effects of a short-term vitamin D (3) and calcium supplementation on blood pressure and parathyroid hormone levels in elderly women. *J Clin Endocrinol Metab* 2001;86:1633–7.

213. Qi D, Nie XL, Wu S, Cai J. Vitamin D and hypertension: prospective study and meta-analysis. *PLoS One* 2017;12(3):e0174298.

214. McMullan CJ, Borgi L, Curhan GC, Fisher N, Forman JP. The effect of vitamin D on renin-angiotensin system activation and blood pressure: a randomized control trial. *J Hypertens* 2017;35(4):822–9.

215. Qi D, Nie X Cai J The effect of vitamin D supplementation on hypertension in non-CKD populations: a systemic review and meta-analysis. *Int J Cardiol* 2017;227:177–86.

216. Yilmaz S, Sen F, Ozeke O, Temizhan A, Topaloglu S, Aras D, Aydogdu S. The relationship between vitamin D levels and nondipper hypertension. *Blood Press Monit* 2015;20(6):330–4.

217. Beveridge LA, Struthers AD, Khan F, Jorde R, Scragg R, Macdonald HM, Alvarez JA, Boxer RS, Dalbeni A, Gepner AD, Isbel NM, Larsen T, NagpalJ, Petchey WG, Stricker H, Strobel F, Tangpricha V, Toxqui L, Vaquero MP, Wamberg L, Zittermann A, Witham MD, D-PRESSURE Collaboration. Effect of vitamin D supplementation on blood pressure: a systematic review and meta-analysis incorporating individual patient data. *JAMA Intern Med* 2015;175(5):745–54.

218. Forman JP, Scott JB, Ng K, Drake BF, Suarez EG, Hayden DL, Bennett GG, Chandler PD, Hollis BW, Emmons KM, Giovannucci EL, Fuchs CS, Chan AT. Effect of vitamin D supplementation on blood pressure in blacks. *Hypertension* 2013;61(4):779–85.

219. Keniston R, Enriquez JI Sr. Relationship between blood pressure and plasma vitamin B_6 levels in healthy middle-aged adults. *Ann N Y Acad Sci* 1990;585:499–501.

220. Aybak M, Sermet A, Ayyildiz MO, Karakilcik AZ. Effect of oral pyridoxine hydrochloride supplementation on arterial blood pressure in patients with essential hypertension. *Arzneimittelforschung* 1995;45:1271–3.

221. Paulose CS, Dakshinamurti K, Packer S, Stephens NL. Sympathetic stimulation and hypertension in the pyridoxine-deficient adult rat. *Hypertension* 1988;11(4):387–91.

222. Dakshinamurti K, Lal KJ, Ganguly PK. Hypertension, calcium channel and pyridoxine (vitamin B 6). *Mol Cell Biochem* 1998;188(1–2):137–48.

223. Noori N, Tabibi H, Hosseinpanah F, Hedayati M, Nafar M. Effects of combined lipoic acid and pyridoxine on albuminuria, advanced glycation end-products, and blood pressure in diabetic nephropathy. *Int J Vitam Nutr Res* 2013;83(2):77–85.

224. Moline J, Bukharovich IF, Wolff MS, Phillips R. Dietary flavonoids and hypertension: is there a link? *Med Hypotheses* 2000;55:306–9.

225. Knekt P, Reunanen A, Järvinen R, Seppänen R, Heliövaara M, Aromaa A. Antioxidant vitamin intake and coronary mortality in a longitudinal population study. *Am J Epidemiol* 1994;139:1180–9.

226. Karatzi KN, Papamichael CM Karatizis EN, Papaioannou TG, Aznaouridis KA, Katsichti PP, Stamatelopuolous KS. Red wine acutely induces favorable effects on wave reflections and central pressures in coronary artery disease patients. *Am J Hypertens* 2005;18(9):1161–7.

227. Biala A, Tauriainen E, Siltanen A, Shi J, Merasto S, Louhelainen M, Martonen E, Finckenberg P, Muller DN, Mervaala E. Resveratrol induces mitochondrial biogenesis and ameliorates Ang II-induced cardiac remodeling in transgenic rats harboring human renin and angiotensinogen genes. *Blood Press* 2010;19(3):196–205.
228. Wong RH, Howe PR, Buckley JD, Coates AM, Kunz L, Berry NM. Acute resveratrol supplementation improves flow-mediated dilatation in overweight obese individuals with mildly elevated blood pressure. *Nutr Metab Cardiovasc Dis* 2010 July 29; 44:33–39 (Epub).
229. Bhatt SR, Lokhandwala MF, Banday AA. Resveratrol prevents endothelial nitric oxide synthase uncoupling and attenuates development of hypertension in spontaneously hypertensive rats. *Eur J Pharmacol* 2011;667(1–3):258–64.
230. Rivera L, Moron R, Zarzuelo A, Galisteo M. Long-term resveratrol administration reduces metabolic disturbances and lowers blood pressure in obese Zucker rats. *Biochem Pharmacol* 2009; 77(6):1053–63.
231. Sahebkar A Ferri C, Giorgini P, Bo S Nachtigal P, Grassi D. Effects of pomegranate juice on blood pressure: a systematic review and meta-analysis of randomized controlled trials. *Pharmacol Res* 2017;115:149–61.
232. Tjelle TE, Holtung L, Bøhn SK, Aaby K, Thoresen M, Wiik SÅ, Paur I, Karlsen AS, Retterstøl K, Iversen PO, Blomhoff R. Polyphenol-rich juices reduce blood pressure measures in a randomised controlled trial in high normal and hypertensive volunteers. *Br J Nutr* 2015;114(7):1054–63.
233. de Jesús Romero-Prado MM, Curiel-Beltrán JA, Miramontes-Espino MV, CardonaMuñoz EG, Rios-Arellano A, Balam-Salazar LB. Dietary flavonoids added to pharmacological antihypertensive therapy are effective in improving blood pressure. *Basic Clin Pharmacol Toxicol* 2015;117(1):57–64.
234. Asgary S, Sahebkar A, Afshani MR, Keshvari M, Haghjooyjavanmard S, Rafieian-Kopaei M Clinical evaluation of blood pressure lowering, endothelial function improving, hypolipidemic and anti-inflammatory effects of pomegranate juice in hypertensive subjects. *Phytother Res* 2014;28(2):193–9.
235. Paran E, Engelhard YN. Effect of lycopene, an oral natural antioxidant on blood pressure. *J Hypertens* 2001;19:S74. Abstract P 1.204.
236. Engelhard YN, Gazer B, Paran E. Natural antioxidants from tomato extract reduce blood pressure in patients with grade-1 hypertension: a double blind placebo controlled pilot study. *Am Heart J* 2006;151(1):100.
237. Paran E, Novac C, Engelhard YN, Hazan-Halevy I. The effects of natural antioxidants form tomato extract in treated but uncontrolled hypertensive patients. *Cardiovasc Durgs Ther* 2009;23(2):145–51.
238. Reid K, Frank OR, Stocks NP. Dark chocolate or tomato extract for prehypertension: a randomized controlled trial. *BMC Complement Altern Med* 2009;9:22.
239. Paran E, Engelhard Y. Effect of tomato's lycopene on blood pressure, serum lipoproteins, plasma homocysteine and oxidative stress markers in grade I hypertensive patients. *Am J Hypertens* 2001;14:141A. Abstract P-333.
240. Ried K, Fakler P. Protective effect of lycopene on serum cholesterol and blood pressure: meta-analyses of intervention trials. *Maturitas* 2011;68(4):299–310.
241. Burton-Freeman B, Sesso HD. Whole food versus supplement: comparing the clinical evidence of tomato intake and lycopene supplementation on cardiovascular risk factors. *Adv Nutr* 2014;5(5):457–85.
242. Langsjoen PH, Langsjoen AM. Overview of the use of Co Q 10 in cardiovascular disease. *Biofactors* 1999;9:273–84.
243. Singh RB, Niaz MA, Rastogi SS, Shukla PK, Thakur AS. Effect of hydrosoluble coenzyme Q10 on blood pressure and insulin resistance in hypertensive patients with coronary heart disease. *J Hum Hypertens* 1999;13(3):203–8.
244. Burke BE, Neustenschwander R, Olson RD. Randomized, double-blind, placebo-controlled trial of coenzyme Q10 in isolated systolic hypertension. *South Med J* 2001;94:1112–7.
245. Rosenfeldt FL, Haas SJ, Krum H, Hadu A. Coenzyme Q 10 in the treatment of hypertension: a meta-analysis of the clinical trials. *J Hum Hypertens* 2007;21(4):297–306.
246. Ankola DD, Viswanas B, Bhardqaj V, Ramarao P, Kumar MN. Development of potent oral nanoparticulate formulation of coenzyme Q10 for treatment of hypertension: can the simple nutritional supplement be used as first line therapeutic agents for prophylaxis/therapy? *Eur J Pharm Biopharm* 2007:67(2):361–9.
247. Ho MJ, Li EC, Wright JM. Blood pressure lowering efficacy of coenzyme Q10 for primary hypertension. *Cochrane Database Syst Rev* 2016;3:CD007435.
248. Ho MJ, Bellusci A, Wright JM. Blood pressure lowering efficacy of coenzyme Q10 for primary hypertension. *Cochrane Database Syst Rev* 2009 Oct 7;4:CD007435.

249. Mikhin VP, Kharchenko AV, Rosliakova EA, Cherniatina MA. Application of coenzyme Q(10) in combination therapy of arterial hypertension. *Kardiologiia* 2011;51(6):26–31.
250. Tsai KL, Huang YH, Kao CL, Yang DM, Lee HC, Chou HY, Chen YC, Chiou GY, Chen LH, Yang YP, Chiu TH, Tsai CS, Ou HC, Chiou SH. A novel mechanism of coenzyme Q10 protects against human endothelial cells from oxidative stress-induced injury by modulating NO-related pathways. *J Nutr Biochem* 2012;23(5):458–68.
251. Sohet FM, Delzenne NM. Is there a place for coenzyme Q in the management of metabolic disorders associated with obesity? *Nutr Rev* 2012;70(11):631–41.
252. Digiesi V, Cantini F, Oradei A, Bisi G, Guarino GC, Brocchi A, Bellandi F, Mancini M, Littarru GP. Coenzyme Q10 in essential hypertension. *Mol Aspects Med* 1994;15:s257–63.
253. Langsjoen P, Langsjoen P, Willis R, Folkers K. Treatment of essential hypertension with coenzyme Q10. *Mol Aspects Med* 1994;15:S265–72.
254. Trimarco V, Cimmino CS, Santoro M, Pagnano G, Manzi MV, Piglia A, Giudice CA, De Luca N, Izzo R. Nutraceuticals for blood pressure control in patients with high-normal or grade 1 hypertension. *High Blood Press Cardiovasc Prev* 2012;19(3):117–22.
255. Young JM, Florkowski CM, Molyneux SL, McEwan RG, Frampton CM, Nicholls MG, Scott RS, George PM. A randomized, double-blind, placebo-controlled crossover study of coenzyme Q10 therapy in hypertensive patients with the metabolic syndrome. *Am J Hypertens* 2012;2:261–70.
256. Kontush A, Reich A, Baum K, Spranger T, Finckh B, Kohlschütter A, Beisiegel U. Plasma ubiquinol-10 is decreased in patients with hyperlipidaemia. *Atherosclerosis* 1997;129(1):119–26.
257. McLachlan J, Beattie E, Murphy MP, Koh-Tan CH, Olson E, Beattie W, Dominiczak AF, Nicklin SA, Graham D. Combined therapeutic benefit of mitochondria-targeted antioxidant, MitoQ10, and angiotensin receptor blocker, losartan, on cardiovascular function. *J Hypertens* 2014;32(3):555–64.
258. Rosenfeldt F, Hilton D, Pepe S, Krum H. Systematic review of effect of coenzyme Q10 in physical exercise, hypertension and heart failure. *Biofactors* 2003;18(1–4):91–100.
259. McMackin CJ. Widlansky ME, Hambury NM, Haung, AL. Effect of combined treatment with alpha lipoic acid and acetyl carnitine on vascular function and blood pressure in patients with coronary artery disease. *J Clin Hypertens* 2007;9:249–55.
260. Salinthone S, Schillace RV, Tsang C, Regan JW, Burdette DN, Carr DW. Lipoic acid stimulates cAMP production via G protein-coupled receptor-dependent and independent mechanisms. *J Nutr Biochem* 2011;22(7):681–90.
261. Rahman ST, Merchant N, Hague T, Wahi J, Bhaheetharan S, Ferdinand KC, Khan BV. The impact of lipoic acid on endothelial function and proteinuria in quinapril-treated diabetic patients with stage I hypertension: results from the quality study. *J Cardiovasc Pharmacol Ther* 2012;17(2):139–45.
262. Huang YD, Li N, Zhang WG, Hu XJ, Wang Q, Wang CC, Xu RW, Uan K, Hou XY, Naer K, Want XL, Yan WL. The effect of oral alpha-lipoic acid in overweight/obese individuals on the brachial-ankle pulse wave velocity and supine blood pressure: a randomized, crossover, double-blind, placebo-controlled trial. *Zhonghua Liu Xing Bing Xue Za Zhi* 2011;32(3):290–6.
263. Morcos M, Borcea V, Isermann B, et al. Effect of alpha-lipoic acid on the progression of endothelial cell damage and albuminuria in patients with diabetes mellitus: an exploratory study. *Diabetes Res Clin Prac* 2001;52(3):175–83.
264. Hosseini S, Lee J, Sepulveda RT, et al. A randomized, double-blind, placebo-controlled, prospective 16 week crossover study to determine the role of pycnogenol in modifying blood pressure in mildly hypertensive patients. *Nutr Res* 2001;21:1251–60.
265. Zibadi S, Rohdewald PJ, Park D, Watson RR. Reduction of cardiovascular risk factors in subjects with type 2 diabetes by pycnogenol supplementation. *Nutr Res* 2008:28(5):315–20.
266. Liu X, Wei J, Tan F, Zhou S, Wurthwein G, Rohdewald P. Pycnogenol French maritime pine bark extract improves endothelial function of hypertensive patients. *Life Sci* 2004;74(7):855–62.
267. Van der Zwan LP, Scheffer PG, Teerlink T. Reduction of myeloperoxidase activity by melatonin and pycnogenol may contribute to their blood pressure lowering effect. *Hypertension* 2010;56(3):e35.
268. Cesarone MR, Belcaro G, Stuard S, Schonlau F, Di Renzo A, Grossi MG, Dugall M, Cornelli U, Cacchio M, Gizzi G, Pellegrini L. Kidney flow and function in hypertension: protective effects of pyconogenol in hypertensive particpants—a controlled study. *J Cardiovasc Pharmacol Ther* 2010;15(1):41–6.
269. Gulati OP. Pycnogenol in metabolic syndrome and related disorders. *Phytother Res.* 2015;29(7):949–68.
270. Hu S, Belcaro G, Cornelli U, Luzzi R, Cesarone M, Dugall M, Feragalli B, Errichi B, Ippolito E, Grossi M, Hosoi M, Gizzi G, Trignani M. Effects of pycnogenol on endothelial dysfunction in borderline hypertensive, hyperlipidemic, and hyperglycemic individuals: the borderline study. *Int Angiol* 2015;34(1):43–52.

271. Enseleit F, Sudano I, Périat D, Winnik S, Wolfrum M, Flammer AJ, Fröhlich GM, Kaiser P, Hirt A, Haile SR, Krasniqi N, Matter CM, Uhlenhut K, Högger P, Neidhart M, Lüscher TF, Ruschitzka F, Noll G. Effects of pycnogenol on endothelial function in patients with stable coronary artery disease: a double-blind, randomized, placebo-controlled, cross-over study. *Eur Heart J* 2012;33(13):1589–97.
272. Luzzi R, Belcaro G, Hosoi M, Feragalli B, Cornelli U, Dugall M, Ledda A. Normalization of cardiovascular risk factors in peri-menopausal women with Pycnogenol®. *Minerva Ginecol* 2017;69(1):29–34.
273. Simons S, Wollersheim H, Thien T. A systematic review on the influence of trial quality on the effects of garlic on blood pressure. *Neth J Med* 2009;67(6):212–9.
274. Reinhard KM, Coleman CI, Teevan C, Vacchani P. Effects of garlic on blood pressure in patients with and without systolic hypertension: a meta-analysis. *Ann Pharmacother* 2008:42(12):1766–71.
275. Reid K, Frank OR, Stocks NP. Aged garlic extract lowers blood pressure in patients with treated but uncontrolled hypertension: a randomized controlled trial. *Maturitas* 2010; 67(2):144–50.
276. Nakasone Y, Nakamura Y, Yamamoto T, Yamaguchi H. Effect of a traditional Japanese garlic preparation on blood pressure in prehypertensive and mildly hypertensive adults. *Exp Ther Med* 2013;5(2):399–405.
277. Ried K, Frank OR, Stocks NP. Aged garlic extract reduces blood pressure in hypertensives: a dose-response trial. *Eur J Clin Nutr* 2013;67(1):64–70.
278. Shouk R, Abdou A, Shetty K, Sarkar D, Eid AH. Mechanisms underlying the antihypertensive effects of garlic bioactives. *Nutr Res* 2014;34(2):106–15.
279. Stabler SN, Tejani AM, Huynh F, Fowkes C. Garlic for the prevention of cardiovascular morbidity and mortality in hypertensive patients. *Cochrane Database Syst Rev* 2012 Aug 15;8:CD007653.
280. Mahdavi-Roshan M, Nasrollahzadeh J, Mohammad Zadeh A, Zahedmehr A. Does garlic supplementation control blood pressure in patients with severe coronary artery disease? A clinical trial study. *Iran Red Crescent Med J* 2016 Aug 24;18(11):e23871.
281. Ried K, Travica N, Sali A. The effect of aged garlic extract on blood pressure and other cardiovascular risk factors in uncontrolled hypertensives: the AGE at Heart Trial. *Integr Blood Press Control* 2016;9:9–21.
282. Varshney R Budoff MJ. Garlic and heart disease. *J Nutr* 2016;146(2):416S–21S.
283. Xiong XJ, Wang PQ Li SJ, Li XK, Zhang YQ, Wang J. Garlic for hypertension: a systematic review and meta-analysis of randomized controlled trials. *Phytomedicine* 2015;22(3):352–61.
284. Suetsuna K, Nakano T. Identification of an antihypertensive peptide from peptic digest of wakame (Undaria pinnatifida). *J Nutr Biochem* 2000;11:450–4.
285. Nakano T, Hidaka H, Uchida J, Nakajima K, Hata Y. Hypotensive effects of wakame. *J Jpn Soc Clin Nutr* 1998;20:92.
286. Krotkiewski M, Aurell M, Holm G, Grimby G, Szczepanik J. Effects of a sodium-potassium ion-exchanging seaweed preparation in mild hypertension. *Am J Hypertens* 1991;4:483–8.
287. Sato M, Oba T, Yamaguchi T, Nakano T, Kahara T, Funayama K, Kobayashi A, Nakano T. Antihypertensive effects of hydrolysates of wakame (Undaria pinnatifida) and their angiotnesin-1-converting inhibitory activity. *Ann Nutr Metab* 2002;46(6):259–67.
288. Sato M, Hosokawa T, Yamaguchi T, Nakano T, Muramoto K, Kahara T, Funayama K, Kobayashi A, Nakano T. Angiotensin I converting enzyme inhibitory peptide derived from wakame (Undaria pinnatifida) and their antihypertensive effect in spontaneously hypertensive rats. *J Agric Food Chem* 2002;50(21):6245–52.
289. Taubert D, Roesen R, Schomig E. Effect of cocoa and tea intake on blood pressure: a meta-analysis. *Arch Intern Med* 2007;167(7):626–34.
290. Grassi D, Lippi C, Necozione S, Desideri G, Ferri C. Short-term administration of dark chocolate is followed by a significant increase in insulin sensitivity and a decrease in blood pressure in healthly persons. *Am J Clin Nutr* 2005;81(3):611–4.
291. Taubert D, Roesen R, Lehmann C, Jung N, Schomig E. Effects of low habitual cocoa intake on blood pressure and bioactive nitric oxide: arandomized controlled trial. *JAMA* 2007;298(1):49–60.
292. Cohen DL, Townsend RR. Cocoa ingestion and hypertension-another cup please? *J Clin Hypertens* 2007;9(8):647–8.
293. Reid I, Sullivan T, Fakler P, Frank OR, Stocks NP. Does chocolate reduce blood pressure? A meta-analysis. *BMC Med* 2010;8:39–46.
294. Egan BM, Laken MA, Donovan JL, Woolson RF. Does dark chocolate have a role in the prevention and management of hypertension? Commentary on the evidence. *Hypertension* 2010;55(6):1289–95.
295. Desch S, Kobler D, Schmidt J, Sonnabend M, Adams V, Sareben M, Eitel I, Bluher M, Shuler G, Thiele H. Low vs higher-dose dark chocolate and blood pressure in cardiovascular high-risk patients. *Am J Hypertens* 2010;23(6):694–700.

296. Desch S, Schmidt J, Sonnabend M, Eitel I, Sareban M, Rahimi K, Schuler G, Thiele H. Effect of cocoa products on blood pressure: systematic review and meta-analysis. *Am J Hypertens* 2010;23(1):97–103.
297. Grassi D, Desideri G, Necozione S, Lippi C, Casale R, Properzi G, Blumberg JB, Ferri C. Blood pressure is reduced and insulin sensitivity increased in glucose intolerant hypertensive subjects after 15 days of consuming high-polyphenol dark chocolate. *J Nutr* 2008;138(9):1671–6.
298. Grassi D, Necozione S, Lippi C, Croce G, Valeri L, Pasqualetti P, Desideri G, Blumberg JB, Ferri C. Cocoa reduces blood pressure and insulin resistance and improved endothelium-dependent vasodilation in hypertensives. *Hypertension* 2005;46(2):398–405.
299. Grassi D, Desideri G, Necozione S, Ruggieri F, Blumberg JB, Stornello M, Ferri C. Protective effects of flavanol-rich dark chocolate on endothelial function and wave reflection during acute hyperglycemia. *Hypertension* 2012;60:827–32.
300. Ried K, Sullivan TR, Fakler P, Frank OR, Stocks NP. Effect of cocoa on blood pressure. *Cochrane Database Syst Rev* 2012;8:CD008893.
301. Scheer FA, Van Montfrans GA, van Someren EJ, Mairuhu G, Buijs RM. Daily nighttime melatonin reduces blood pressure in male patients with essential hypertension. *Hypertension* 2004;43(2):192–7.
302. Cavallo A, Daniels SR, Dolan LM, Khoury JC, Bean JA. Blood pressure response to melatonin in type I diabetes. *Pediatr Diabetes* 2004;5(1):26–31.
303. Cavallo A, Daniels SR, Dolan LM, Bean JA, Khoury JC. Blood pressure-lowering effect of melatonin in type 1 diabetes. *J Pineal Res* 2004;36(4):262–6.
304. Cagnacci A, Cannoletta M, Renzi A, Baldassari F, Arangino S, Volpe A. Prolonged melatonin administration decreases nocturnal blood pressure in women. *Am J Hypertens* 2005;18(12 Pt 1):1614–8.
305. Grossman E, Laudon M, Yalcin R, Zengil H Peleg E, Sharabi Y, Kamari Y, Shen-Orr Z, Zisapel N. Melatonin reduces night blood pressure in patients with nocturnal hypertension. *Am J Med* 2006;119 (10):898–902.
306. Rechcinski T, Kurpese M, Trzoa E, Krzeminska-Pakula M. The influence of melatonin supplementation on circadian pattern of blood pressure in patients with coronary artery disease-preliminary report. *Pol Arch Med Wewn* 2006;115(6):520–8.
307. Merkureva GA, Ryzhak GA. Effect of the pineal gland peptide preparation on the diurnal profile of arterial pressure in middle-aged and elderly women with ischemic heart disease and arterial hypertension. *Adv Gerontol* 2008;21(1):132–42.
308. Zaslavskai RM, Scherban EA, Logvinenki SI. Melatonin in combined therapy of patients with stable angina and arterial hypertension. *Klin Med (Mosk)* 2009;86:64–7.
309. Zamotaev IuN, Enikeev AKh, Kolomets NM. The use of melaxen in combined therapy of arterial hypertension in subjects occupied in assembly line production. *Klin Med (Mosk)* 2009;87(6):46–9.
310. Rechcinski T, Trzos E, Wierzbowski-Drabik K, Krzeminska-Pakute M, Kurpesea M. Melatonin for nondippers with coronary artery disease: assessment of blood pressure profile and heart rate variability. *Hypertens Res* 2002;33(1):56–61.
311. Kozirog M, Poliwczak AR, Duchnowicz P, Koter-Michalak M, Sikora J, Broncel M. Melatonin treatment improves blood pressure, lipid profile and parameters of oxidative stress in patients with metabolic syndrome. *J Pineal Res* 2011;50(3):261–6.
312. Zeman M, Dulkova K, Bada V, Herichova I. Plasma melatonin concentrations in hypertensive patients with the dipping and nondipping blood pressure profile. *Life Sci* 2005;75(16):1795–803.
313. Jonas M, Garfinkel, D, Zisapel N, Laudon M, Grossman E. Impaired nocturnal melatonin secretion in non-dipper hypertensive patients. *Blood Pressure* 2003;12(1):19–24.
314. Simko F, Pechanova O. Potential roles of melatonin and chronotherapy among the new trends in hypertension treatment. *J Pineal Res* 2009;47(2):127–33.
315. Cui HW, Zhang ZX, Gao MT, Liu Y, Su AH, Wang MY. Circadian rhythm of melatonin and blood pressure changes in patients with essential hypertension. *Zhonghua Xin Xue Guan Bing Za Zhi* 2008;36(1):20–3.
316. Ostrowska Z, Kos-Kudla B, Marek B, Kajdaniuk D, Wolkowska K, Swietochowska E, Gorski J, Szapska B. Circadian rhythm of melatonin in patients with hypertension. *Pol Merkur Lekarski* 2004;17(97):50–4.
317. Shatilo VB, Bondarenke EV, Amtoniuk-Shcheglova IA. Pineal gland melatonin-producing function in elderly patients with hypertensive disease: age peculiarities. *Adv Gerontol* 2010;23(4):530–42.
318. Forman JP, Curhan GC, Schemhammer ES. Urinary melatonin and risk of incident hypertension among young women. *J Hypertens* 2010;28(3):336–51.
319. Li HL, Kang YM, Yu L, Xu HY, Zhao H. Melatonin reduces blood pressure in rats with stress-induced hypertension via GABAA receptors. *Clin Exp Pharmacol* 2009;36(4):436–40.
320. Simko F, Paulis L. Melatonin as a potential antihypertensive treatment. *J Pineal Res* 2007;42(4):319–22.

321. Irmak MK, Sizlan A. Essential hypertension seems to result from melatonin-induced epigenetic modifications in area postrema. *Med Hypthesis* 2006;66(5):1000–7.
322. De-Leersnyder H, de Biois MC, Vekemans M, Sidi D, Villain E, Kindermans C, Munnich A. Beta (1) adrenergic antagonists improve sleep and behavioural disturbances in a circadian disorder, Smith-Magenis syndrome. *J Med Genet* 2010;38(9):586–90.
323. Rodella LF, Favero G, Foglio E, Rossini C, Castrezzati S, Lonati C, Rezzani R. Vascular endothelial cells and dysfunctions: role of melatonin. *Front Biosci* 2013;5:119–29.
324. Grossman E, Laudon M, Zisapel N. Effect of melatonin on nocturnal blood pressure: meta-analysis of randomized controlled trials. *Vasc Health Risk Manag* 2011;7:577–84.
325. Scheer FA, Morris CJ, Garcia JI, Smales C, Kelly EE, Marks J, Malhotra A, Shea SA. Repeated melatonin supplementation improves sleep in hypertensive patients treated with beta-blockers: a randomized controlled trial. *Sleep* 2012;35:1395–402.
326. Zaslavskaya RM, Lilitsa GV, Dilmagambetova GS, Halberg F, Cornélissen G, Otsuka K, Singh RB, Stoynev A, Ikonomov O, Tarquini R, Perfetto F, Schwartzkopff O, Bakken EE. Melatonin, refractory hypertension, myocardial ischemia and other challenges in nightly blood pressure lowering. *Biomed Pharmacother* 2004;58(S1):S129–34.
327. Sun H, Gusdon AM, Qu S. Effects of melatonin on cardiovascular diseases: progress in the past year. *Curr Opin Lipidol.* 2016 Aug;27(4):408–13.
328. Feringa HH, Laskey DA, Dickson JE, Coleman CI. The effect of grape seed extract on cardiovascular risk markers: a meta-analysis of randomized controlled trials. *J Am Diet Assoc* 2011;111(8):1173–81.
329. Sivaprakasapillai B, Edirsinghe K, Randolph J, Steinberg F, Kappagoda T. Effect of grape seed extract on blood pressure in subjects with the metabolic syndrome. *Metabolism* 2009;58(12):1743–6.
330. Edirisinghe I, Burton-Freeman B, Tissa Kappagoda C. Mechanism of the endothelium-dependent relaxation evoked by grape seed extract. *Clin Sci (Lond)* 2008;114(4):331–7.
331. Zhang H, Liu S, Li L, Liu S, Liu S, Mi J, Tian G. The impact of grape seed extract treatment on blood pressure changes: a meta-analysis of 16 randomized controlled trials. *Medicine (Baltimore)* 2016;95(33):e4247.
332. Park E, Edirisinghe I, Choy YY, Waterhouse A, Burton-Freeman B. Effects of grape seed extract beverage on blood pressure and metabolic indices in individuals with pre-hypertension: a randomised, double-blinded, two-arm, parallel, placebo-controlled trial. *Br J Nutr* 2016 Jan 28;115(2):226–38.
333. Clements WT, Lee SR, Bloomer RJ. Nitrate ingestion: a review of the health and physical performance effects. *Nutrients* 2014;6:5224–64.
334. Kapil V, Milsom AB, Okorie M, Maleki-Toyserkani S, Akram F, Rehman F, Arghandawi S, Pearl V, Benjamin N, Loukogeorgakis S, Macallister R, Hobbs AJ, Webb AJ, Ahluwalia A. Inorganic nitrate supplementation lowers blood pressure in humans: role for nitrite-derived NO. *Hypertension* 2010;56:274–81.
335. Kapil V, Khambata RS, Robertson A, Caulfield MJ, Ahluwalia A. Dietary nitrate provides sustained blood pressure lowering in hypertensive patients: a randomized, phase 2, double-blind, placebo-controlled study. *Hypertension* 2015;65(2):320–7.
336. Coles LT, Clifton PM. Effect of beetroot juice on lowering blood pressure in free-living, disease-free adults: a randomized, placebo-controlled trial. *Nutr J* 2012;11:106.
337. Siervo M, Lara J, Ogbonmwan I, Mathers JC. Inorganic nitrate and beetroot juice supplementation reduces blood pressure in adults: a systematic review and meta-analysis. *J Nutr* 2013;143:818–26.
338. Houston M. Acute effects of an oral nitric oxide supplement on blood pressure, endothelial function, and vascular compliance in hypertensive patients. *J Clin Hypertens (Greenwich)* 2014;16(7):524–9.
339. Hobbs DA, Kaffa N, George TW, Methven L, Lovegrove JA. Blood pressure-lowering effects of beetroot juice and novel beetroot-enriched bread products in normotensive male subjects. *Br J Nutr* 2012;108(11):2066–74.
340. Kapil V, Pearl V, Ghosh S, Ahluwalia A. Inorganic nitrate ingestion improves vascular compliance but does not alter flow-mediated dilatation in healthy volunteers. *Nitric Oxide* 2012;26(4):197–202.
341. Asgary S, Afshani MR, Sahebkar A, Keshvari M, Taheri M, Jahanian E, Rafieian-Kopaei M, Malekian F, Sarrafzadegan N. Improvement of hypertension, endothelial function and systemic inflammation following short-term supplementation with red beet (Beta vulgaris L.) juice: a randomized crossover pilot study. *J Hum Hypertens* 2016;30(10):627–32.
342. Bryan NS. Application of nitric oxide in drug discovery and development. *Expert Opin Drug Discov* 2011 Nov;6(11):1139–54.
343. Machha A, Schechter AN. Inorganic nitrate: a major player in the cardiovascular health benefits of vegetables? *Nutr Rev* 2012 Jun;70(6):367–72.

344. Liu G, Mi XN, Zheng XX, Xu YL, Lu J, Huang XH. Effects of tea intake on blood pressure: a meta-analysis of randomised controlled trials. *Br J Nutr* 2014;112:1043–54.

345. Hodgson JM, Puddey IB, Burke V, Beilin LJ, Jordan N. Effects on blood pressure of drinking green and black tea. *J Hypertens* 1999;17:457–63.

346. Kurita I, Maeda-Yamamoto M, Tachibana H, Kamei M. Anti-hypertensive effect of Benifuuki tea containing O-methylated EGCG. *J Agric Food Chem* 2010;58(3):1903–8.

347. McKay DL, Chen CY, Saltzman E, Blumberg JB. Hibiscus sabdariffa L tea (tisane) lowers blood pressure in pre-hypertensive and mildly hypertensive adults. *J Nutr* 2010;140(2):298–303.

348. Bogdanski P, Suliburska J, Szulinska M, Stepien M, Pupek-Musialik D, Jablecka A. Green tea extract reduces blood pressure, inflammatory biomarkers, and oxidative stress and improves parameters associated with insulin resistance in obese, hypertensive patients. *Nutr Res* 2012 Jun;32(6):421–7.

349. Hodgson JM, Woodman RJ, Puddey IB, Mulder T, Fuchs D, Croft KD. Short-term effects of polyphenol-rich black tea on blood pressure in men and women. *Food Funct* 2013 Jan 19;4(1):111–5.

350. Medina-Remón A, Estruch R, Tresserra-Rimbau A, Vallverdú-Queralt A, Lamuela-Raventos RM. The effect of polyphenol consumption on blood pressure. *Mini Rev Med Chem* 2013;13:1137–49.

351. Jiménez R, Duarte J, Perez-Vizcaino F. Epicatechin: endothelial function and blood pressure. *J Agric Food Chem* 2012;60(36):8823–30.

352. Nogueira LP, Nogueira Neto JF, Klein MR, Sanjuliani AF. Short-term effects of green tea on blood pressure, endothelial function, and metabolic profile in obese prehypertensive women: a crossover randomized clinical trial. *J Am Coll Nutr* 2017;36(2):108–15.

353. Wasilewski R, Ubara EO, Klonizakis M. Assessing the effects of a short-term green tea intervention in skin microvascular function and oxygen tension in older and younger adults. *Microvasc Res* 2016;107:65–71.

354. Yarmolinsky J, Gon G, Edwards P. Effect of tea on blood pressure for secondary prevention of cardiovascular disease: a systematic review and meta-analysis of randomized controlled trials. *Nutr Rev* 2015;73(4):236–46.

355. Houston MC. Treatment of hypertension with nutraceuticals, vitamins, antioxidants and minerals. *Expert Rev Cardiovasc Ther* 2007;5:681–91.

356. Miguel-Carrasco JL, Monserrat MT, Mate A, Vázquez CM. Comparative effects of captopril and L-carnitine on blood pressure and antioxidant enzyme gene expression in the heart of spontaneously hypertensive rats. *Eur J Pharmacol* 2010;632(1–3):65–72.

357. Zambrano S, Blanca AJ, Ruiz-Armenta MV, Miguel-Carrasco JL, Arévalo M, Vázquez MJ, Mate A, Vázquez CM. L-Carnitine protects against arterial hypertension-related cardiac fibrosis through modulation of PPAR-γ expression. *Biochem Pharmacol* 2013 Jan 4;16:88–97 (Epub).

358. Vilskersts R, Kuka J, Svalbe B, Cirule H, Liepinsh E, Grinberga S, Kalvinsh I, Dambrova M. Administration of L-carnitine and mildronate improves endothelial function and decreases mortality in hypertensive Dahl rats. *Pharmacol Rep* 2011;63(3):752–62.

359. Mate A, Miguel-Carrasco JL, Monserrat MT, Vázquez CM. Systemic antioxidant properties of L-carnitine in two different models of arterial hypertension. *J Physiol Biochem* 2010 Jun;66(2):127–36.

360. Digiesi V, Cantini F, Bisi G, Guarino G, Brodbeck B. L-carnitine adjuvant therapy in essential hypertension. *Clin Ter* 1994;144:391–5.

361. Ghidini O, Azzurro M, Vita G, Sartori G. Evaluation of the therapeutic efficacy of L-carnitine in congestive heart failure. *Int J Clin Pharmacol Ther Toxicol* 1988;26(4):217–20.

362. Digiesi V, Palchetti R, Cantini F. The benefits of L-carnitine therapy in essential arterial hypertension with diabetes mellitus type II. *Minerva Med* 1989;80(3):227–31.

363. Ruggenenti P, Cattaneo D, Loriga G, Ledda F, Motterlini N, Gherardi G, Orisio S, Remuzzi G. Ameliorating hypertension and insulin resistance in subjects at increased cardiovascular risk: effects of acetyl-L-carnitine therapy. *Hypertension* 2009;54(3):567–74.

364. Martina V, Masha A, Gigliardi VR, Brocato L, Manzato E, Berchio A, Mate A, Miguel-Carrasco JL, Vázquez CM. The therapeutic prospects of using L-carnitine to manage hypertension-related organ damage. *Drug Discov Today* 2010;15(11–12):484–92.

365. Korkmaz S, Yıldız G, Kılıçlı F, Yılmaz A, Aydın H, Içağasıoğlu S, Candan F. Low L-carnitine levels: can it be a cause of nocturnal blood pressure changes in patients with type 2 diabetes mellitus? *Anadolu Kardiyol Derg* 2011;11(1):57–63.

366. Velasquez MT, Ramezani A, Manal A, Raj DS. Trimethylamine N-oxide: the good, the bad and the unknown. *Toxins (Basel)* 2016;8(11):1–12.

367. He J, Whelton PK. Effect of dietary fiber and protein intake on blood pressure: a review of epidemiologic evidence. *Clin Exp Hypertens* 1999;21:785–96.

368. Pruijm M, Wuerzer G, Forni V, Bochud M, Pechere-Bertschi A, Burnier M. Nutrition and hypertension: more than table salt. *Rev Med Suisse* 2010;6(282):1715–20.

369. Cicero AF, Derosa G, Manca M, Bove M, Borghi C, Gaddi AV. Different effect of psyllium and guar dietary supplementation on blood pressure control in hypertensive overweight patients: a six-month, randomized clinical trial. *Clin Exp Hypertens* 2007;29:383–94.

370. Pal S, Khoussousi A, Binns C, Dhaliwal S, Radavelli-Bagatini S. The effects of 12-week psyllium fibre supplementation or healthy diet on blood pressure and arterial stiffness in overweight and obese individuals. *Br J Nutr* 2012;107:725–34.

371. Houston MC. Nutrition and nutraceuticals supplements in the treatment of hypertension. *Prog Cardiovasc Dis* 2005;47:396–449.

372. Caligiuri SP, Edel AL, Aliani M, Pierce GN. Flaxseed for hypertension: implications for blood pressure regulation. *Curr Hypertens Rep* 2014;16:499.

373. Sankar D, Sambandam G, Ramskrishna Rao M, Pugalendi KV. Modulation of blood pressure, lipid profiles and redox status in hypertensive patients taking different edible oils. *Clin Chim Acta* 2005;355(1–2):97–104.

374. Sankar D, Rao MR, Sambandam G, Pugalendi KV. Effect of sesame oil on diuretics or beta-blockers in the modulation of blood pressure, athropometry, lipid profile and redox status. *Yale J Biol Med* 2006;79(1):19–26.

375. Miyawaki T, Aono H, Toyoda-Ono Y, Maeda H, Kiso Y, Moriyama K. Anti-hypertensive effects of sesamin in humans. *J Nutr Sci Vitaminol (Toyko)* 2009;55(1):87–91.

376. Wichitsranoi J, Weerapreeyakui N, Boonsiri P, Settasatian N, Komanasin N, Sirjaichingkul S, Teerajetgul Y, Rangkadilok N and Leelayuwat N. Antihypertensive and antioxidant effects of dietary black sesame meal in pre-hypertensive humans. *Nutr J* 2011;10(1):82–88.

377. Sudhakar B, Kalaiarasi P, Al-Numair KS, Chandramohan G, Rao RK and Pugalendi KV. Effect of combination of edible oils on blood pressure, lipid profile, lipid peroxidative markers, antioxidant status, and electrolytes in patients with hypertension on nifedipine treatment. *Saudi Med J* 2011;32(4):379–85.

378. Sankar D, Rao MR, Sambandam G, Pugalendi KV. A pilot study of open label sesame oil in hypertensive diabetics. *J Med Food* 2006;9(3):408–12.

379. Harikumar KB, Sung B, Tharakan ST, Pandey MK, Joy B, Guha S, Krishnan S, Aggarwai BB. Sesamin manifests chemopreventive effects through the suppression of NF-kappa-B-regulated cell survival, proliferation, invasion and angiogenic gene products. *Mol Cancer Res* 2010;8(5):751–61.

380. Nakano D, Ogura K, Miyakoshi M, Ishii F, Kawanishi H, Kuramazuka D, Kwak CJ, Ikemura K, Takaoka M, Moriguchi S, Ling T, Kusomoto A, Asami S, Shibata K, Kis Y, Matsumura Y. Antihyptensive effect of angiotensin–I–converting enzyme inhibitory peptides from a sesame protein hydrolysate in spontaneously hypertensive rats. *Biosci Biotechnol Biochem* 2006;70(5):1118–26.

381. Karatzi K, Stamatelopoulos K, Lykka M, Mantzouratou P, Skalidi S, Manios E, Georgiopoulos G, Zakopoulos N, Papamichael C, Sidossis LS. Acute and long-term hemodynamic effects of sesame oil consumption in hypertensive men. *J Clin Hypertens (Greenwich)* 2012;14(9):630–6.

382. Morand C, Dubray C, Milenkovic D, Lioger D, Martin JF, Scalber A, Mazur A. Hesperidin contributes to the vascular protective effects of orange juice: a randomized crossover study in healthy volunteers. *Am J Clin Nutr* 2011;93(1):73–80.

383. Jiang B, Haverty M, Brecher P. N-acetyl-L-cysteine enhances interleukin-1beta-induced nitric oxide synthase expression. *Hypertension* 1999;34(4 Pt 1):574–9.

384. Vasdev S, Singal P, Gill V. The antihypertensive effect of cysteine. *Int J Angiol* 2009;18(1):7–21.

385. Meister A, Anderson ME, Hwang O. Intracellular cysteine and glutathione delivery systems. *J Am Coll Nutr* 1986;5(2):137–51.

386. Asher GN, Viera AJ, Weaver MA, Dominik R, Caughey M, Hinderliter AL. Effect of hawthorn standardized extract on flow mediated dilation in prehypertensive and mildly hypertensive adults: a randomized, controlled cross-over trial. *BMC Complement Altern Med* 2012;12:26–30.

387. Koçyildiz ZC, Birman H, Olgaç V, Akgün-Dar K, Melikoğlu G, Meriçli AH. Crataegus tanacetifolia leaf extract prevents L-NAME-induced hypertension in rats: a morphological study. *Phytother Res* 2006;20(1):66–70.

388. Schröder D, Weiser M, Klein P. Efficacy of a homeopathic Crataegus preparation compared with usual therapy for mild (NYHA II) cardiac insufficiency: results of an observational cohort study. *Eur J Heart Fail* 2003;5(3):319–26.

389. Walker AF, Marakis G, Simpson E, Hope JL, Robinson PA, Hassanein M, Simpson HC. Hypotensive effects of hawthorn for patients with diabetes taking prescription drugs: a randomised controlled trial. *Br J Gen Pract* 2006;56(527):437–43.

390. Walker AF, Marakis G, Morris AP, Robinson PA. Promising hypotensive effect of hawthorn extract: a randomized double-blind pilot study of mild, essential hypertension. *Phytother Res* 2002;16(1):48–54.
391. Larson A, Witman MA, Guo Y, Ives S, Richardson RS, Bruno RS, Jalili T, Symons JD. Acute, quercetin-induced reductions in blood pressure in hypertensive individuals are not secondary to lower plasma angiotensin-converting enzyme activity or endothelin-1: nitric oxide. *Nutr Res* 2012;32(8):557–64.
392. Edwards RL, Lyon T, Litwin SE, Rabovsky A, Symons JD, Jalili T. Quercetin reduces blood pressure in hypertensive subjects. *J Nutr* 2007;137(11):2405–11.
393. Egert S, Bosy-Westphal A, Seiberl J, Kürbitz C, Settler U, Plachta-Danielzik S, Wagner AE, Frank J, Schrezenmeir J, Rimbach G, Wolffram S, Müller MJ. Quercetin reduces systolic blood pressure and plasma oxidised low-density lipoprotein concentrations in overweight subjects with a high-cardiovascular disease risk phenotype: a double-blinded, placebo-controlled cross-over study. *Br J Nutr* 2009;102(7):1065–74.
394. Khalesi S, Sun J, Buys N, Jayasinghe R. Effect of probiotics on blood pressure: a systematic review and meta-analysis of randomized, controlled trials. *Hypertension* 2014;64:897–903.
395. Hendijani F, Akbari V. Probiotic supplementation for management of cardiovascular risk factors in adults with type II diabetes: a systematic review and meta-analysis. *Clin Nutr* 2017 Feb 24. pii: S0261-5614(17)30065-1. doi:10.1016/j.clnu.2017.02.015 [Epub ahead of print].
396. Robles-Vera I, Toral M, Romero M, Jiménez R, Sánchez M, Pérez-Vizcaíno F, Duarte J. Antihypertensive effects of probiotics. *Curr Hypertens Rep* 2017;19(4):26.
397. de Sousa VP, Cavalcanti Neto MP, Magnani M, Braga VA, da Costa-Silva JH, Leandro CG, Vidal H, Pirola L. New insights on the use of dietary polyphenols or probiotics for the management of arterial hypertension. *Front Physiol* 2016;7:448–60.
398. Dairi EBM, Lee BH, Oh DH. Current perspectives on antihypertensive probiotics. *Probiotics Antimicrob Proteins* 2016 Nov 29;67:43–49 [Epub ahead of print].
399. Whelton PK, Carey RM, Aronow WS, Casey DE Jr, Collins KJ, Dennison Himmelfarb C, DePalma SM, Gidding S, Jamerson KA, Jones DW, MacLaughlin EJ, Muntner P, Ovbiagele B, Smith SC Jr, Spencer CC, Stafford RS, Taler SJ, Thomas RJ, Williams KA Sr, Williamson JD, Wright JT Jr. ACC/AHA/AAPA/ABC/ACPM/AGS/APhA/ASH/ASPC/NMA/PCNA guideline for the prevention, detection, evaluation, and management of high blood pressure in adults: a report of the American College of Cardiology/American Heart Association Task Force on clinical practice guidelines. *Hypertension* 2018 Jun;71(6):e13–115. doi:10.1161/HYP.0000000000000065 [Epub 2017 Nov 13].
400. Wright JM, Musini VM, Gill R. First-line drugs for hypertension. *Cochrane Database Syst Rev* 2018 Apr 18;4:CD001841. doi:10.1002/14651858.CD001841.pub3.
401. Trovato A, Nuhlicek DN, Midtling JE. Drug-nutrient interactions. *Am Fam Physician* 1991;44(5):1651–8.
402. McCabe BJ, Frankel EH, Wolfe JJ. Eds. *Handbook of Food-Drug Interactions.* CRC Press, Boca Raton, FL. 2003.
403. Houston MC. The role of cellular micronutrient analysis and minerals in the prevention and treatment of hypertension and cardiovascular disease. *Ther Adv Cardiovasc Dis* 2010;4:165–83.

8 Metabolic Cardiology
Management of Congestive Heart Failure

Stephen T. Sinatra

CONTENTS

Takeaways and Key Concepts...189
The Secrets of the Cell...193
Energy Starvation in the Failing Heart...196
Energy Nutrients for Congestive Heart Failure..199
      D-Ribose (Ribose) 199
Coenzyme Q10 and the Heart..202
CoQ10 – Inflammatory Coronary Heart Disease/Diabetes..205
Coenzyme Q10 Varietals – Ubiquinone, Ubiquinol and MitoQ 205
Levocarnitine (L-Carnitine or Carnitine)..206
Magnesium – Switching on the Energy Enzymes 209
Taurine 209
Summary 209
Conclusion 210
References... 211

TAKEAWAYS AND KEY CONCEPTS

1. Congestive heart failure (CHF) affects 23,000,000 people per year worldwide.
2. Mitochondrial and intrinsic stem cell support offers new therapeutic strategies.
3. Metabolic therapy involves the administration of a substance normally found in the body to enhance a metabolic reaction within the cell.
4. Such a therapy may be utilized in two ways. A substance can be given to correct a deficiency of a cellular component or a substance can be given to achieve greater than normal levels in the body to drive an enzymatic reaction in a preferential direction.
5. In this chapter, four metabolic substances that support cardiac metabolism will be reviewed:
    a. Magnesium involves 300 enzymatic reactions.
    b. Coenzyme Q10, a lipid-soluble antioxidant, plays a vital role in oxidative phosphorylation.
    c. L-carnitine supports beta-oxidation of fatty acids in mitochondria while removing toxic metabolic byproducts at the same time.
    d. D-ribose is the energy-limiting substrate that supports ATP production in the myocyte.
6. Metabolic cardiology supports biochemical reactions that improve energy substrates in heart cells.
7. CHF is literally an "energy-starved" heart, and compounds that enhance energy supply must be given to make a positive impact on heart function.

DOI: 10.1201/9781003137849-8

8. Diastolic dysfunction occurs when ATP levels fall and is the most important precursor of systolic dysfunction and therefore, CHF.
9. Metabolic cardiology is a unique strategy to energize diastole and perhaps will become the standard of care for the treatment of heart failure.

Heart failure (HF) is defined by the American Heart Association (AHA) and the American College of Cardiology (ACC) as a complex clinical syndrome that can result from any structural or functional cardiac disorder that impairs the ability of the ventricle to fill (diastole) or eject (systole) blood.[1,2] This common pathological situation for physicians remains the leading cause of hospitalization in the United States. It affects 23,000,000 worldwide[3] and 5,000,000 in the United States alone.[4] Since its prevalence continues to increase as the population ages, the amount of human suffering associated with HF is staggering and the financial burden placed on society is remarkable. Although there has been some considerable progress in the treatment of HF over the past 20 years with diuretics, angiotensin-converting enzyme (ACE) therapies,[5,6] beta-receptor blockade[7,8] and resynchronization therapy,[9–11] HF is still associated with an annual mortality of 10%, and 30%–40%[12,13] of patients die within one year of diagnosis.

Mitochondrial dysfunction is believed to be the essence of HF with an adenosine triphosphate (ATP) myocardial deficit, dysfunctional calcium dynamics, and an increase in reactive oxygen species (ROS) resulting in endothelial dysfunction.[14–16]

The search for more novel and effective treatments such as mitochondrial support and stem cell therapy is becoming one of the most interesting areas of modern investigative cardiology. Adipose-derived stem cell therapy has recently offered new therapeutic strategies and may be an attractive missing link in the future treatment of congestive heart failure (CHF).[17]

Treating the heart at metabolic and cellular levels in HF is acquiring increasing popularity. The preservation of mitochondrial function and optimization of energy substrates in the heart is gaining considerable momentum as a contemporary therapy.[18,19] Because the failing myocardium is "viable but dysfunctional,"[18] and not irreversibly damaged, treatment options that target the cardiomyocyte itself should be instituted as vulnerable and dysfunctional heart cells can still be rescued.[20] If we consider the evidence for cardiomyocyte renewal in humans,[21] it makes even more sense to treat the myocardium at cellular and metabolic levels to help bolster progress in assisting the body's intrinsic stem cell wisdom in the direction of regenerative therapy.[21,22]

Although the genesis of HF includes multiple factors and many mechanisms, the essence of HF as an energy-starved heart running out of fuel identifies the myocardial energetics of the failing heart.[23,24] There is a definite energy disequilibrium between the available energy the heart has and the required energy to fulfill its needs.

Thus, supporting energy substrates in heart cells will be a new cardiological approach that focuses on the biochemistry of cellular energy as "metabolic cardiology."[25] Many physicians are not trained to look at heart disease in terms of cellular biochemistry; therefore, the challenge in any metabolic cardiology discussion is in taking the conversation from the "bench to bedside."[25–27]

Bioenergetics is the study of energy transformation in living organisms used in the field of biochemistry to reference cellular energy. The concentration of adenosine triphosphate (ATP) in the cell and the efficiency of ATP turnover and recycling are central to our appreciation of cellular bioenergetics as a new form of non-pharmaceutical therapy.

Once an understanding of how ATP repairs and restores heart cells is realized, targeted biochemical interventions to support ATP production and turnover will be strongly considered by physicians. For example, coenzyme Q10 (CoQ10) has not only shown to improve ATP dynamics but also facilitates endothelial function while mediating epigenetic gene regulation of cell signaling[28] at the same time. We will discuss the profound clinical implications of CoQ10's remarkable abilities on myocardial function later in the chapter.

Metabolic therapies that help cardiomyocytes meet their absolute need for ATP fulfill a major clinical challenge of preserving pulsatile cardiac function while maintaining mitochondrial, cellular, and tissue viabilities. D-ribose, L-carnitine and CoQ10 work in synergy to help the ischemic or hypoxic heart preserve its energy charge.

We shall learn that the bottom line in the treatment of any form of cardiovascular disease and especially in CHF, is the restoration of the heart's supply of ATP. Cardiac conditions like angina, CHF, silent ischemia and diastolic dysfunction all cause an ATP deficit. These conditions are both the cause and the result of chronic energy demand in the compromised heart. Over the years, it has been quite clear to many of our colleagues that the concept of metabolic cardiology is the missing link that has been eluding health professionals for years. It is also the solution that improves quality of life for those struggling with symptoms of CHF.

Although I struggled early in my career using conventional methodologies to treat HF, my new journey into metabolic cardiology commenced in 1982 when I successfully treated a 30-year-old female with congestive post-partum cardiomyopathy utilizing CoQ10. For the next 40 years, I continued to use CoQ10 while adding magnesium and later L-carnitine to the mix. Then in 2004, the missing link I have been searching for suddenly materialized in a heartbeat!

I was attending a lecture at a symposium on anti-aging medicine, when another like-minded, board-certified cardiologist started his sizzling presentation on a new nutrient, D-ribose. Jim Roberts, an integrative cardiologist like myself, practices in the Midwest, Ohio to be specific. Within the first 15 minutes of his spellbinding lecture, I felt an enormous connection with him. I was inspired by his enthusiasm for treating people! Then, when I least expected it, I had an extraordinary epiphany, an "aha" moment. The metaphorical "light bulb" went off in my head, as I listened to him describe how this new nutrient was working for his patients. Had I at last found the final puzzle piece for my metabolic approach to heart diseases? "Yes, this is it!" I realized excitedly.

I had been combining traditional medical approaches to heart disease including pharmaceutical drugs, procedures and surgeries with several targeted nutritional supplements to support and strengthen the heart, and at least 85%–90% of my patients were improving, recovering and maintaining those strides on my approach.

But at the end of the day, it was the other 10%–15% who still struggled in compromised bodies despite being faithful to my instructions that challenged me. I knew that there must be another piece to the treatment puzzle in those cases, many of them with chronic CHF and/or hypertensive cardiovascular disease with significant mitral regurgitation. The final "missing link" had eluded me for decades.

It came as a flash in my mind as I sat there in my seat; my mental wheels were spinning wildly, adding Roberts' theory of how D-ribose contributed to the core program I had been using. I saw the heart as a busy network of vibrating cells and realized that it was all about treating the energy in each and every cardiac cell. The concept of metabolic cardiology is built on the premise that supporting cellular energy is the key to unlocking the heart's innate potential and it unfolded in my mind as if it had always been there, just waiting for me to get it!

Adding D-ribose to my basic foundation nutrient program started turning around that subgroup of people in my practice who needed something more, and even put new life into those who were doing well on the other core nutrients like CoQ10, L-carnitine and magnesium. As my patients reported progress about having extraordinary symptom relief in their own words, it became clear that we needed to spread the news. In 2005, I wrote *The Sinatra Solution: Metabolic Cardiology*[26] with a fitting introduction by Dr. Jim Roberts. Later, we would coauthor a book together entitled *Reverse Heart Disease Now* (Wiley, 2007);[27] and *The Sinatra Solution/Metabolic Cardiology* was updated and republished in April 2008 and again in 2011.

The concept of metabolic cardiology is no fluke. Over the years, I have heard from hundreds of patients and physicians, even cardiovascular pediatric surgeons and electrophysiologists, who shared enough positive experiences with me that it's obvious this approach in healing the heart absolutely works. Even the most complex congenital cardiac cases such as tetralogy of Fallot and single-outlet left ventricle have improved considerably on a metabolic cardiology program.

Once I understood how D-ribose would intertwine with the other key nutrients in my plan, it made perfect sense that this missing link could build and magnify the generation of energy within the heart cells. Once I saw the heart muscle as "energy-starved," how to promote energy recovery became clearer. It is all about supporting those energy-starved hearts and maintaining that support on a cellular level.

D-ribose is a building block of adenosine triphosphate (ATP) – the energy of life. Almost 40 years ago, I first started my patients, and myself, on the vitamin-like/antioxidant/nutrient called CoQ10 (ubiquinone). CoQ10 is effective on almost everything cardiac: blood pressure stabilization, oxygen utilization, angina, valvular problems, arrhythmias and chronic HF. One of the first articles that caught my attention on CoQ10 was an investigation in the *Annals of Thoracic Surgery* in 1982[29] where Japanese researchers showed that patients came off heart-lung bypass machines more easily post-operatively when CoQ10 was taken for the month before heart surgery. It reduced pulmonary wedge pressure and increased cardiac index.[29] As an antioxidant and membrane stabilizer, it helped to prevent the oxidation of LDL. I even tracked some heart transplant candidates who were able to come off the transplant list if they maintained the higher CoQ10 blood levels that I monitored for them.

I learned enough about the carnitines more than 25 years ago when I wrote *L-Carnitine and The Heart*, 1999, Keats Publishing. I then added them to my basic game plan, which of course always included a solid multivitamin/multimineral at its base. The carnitines are effective in the beta-oxidation of fats as well as transporting toxic metabolites safely out of the mitochondria, the powerhouses of the cells that generate ATP.

I added in magnesium supplementation because, like CoQ10, the nutrient does so many things right for the heart. An essential component for over 300 of the body's enzymatic reactions, magnesium helps increase ATP turnover in the energy-starved heart.

Despite all my successes, there was still something sticking in my craw; something was amiss. I had doubts because not everyone with angina or HF got better on my program. Even though I was able to reduce suffering and pain for most, just one clinical failure could keep me up at night. Like most physicians and healthcare providers, it's that one case where all your best efforts just aren't good enough, or helped only a little, that gets you obsessing. One failure means more than nine successes. It was the failures that kept me going; drove me, in fact. I kept reading, rereading and trying multiple nutraceutical supports. So, the day I heard of D-ribose – the pivotal pentose sugar/nutrient that forms the basic molecule generating adenosine triphosphate (ATP), I knew in my own mind that we were on to something big in terms of helping more people get well.

In 2005, I coined the term metabolic cardiology – after I sent a Letter to the Editor of the *Journal of Clinical Cardiology*[30] commenting on the use of CoQ10 for patients awaiting heart transplantation. In essence, metabolic cardiology describes the biochemical interventions we are learning to employ to directly improve energy metabolism in heart cells.

Metabolic cardiology offers the greatest hope for the largest number of patients with cardiovascular disease. My 40+ years as a board-certified cardiologist has afforded me time and experience to add what had previously been considered alternatives to the pharmaceutical and technical standard-of-care treatments that were basic to my studies in post-graduate training of cardiology. However, this specialty I hold so close to my heart still has considerable limitations that need to be addressed before any explanation or discussion on how to implement metabolic cardiology into clinical practice can take place.

Pharmaceutical drugs, bypass surgery, angioplasty, stent placements, pacemakers and implantable defibrillators all have their place, and many lives would be lost without these high-tech interventions. Cardiologists face a daily dilemma concerning the best diagnostic procedures to recommend to their patients, and then, based on those test results, which surgical and/or pharmaceutical interventions to select. To complicate the choice, the evaluations we order and the treatments we select may create unnecessary risks for patients – risks that are out of proportion to the benefits they will experience. For example, we recommend angioplasty and stent procedures for too many patients who are asymptomatic. Continuing technological advances, although necessary, add to the complexity of the decision-making process.

Cardiologists have grown reliant upon these sophisticated medical processes, but somewhere along the way, something has gone amiss. Recently, there has been much mistrust and skepticism among the public toward the conventional medical model. Starving for new information, massive numbers of patients are consulting alternative therapy practitioners, visiting book and health food stores in record numbers, searching the internet for advice, and creating a multibillion-dollar industry outside of the mainstream medical community.

What is driving even our most conservative patients to look at other forms of therapies? There are many reasons for the increased popularity of alternative medicine, including patient dissatisfaction with ineffective conventional treatments, pharmacologic drug side effects, drug errors and the high price of medications.

Many patients are now questioning the need for potentially life-threatening drugs and invasive interventions that carry considerable side effects, complications and even mortality.

Recent research reviews and an analysis of peer-reviewed medical journals, as well as government health statistics, demonstrate that our trusted medical model can cause more harm than good. Complications from standard-of-care interventions, medical errors and the overuse of antibiotics are increasing at an alarming rate. When we consider that the fourth leading cause of death in the United States is properly prescribed medications[31] in a hospital setting, something has got to give.

For some patients, traditional medicine and the use of prescription medication can be immensely helpful in alleviating symptoms. For others, the side effects of strong drugs can be almost as problematic as the initial symptoms. In other cases, the drugs simply aren't providing enough relief. You feel better, but not up to par.

Natural therapies, which are virtually side-effect free, can reduce our reliance on conventional medicines. They are being utilized, and even preferred, by more and more people. In many cases, alternative therapies can augment traditional medicines and provide the final measure of relief that was lacking with drug therapy alone. Many patients benefit greatly from blending conventional and alternative therapies – a strategy I call "smart medicine." But before discussing any therapeutic interventions, we must first focus on why we become ill.

I've spent decades analyzing the body's electrical potential in electrocardiograms (ECGs or EKGs), watching its ultrasonic synchronous vibrations on echocardiograms, and studying its pulsating structure in invasive procedures like angiography of the great vessels and heart chambers. I've come to appreciate the complexity and perfection of the human body and also the key importance of cellular and vibrational energy.

Every cell generates its own energy through enzymatic reactions in the mitochondria that generate ATP, but in order to understand pathology and illness, we need to focus on the damage that happens to the repair loops in each cell.

The health of the cell is negatively impacted by bodily trauma, emotional blocks, environmental toxins, pharmaceutical drugs, trans-fats and most recently, electromagnetics. When the cells are bombarded with one or more of these agents, a departure from their healthy electrical potential occurs and asynchronous vibration often is the result. For example, both atrial fibrillation and congestive cardiomyopathy may occur because of mercury toxicity, and disturbed heart rate variability may become apparent as a result of chaotic electromagnetic fields (EMFs).

THE SECRETS OF THE CELL

It is my firm belief that the reason we become ill – whether it be heart disease or any other condition – is more about the jeopardized integrity of the cellular membrane of each and every cell than anything else. Whatever the target organ(s), when the cell membrane is threatened, normal functioning is impaired. Simply stated, a healthy, semi-permeable cell wall (membrane) allows nutrients in and toxins out. To be healthy, the cell's membrane must be able to breathe as it ushers in the nutrients that support its metabolism and safely transports out the waste products of those chemical reactions to be excreted. In other words, the cellular membrane must be able to take in oxygen, water, glucose, nutrients, hormones and so forth and excrete waste and toxic byproducts. Essentially, the cell must have an energy gain.

When the integrity of the cell membrane is impaired, microbial production increases. The invasion of microbes initiates and provokes degenerative processes that eventually cause insidious and relentless inflammation, a cycle that, unchecked, continuously damages the cell and causes an energy drain.

Cellular energy levels can be measured. Healthy cells pulsate at higher frequencies and have more ATP than diseased cells. Using a cutting-edge imaging technique, MIT researchers demonstrated this by studying red blood cells. When researchers compared the vibration of healthy cells against the vibration of unhealthy cells (which were depleted of ATP), they found that the frequencies of the unhealthy cells were 20% lower than the healthy cells. The researchers also noted that when ATP was re-introduced into the unhealthy cells, the vibrations increased back to normal.[32,33]

I was excited to read about these experiments at MIT, but – admittedly – not surprised, as I treated hundreds of patients using a metabolic approach that is specifically designed to replenish ATP supplies in the body, especially the heart. Countless times, I witnessed the profound healing that happens when you give the body the key nutrients it needs to make ATP molecules. Many of my patients who were on heart transplant lists no longer needed donor hearts after a few months or even weeks of treatment, and several were successfully weaned from life support. Hundreds of others improved their cardiovascular health and quality of life, and many even extended their lifespans – all by supporting natural energy production in their own compromised cardiomyocytes.

As the MIT experiment demonstrates, the free energy of hydrolysis of ATP – or the amount of chemical energy available to fuel cellular function – is vitally important. We shall soon see that in heart disease, the bioenergetic property of cardiac cells is impaired because of the faulty metabolism of ATP, especially in situations of coronary ischemia. To maintain the heart's pulsatory and vibratory energy levels, supporting the mitochondrial production of ATP is critical.

Every cell has the same basic structures, in addition to being specialized. Unlike well-armored nuclear DNA (the genetic material in the nucleus of the cell), mitochondrial DNA has minimal defense mechanisms. The mitochondria generate the chemical energy (ATP) that is transferred to mechanical energy. In the heart muscle cell, that means managing cellular respiration, calcium, and sodium pumps, contracting and relaxing, conducting impulses, and so on.

In the process of mitochondrial respiration and the genesis of ATP, not all the oxygen is converted to carbon dioxide and water. Three to five percent of the oxygen is generated from breakdown products known as free radicals. Because mitochondrial DNA has sparse defensive mechanisms, it is vulnerable to these unstable, unpaired electrons typical of free radical oxidative stress. So, it is essential to repair and support vulnerable mitochondrial activity from the relentless free radical stress of mitochondrial respiration that can negatively impact tissue and organ function.

In cardiology, solving the heart's energy crisis is essential to optimizing cardiovascular function. For decades, heart disease prevention has inappropriately and inadvertently been focused on lowering lipids (cholesterol) to prevent or slow coronary artery disease. Rather, it behooves us to shift the focus to the mitochondria and employ nutritional strategies targeting improved ATP synthesis and, therefore, heart function. Metabolic cardiology, a form of metabolic medicine, highlights the importance of sustaining key enzymatic and biochemical reactions in a preferential direction to revitalize the life of the cells in the heart and body. It is now widely accepted that one characteristic of the failing heart is the persistent and progressive loss of energy. The requirement for energy to support the systolic and diastolic work of the heart is absolute. Therefore, a disruption in cardiac energy metabolism, and the energy supply/demand mismatch that results, can be identified as the pivotal factor contributing to the inability of failing hearts to meet the hemodynamic requirements of the body. In her landmark book, *ATP and the Heart*, Joanne Ingwall, Ph.D.,[34] describes the metabolic process associated with the progression of CHF and identifies the mechanisms that lead to a persistent loss of cardiac energy reserves as the disease process unfolds.

The heart contains approximately 700 mg of ATP, enough to fuel about 10 heartbeats. At a rate of 60 beats per minute, the heart will beat 86,400 times in the average day, forcing the heart to produce and consume an amazing 6,000 g of ATP daily, and causing it to recycle its ATP pool 10,000 times every day. This process of energy recycling occurs primarily in the mitochondria of the myocyte. These organelles produce more than 90% of the energy consumed in the healthy heart, and in the heart cell, the 3,500–5,000 mitochondria fill about 35% of the cell volume. Disruption in mitochondrial function significantly restricts the energy-producing processes of the heart, causing a clinically relevant impact on heart function that translates to peripheral tissue involvement.

The heart consumes more energy per gram than any other organ, and the chemical energy that fuels the heart comes primarily from adenosine triphosphate, or ATP (Figure 8.1).

The chemical energy held in ATP is resident in the phosphoryl bonds, with the greatest amount of energy residing in the outermost bond holding the ultimate phosphoryl group to the penultimate group. When energy is required to provide the chemical driving force to a cell, this ultimate phosphoryl bond is broken, and chemical energy is released. The cell then converts this chemical energy to mechanical energy to do its work.

In the case of the heart, this energy is used to sustain stretching and contracting, drive ion pump function, synthesize large and small molecules, and perform other necessary activities of the cell. The consumption of ATP in the enzymatic reactions that release cellular energy yields the metabolic byproducts adenosine diphosphate (ADP) and inorganic phosphate (Pi) (Figure 8.2).

A variety of metabolic mechanisms have evolved within the cell to provide rapid re-phosphorylation of ADP to restore ATP levels and maintain the cellular energy pool. These metabolic mechanisms are disrupted in CHF, tipping the balance in a manner that creates a chronic energy supply/demand mismatch that results in an energy deficit or energy drain.

The normal non-ischemic heart can maintain a stable ATP concentration despite large fluctuations in workload and energy demand. In a normal heart, the rate of cellular ATP synthesis via re-phosphorylation of ADP closely matches ATP utilization. The primary site of cellular ATP re-phosphorylation is the mitochondria, where fatty acid and carbohydrate metabolic products flux

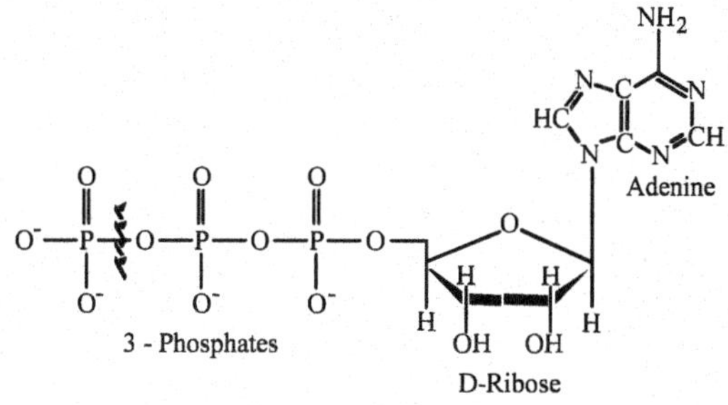

FIGURE 8.1   ATP is composed of D-ribose, adenine and three phosphate groups. Breaking the chemical bond attaching the last phosphate group to ATP releases the chemical energy that is converted to mechanical energy to perform cellular work.

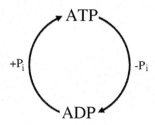

FIGURE 8.2   When ATP is used, the remaining byproducts are adenosine diphosphate (ADP) and inorganic phosphate (Pi). ADP and Pi can then recombine to form ATP in the cellular processes of energy recycling. When oxygen and food (fuel) are available, energy recycling occurs unimpeded millions of times per second in every cell in the body. Lack of oxygen or mitochondrial dysfunction severely limits the cell's ability to recycle its energy supply.

down the oxidative phosphorylation pathways. ATP recycling can also occur in the cytosol via the glycolytic pathway of glucose metabolism, but in normal hearts, this pathway accounts for only about 10% of ATP turnover.

ATP levels are also maintained through the action of creatine kinase in a reaction that transfers a high-energy phosphate creatine phosphate (PCr) to ADP to yield ATP and free creatine. Because the creatine kinase reaction is approximately 10-fold faster than ATP synthesis via oxidative phosphorylation, creatine phosphate acts as a buffer to assure a consistent availability of ATP in times of acute high metabolic demand. Although there is approximately twice as much creatine phosphate in the cell as ATP, there is still only enough to supply energy to drive about 10 heartbeats, making the maintenance of high levels of ATP availability critical to cardiac function.

The content of ATP in heart cells progressively falls in CHF, frequently reaching and then stabilizing at levels that are 25%–30% lower than normal.[23,35] The fact that ATP falls in the failing heart means that the metabolic network responsible for maintaining the balance between energy supply and demand is no longer functioning normally in these hearts. It is well established that oxygen deprivation in ischemic hearts contributes to the depletion of myocardial energy pools, but the loss of energy substrates in the failing heart is a unique example of chronic metabolic failure in the well-oxygenated myocardium.

The mechanism explaining energy depletion in HF is the loss of energy substrates and the delay in their re-synthesis. In conditions where energy demand outstrips supply, ATP is consumed at a rate that is faster than it can be restored via oxidative phosphorylation or the alternative pathways of ADP re-phosphorylation. The cell has a continuing need for energy, so it will use all its ATP stores and then break down the byproduct, adenosine diphosphate (ADP), to pull the remaining energy out of this compound as well. What's left is adenosine monophosphate (AMP).

Since a growing concentration of AMP is incompatible with sustained cellular function, it is quickly broken apart and the byproducts are washed out of the cell. The net result of this process is a depletion of the cellular pool of energy substrates. When the byproducts of AMP catabolism are washed out of the cell, they are lost forever (Figure 8.3).

It takes a long time to replace these lost energy substrates even if the cell is fully perfused with oxygen again. This reduction in energy is like a depleted car battery struggling to start your engine. In diseased hearts, the energy pool depletion via this mechanism can be significant, reaching levels that exceed 40% in ischemic heart disease and 30% in HF. Making up this profound ATP deficit is the hallmark of metabolic cardiology!

Under high-workload conditions, even normal hearts display a minimal loss of energy substrates. These substrates must be restored via the de novo pathway of ATP synthesis. This pathway is slow and energy costly, requiring consumption of six high-energy phosphates to yield one newly synthesized ATP molecule. The slow speed and high energy cost of de novo synthesis highlight the importance of cellular mechanisms designed to preserve energy pools. In normal hearts, the salvage pathways are the predominant means by which the ATP pool is maintained.

While de novo synthesis of ATP proceeds at a rate of approximately 0.02 nM/min/g in the heart, the salvage pathways operate at a 10-fold higher rate.[36] The function of both the de novo and salvage pathways of ATP synthesis is limited by the cellular availability of 5-phosphoribosyl-1-pyrophosphate, or PRPP (Figure 8.4).

PRPP initiates these synthetic reactions and is the sole compound capable of donating the D-ribose-5-phosphate moiety required to re-form ATP and preserve the energy pool. In muscle tissue, including that of the heart, formation of PRPP is slow and rate limited, impacting the rate of ATP restoration via the de novo and salvage pathways.

ENERGY STARVATION IN THE FAILING HEART

The chronic mechanism explaining the loss of ATP in CHF is decreased capacity for ATP synthesis relative to ATP demand. In part, the disparity between energy supply and demand in hypertrophied

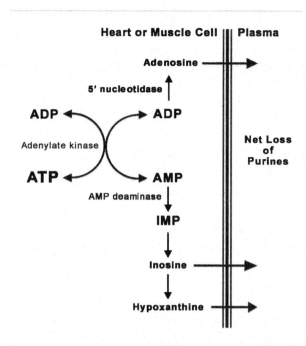

FIGURE 8.3 When the cellular concentration of ATP falls and ADP levels increase, two molecules of ADP can combine. This reaction provides one ATP, giving the cell additional energy, and one AMP. The enzyme adenylate kinase (also called myokinase) catalyzes this reaction. The AMP formed in this reaction is then degraded, and the byproducts are washed out of the cell. The loss of these purines decreases the cellular energy pool and is a metabolic disaster to the cell.

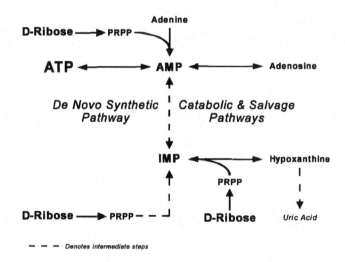

FIGURE 8.4 Replacing lost energy substrates through the de novo pathway of energy synthesis begins with D-ribose. D-ribose can also "salvage" AMP degradation products by capturing them before they can be washed out of the cell. Both the de novo and salvage pathways of energy synthesis are rate limited by the availability of D-ribose in the cell.

and failing hearts is associated with a shift in relative contribution of fatty acid versus glucose oxidation to ATP synthesis. The major consequence of the complex readjustment toward carbohydrate metabolism is that the total capacity for ATP synthesis decreases. At the same time, the demand for ATP continually increases as hearts work harder to circulate blood in the face of the increased filling pressures that are associated with CHF and hypertrophy of the left ventricle.

The net result of this energy supply/demand mismatch is a decrease in the absolute concentration of ATP in the failing heart, and this decrease in absolute ATP level is reflected in a lower energy reserve in the failing and hypertrophied or dilated heart. A declining energy reserve is directly related to heart function, with diastolic function being the first to be affected, followed by systolic function, and finally global performance (Figure 8.5).

In ischemic or hypoxic hearts, the cell's ability to match ATP supply and demand is disrupted, leading to both depletion of the cardiac energy pool and dysfunction in mitochondrial ATP turnover mechanisms. When ATP levels drop, diastolic heart function deteriorates. This is the most critical occurrence that requires a metabolic cardiology program.

Diastolic dysfunction (DD) is an early sign of myocardial failure despite the presence of normal systolic function and preserved ejection fraction. Higher concentrations of ATP are required to activate calcium pumps necessary to facilitate cardiac relaxation and promote diastolic filling. This observation leads to the conclusion that, in absolute terms, more ATP is needed to fill the heart than to empty it, consistent with Starling's law that requires more energy in diastole than in systole. The absolute requirement for ATP in the context of cardiac conditions in which energy is depleted again is what makes a metabolic therapeutic approach such a reasonable intervention.

LaPlace's law confirms that pressure overload increases energy consumption in the face of abnormalities in energy supply. In failing hearts, these energetic changes become more profound as left ventricle remodeling proceeds,[37-39] but they are also evident in the early development of the disease.[40] It has additionally been found that similar adaptations occur in the atrium, with energetic abnormalities constituting a component of the substrate for atrial fibrillation in CHF.[41] Atrial fibrillation following CABS has also been identified as a sequelae of DD.[42]

Left ventricular hypertrophy is initially an adaptive response to chronic pressure overload, but it is ultimately associated with a 10-fold greater likelihood of subsequent chronic CHF. While metabolic abnormalities are persistent in CHF and left ventricular hypertrophy, at least half of all patients with left ventricular hypertrophy-associated HF have preserved systolic function, with components of diastolic HF.

Oxidative phosphorylation is directly related to oxygen consumption, which is not decreased in patients with pressure-overload left ventricular hypertrophy. Metabolic energy defects instead relate to the absolute size of the energy pool and the kinetics of ATP turnover through oxidative

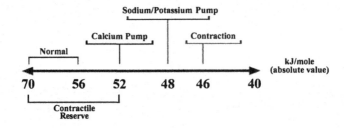

FIGURE 8.5 Cellular energy levels can be measured as the free energy of hydrolysis of ATP, or the amount of chemical energy available to fuel cellular function. Healthy, normal hearts contain enough energy to fuel all the cellular functions with a contractile reserve for use in emergency. Cellular mechanisms used in calcium management and cardiac relaxation require the highest level of available energy. Sodium/potassium pumps needed to maintain ion balance are also significant energy consumers. The cellular mechanisms associated with contraction require the least amount of cellular energy. (Adapted from several sources.)

phosphorylation and creatine kinase. Dysfunctional ATP kinetics is similar in both systolic and diastolic heart failures and may be both an initiating event and a consequence.

Inadequate ATP availability would be expected to initiate and accentuate the adverse consequences of abnormalities in energy-dependent pathways. Factors that increase energy demand, such as adrenergic stimulation and systolic overload, exaggerate the energetic deficit. Consequently, the hypertrophied heart is more metabolically susceptible to stressors such as increased chronotropic and inotropic demand, and ischemia.

In humans, this metabolic deficit is shown to be greater in compensated left ventricular hypertrophy (with or without concomitant CHF) than in dilated cardiomyopathy.[43,44] Hypertensive heart disease alone was not shown to contribute to alterations in high-energy phosphate metabolism, but it can contribute to left ventricular hypertrophy and DD that can later alter cardiac energetics.[45,46] Further, for a similar clinical degree of HF, volume overload hypertrophy does not, but pressure overload does, induce significant high-energy phosphate impairment.[47,48] This explains why hypertensive patients or patients with aortic valvular disease are so much more vulnerable in the setting of even mild CHF.

Type 2 diabetes has also been shown to contribute to altering myocardial energy metabolism early in the onset of diabetes, and these alterations in cardiac energetics may contribute to left ventricular functional changes.[49] The effect of age on progression of energetic altering has also been reviewed, with results of both human[50] and animal[51] studies suggesting that increasing age plays a moderate role in the progressive changes in cardiac energy metabolism that correlates to DD, left ventricular mass and ejection fraction.

Cardiac energetics also provide important prognostic information in patients with HF, and determining the myocardial contractile reserve has been suggested as a method of differentiating which patients seeking to reverse LV remodeling[52] would most likely respond to cardiac resynchronization therapy (CRT). Patients with a positive contractile reserve are more likely to respond to CRT and reverse remodeling of the left ventricle. Non-responders show a negative contractile reserve, suggesting increased abnormality in cardiac energetics.

Taken together, results of clinical and laboratory studies confirm that energy metabolism in CHF and left ventricular hypertrophy is of vital clinical importance. Impaired diastolic filling and stroke volume limit the delivery of oxygen-rich blood to the periphery. This chronic oxygen deprivation forces peripheral muscles to adjust and down-regulate energy turnover mechanisms, a contributing cause of symptoms of fatigue, dyspnea and muscle discomfort associated with CHF. To summarize, the key points of HF include cellular dysfunction, increase in ROS, mitochondrial dysfunction and decreased production of ATP with often poor or compromised quality-of-life issues.[14,15,53]

Treatment options that include a metabolic intervention with therapies shown to preserve energy substrates or accelerate ATP turnover are indicated for at-risk populations or patients at any stage of disease. D-ribose, CoQ10, L-carnitine and magnesium provide critical energy support to the compromised heart.

ENERGY NUTRIENTS FOR CONGESTIVE HEART FAILURE

D-RIBOSE (RIBOSE)

The effect of the pentose monosaccharide, D-ribose, in cardiac energy metabolism has been studied since the 1970s, with clinical studies describing its value as an adjunctive therapy in ischemic heart disease first appearing in 1991. Ribose is a naturally occurring simple carbohydrate that is found in every living tissue, and natural synthesis is via the oxidative pentose phosphate pathway of glucose metabolism. Remember, from high school biology or college chemistry, ribose is produced via the hexose monophosphate shunt for the sole purpose of making ATP.

But the poor expression of gatekeeper enzymes glucose-6-phosphate dehydrogenase and 6-phosphogluconate dehydrogenase limits its natural production in the heart and muscle tissue.

The primary metabolic fate of ribose is the formation of 5-phosphoribosyl-1-pyrophosphate (PRPP) required for purine synthesis and salvage via the purine nucleotide pathway. PRPP is rate limiting in purine synthesis and salvage, and concentration of the PRPP in tissue defines the rate of flux down this pathway. In this way, ribose is rate limiting for preservation of the cellular adenine nucleotide pool.

As a pentose, ribose is not used by cells as a primary energy fuel. Unlike glucose which will provide a rapid energy source, ribose is preserved for the important metabolic task of stimulating purine nucleotide synthesis and salvage to produce ATP. Approximately 98% of consumed ribose is quickly absorbed into the bloodstream and is circulated to remote tissue with no first pass effect by the liver. As ribose passes through the cell membrane, it is phosphorylated by membrane-bound ribokinase before entering the pentose phosphate pathway downstream of the gatekeeper enzymes. In this way, administered ribose can increase intracellular PRPP concentration and initiate purine nucleotide synthesis and salvage.

The study of ribose in CHF was first reported in the *European Journal of Heart Failure* in 2003.[54] Until that time, the clinical benefit of ribose in cardiovascular disease was largely confined to its increasing role in treating coronary artery disease and other ischemic heart diseases, where its benefit had been well established. The reported double-blind, placebo-controlled, crossover study included patients with chronic coronary artery disease and NYHA Class II/III CHF. Patients underwent two treatment periods of 3 weeks each, during which either oral ribose (5 g t.i.d.) or placebo (glucose; 5 g t.i.d.) was administered. Following a 1-week washout period, the alternate test supplement was administered for a subsequent 3-week test period. Before and after each 3-week trial period, assessment of myocardial function was made by echocardiography, and the patient's exercise capacity was determined using a stationary exercise cycle. Participants also completed a quality-of-life questionnaire. Ribose administration significantly enhanced all indices of diastolic heart function and exercise tolerance, and was also associated with improved quality-of-life score. By comparison, none of these parameters were changed with glucose (placebo) treatment.

Indeed, in my experience, the magic of D-ribose is its efficacy in DD. In a recent review article, the clinical benefits of D-ribose in ischemic cardiovascular disease were revealed. Since myocardial ischemia lowers ATP levels and is reflected in increasing DD, D-ribose as a pentose support has been shown in pilot clinical studies to enhance the recovery of ATP levels while improving DD at the same time.[55]

In another small cohort study using D-ribose, an improvement in tissue Doppler velocity (E′) demonstrated a beneficial trend with 64% of the participants suggesting that D-ribose supports patients with DD.[56]

In addition to impaired pump function, CHF patients exhibited compromised ventilation and oxygen uptake efficiency that presents as dyspnea. Ventilation efficiency slope and oxygen uptake efficiency slope are extremely sensitive predictors of CHF patient survival that can be measured using sub-maximal exercise protocols that include pulmonary assessment of oxygen and carbon dioxide levels. In one study, ribose administration (5 g, t.i.d.) to NYHA Class III/IV CHF patients significantly improved ventilation efficiency, oxygen uptake efficiency and stroke volume, as measured by oxygen pulse.[57]

A second study[58] showed that in NYHA Class II/III CHF patients, ribose administration significantly maintained VO2max when compared to placebo and improved ventilatory efficiency to the respiratory compensation point. A third[59] similar study involving patients with NYHA Class III CHF investigated the effect of ribose on Doppler Tei myocardial performance index (MPI), VO2max and ventilatory efficiency, all-powerful predictors of HF survival in a Class III HF population. Results showed that ribose improved MPI and ventilatory efficiency while preserving VO2max. Results of these studies show that ribose stimulates energy metabolism along the cardiopulmonary axis, thereby improving gas exchange.

Increased cardiac load produces unfavorable energetics that deplete myocardial energy reserves. Because ribose is the rate-limiting precursor for adenine nucleotide metabolism, its role in preserving energy substrates in remote myocardium following infarction was studied in a rat model.[60] In this study, male Lewis rats received continuous venous infusion of ribose or placebo via an osmotic mini-pump for 14 days. One to two days after pump placement, animals underwent ligation of the left anterior descending coronary artery to produce an anterior wall myocardial infarction (MI). Echocardiographic analyses performed preoperatively and at 2 and 4 weeks following infarction were used to assess functional changes as evidenced by ejection indices, chamber dimensions and wall thickness.

All three measured indices shows that ribose administration better maintained the myocardium. Contractility and wall thickness was increased, while less ventricular dilation occurred. This study showed that the remote myocardium exhibits a significant decrease in function within 4 weeks following myocardial infarction, and that ribose administration attenuates this dysfunction to a significant degree.

This is an important clinical concept as I have seen many patients experience typical and atypical chest symptoms as well as generalized weakness following stent and angioplasty procedures. When temporary ischemia occurs in the myocardium following balloon inflation, ATP levels drop. It may take for the body several days to make up the deficit with de novo ATP synthesis. In my experience, ribose has been a significant factor in supporting energy substrate levels that enhance ATP production, thus alleviating symptoms in these patients. Temporary or prolonged ischemia results in lower myocardial energy levels. Increasing the cardiac energy level not only improves symptoms and function but may also delay vulnerable changes in a variety of CHF conditions. This therapeutic advantage ribose provides in improving cardiac index and left ventricular function suggests its value as an adjunct to traditional therapy for ischemia and CHF.

Since D-ribose administration creates favorable physiological parameters on cardiac function and has been shown to enhance the recovery of high-energy phosphates following myocardial ischemia, it was hypothesized that D-ribose could improve cardiological indices for off-pump coronary artery bypass procedures.[61] In a retrospective analysis of 366 patients undergoing off-pump CABS, 308 patients received D-ribose as a peri-operative metabolic protocol. D-ribose patients had a greater improvement in cardiac index post-revascularization compared with non-D-ribose patients (37% vs 17% $p < 0.0001$). The research has suggested that a larger randomized placebo-controlled prospective trial be evaluated to further test the hypothesis that ribose be considered standard management in myocardial ischemia. This concept was again suggested in a study indicating that D-ribose will replenish cellular energy in ischemic myocardium.[62]

Researchers and practitioners using ribose in cardiology practice recommend a dose range of 10–15 g/day as metabolic support for CHF or other heart diseases. In my practice, patients are placed on a regimen of 5 g/dose three times per day for any form of CHF and/or myocardial ischemia. Individual doses of greater than 10 g are not recommended because high single doses of a hygroscopic carbohydrate may cause mild gastrointestinal discomfort or transient lightheadedness. Since ribose has a lower glycemic index, it should be administered with meals or mixed in beverages containing a secondary carbohydrate source when administered to diabetic patients prone to hypoglycemia. I also frequently recommend ribose in fruit juices to these patients or in diabetic patients taking insulin.

In conclusion, D-ribose has been instrumental in alleviating symptoms of shortness of breath and easy fatigability in my patients experiencing CHF and hypertensive cardiovascular disease with and without left ventricular hypertrophy. D-ribose along with CoQ10, L-carnitine and magnesium (awesome foursome) has reduced considerable suffering in our patients. Since the clinical efficacy of these nutraceuticals has been appreciated by many healthcare practitioners, the University of Kansas Medical Center is participating in a 153-patient randomized, double-blind, placebo-controlled trial that will evaluate the clinical benefits of D-ribose and CoQ10 in improving mitochondrial bioenergetics.[63] The trial, which has already presented some impressive data regarding myocardial dysfunction in a 2020 publication, is still ongoing and should be completed in 2021. This trial is supported by an NIH grant that is evaluating the clinical benefits of D-ribose and ubiquinol in patients with HF and preserved ejection fraction.

COENZYME Q10 AND THE HEART

Coenzyme Q10, so named for its ubiquitous nature in cells, is a fat-soluble compound that functions as an antioxidant and coenzyme in the energy-producing pathways. Ubiquinol – known as the reduced form – and ubiquinone – the oxidized form – both coexist in the body and regenerate each other in our cells through sequential redox reactions. As an antioxidant, the reduced form of CoQ10 inhibits lipid peroxidation in both cell membranes and serum low-density lipoprotein, and protects proteins and DNA from oxidative damage. In vitro, CoQ10 inhibits LDL oxidation more than beta-carotene and alpha-tocopherol.[64] CoQ10 also has membrane-stabilizing activity. However, its bioenergetic activity and electron transport function for its role in oxidative phosphorylation are probably its most important functions.

The electron transport chain is a series of oxidation-reduction (REDOX) chemical reactions that allow the mitochondria to transform the food you eat into energy (ATP). The electrons need CoQ10 to make their way down the electron transport chain or ATP production slows, causing a decrease in energy production, an increase in free radicals, and potentially disease or even death.

In CHF, oxidative phosphorylation slows due to a loss of mitochondrial protein and lack of expression of key enzymes involved in the cycle. Disruption of mitochondrial activity may lead to a loss of CoQ10 that can further depress oxidative phosphorylation. In patients taking statin-like drugs, the mitochondrial loss of CoQ10 may be exacerbated by restricted CoQ10 synthesis resulting from HMG-CoA reductase inhibition (Figure 8.6).

One study on this association was reported by Japanese researchers in the *International Heart Journal*.[65] In essence, long-term treatment with atorvastatin may increase plasma levels of brain natriuretic peptide (BNP) in coronary artery disease when associated with a greater reduction in plasma CoQ10.

Thus, this favorable effect of CoQ10 on statin-induced myopathy just makes good clinical sense. Although statins and other pharmaceutical drugs appear to be the most significant source of CoQ10 deficiency in the general population, other sources of CoQ10 decline appear in tissues that are highly metabolically active, such as those of the heart, immune system, inflamed gingiva and overactive thyroid gland. As we age, the levels of CoQ10 in our body also decrease.[66] This may be due to decreased endogenous production, an insufficiency in the diet, or the cumulative effects of stress and free radicals. While there is no evidence that healthy individuals need to supplement with CoQ10, tissues will benefit from CoQ10 support during times of metabolic stress.

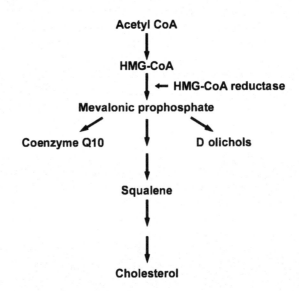

FIGURE 8.6   Statin drugs (HMG-CoA reductase inhibitors) can reduce natural CoQ10 synthesis in the body.

Although CoQ10 is found in relatively high concentrations in the liver, kidney, and lung, the heart requires the highest levels of ATP activity because it is continually aerobic and contains more mitochondria per gram than any other tissue in the body. Cardiomyocytes, for example, contain more than 3,500 mitochondria per cell compared to a biceps muscle cell that houses approximately 200 mitochondria per cell.

As a high-energy-efficient transfer molecule supporting high metabolic reactions, the heart must have adequate levels of this compound in its cells.[67] CoQ10's potent antioxidant action will not only help prevent free radical damage by regulating transcriptional pathways but will also help to deactivate inflammatory processes.[68] Its clinical use in reducing inflammatory markers will help support healing in pathogenic situations.[69]

Tissue deficiencies and low serum blood levels of CoQ10 have been reported across a wide range of cardiovascular diseases, including DD, CHF, hypertension, aortic valvular disease and coronary artery disease, and research suggests that CoQ10 support may be indicated in these disease conditions.[70,71]

Although the medical literature generally supports the use of CoQ10 in CHF, the evaluated dose-response relationships for this nutrient have been confined to a narrow dose range, with most clinical studies having been conducted on subjects who were taking only 90–300 mg daily. At such doses, some patients have responded, while others have not. In more than two dozen controlled trials of supplemental CoQ10 in CHF, only three investigations[72-74] which failed to show improvement in any significant cardiovascular function had major limitations.

In the well-known study conducted by Permanetter et al.,[72] a 100 mg dose of CoQ10 failed to show improvement. However, actual blood levels of CoQ10 were not obtained in this investigation; thus, it is impossible to know if a therapeutic blood level was ever achieved. In the second trial by Watson et al.,[73] a mean treatment plasma CoQ10 level of only 1.7 μg/mL was obtained with only 2 of the 30 patients having a plasma level greater than 2.0μg/mL.

The third study performed by Khatta et al.[74] demonstrated a mean treatment plasma CoQ10 level of 2.2±1.1 μg/mL, and indicated that approximately half of the patients had treatment levels as low as 1.0μg/mL. Unfortunately, these last two clinical trials are frequently quoted as CoQ10 failures, even though a bio-sensitive result was not achieved.

In patients with CHF or dilated cardiomyopathy, I generally use higher doses of CoQ10 in ranges of at least 300 mg or more to get a bio-sensitive result requiring a blood level at least greater than 2.5 μg/mL and preferably 3.5 μg/mL.[75] In a previous analysis in three patients with refractory CHF, such higher doses of CoQ10 were required in order to get such a bio-sensitive or therapeutic result.[76] In an investigation at the Lancisi Heart Institute in Italy, researchers studied 23 patients with a mean age of 59, using a double-blind, placebo-controlled, crossover design. Patients were assigned to receive 100 mg of oral CoQ10 three times per day, plus supervised exercise training. The study concluded that CoQ10 supplementation improved functional capacity, endothelial function and left ventricular contractility in CHF without any side effects.[77]

In a previous long-term study of 424 patients with systolic and/or DD in the presence of CHF, dilated cardiomyopathy, or hypertensive heart disease, a dose of 240 mg/day maintained blood levels of CoQ10 above 2.0μg/mL, and allowed 43% of the participants to discontinue one to three conventional drugs over the course of the study.[78] Patients were followed for an average of 17.8 months, and during that time, a mild case of nausea was the only reported side effect. This long-term study clearly shows CoQ10 to be a safe and effective adjunctive treatment for patients with systolic and/or diastolic left ventricular dysfunction with or without CHF, dilated cardiomyopathy or hypertensive heart disease.

These results are further confirmed by an investigation involving 109 patients with hypertensive heart disease and isolated DD showing that CoQ10 supplementation resulted in clinical improvement, lowered elevated blood pressure, enhanced diastolic cardiac function and decreased myocardial thickness in 53% of study patients.[79] A meta-analysis of 17 randomized controlled trials of 684 patients showed that CoQ10 possibly reduced systolic blood pressure via promoting endothelial vasodilatation through enhancing nitric oxide bioavailability.[80]

A study on the longevity merits of CoQ10 in HF was published in a fall 2008 issue of the *Journal of the American College of Cardiology*.[81] New Zealand researchers studied the relationship between plasma CoQ10 levels and survival in patients with chronic HF. In their cohort of 236 patients (mean age 77 years), they concluded that plasma CoQ10 concentrations were an independent predictor of mortality. The higher blood levels were the best predictors for survival. Researchers suggested that lower concentrations of plasma CoQ10 might be detrimental in the long-term prognosis of CHF. Since CoQ10 depletion is associated with worse outcomes in CHF, they suggest further controlled intervention studies on CoQ10 supplementation.

Several years later, the most impressive analysis of CoQ10 and survival in patients with severe HF was reproduced in the Q-SYMBIO study.[82] In this double-blind, placebo-controlled trial involving 420 patients with moderate to severe HF, subjects treated with 300 mg of CoQ10 supplementation (ubiquinone) or placebo were evaluated. While there were no changes in short-term end points, the long-term benefits were considerable. There was a significant reduction in the incidence of major adverse cardiovascular events in the CoQ10 group: 15% in the CoQ10 group versus 26% in the placebo group. There was also a significant reduction in overall mortality: 9% in the CoQ10 group versus 16% in the placebo group. The study strongly suggests that CoQ10 is a major nutraceutical to improve survival in chronic HF. Although ACE inhibitors and beta-blockers have shown to have efficacy in HF, CoQ10 is the non-pharmaceutical nutrient of choice in chronic CHF or the energy-starved heart.

This effect of CoQ10 administration on 32 heart transplant candidates with end-stage CHF and cardiomyopathy was reported in 2004.[83] The study was designed to determine if CoQ10 could improve the pharmacological bridge to transplantation, and the results showed three significant findings. First, following 6 weeks of CoQ10 therapy, the study group showed elevated blood levels from an average of 0.22 mg/L to 0.83 mg/L*, an increase of 277% (*Please note that different labs in other countries have different standardizations of CoQ10). By contrast, the placebo group measured 0.18 mg/L at the onset of the study and 0.178 mg/L at 6 weeks. Second, the study group showed significant improvement in 6-minute walk test distance, shortness of breath, NYHA functional classification, fatigue and episodes of waking for nocturnal urination. No such changes were found in the placebo group. These results strongly show that CoQ10 therapy may augment pharmaceutical treatment of patients with end-stage CHF and cardiomyopathy.

Recently, three CoQ10 studies were published suggesting even more evidence for its consideration in LV dysfunction. In one small study of 28 patients with ischemic left ventricular systolic dysfunction, taking 300 mg of CoQ10 supplement per day versus 28 placebo controls, 8 weeks of supplementation improved mitochondrial functioning and brachial flow-mediated dilatation (FMD).[84] The researchers concluded that CoQ10 improved endothelial function via reversal of mitochondrial dysfunction in patients with diminished ejection fraction.

In a more recent analysis of the Q-SYMBIO study,[85] the subgroup analysis data of 231 patients after two more years showed continued significant improvements in hospitalizations as well as all-cause mortality. Once again, the investigators concluded that CoQ10 should strongly be considered as part of the maintenance treatment of CHF. Previously, this trend of decreased mortality was also revealed in a 2017 meta-analysis of clinical trials in patients with CHF. Lei et al. demonstrated that CoQ10 supplementation decreased mortality vs placebo while improving exercise capacity at the same time.[86]

In another double-blind, placebo-controlled trial[87] among elderly Swedish citizens, selenium and CoQ10 were administered vs placebo to 443 patients aged 77–88. There was a significant reduction in mortality in the active group 5.9% vs 12.6% controls. In addition, N-terminal pro-B-type natriuretic peptide (NT-proBnp) and echocardiographic measurements were significantly improved.

Finally, in a 2021 issue of the *Journal of the American College of Cardiology*, a connection between statin-related CoQ10 deficiency and diastolic HF was strongly suggested. Although more research is warranted, the application of CoQ10 in patients suffering from DD previously treated with statins in my opinion is simply good medicine.[87A]

COQ10 – INFLAMMATORY CORONARY HEART DISEASE/DIABETES

CoQ10 has also demonstrated a considerable impact on the lipid marker lipoprotein (a) – Lp(a) which is perhaps one of the major risk factors in the development of inflammatory coronary artery disease. In a meta-analysis of six small trials, including subjects with type 2 diabetes, coronary artery disease, obesity, hypertriglyceridemia, hemodialysis patients and systolic dysfunction, CoQ10 supplementation 100–300 mg a day was associated with an Lp(a) reduction of 3.54 mg/dL, $P<0.001$ with the effect being more pronounced in patients with the highest Lp(a) levels.[88] In another meta-analysis, patients with coronary artery disease presented increased HDL levels with CoQ10.[89] In another review on lipid profiles, a reduction in total cholesterol and triglycerides was realized.[90]

Additionally, a recent meta-analysis of randomized trials observed the effect of CoQ10 supplementation on another inflammatory marker, high-sensitivity C-reactive protein (hs-CRP).[91] In cardiovascular disease patients who took CoQ10 for more than 12 weeks with baseline serum levels of hs-CRP of greater than 3 mg/L, a beneficial effect was realized. Thus, it makes sense to utilize CoQ10 to assuage biomarkers of inflammation including interleukin-6 (IL-6)[92] in patients with any form of cardiovascular disease including CHF.

In extreme insulin resistance rendering type 2 diabetes, the consumption of less than 200 mg of CoQ10 daily reduced fasting glucose, triglycerides and HbA1c. Since diminished levels of CoQ10 are often found in plasma levels of diabetics when compared to healthy controls, it makes sense to include CoQ10, exercise and a prudent carbohydrate diet in any overweight type 2 diabetic and especially if there is any degree of diabetic nephropathy (DN). CoQ10 may also offer a supportive Rx in patients with DN. Lower CoQ10 blood levels found in insulin-resistant rats with higher ROS concentrations were perhaps the contributing factors in DN. CoQ10 might be an early Rx for DN by increasing insulin sensitivity while neutralizing mitochondrial oxidants at the same time.[93,94]

COENZYME Q10 VARIETALS – UBIQUINONE, UBIQUINOL AND MITOQ

Ever since CoQ10 was first isolated by Dr. Frederick Crane and colleagues in 1957,[95] scientists have been conducting hundreds of clinical studies on this intriguing nutrient. Over the last few years, there has been some considerable debate about which form of CoQ10 should be utilized in clinical practice as the ubiquinol/ubiquinone controversy continues. Quite frankly, the use of a high quality ubiquinone versus ubiquinol does not really matter, as many people prefer ubiquinol while others like ubiquinone.

In a recent study, looking into the bioavailability of CoQ10 supplements, carrier lipids and solubilization were strong considerations. In a small study involving 14 volunteers in a double-blind crossover design with a four-week washout between intakes, the best absorbable formulations were soft-gel capsules containing ubiquinone or ubiquinol.[96] I conducted an unpublished study in 12 patients with a crossover design involving ubiquinone vs ubiquinol in which blood levels were slightly higher on ubiquinol. However, a Connecticut female weightlifter had such profound fatigue and diminished ability in competition on ubiquinol she literally wanted to drop out of the study. When I convinced her that it was only a few more weeks for the washout to be completed, she agreed to go back on ubiquinone in which she reported profound energy and stamina. We really cannot explain why there is such a discrepancy in energy and endurance in these competitive endeavors. However, since most clinical trials have been conducted with ubiquinone over ubiquinol, it makes sense to utilize ubiquinone as ubiquinol is considerably more costly both to the manufacturer and the patient. Since ubiquinone and ubiquinol shift from one form to another inside the body, the most important aspect is clinical response. This was obviously demonstrated in the last two statistically significant major trials on CoQ10 (Q-SYMBIO and KiSEL).[85,87] If a clinical benefit is not realized with the reduced or the oxidative varietal of CoQ10 despite an optimal blood level analysis, switching the compound should strongly be considered. Ubiquinol was the CoQ10 varietal in the previously mentioned Kansas study,[63] and the preliminary data shows promise in mitochondrial support as well as left ventricular function.

To complicate the ubiquinone/ubiquinol controversy, another form of CoQ10 referred to as MitoQ surfaced within the last several years. MitoQ is a mitochondrial-Quinol ROS moiety linked to triphenyl phosphonium (TPP), a lipophilic compound that easily crosses the membranes and accumulates in the mitochondrial matrix as a function of membrane potential.

Since CoQ10 has been utilized in clinical practice for almost 50 years, it is reasonable that multiple varietals of CoQ10 preparations have been studied. Massive marketing campaigns for ubiquinone, ubiquinol and MitoQ may have caused confusion for both clinicians and their patients about what form of the compound to consider. Again, I feel that a high-quality ubiquinone that has demonstrated superior bioavailability in blood analysis studies is the most logical and ethical option to consider. In the final analysis, since different forms of CoQ10 can be converted to one form or another, it makes sense to consider the most affordable and bioavailable compound available. Certainly, more research regarding MitoQ and other forms of Q10 is reasonable and it may take a considerable amount of study to see if one compound is indeed clinically better than another.

To complicate the confusion regarding different forms of Q10, a recent investigation suggested that the gamma cyclodextrin complex form of CoQ10 is a powerful nutraceutical for additional anti-aging and health improvements.[97] Certainly the most important aspect of CoQ10 is its bioavailability, and the CoQ10 gamma cyclodextrin complex has major improvements in plasma concentrations of CoQ10. Thus, any CoQ10 formulation with a gamma cyclodextrin complex may perhaps be the most bioavailable form of Q10 to consider.

To summarize, CoQ10 is one of the body's most important endogenous compounds as a powerful antioxidant and membrane stabilizer as well as a critical electron donor for mitochondrial cellular production. Multiple controlled studies have confirmed my observation over almost four decades of CoQ10 applications in thousands of patients. It is the most efficacious, bioenergetic and therapeutic compound I have ever discovered in the treatment and management of CHF.

LEVOCARNITINE (L-CARNITINE OR CARNITINE)

Carnitine is derived naturally in the body from the amino acids lysine and methionine. Biosynthesis occurs in a series of metabolic reactions involving these amino acids, complemented with niacin, vitamin B6, vitamin C and iron. Although carnitine deficiency is rare in a healthy, well-nourished population consuming adequate protein, CHF, left ventricular hypertrophy, and other cardiac conditions causing renal insufficiency can lead to cellular depletion and conditions of carnitine deficiency.

The principal role of carnitine is to facilitate the transport of fatty acids across the inner mitochondrial membrane to initiate beta-oxidation. The inner mitochondrial membrane is normally impermeable to activated coenzyme A (Co A) esters. To affect transfer of the extracellular metabolic byproduct acyl-Co A across the cellular membrane, the mitochondria deliver its acyl unit to the carnitine residing in the inner mitochondrial membrane. Carnitine (as acetyl-carnitine) then transports the metabolic fragment across the membrane and delivers it to coenzyme A residing inside the mitochondria. This process of acetyl transfer is known as the carnitine shuttle, and the shuttle also works in reverse to remove excess acetyl units from the inner mitochondria for disposal. Excess acetyl units that accumulate inside the mitochondria disturb the metabolic burning of fatty acids.

Nature created carnitine to serve as a freight train or ferry boat to carry fatty acids into the mitochondria. More importantly, it is not only the burning of fat in the mitochondria that fuels the energy for ATP, but as high-energy organisms, we humans produce a lot of toxic waste as well. This is where the carnitines are so phenomenal and instrumental – especially in cardiac health. Not only do these carnitines shuttle in the fatty acids to be burned in the mitochondria as fuel, but they shuttle out the toxic metabolites as well. In essence, L-carnitine promotes a balanced cardiac energy metabolism and regulation of calcium influx.[98]

Other crucial functions of intracellular carnitine include the metabolism of branched-chain amino acids, ammonia detoxification and lactic acid clearance from tissue. Carnitine also exhibits antioxidant and free radical scavenger properties, reducing oxidative stress as well as assuaging inflammation and necrosis of cardiac cells at the same time.[98]

Although the role of carnitine in the utilization of fatty acids and glucose in cardiac metabolism has been known for decades, the relationship between carnitine availability in heart tissue, carnitine metabolism in the heart, and carnitine's impact on left ventricular function has been elucidated only recently. Two independent studies have investigated the relationship between tissue carnitine levels and heart function, and whether plasma or urinary carnitine levels might serve as markers for impaired left ventricular function in patients with CHF.

In the first study of carnitine tissue levels and CHF, the myocardial tissue from 25 cardiac transplant recipients with end-stage CHF and 21 control donor hearts was analyzed for concentrations of total carnitine, free carnitine and carnitine derivatives. Compared to controls, the concentration of carnitines in the heart muscle of heart transplant recipients was significantly lower in patients, and the level of carnitine in the tissue was directly correlated to ejection fraction. This study concluded that carnitine deficiency in the heart tissue might be directly related to heart function.[99]

The second study measured plasma and urinary levels of L-carnitine in 30 patients with CHF and cardiomyopathy and compared them to 10 control subjects with no heart disease.[100] Results showed that patients with CHF had higher plasma and urinary levels of carnitine, suggesting that carnitine was being released from the challenged heart muscle cells. Similarly, the results showed that the level of plasma and urinary carnitine was related to the degree of left ventricular systolic dysfunction and ejection fraction, showing that elevated plasma and urinary carnitine levels – indices of carnitines being leeched out of compromised cardiomyocytes – might represent measurable physiological markers for myocardial damage and impaired left ventricular function.

Free L-carnitine levels and its derivative palmitoyl-L-carnitine were increased in CHF patients and correlated with NT-proBnp and NYHA functional class status. In this study of 183 HF patients and 111 healthy controls, higher levels of palmitoyl-L-carnitine were also associated with more adverse outcomes. The authors believed these findings suggested prognostic value and recommended additional investigational analysis of L-carnitine administration in HF candidates.[101] More recently, L-carnitine has shown favor in cardiomyopathy and especially in dilated cardiomyopathy. In a previous meta-analysis of 23 RCTs conducted in China in 1,455 DCM patients, L-carnitine therapy significantly decreased left ventricular end diastolic dimensions (LVEDD), BNP and transforming growth factor-beta (TGF-Beta1), while increasing left ventricular ejection fraction (LVEF) and cardiac output at the same time.[102] In another previous study of 28 patients, a reduction in systolic and diastolic diameters with an increase in LVEF was realized.[103]

A previous investigation examined the effect of long-term carnitine administration on mortality in patients with CHF and dilated cardiomyopathy. This study followed 80 patients with moderate to severe HF (NYHA class III/IV) for 3 years. After a 3-month period of stable cardiac function on normal medication, patients were randomly assigned to receive either 2 g of carnitine per day or a matched placebo. After an average of 33.7 months of follow-up, 70 patients remained in the study (33 taking placebo and 37 supplementing with carnitine), and at the end of the study period, 63 had survived (27 placebo and 36 carnitine). This study determined that carnitine provided a benefit to longer-term survival in late-stage HF in dilated cardiomyopathy.[104]

A similar placebo-controlled study evaluated 160 myocardial infarction survivors for 12 months.[105] Eighty subjects were included in each group; the study group received a daily dose of 4 g of L-carnitine and the controls a placebo. Both the carnitine and control groups continued their conventional therapeutic regimen while on the test substance. Subjects in both groups showed improvement in arterial blood pressure, cholesterol levels, rhythm disorders, and signs and symptoms of CHF over the study period, but all-cause mortality was significantly lower in the carnitine group than the placebo group (1.2% and 12.5%, respectively). A further double-blind, placebo-controlled trial by Singh and coworkers studied 100 patients with suspected myocardial infarction. Patients taking carnitine (2 g/day for

28 days) showed improvement in arrhythmia, angina, onset of HF and mean infarct size, as well as a reduction in total cardiac events. There was a significant reduction in cardiac death and non-fatal infarction in the carnitine group versus the placebo group (15.6% vs. 26%, respectively).[106]

In a European study of 472 patients published in the *Journal of the American College of Cardiology*, 9 g/day of carnitine was administered intravenously for 5 days followed by 6 g/day orally for the next 12 months.[107] The study validated previous findings, demonstrating an improvement in ejection fraction and a reduction in left ventricular size in carnitine-treated patients. Although the European study was not designed to demonstrate outcome differences, the combined incidence of CHF death after discharge was lower in the carnitine group than placebo group (6.0% vs. 9.6%, respectively), a reduction of more than 30%.

In a later study, only 1,500 mg of L-carnitine in 29 patients with NYHA Class II symptoms and preserved left ventricular function demonstrated not only an improvement of shortness of breath in the carnitine group but also improved diastolic relationships on echocardiographic analysis after only 3 months of treatment.[108]

A thorough review of the benefits of L-carnitine and cardiovascular function was reported as a meta-analysis in the Mayo Clinic's proceedings 2013.[109] Thirteen clinical trials involving 3,629 patients post MI were evaluated. L-Carnitine benefits were attributed to the ability of L-carnitine to limit infarct size, stabilize membranes and improve compromised cellular energy production. The major improvements in these vulnerable post-MI patients not only showed a reduction of angina symptoms by 40% and reduced arrhythmia by 60%, but a striking reduction in all-cause death by 27%.[109] Indeed, L-carnitine has been instrumental and extremely favorable in improving the quality of life in the cardiovascular population with HF and angina. However, L-carnitine may have been tarnished over the last few years as trimethylamine-N-oxide (TMAO) investigations have placed carnitine into somewhat of a controversy, suggesting that L-carnitine may enhance the pro-atherogenic metabolites TMAO which could adversely affect the gut microbiome and have a negative impact on coronary artery disease. In a recent review in the *Journal of the American College of Cardiology*, an increase in TMAO in the plasma over a 10-year period demonstrated a higher risk of coronary artery disease.[109A]

However, other TMAO investigations that have emerged in the medical literature over the past few years suggest opposite correlations. In a very recent rodent model, low-dose TMAO Rx reduced DD and heart fibrosis in hypertensive rats.[110] Indeed, the TMAO hypothesis may be in a crossfire and the research needs further investigation.[111] Perhaps TMAO may just be a mere compensatory mechanism as a marker or a response to pathology.[112] When one considers the longevity merits of the Mediterranean and Okinawan diets, abundant in proteins, sea foods and other TAMO-raising properties, it just doesn't make sense to restrict and modify the diet over controversial evidence. A healthy diet will be the most cost-effective way to positively affect the gut microbiota while treating and preventing HF at the same time.[112A]

The Mediterranean diet perhaps addresses the possible pathological sequelae of TMAO as a few constituents tend to reduce it. Let me explain. For example, extra virgin olive oil, or EVOO – the secret sauce of the Mediterranean diet – contains DMB (3,dimethyl-1-butanol) which reduces TMAO.[112B] In addition, allicin,[112C] the active ingredient in garlic, reduces TMAO, and resveratrol found in red wines helps to shift the gut microbiota composition, reducing TMAO and bile acid synthesis.[112D] Although the Mediterranean diet has demonstrated longevity, perhaps these TMAO-reducing constituents in the diet make it even more favorable, especially if continued research brings clarity into the controversial TMAO concept. However, currently there is still no evidence showing that reducing TMAO levels is beneficial.[112A]

A newer form of carnitine called glycine propionyl L-carnitine (GPLC) has demonstrated significant advantages in the production of nitric oxide and lower malondialdehyde (MDA) – a marker of lipid peroxidation and oxidative damage. This form of carnitine has demonstrated the important property of vasodilation via a nitric oxide mechanism. GPLC also blocked key steps in the process of platelet aggregation and adhesion, as well as reducing levels of lipid peroxidation and oxidative damage.[113]

To summarize, without carnitine, fats which are a high-energy fuel for the heart cannot be converted to ATP. The heart uses free-fatty acids as its main energy source, and the only way for long-chain fatty acids to get to the inner mitochondrial membrane where energy is produced is via the carnitine shuttle. Thus, the addition of L-carnitine is a particularly important contribution in the synergy of metabolic cardiology.

MAGNESIUM – SWITCHING ON THE ENERGY ENZYMES

Magnesium is an essential mineral that is critical for energy-requiring processes in protein synthesis, membrane integrity, nervous tissue conduction, neuromuscular excitation, muscle contraction, hormone secretion, maintenance of vascular tone and in intermediary metabolism. Magnesium deficiency may lead to changes in neuromuscular, cardiovascular, immune and hormonal functions, impaired energy metabolism and reduced capacity for physical work. Its deficiency is now considered to contribute to many diseases, and the role for magnesium as a therapeutic agent is expanding. A published German study[114] brings this point into focus.

Researchers in this study evaluated a random population of about 16,000 people, who were assigned to subgroups based on gender, age and state of health. Low blood levels of magnesium, or hypomagnesemia, were identified in 14.5% of all persons examined, and suboptimal levels were found in yet another 33.7% – a total of 58.2% – more than half of those evaluated.[114] Thus, low-magnesium situations are more common than we think.

Magnesium deficiency reduces the activity of important enzymes used in energy metabolism. Hypomagnesemia can result in progressive vasoconstriction, coronary spasm and even sudden death.[115] In anginal episodes due to coronary artery spasm, treatment with magnesium has been shown to be efficacious.[116]

Magnesium deficiency, which is better detected by mononuclear blood cell magnesium than the standard serum level performed at most hospitals, predisposes to excessive mortality and morbidity in patients with acute MI.[117]

Unless we have adequate levels of magnesium in our cells, the cellular processes of energy metabolism cannot function. Small changes in magnesium levels can have a large effect on heart and blood vessel functions. While magnesium is found in most foods – particularly beans, figs and vegetables – its deficiency is increasing. Softened water, depleted soils and a trend toward lower vegetable consumption are the culprits contributing to these rising deficiencies. Thus, supplementation of magnesium is a good idea! I personally take 200–400 mg of magnesium at bedtime of a mixed Krebs cycle broad-spectrum complex containing citrate, glycinate, orotate and taurinate. I especially like the orotate formulation, as Australian thoracic surgeons using this varietal had better outcomes in their patients as the orotate varietal helps drive ATP in a preferential direction.

TAURINE

The use of taurine in CHF may help to reduce human suffering, especially if a traditional metabolic cardiology approach is not ideal. Taurine is a non-essential amino acid that stabilizes cellular membranes in the heart. Several citations on taurine came out in the 1980s by Japanese researchers suggesting that 2 g three times a day may have benefit in CHF.[118] If a basic metabolic program of CoQ10, D-ribose, L-carnitine and magnesium offers little clinical improvement, the addition of taurine is certainly warranted.

SUMMARY

The energy-starved heart is often not considered by physicians who treat cardiac disease on a day-to-day basis. Angiotensin-converting enzyme inhibitors and angiotensin receptor II blockers improve survival in ischemic and non-ischemic HFs and should be considered as a conventional approach in any patient with heart failure. However, therapies that target the cardiomyocyte itself must also be employed as it has been shown that cardiomyocytes in the failing heart, although metabolically compromised, and their function can be potentially improved and restored. Therapies that go beyond symptomatic relief (diuretics), and the neurohormonal axis, must also be considered that target the cellular, mitochondrial and metabolic defects. Metabolic support with D-ribose, CoQ10, L-carnitine and magnesium is critical for the maintenance of contractile reserve and energy charge in minimally oxidative ischemic or hypoxic hearts. Preservation of cellular energy charge provides the chemical driving force required to complete ATPase reactions needed to maintain cell and tissue viability and function. D-ribose, CoQ10, L-carnitine and magnesium exert a physiological benefit that has a positive impact on cardiac function.

A metabolic cardiology approach using these components is suggested below: When taking the suggested amounts, it is recommended that the total dose be given in divided doses after breakfast and after dinner. For D-ribose, take 5 g (1 scoop) dose, three times a day.

Mild to Moderate Congestive Heart Failure
   Multivitamin/mineral foundation program with 1 g of fish oil
   Coenzyme Q10: 300–400 mg
   L-carnitine: 1,000–1,500 mg
   D-ribose: 15 g
   Magnesium: 400–800 mg

Severe Congestive Heart Failure, Dilated Cardiomyopathy, Patients Awaiting Heart Transplantation
   Multivitamin/mineral foundation program with 1 g of fish oil
   Coenzyme Q10: 360–600 mg
   L-carnitine: 2,000–2,500 mg
   D-ribose: 15 g
   Magnesium: 400–800 mg
   Note: If quality of life is still not satisfactory, add 1,500 mg of Hawthorn Berry and 2–3 g of taurine, as the addition of these two nutraceuticals has helped many of my patients with severe refractory CHF.

CONCLUSION

Cardiovascular function depends on the operational capacity of myocardial cells to generate the energy to expand and contract. Insufficient myocardial energy contributes significantly to CHF. Literally, HF is an "energy-starved heart."

Although there may be several causes of myocardial dysfunction, the energy deficiency in cardiac myocytes plays a significant role and is probably the major factor in CHF. It is no longer enough that physicians focus on the fluid retention aspects of "pump failure". For instance, diuretic therapies target the kidneys indirectly to relieve the sequelae of CHF without addressing the root cause. Inotropic agents attempt to increase contractility directly yet fail to offer the extra energy necessary to assist the weakened heart muscle. Metabolic solutions, on the other hand, treat the heart muscle cells directly.

Physicians must consider the biochemistry of "pulsation". It is critically important to treat both the molecular and cellular components of the heart when managing CHF. Remember, one characteristic of the failing heart is the persistent and progressive loss of cellular energy substrates and abnormalities in cardiac bioenergetics that directly compromise diastolic performance, with the capacity to impact global cardiac function. It took me 30 years of cardiology practice to learn that the heart is all about ATP, and the bottom line in the treatment of any form of cardiovascular disease, and especially CHF and cardiomyopathy, is restoration of the heart's energy reserve.

"Metabolic Cardiology" addresses the biochemical interventions that directly improve energy substrates and therefore energy metabolism in heart cells. In simple terms, sick hearts leak out and lose vital ATP, and the endogenous restoration of ATP cannot keep pace with the relentless depletion of energy substrates, especially in situations of ischemia. When ATP levels drop, diastolic function – the most important precursor of CHF – deteriorates. Since epidemiological studies suggest that DD is present in more than half of patients admitted to hospitals with CHF,[119] it makes sense to target myocardial energetics with effective modalities that truly work.

D-ribose, CoQ10, L-carnitine and magnesium all act to promote cardiac energy metabolism and help normalize myocardial adenine nucleotide concentrations. These naturally occurring compounds exert a physiological benefit that positively impacts diastolic heart function. All are recommended as adjunctive metabolic therapies in the treatment of HF and cardiomyopathy.

Acknowledging this metabolic support for the heart provides the missing link that has been eluding cardiologists for decades and offers hope for the future treatment of cardiovascular disease. Energizing diastole and myocyte metabolism is the most effective therapy for diastolic HF and some day may be the standard of care for all forms of heart disease,[119] and especially CHF. Such potential treatment strategies are currently being modulated from the bench to the bedside.[25,26,76]

In final analysis, CoQ10 unequivocally supports cardiac function, and recent investigations have also demonstrated a wide application in other illness and pathological situations. For instance, a recent review of CoQ10 in a November 2020 publication[120] highlights a wide applicability for the compound. As a potent mitochondrial support, traditional applications in arthrosclerosis, ischemia and CHF are well documented. However, investigations in Down's syndrome, cancer, diabetes, epilepsy palliation, protection from UV radiation and even glaucoma have all shown clinical improvement with CoQ10. In fact, the effect of CoQ10 supplementation in patients admitted to the intensive care unit demonstrated an overwhelming reduction in intensive care unit length of stay, hospital length of stay and days on mechanical ventilation. In this day and age of killer respiratory viruses frequently resulting in mechanical ventilation, this clinical study may prove very fruitful in hospitalized patients on mechanical ventilatory support.[121] These non-cardiac clinical applications of CoQ10 are astonishing! In the future, this remarkable vitamin-like compound will perhaps be the most utilized nutraceutical for improving clinical and therapeutic outcomes by the health professional community.

REFERENCES

1. Bozkurt B. 2018. What is new in heart failure management in 2017? Update on ACC/AHA heart failure guidelines. *Curr Cardiol Rev* 20:39.
2. Jessup M, Marwick TH, Ponikowski P, et al. 2016. ESC and ACC/AHA/heart failure guideline update – What is new and why is it important? *Nat Rev Cardiol* 13:623–628.
3. Liu L, Eisen HJ. 2014. Epidemiology of heart failure and scope of the problem. *Cardiol Clin* 32:1–8.
4. Mozaffarian D, Benjamin EJ, Go AS, et al. 2016. American Heart Association Statistics Committee; Stroke Statistics Subcommittee. Heart disease and stroke-2016 Update: A report from the American Heart Association. *Circulation* 133:e38–e360.
5. The CONSENSUS Trial Study Group. 1987. Effects of enalapril on mortality on mortality in severe congestive heart failure: Results of the Cooperative North Scandinavian Enalapril Survival Study (CONSENSUS). *N Engl J Med* 316:1429–1435.
6. Pfeffer MA, Braunwalk E, Moye LA, et al. 1992. Effect of captopril on mortality and morbidity in patients with left ventricular dysfunction after myocardial infarction: Results of the Survival and Ventricular Enlargement Trial. *N Engl J Med* 327:669–677.
7. CIBIS Investigators and Committees. 1994. A randomized trial of B-blockade in heart failure: The Cardiac Bisoprolol Insufficiency Study (CIBIS). *Circulation* 90:1765–1773.
8. Packer M, Bristow MR, Cohn JN, et al. 1996. The effect of carvedilol on morbidity and mortality in patients with chronic heart failure. *N Engl J Med* 334:1349–1355.
9. Agnetti N, Kaludercic LA, Kane ST, et al. 2010. Modulation of mitochondrial proteome and improved mitochondrial function by biventricular pacing of dyssynchronous failing hearts. *Circ Cardiovasc Genet* 3:78–87.

10. Kitaizumi K, Yukiiri K, Masugata H, et al. 2008. Positron emission tomographic demonstration of myocardial oxidative metabolism in a case of left ventricular restoration after cardiac resynchronization therapy. *Circ J* 72:1900–1903.

11. Christenson SD, Chareonthaitawee P, Burnes JE, et al. 2008. Effects of simultaneous and optimized sequential cardiac resynchronization therapy on myocardial oxidative metabolism and efficiency. *J Cardiovasc Electrophysiol* 19:125–132.

12. McMurray JJ, Pfeffer MA. 2005. Heart failure. *Lancet* 365:1877–1889.

13. Gheorghiade M, Peterson ED. 2011. Improving post discharge outcomes in patients hospitalized for acute heart failure syndromes. *JAMA* 305:2456–2457.

14. Aimo A, Castiglione V, Borrelli C, et al. 2019. Oxidative stress and inflammation in the evolution of heart failure: From pathophysiology to therapeutic strategies. *Eur J Prev Cardiol* 27:494–510.

15. Kumar AA, Kelly DP, Chirinos JA. 2019. Mitochondrial dysfunction in heart failure with preserved ejection fraction. *Circulation* 139:1435–1450.

16. Chaanine AH, Joyce LD, Stulak JM, et al. 2019. Mitochondrial morphology, dynamics, and function in human pressure overload or ischemic heart disease with preserved or reduced ejection fraction. *Circ Hear Fail* 12:e005131.

17. Ma T, Sun J, Zhao Z, et al. 2017. A brief review: Adipose-derived stem cells and their therapeutic potential in cardiovascular disease. *Stem Cell Res Ther* 8(1):124.

18. Stanley WC, Hoppel CL. 2000. Mitochondrial dysfunction in heart failure: Potential for therapeutic interventions? *Cardiovasc Res* 45:805–806.

19. Bayeva M, Gheorghiade M, Ardehali H. 2013. Mitochondria as a therapeutic target in heart failure. *J Am Coll Cardiol* 61(6):599–610.

20. Ardehali H, Sabbah HN, Burke MA, et al. 2012. Targeting myocardial substrate metabolism in heart failure: Potential for new therapies. *Eur J Heart Fail* 14:120–9.

21. Bergmann O, Bhardwaj RD, Bernard S, et al. 2009. Evidence for cardiomyocyte renewal in humans. *Science* 324:98–102.

22. Parmacek MS, Epstein JA. 2009. Cardiomyocyte renewal. *N Engl J Med* 361(1):86–88.

23. Ingwall JS, Weiss RG. 2004. Is the failing heart energy starved? On using chemical energy to support cardiac function. *Circ Res* 95:135–145.

24. Neubauer S. 2007. The failing heart – An engine out of fuel. *N Engl J Med* 356(11):1140–1151.

25. Sinatra ST. 2009. Metabolic Cardiology: The missing link in cardiovascular disease. *Altern Ther Health Med* 15(2):48–50.

26. Sinatra ST. 2005, 2008, 2011. *The Sinatra Solution/Metabolic Cardiology.* Laguna Beach: Basic Health Publications.

27. Sinatra ST, Roberts JC. 2007. *Reverse Heart Disease Now.* Hoboken, NJ: John Wiley & Sons, Inc.

28. De Barcelos IP, Haas RH. 2019. CoQ10 and aging. *Biology* 8:28.

29. Tanaka J, Tominaga R, Yoshitoshi M, et al. 1982. Coenzyme Q10: The prophylactic effect on low cardiac output following cardiac valve replacement. *Ann Thorac Surg* 33:145–151.

30. Sinatra ST. 2004. Letter to the Editor: Coenzyme Q10 in patients with end-stage heart failure awaiting cardiac transplantation: A randomized, placebo-controlled study. *Clin Cardiol* 27(10):A26.

31. Lazaron J, Pomeranz B, Corey P. 1998. Incidence of adverse drug reaction in hospitalized patients. *JAMA* 279:1200–1205.

32. Fitzgerald M. 2008. Vibrating cells disclose their ailments. MIT Technology Review Sept 9 Accessed Dec 26, 2017, at https://www.technologyreview.com/s/410793/vibrating-cells-disclose-their-ailments/.

33. Trafton A. 2009. Chemical energy influences tiny vibrations of red blood cell membranes. *Phys Org* Dec 21, 2009. Accessed Dec 26, 2017, at https://phys.org/news/2009-12-chemical-energy-tiny-vibrations-red.html.

34. Ingwall JS. 2002. *ATP and the Heart.* Boston, MA: Kluwer Academic Publishers.

35. Ingwall JS. 2006. On the hypothesis that the failing heart is energy starved: Lessons learned from the metabolism of ATP and creatine. *Cur Hypertens Rev* 8:457–464.

36. Manfredi JP, Holmes EW. 1985. Purine salvage pathways in myocardium. *Ann Rev Physiol* 47:691–705.

37. Gourine AV, Hu Q, Sander PR, et al. 2004. Interstitial purine metabolites in hearts with LV remodeling. *Am J Physiol Heart Circ Physiol* 286:H677–H684.

38. Hu Q, Wang Q, Lee J, et al. 2006. Profound bioenergetics abnormalities in peri-infarct myocardial regions. *Am J Physiol Heart Circ Physiol* 291:H648–H657.

39. Ye Y, Gong G, Ochiai K, et al. 2001. High-energy phosphate metabolism and creatine kinase in failing hearts: A new porcine model. *Circulation* 103:1570–1576.

40. Maslov MY, Chacko VP, Stuber M, et al. 2007. Altered high-energy phosphate metabolism predicts contractile dysfunction and subsequent ventricular remodeling in pressure-overload hypertrophy mice. *Am J Physiol Heart Circ Physiol* 292:H387–H391.
41. Cha Y-M, Dzeja PP, Shen WK, et al. 2003. Failing atrial myocardium: Energetic deficits accompany structural remodeling and electrical instability. *Am J Physiol Heart Circ Physiol* 284:H1313–H1320.
42. Melduni R, Suri RM, Seward JB, et al. 2011. Diastolic dysfunction in patients undergoing cardiac surgery: A pathophysiological mechanism underlying the initiation of new-onset post-operative atrial fibrillation. *J Am Coll Cardiol* 58(9):953–961.
43. Bache RJ, Zang J, Murakami Y, et al. 1999. Myocardial oxygenation at high work states in hearts with left ventricular hypertrophy. *Cardiovasc Res* 42(3):567–570.
44. Smith CS, Bottomley PA, Schulman SP, et al. 2006. Altered creatine kinase adenosine triphosphate kinetics in failing hypertrophied human myocardium. *Circulation* 114:1151–1158.
45. Weiss RG, Gerstenblith G, Bottomley PA. 2005. ATP flux through creatine kinase in the normal, stressed, and failing human heart. *Proc Natl Academy Sci USA* 102(3):808–813.
46. Beer M, Seyfarth T, Sandstede J, et al. 2002. Absolute concentrations of high-energy phosphate metabolites in normal, hypertrophied, and failing human myocardium measured noninvasively with (31) P-Sloop magnetic resonance spectroscopy. *JACC* 40(7):1267–1274.
47. Lamb HJ, Beyerbacht HP, van der Laarse A, et al. 1999. Diastolic dysfunction in hypertensive heart disease is associated with altered myocardial metabolism. *Circulation* 17:2261–2267.
48. Neubauer S, Horn M, Pabst T, et al. 1997. Cardiac high-energy phosphate metabolism in patients with aortic valve disease assessed by 31P-magnetic resonance spectroscopy. *J Investig Med* 45(8):453–462.
49. Diamant M, Lamb HJ, Groeneveld Y, et al. 2003. Diastolic dysfunction is associated with altered myocardial metabolism in asymptomatic normotensive patients with well-controlled type 2 diabetes mellitus. *JACC* 41(2):328–335.
50. Schocke MF, Metzler B, Wolf C, et al. 2003. Impact of aging on cardiac high-energy phosphate metabolism determined by phosphorous-31 2-dimensional chemical shift imaging (31P 2D CSI). *Magn Reson Imaging* 21(5):553–559.
51. Perings SM, Schulze K, Decking U, et al. 2000. Age-related decline of PCr/ATP-ratio in progressively hypertrophied hearts of spontaneously hypertensives rats. *Heart Vessels* 15(4):197–202.
52. Ypenburg C, Sieders A, Bleeker GB, et al. 2007. Myocardial contractile reserve predicts improvement in left ventricular function after cardiac resynchronization therapy. *Am Heart J* 154(6):1160–1165.
53. Polanczyk CA, Ruschel KB, Castilho FM, et al. 2019. Quality measures in heart failure: The past, the present and the future. *Curr Heart Fail Rep* 16(1):1–6.
54. Omran H, Illien S, MacCarter D, et al. 2003. D-ribose improves diastolic function and quality of life in congestive heart failure patients: A prospective feasibility study. *Eur J Heart Failure* 5:615–619.
55. Shecterle LM, Terry KR, St Cyr JA. 2018. Potential clinical benefits of D-ribose in ischemic cardiovascular disease. *Cureus* 10(3):e2291.
56. Bayram M, St Cyr JA, Abraham WT. 2015. D-ribose aids heart failure patients with preserved ejection fraction and diastolic dysfunction – a pilot study. *Ther Adv Cardiovasc Dis* 9(3):56–65.
57. Vijay N, MacCarter D, Washam M, et al. 2005. Ventilatory efficiency improves with D-ribose in congestive heart failure patients. *J Mol Cell Cardiol* 38(5):820.
58. Carter O, MacCarter D, Manneback S, et al. 2005. D-ribose improves peak exercise capacity and ventilatory efficiency in heart failure patients. *JACC* 45(3 Suppl A):185A.
59. Sharma R, Munger M, Litwin S, et al. 2005. D-ribose improves Doppler TEI myocardial performance index and maximal exercise capacity in stage C heart failure. *J Mol Cell Cardiol* 38(5):853.
60. Befera N, Rivard A, Gatlin G, et al. 2007. Ribose treatment helps preserve function of the remote myocardium after myocardial infarction. *J Surg Res* 137(2):156.
61. Perkowski DJ, Wagner S, Schneider JR. 2011. A targeted metabolic protocol with D-ribose for off-pump coronary artery bypass procedures: A retrospective analysis. *Ther Adv Cardiovasc Dis* 5(4):185–192.
62. Hiebert JB, Shen Q, Thimmesch A, et al. 2016. Impaired myocardial bioenergetics in HFpEF and the role of antioxidants. *Open Cardiovasc Med J* 10:158–162.
63. Pierce JD, Shen Q, Vacek J, et al. 2020. Potential use of ubiquinol and D-ribose in patients with heart failure with preserved ejection fraction. *Ann Med Surg (Lond)* 55:77–80.
64. Malekmohammad K, Sewell RDE, Rafieian-Kopaei M. 2019. Antioxidants and atherosclerosis: Mechanistic aspects. *Biomolecules* 9:301.
65. Suzuki T, Nozawa T, Sobajima M. 2008. Atorvastatin-induced changes in plasma coenzyme Q10 and brain natriuretic peptide in patients with coronary artery disease. *Int Heart J* 49(4):423–433.
66. Lass A. 1999. Mitochondrial coenzyme Q content and aging. *Biofactors* 9(2–4):199–205.

67. Boroujeni MB, Khayat ZK, Anbari K, et al. 2017. Coenzyme Q10 protects skeletal muscle from isch-emia-reperfusion through the NF-kappa B pathway. *Perfusion* 32:372–377.

68. Zhai J, Bo Y, Lu Y, et al. 2017. Effects of coenzyme Q10 on markers of inflammation: A systematic review and meta-analysis. *PLoS One* 12:e0170172.

69. Mantle D, Hargreaves I. 2019. Coenzyme Q10 and degenerative disorders affecting longevity: An over-view. *Antioxidants* 8(2):44.

70. Langsjoen PH, Langsjoen AM. 1999. Overview of the use of CoQ10 in cardiovascular disease. *Biofactors* 9(2–4):273–284.

71. Langsjoen PH, Littarru GP, Silver MA. 2005. Role of concomitant coenzyme Q10 with statins for patients with hyperlipidemia. *Curr Topics Nutr Res* 3(3):149–158.

72. Permanetter B, Rossy W, Klein G, et al. 1992. Ubiquinone (coenzyme Q10) in the long-term treatment of idiopathic dilated cardiomyopathy. *Eur Heart J* 13(11):1528–1533.

73. Watson PS, Scalia GM, Gaibraith AJ, et al. 2001. Is coenzyme Q10 helpful for patients with idiopathic cardiomyopathy? *Med J Aust* 175(8): 447–448.

74. Khatta M, Alexander BS, Krichten CM, et al. 2000. The effect of coenzyme Q10 in patients with con-gestive heart failure. *Ann Intern Med* 132(8):636–640.

75. Sinatra ST. 1996. Comments made in presentation by Dr. Sinatra at the *Proceedings of the International Conference on coenzyme Q10* in Ancona, Italy.

76. Sinatra ST. 1997. Coenzyme Q10: A vital therapeutic nutrient for the heart with special application in congestive heart failure. *Conn Med* 61(11):707–711.

77. Belardinelli R, Mucaj A, Lacalaprice F, et al. 2006. Coenzyme Q10 and exercise training in chronic heart failure. *Eur Heart J* 27(22):2675–2681.

78. Langsjoen PH, Langsjoen P, Willis R, et al. 1994. Usefulness of coenzyme Q10 in clinical cardiology: A long-term study. *Mol Aspects Med* 15:S165–S175.

79. Langsjoen P, Willis R, Folkers K. 1994. Treatment of essential hypertension with coenzyme Q10. *Mol Aspects Med* 15:265–272.

80. Tabrizi R, Akbari M, Sharifi N, et al. 2018. The effects of coenzyme Q10 supplementation on blood pressures among patients with metabolic diseases: A systematic review and meta-analysis of random-ized controlled trials. *High Blood Press Cardiovasc Prev* 25:41–50.

81. Molyneux S, Florkowski C, George P, et al. 2008. Coenzyme Q10: An independent predictor of mortal-ity in chronic heart failure. *JACC* 52(18):1435–1441.

82. Mortensen SA. 2014. The effect of coenzyme Q10 on morbidity and mortality in chronic heart failure: Results from Q-SYMBIO: A randomized double-blind trial. *JACC-Heart Failure* 2(6):641–649.

83. Berman M, Erman A, Ben-Gal T, et al. 2004. Coenzyme Q10 in patients with end-stage heart failure awaiting cardiac transplantation: A randomized, placebo-controlled study. *Clin Cardiol* 27:295–299.

84. Dai YL, Luk TH, Yiu KH, et al. 2011. Reversal of mitochondrial dysfunction by coenzyme Q10 supple-ment improves endothelial function in patients with ischemic left ventricular systolic dysfunction: A randomized controlled trial. *Atherosclerosis* 216(2):395–401.

85. Mortensen AL, Rosenfeldt F, Filipiak KJ. 2019. Effect of coenzyme Q10 in Europeans with chronic heart failure: A sub-group analysis of the Q-SYMBIO randomized double-blind trial. *Cardiol J* 26:147–156.

86. Lei L, Liu Y. 2017. Efficacy of coenzyme Q10 in patients with cardiac failure: A meta-analysis of clini-cal trials. *BMC Cardiovasc Disord* 17:196.

87. Alehagen U, Johansson P, Bjornstedt M, et al. 2013. Cardiovascular mortality and N-terminal-proBNP reduced after combined selenium and coenzyme Q10 supplementation: A 5-year prospective ran-domized double-blind placebo-controlled trial among elderly Swedish citizens. *Int J Cardiol* 167(5): 1860–1866.

87a. Raizner AE, Quinones MA. 2021. Coenzyme Q10 for patients with cardiovascular disease. *JACC* 77(5):609–619.

88. Sahebkar A, Simental-Mendia LE, Stefanutti C, et al. 2016. Supplementation with coenzyme Q10 reduces plasma lipoprotein(a) concentrations but not other lipid indices: A systematic review and meta-analysis. *Pharmacol Res* 105:198–209.

89. Jorat MV. 2018. The effects of coenzyme Q10 supplementation on lipid profiles among patients with coronary artery disease: A systematic review and meta-analysis of randomized controlled trials. *Lipids Health Dis* 17(1):230.

90. Sharifi N. 2018. The effects of coenzyme Q10 supplementation on lipid profiles among patients with metabolic diseases: A systematic review and meta-analysis of randomized controls trials. *Curr Pharm Des* 24(23):2729–2742.

91. Aslani Z, Shab-Bidar S, Fatahi S, et al. 2018. Effect of coenzyme Q10 supplementation on serum of high sensitivity c-reactive protein level in patients with cardiovascular diseases: A systematic review and meta-analysis of randomized controlled trials. *Int J Prev Med* 9:82.

92. Lee B, Huang Y, Chen S, et al. 2012. Effects of coenzyme Q10 supplementation on inflammatory markers (high-sensitivity C-reactive protein, interleukin-6, and homocysteine) in patients with coronary artery disease. *Nutrition* 28(7–8):767–772.

93. Ates O, Biden H, Keles S, et al. 2013. Plasma coenzyme Q10 levels in type 2 diabetic patients with retinopathy. *Int J Ophthalmol* 6:675–679.

94. Huang H, Chi H, Liao D, et al. 2018. Effects of coenzyme Q10 on cardiovascular and metabolic biomarkers in overweight and obese patients with type 2 diabetes mellitus: A pooled analysis. *Diabetes Metab Syndr Obes* 11:875–886.

95. Crane FL, Hatefi Y, Lester RL, et al. 1957. Isolation of a quinone from beef heart mitochondria. *Biochim Biophys Acta* 25(1):220–221.

96. Lopez G, del Ponzo-Cruz J, Sanchez-Cuesta A, et al. 2019. Bioavailability of coenzyme Q10 supplements depends on carrier lipids and solubilization. *Nutrition* 57:133–140.

97. Uekaji Y, Terao K. 2017. Coenzyme Q10 – gamma cyclodextrin complex is a powerful nutraceutical for anti-aging and health improvements. *Biomed Res Clin Prac* 2(1):1–5.

98. Wang Z, Liu Y, Liu G, et al. 2018. L-carnitine and heart disease. *Life Sci* 194:88–97.

99. El-Aroussy W, Rizk A, Mayhoub G, et al. 2000. Plasma carnitine levels as a marker of impaired left ventricular functions. *Mol Cell Biochem* 213(1–2):37–41.

100. Narin F, Narin N, Andac H, et al. 1997. Carnitine levels in patients with chronic rheumatic heart disease. *Clin Biochem* 30(8):643–645.

101. Ueland T, Svardal A, Oie E, et al. 2013. Disturbed carnitine regulation in chronic heart failure—increased plasma levels of palmitoyl-carnitine are associated with poor prognosis. *Int J Cardiol* 167(5):1892–1899.

102. Weng Y, Zhang S, Huang W, et al. 2021. Efficacy of L-carnitine for dilated cardiomyopathy: A meta-analysis of randomized controlled trials. *Biomed Res Int* 2021:9491615.

103. da Silva Guimaraes S, de Souza Crus W, da Silva L, et al. 2017. Effect of L-carnitine supplementation on reverse remodeling in patients with ischemic heart disease undergoing coronary artery bypass grafting: A randomized, placebo-controlled trial. *Ann Nutr Metab* 70(2):106–110.

104. Rizos I. 2000. Three-year survival of patients with heart failure caused by dilated cardiomyopathy. *Am Heart J* 139(2 Pt 3):S120–S123.

105. Davini P, Bigalli A, Lamanna F, et al. 1992. Controlled study on L-carnitine therapeutic efficacy in post-infarction. *Drugs Exp Clin Res* 18:355–365.

106. Singh RB, Niaz MA, Agarwal P, et al. 1996. A randomized, double-blind, placebo-controlled trial of L-carnitine in suspected acute myocardial infarction. *Postgrad Med* 72:45–50.

107. Iliceto S, Scrutinio D, Bruzzi P, et al. 1995. Effects of L-carnitine administration on left ventricular remodeling after acute anterior myocardial infarction: The L-carnitine Eocardiografia Digitalizzata Infarto Miocardioco (CEDIM) Trial. *JACC* 26(2):380–387.

108. Serati AR, Motamedi MR, Emami S, et al. 2010. L-carnitine treatment in patients with mild diastolic heart failure is associated with improvement in diastolic function and symptoms. *Cardiology* 116:178–182.

109. DiNicolantonio JD. 2013. L-carnitine in the secondary prevention of cardiovascular disease: Systemic review and meta-analysis. *Mayo Clinic Proceed* 88(6):544–551.

109a. Heianza Y, Ma W, DiDonato J, et al. 2020. Long-term changes in gut microbial metabolite trimethylamine N-oxide and coronary heart disease risk. *JACC* 75(7):763–772.

110. Huc T, Drapala A, Gawrys M, et al. 2018. Chronic, low-dose TMAO treatment reduces diastolic dysfunction in heart fibrosis in hypertensive rats. *Am J Physiol Heart Circ Physiol* 315(6):H1805–H1820.

111. Cho CE, Caudill MA. 2017. Trimethylamine-N-Oxide: Friend, foe, or simply caught in the crossfire? *Trends Endocrinol Metab* 28(2):121–130.

112. Papandreou C, More M, Bellamine A. 2020. Trimethylamine N-oxide in relation to cardiometabolic health – cause or effect? *Nutrients* 12(5):1330.

112a. Zhang Y, Wang Y, Ke B, et al. 2021. TMAO: How gut microbiota contributes to heart failure. *J Lab Clin Med* 228:109–126.

112b. Wang G, Kong B, Shuai W, et al. 2020. 3,3-Dimethyl-l-butanol attenuates cardiac remodeling in pressure-overload induced heart failure in mice. *J Nutr Biochem* 78:108–341.

112c. Wu WK, Ho CT, Kuo CH, et al. 2015. Dietary allicin reduces transformation of L-carnitine to TMAO through impact on the gut microbiota. *J Funct Foods* 15:408–417.

112d. Chen ML, Yi L, Zhang Y, et al. 2016. Resveratrol attenuations TMAO induced arthrosclerosis by regulating TMAO synthesis and bile acid metabolism via remodeling of the gut microbiota. *M Bio* 7:e00210–e02215.

113. Bloomer RJ, Smith WA, Fisher-Wellman KH. 2007. Glycine propionyl-L-carnitine increases plasma nitrate/nitrite in resistance trained men. *J Int Soc Sports Nutr* 4:22.

114. Schimatschek HF, Rempis R. 2001. Prevalence of hypomagnesemia in an unselected German population of 16,000 individuals. *Magnes Res* 14(4):283–290.

115. Turlapaty PDMV, Altura BM. 1980. Magnesium deficiency produces spasms of coronary arteries: Relationship to etiology of sudden death ischemic heart disease. *Science* 208:198.

116. McLean RM. 1994. Magnesium and its therapeutic uses: A review. *Am J Med* 96:63.

117. Elin RJ. 1998. Magnesium metabolism in health and disease. *Dis* Mon 34:161.

118. Azuma J, Sawamura A, Awata N, et al. 1985. Therapeutic effect of taurine in congestive heart failure: A double-blind crossover trial. *Clin Cardiol* 8(5):276–282.

119. Baliga RR, Young JB. 2008. Energizing diastole. *Heart Fail Clin* 4(1):9–13.

120. Pastor-Maldonado CJ, Suarez-Rivero JM, Povea-Cabello S, et al. 2020. Coenzyme Q10: Novel formulations and medical trends. *Int J Mol Sci* 21(22):8432.

121. Hasanloei M, Zeinaly A, Rahimlou M, et al. 2021. Effect of coenzyme Q10 supplementation on oxidative stress and clinical outcomes in patients with low levels of coenzyme Q10 admitted to the intensive care unit. *J Nutr Sci* 10. https://www.cambridge.org/core/journals/journal-of-nutritional-science/article/effect-of-coenzyme-q10-supplementation-on-oxidative-stress-and-clinical-outcomes-in-patients-with-low-levels-of-coenzyme-q10-admitted-to-the-intensive-care-unit/A0CD43D74149B86769D66D553A12ED41#.

9 Cardiovascular Disease in Women

Stephen T. Sinatra

Sara Gottfried

CONTENTS

Case: 60-Year-Old Female with Nausea and Vomiting... 218
Sex Differences 218
Gender Differences 219
Racial Disparities 220
Defining the Problem in Women... 220
    Diastolic Dysfunction 221
    Hypertension.. 223
    Mitral Valve Prolapse.. 224
    Peripheral Artery Disease 225
Summary... 226
References... 227

One woman dies of cardiovascular disease (CVD) every 80 seconds in the United States, a tragedy driven primarily by coronary heart disease and stroke.[1] Mortality from coronary heart disease is higher in women than men, even though the prevalence is higher in men for all age groups except 20–39. Women experience delays in receiving care,[2-5] poorer outcomes when treated by male physicians[6] and lower rates of guideline-based medical therapy than men.[7] These data confirm a sex and gender gap in the cardiovascular care of women. Why? What can be done?

Both pre-disease and disease are under-recognized and underdiagnosed in women. Half of women in developed countries will die of mostly preventable heart disease or stroke. While it was previously believed that men and women share the same cardiovascular risk factors, we now know that there are dozens of risk factors that affect women exclusively. Traditional risk factors, such as insulin resistance, hypertension and tobacco use are more deleterious in women—and at equal age, women have more cardiovascular risk factors than men. When considered along with sex differences in the manifestations and clinical presentation of CVD, a discrepancy emerges that is not sufficiently captured in recent guidelines such that the cardiovascular risk of women remains underestimated.

Moreover, awareness among women is declining. Recent evidence highlights that women are less aware of their risk of CVD than they were one decade ago, despite public service campaigns such as "Go Red for Women."[8] Overall, less than half of women identify CVD as the leading cause of death. They are not alone: only half of primary care physicians identify CVD as a top concern after breast health and weight.

In this chapter, we will cover the putative mechanisms for sex and gender differences that result in greater mortality from CVD in women, how the mechanisms translate into differential signs and

DOI: 10.1201/9781003137849-9

symptoms, racial disparities among women patients, and potential solutions to close the sex and gender gap.

CASE: 60-YEAR-OLD FEMALE WITH NAUSEA AND VOMITING

A female colleague had a recent, unexpected myocardial infarction (MI) at age 60. She had been awakened in the middle of the night with profound nausea and vomiting. The unexplained symptoms dissipated. She realized that there was no apparent reason for the onset of symptoms, such as food poisoning or stomach flu. So, she went back to bed. A few days later, she awoke again at night with profuse sweating accompanied by ill-defined chest discomfort. She experienced extreme dread, an important hallmark sign.

Dangerously, she drove herself to an urgent care center where both her electrocardiogram and blood tests confirmed the diagnosis of MI. The damage was caused by a blockage in her circumflex coronary artery, a location much preferable to the left anterior descending which would have resulted in more significant muscle damage. She was successfully stented, and fortunately had a happy ending.

Although her prognosis remained good for the future, she was also placed on statin therapy, despite the fact that she had a cholesterol level within normal limits. Generally speaking, we are less likely to prescribe stain drugs to women because the risk/benefit ratio is just not in their favor.

SEX DIFFERENCES

Sex differences are based on biology and are specific to one sex, whereas gender differences are socially constructed. Sex differences in CVD include conditions that differ in prevalence, incidence, pathophysiology, symptomatology, diagnosis, treatment response, morbidity and mortality. They are believed to be a product of genetic and hormonal differences between males and females and how they interact with the environment, and they are important to understand for management of diagnostic subtleties in women. Here are the sex differences relevant to our discussion in this chapter, adapted from Saeed et al.:[9]

- **Hormonal**: Endogenous estrogen provides a protective cardiovascular effect in women, and endogenous testosterone in men. Women are exposed to other hormonal transitions that men do not experience, such as pregnancy and the marked hormonal changes of perimenopause and menopause. Increasingly, pregnancy is emerging as a stressor that may unmask underlying vascular and metabolic abnormalities, given that 10%–20% of women experience adverse pregnancy outcomes, such as hypertensive disorders of pregnancy, gestational diabetes, preterm birth and small for gestational age at birth, all conditions associated with a greater risk of future cardiovascular events.
- **Anatomical**: Women have smaller vessel size and smaller left ventricular size. In the coronary circulation, their smaller arteries may be more difficult to navigate with stents and even bypass grafting. This is probably why they have an increased mortality following acute MI, stent and coronary artery bypass surgery interventions.
- **Functional**: Women have 10% less stroke volume than men. Females have lower sympathetic activity and higher parasympathetic activity than men. Overall, women have greater systolic function and less diastolic compliance than men. Men generally have higher blood pressure than women. However, when a woman enters menopause, blood pressure elevations are similar to their male counterparts.[10]
- **EKG**: Women have a longer corrected QT interval and shorter PR interval than men.
- **Under Stress**: Women have increased heart rate with increased cardiac output. Women have more white-coat hypertension[11] and demonstrate more microvascular dysfunction after stress. Women show higher rates of mental stress-induced myocardial ischemia (MSIMI), and the sex difference is not explained by psychosocial or clinical risk factors.[12,13]

- **Risk Factors**: Women experience unique risk factors and higher prevalence of certain risk factors, and even the more traditional factors are more deleterious in women.
  - Unique risk factors include adverse pregnancy outcomes, endometriosis, hormonal contraception, polycystic ovary syndrome, perimenopause and menopause.
  - Higher prevalence risk factors include adverse childhood experiences, autoimmune disease, breast cancer treatment, migraine with aura, and mental health conditions such as anxiety and post-traumatic stress disorder. Women have more physical inactivity and obesity.
  - Traditional risk factors that cause more harm to women include insulin resistance, diabetes, smoking, dyslipidemia and depression.
- **Conditions**: Women have less obstructive coronary artery disease and higher prevalence of the following: coronary microvascular dysfunction, spontaneous coronary artery dissection, diseases of the cardiac muscle including heart failure and Takotsubo cardiomyopathy, diastolic dysfunction, mitral valve prolapse, peripheral artery disease, and problems related to neurovascular dysregulation including hot flashes and night sweats associated with perimenopause and menopause. In fact, untreated vasomotor symptoms are now considered a potential biomarker of CVD risk, such as an adverse CVD risk factor profile, greater subclinical CVD and, in emerging work, CVD events.[14–18] Hypertension is the number one cause of CVD, and while it is more prevalent in men until age 50, women have more serious sequelae.
- **Environmental**: Women may be more sensitive to mercury than men, and exposure may lead to a greater risk of hypertension and autoimmune disease.[19,20]

GENDER DIFFERENCES

Not only are there sex differences, but also multiple streams of evidence suggest a gender gap. For years, it has been generally thought that women are not at serious risk for coronary artery disease.

- Women with MI presenting to an emergency room have increased mortality when treated by male physicians compared with female physicians. No such gap was found for female physicians: outcomes for male and female patients were the same.[6] Certainly, more research is needed to study gender concordance and outcomes.
- Feminine personality traits and roles are associated with higher rates of recurrent acute coronary syndrome (ACS) and major adverse cardiac events (MACE) compared to traditional masculine characteristics.[21]
- There are delays in care for women. The difference in the use of percutaneous coronary artery (PTCA) intervention in acute MI in women demonstrated delay as the women in this study waited approximately 37 minutes longer before contacting emergency medical services.[22] In this study of 4,360 patients (967 females) from 2006 to 2016, the 37-minute delay was costly in that the mortality in women was 5.9% vs. the men at 4.5%. Any invasive cardiologist knows that every minute counts when the blood supply in an area of the myocardium is obstructed.
- Pharmaceutical under-treatment in women can be complex. In the Study of Women Across the Nation (SWAN), there were low statin prescription rates in women who might benefit, with the lowest rates in Black women. In 2,399 women included, 234 had a diagnosis of atherosclerotic disease, statins were used by 49.6% of women with CVD, and 42.3% of women with an LDL ≥ 190 mg/dL.[23] On the other hand, we (Drs. Sinatra and Gottfried – the authors) are not strong advocates of statin use in women. In other words, while there are sex and gender differences in how women are treated, some prescribing clinicians may use less statins not based on discrimination but rather thoughtful consideration of the evidence.

Even though research urges that more consideration be given to women with heart disease symptoms, it takes time to help eradicate so many years of bias.

RACIAL DISPARITIES

Significant racial disparity persists. Black women have double the rates of chronic hypertension compared with White women, and female blood pressure Rx goals especially among Black and Hispanic females have not been established.[24] As a consequence, heart failure prevalence is higher in Black women and continues to rise. While in-hospital mortality is higher for women, race matters too: for 194,071 patients aged <65 hospitalized with acute MI, mortality was highest for Latinx women (3.7%), followed by Black women (3.1%), and then by White women (2.5%). At 65 and older, mortality is highest for White women.[25] Adverse pregnancy outcomes represent interdependent conditions that are associated with higher maternal mortality, which again disproportionately affects Black women, as well as greater future maternal and offspring cardiometabolic outcomes, including coronary heart disease, stroke and heart failure.

Hypertensive disorders of pregnancy—including pre-eclampsia, chronic hypertension and gestational hypertension—are similarly increasing in prevalence. Black women experience not only higher prevalence but also greater risk of preterm birth, intrauterine fetal death, more severe hypertension, antepartum hemorrhage and mortality, in addition to preexisting conditions such as systemic lupus erythematosus and sickle cell disease in the mother.[26] Gestational diabetes is rising in prevalence overall with Asian females at the greatest risk (11.1%), followed by Latinx (6.6%), White (5.3%) and Black women (4.8%).[27]

DEFINING THE PROBLEM IN WOMEN

The sex and gender gaps in cardiovascular medicine have not improved despite decades of attention, impassioned entreaties and effort. In the face of so many challenges, many have called upon the field of Cardiology to develop gender-specific medicine. Over 20 years ago, one of us (SS) published the book *Heart Sense for Women* and described the differential symptoms and presentation of heart disease in women, for whom we previously thought were the same as they are for men.[28] The sexes are different not only in clinical presentation, pathophysiology, diagnosis and treatment, but prognosis as well.[29]

Although women are generally better in touch with their physical and emotional pain than men, they tend to experience more subtle and/or vague physical symptoms of heart disease compared to their male counterparts. As myocardial ischemia may be manifested as both typical and atypical symptoms in women, making the diagnosis of angina or coronary heart disease is a more complex and a poorly understood process. In general, most men experience a dramatic crushing substernal pain in their chest, with or without radiation to the left shoulder and/or left elbow area, or extreme shortness of breath when having a MI.

Symptoms: Women's symptoms may be vaguer and include the following:

- Discomfort, pressure or pain in the chest, arm and/or back
- Tingling or pain in the jaw, elbow or arm (both men and women collectively tend to feel pain in the left elbow or arm when having ischemia)
- Profound shortness of breath and/or dizziness with exertion
- Profound sudden fatigue
- Tightness or a strangling sensation in the throat
- Dizziness and/or vertigo
- Nausea and/or vomiting
- Indigestion (women often feel if they just "burp", they would feel better).

While some men may have any of these symptoms as well, they are more subtle in presentation for women.

Side Effects with Statin Treatment: Although the blood-thinning and antioxidant properties of statins may be beneficial to some women, many more women compared to men develop intolerable side effects in the musculoskeletal system, including weakness and myalgias.[30] In addition, calcification of the coronaries[31] and diabetes[32–34] may be problematic for women on long-term statin therapy. Risk of prediabetes and diabetes with statin therapy varies depending upon baseline glucose and insulin pathways, dose and statin potency, though many of the studies on statin use do not report sex-specific results.[34–37] In fact, a 2010 meta-analysis found that statin therapy actually increased rather than decreased coronary artery disease (CAD) risk in women.[38] However, efficacy in women versus men continues to be debated. Coronary intravascular ultrasound, used to image plaque burden and predict incident cardiovascular events, has shown that use of rosuvastatin over 24 months is associated with greater coronary atheroma regression in women compared with men.[39]

The use of statins warrants careful scrutiny as a gender-specific intervention, but baseline phenotyping is important. In the most recent study on statin therapy in the primary prevention of CAD, statin medications provided no clinical benefit when prior coronary artery calcium score was zero in a retrospective analysis of 13,644 patients.[40] However, in men under the age of 75 with proven CAD, we prefer a low-dose statin in combination with coenzyme Q10 (CoQ10) therapy. Like CoQ10, statins have favorable antioxidant and blood-thinning properties which appear promising for younger men.[41] In our experience, the benefits may be worth the possible side effects, which is less deleterious than in women.

To further complicate the diagnosis and prognosis of heart disease in women, women physicians do a better job assessing other women presenting in urgent care centers who are experiencing chest pain compared to their male counterparts. As mentioned previously, women patients are more likely to survive a heart attack if their treatment is administered and overseen by female doctors.[6] In ambulatory medicine, the prevalence of chest pain is similar for women and men, but men are more than twice as likely to be referred to a cardiologist.[42] Are women physicians better at listening to female patients, and/or have a higher index of suspicion with nonspecific symptoms? Certainly, more research is needed to assess outcomes with female gender concordance between patients and physicians. Currently, models for assessment of non-acute chest pain are being tested in cardiology clinics that improve outcomes in women and could help us close the sex and gender gap.[43]

Even though studies demonstrate that more consideration be given to women with heart disease symptoms, it will take time to eradicate the so many years of bias. For decades, it has been generally thought that women are not serious candidates for CAD. However, in the last 5–10 years, the data is confirming the direct opposite.[44]

Since a women's coronary anatomy is also smaller, PTCA and stenting may be more problematic with additional morbidity and mortality. These smaller anatomical coronary artery issues present a major consideration in the overall assessment of women. In addition to realizing these gender-specific differences in myocardial ischemia between women and men, other major female cardiovascular concerns in this day and age include diastolic dysfunction (DD), hypertension, mitral valve prolapse (MVP) and peripheral artery disease (PAD).

DIASTOLIC DYSFUNCTION

DD is one of the most poorly understood pathological situations affecting both men and women, and a key predisposing factor leading to systolic and eventually global left ventricular dysfunction. Most patients, women more than men, with DD have normal or near-normal left ventricular ejection fractions.[45,46] Many of these patients experience the same signs and symptoms as patients with heart failure and reduced ejection fraction. Symptomatic suffering and unacceptable quality of life are reported in many of these patients.[47,48] Overall, the prevalence of DD is increasing,[49] and associated with 3.5-fold increased risk of cardiovascular events or mortality.[50]

Diastolic heart failure results from compliance issues or a "stiffening of heart muscle." When the left ventricle does not relax fully, the cavity inside the heart is unable to fill properly with blood. In essence, during diastole, the filling cycle struggles and the heart is compromised. Patients may feel shortness of breath and fatigue, and some even experience chest discomfort as well as peripheral edema. Their symptoms and physical findings are similar to patients with systolic heart failure caused by a weakened heart, and their prognosis remains guarded.[50,51] The connection between DD and cirrhosis of the liver[52] is now receiving more attention from healthcare providers as is the more common relationship of DD to hypertension.[51] Thus, DD must be on the radar of not only cardiologists but any physician caring for patients and especially women on a day-to-day basis. The mortality and morbidity caused by DD, which is also referred to as heart failure with preserved systolic function, is very similar to systolic heart failure. Estimated healthcare costs are approximately $30 billion in the United States alone; thus, DD and systolic dysfunction place a great burden on our healthcare system.[53]

The identification of effective treatments remains an important area of investigation given the predominance of women with diastolic heart failure,[54–56] lack of specific therapies,[57–59] and high mortality and morbidity associated with this affliction.[46,47,50] Prevalence is estimated to be 20% in those over the age of 40 and continues to be underdiagnosed.[47,60,61] Multiparity increases risk in women.[62]

The treatment for DD continues to be disappointedly limited as pharmaceutical drugs have been shown to be of little benefit in randomized clinical studies.[63] The Women's Health Coalition Report documented the lack of effective treatments for DD and indicated that the prognosis has not changed for the past few decades.[63]

However, since the advent of the Treatment of Preserved Cardiac Function Heart Failure (TOPCAT) trial,[64] new pharmaceutical enthusiasm for spironolactone has emerged. Although treatment did not significantly reduce deaths for preserved ejection fraction,[65] in those patients at the lower end of the left ventricular ejection fraction (LVEF) spectrum (LVEF of 40%–50%), the effect of spironolactone was somewhat significant.[66]

Similar findings were seen in a *post hoc* subgroup in the PEACE trial in which ACE inhibitors resulted in a benefit in patients with ischemic cardiomyopathy and a midrange LVEF of 40%–50%.[67] In another analysis of TOPCAT, mineralocorticoid receptor antagonists can be considered to reduce the risk of heart failure hospitalization in selected patients with preserved ejection fraction (HFpEF).[68] Although these recent trials suggest some benefit from pharmaceutical therapies on patient outcomes, clearly a more suitable alternative metabolic approach is needed to treat any patient with DD and/or systolic dysfunction.

An understanding of cardiac energetics and metabolic support with a focus on adenosine triphosphate (ATP) must be considered as a form of therapy for DD as well as global left ventricular failure.[69] Since muscle biopsies of cardiac tissues in heart failure patients reveal diminished quantities of ATP in their mitochondria,[70] investigating therapies that promote cellular energetics and metabolism must be utilized. Myocytes contain the highest concentrations of mitochondria organelles necessary to generate the huge amounts of ATP required to fuel the high-energy demand of cardiac energetics.[69,71]

The energetic imbalance of heart failure is characterized by an increase in energy demand and a decrease in energy production, transfer and substrate utilization resulting in an ATP deficit. DD is the result of the heart muscle's inability to relax sufficiently after contraction because it cannot maintain the higher concentrations of ATP required to effectively activate the calcium pumps necessary to facilitate cardiac relaxation and diastolic filling.[69,71] All patients with heart failure have DD to some degree.

Since the requirements of myocytes for ATP are absolute,[71] incorporating a metabolic approach with nutritional biochemical interventions that preserve and promote myocardial support and ATP production must be considered. In a randomized, controlled trial, 300 mg of CoQ10 reduced plasma pyruvate lactate ratios and improved endothelial function via reversal of mitochondrial dysfunction in patients with ischemic left ventricular systolic dysfunction.[72] Metabolic approaches do not create significant adverse effects and can be supportive in patients with DD.

Recent evidence suggests that blood and tissue deficiency of CoQ10 may be linked to statin-associated muscle symptoms as well as other features seen in patients with heart failure, suggesting that the use of exogenous CoQ10 may be beneficial.[73]

In our opinion, the most effective solution for failing ATP production involves nutraceutical support with CoQ10, L-carnitine, magnesium and D-ribose. When given on a daily basis, they provide essential raw materials that support cellular energy substrates needed by mitochondria to rebuild diminishing ATP levels. Treatment options that incorporate these metabolic interventions targeted to preserve ATP energy substrates (D-ribose) or accelerate ATP turnover (L-carnitine and CoQ10 or ubiquinol) are indicated for at-risk populations and patients undergoing cardiovascular surgery.[69] This metabolic approach does not create any adverse effects and may be also supportive in preventing atrial fibrillation occasionally seen in patients with DD after undergoing cardiac surgery as well as in patients with hypertension where DD is also frequently seen.[74]

HYPERTENSION

Earlier in our careers, we treated men and women similarly regarding blood pressure issues. However, gender-specific issues exist and blood pressure concerns are one of them. More recently, a review article in the *Journal of Hypertension Research* made this consideration very clear.[75] Here are some of the conclusions from the article:

- After smoking cessation, hypertension control is the single-most important intervention to reduce the risk of future cardiovascular events in women.
- Total life expectancy is almost 5 years less for women of 50 years with high blood pressure compared to those without it.
- In the elderly, high blood pressure affects more women than men, and in general, elderly women are underdiagnosed and undertreated.

The authors also indicated that the prevention of cardiovascular events by blood pressure control is "30 to 100% higher in women than in men," and that a mere 15-point rise in systolic blood pressure raises the risk of CVD by 56% in women compared with only 32% in men.[75] A few years later, the SPRINT trial[76] provided key findings in hypertension research. The investigators included 9,361 adults aged 50 or older with a systolic blood pressure of 130 mm/Hg or higher. More aggressive treatment with target blood pressures less than 120 mm/Hg not only reduces cardiovascular events but the risk of death as well. The investigators confirmed that we should aim for lower blood pressures in both men and women.

Another important sex difference is the effect of non-narcotic pain medications on the risk of incident hypertension.[77] The study found that women aged 51–77 years who took an average daily dose of 500 mg of acetaminophen had about double the risk of developing high blood pressure in 3 years. Women in the same age range who took more than 400 mg of nonsteroidal anti-inflammatory drugs (NSAIDs), equal to about two ibuprofen, had a 78% risk of developing high blood pressure over those who did not take any nonsteroidal medications. Younger women, aged 34–53, who took an average of 500 mg of acetaminophen a day had a twofold higher risk of developing high blood pressure. Similar aged women who took 400 mg of NSAIDs had a 60% risk increase over those who did not take the meds. The study also demonstrated that aspirin did not increase these risks. The study involved 5,123 women participating in the Nurses' Health Study at Harvard Medical School and Brigham and Women's Hospital in Boston.[77] Although none of the women had high blood pressure when the study began, higher doses of acetaminophen and NSAIDs independently increased the risk of hypertension in these women. Although NSAIDs increase renal sodium absorption, both acetaminophen and NSAIDs may impair endothelial function which may explain why blood pressure increases. Because the results of this study have confirmed previous investigations, it makes sense to educate women about excess use of these analgesics.

Pregnancy may create an undesirable situation for many women as hypertension can be observed in 6%–8% of cases.[78] Eclampsia or high blood pressure during pregnancy can increase the risk of maternal as well as fetal mortality. Any pregnant woman needs to get her blood pressure evaluated as eclampsia can develop rapidly especially in the last trimester of pregnancy. Some women need Rx following delivery—in the year post-delivery, women with a hypertensive disorder of pregnancy demonstrate a 12- to 25-fold greater rate of hypertension than women with normal blood pressure in pregnancy.[79]

Menopause is another phase in which women need to have blood pressure evaluations especially if they are on menopausal hormone therapy.[80] One of us (SS) remembers a striking case of a female in her late 50s who developed significant mitral regurgitation following a sudden increase in blood pressure. Although she had no prior history of high blood pressure, she became hypertensive following a treatment plan for menopausal symptoms with Premarin and medroxyprogesterone. After several months of treatment with hormone replacement therapy (HRT), her shortness of breath increased significantly and her quality of life was severely limited. After seeing several physicians and taking multiple medications, she saw Dr. Sinatra in cardiovascular consultation as she was considering valvular replacement. Fortunately, the surgeon wanted her evaluated by a cardiologist prior to surgery. She indeed was hypertensive, and Dr. Sinatra realized she was consuming medroxyprogesterone which is known to cause coronary artery constriction. After he suggested coming off hormone therapy, he strongly advised that she delay surgery for the next few weeks. The blood pressure came down significantly, and the mitral regurgitation by echocardiographic analysis was significantly less. Several weeks after cessation of the hormonal therapy, she completely normalized with no quality-of-life issues. Her mitral regurgitation significantly decreased. She certainly did not need valvular surgery. It was a dramatic case to say the least. Hormonal therapy may be appropriate for many women; however, the side effects can overshadow situations in the myocardium that could result in limitation and quality-of-life issues. DD resulting from hypertension is something that we must consider in any woman who has shortness of breath or in women who have MVP where DD is also frequently seen.

MITRAL VALVE PROLAPSE

MVP is relatively benign condition of the mitral valve. Sometimes, the mitral valve leaflets become thickened, stretched or even voluminous, which may cause a slight to even a profound leakage of the valve. Many times on physical evaluation, a mid- to late systolic click may be heard followed by a late systolic murmur in most cases or a mid-systolic murmur in some. While most patients may not even know they have MVP, a few are particularly bothered by symptoms of atypical chest discomfort, shortness of breath, irregular heartbeats or even fatigue. In rare cases, spontaneous rupture of the chordae tendineae may occur resulting in symptoms of severe shortness of breath, significant mitral regurgitation and even left ventricular dysfunction or failure.

Most people with MVP are asymptomatic, and they don't know they have the problem. Although arrhythmias, atypical chest pain, clicks and murmurs were present, several patients in Dr. Sinatra's hospital had shortness of breath as their only symptom. This was both confusing and perplexing, so he proceeded to investigate and report clinical findings. After studying 20 patients with severe shortness of breath with MVP, pulmonary function studies were essentially normal. Although the clinical analysis was published in the pulmonary journal *Chest* in 1979,[81] Dr. Sinatra was unable to come up with a definitive reason why these patients with MVP had shortness of breath despite negative pulmonary function studies.

It would take almost 20 years before sophisticated echocardiographic techniques were able to point out the phenomena of DD.[82] Looking back, he suspected that many of these patients had shortness of breath because of DD. Although many patients with mitral valve prolapse symptoms were treated with beta-blockers, his interest in metabolic cardiology was actually the most effective and therapeutic treatment in patients with MVP as many patients did not respond well on beta-blocking meds. Interestingly, the conventional literature attests to the efficacy of magnesium.

Magnesium has shown efficacy in relieving symptoms of MVP. In a double-blind study of 181 participants, 80 serum magnesium levels were assessed in 141 patients with symptomatic MVP and compared to those of 40 healthy controls. While decreased magnesium levels were found in more than half (60%) of the patients with MVP, only 5% of the controlled subjects showed similar decreases.[83]

Participants with magnesium deficits were randomly assigned to receive magnesium supplement or placebo, and the results for the magnesium group were noteworthy. The mean (average) number of symptoms per patient was significantly reduced with magnesium supplementation. Weakness, chest pain, shortness of breath, palpitations and even anxiety were assuaged. Laboratory analysis also demonstrated decreases in the amount of adrenalin-like substances in the urine. The researchers concluded that many patients with MVP may have symptoms related to low magnesium levels. Additionally, with supplementation of the mineral, an improvement in symptoms and a decrease in adrenalin-like substances in the urine were realized.[83]

In Dr. Sinatra's experience, treating the symptomatic patient with MVP with pharmaceutical drugs can be problematic. He especially sees this with beta-blockers when many of patients complained about side effects, especially fatigue. When he started to utilize nutraceutical treatments including magnesium and CoQ10, many of his patients were able to experience an excellent quality of life despite echocardiographic correlations of moderate to severe MVP. On occasion, with some of his most refractory patients with MVP, the addition of 5 g of D-ribose and 1–2 g of L-carnitine was significant in the control of their symptoms. This metabolic approach has also been significant in the treatment of PAD.

PERIPHERAL ARTERY DISEASE

PAD is the third leading cause of arteriosclerotic cardiovascular morbidity followed by CAD and stroke. In a broad-based review of the literature involving 34 studies worldwide,[84] PAD has become a global problem involving over 200 million people, with smoking, diabetes and hypertension being the prevalent risk factors. In fact, when Dr. Sinatra was performing cardiac catheterization and saw plaque in the coronary arteries, he always knew it would show up elsewhere in the body. Frequently, it would show up in the arteries of the lower legs (PAD).

PAD has received very little public recognition, and it has always been considered a man's disease. In our practices, we see many more men than women with PAD symptoms, most typically cramping and pain in the calves when walking (called intermittent claudication). Women don't seem to develop those symptoms as often unless they are smokers. They usually complain more of fatigue and functional decline in the legs. But the following revelations from a recent American Heart Association (AHA) "call to action" article published in the journal *Circulation* clearly illustrate how prevalent and serious a problem of PAD appears to be for women.[85]

PAD increases with age for both men and women yet evidence suggests that over 40 years of age more women than men are affected. The summary statements by the authors indicate the following:[85]

- Most women with PAD, unlike men, do not have classic symptoms of intermittent claudication.
- Women with PAD have greater functional impairment and a more rapid functional decline than women without PAD.
- Women (and particularly Black women) are more likely than men to experience graft failure or limb loss.
- There is a need to identify women with or at risk for PAD, especially Black women, to lower cardiovascular ischemic event rates, loss of independent functional capacity and ischemic amputation rates.

The evaluation of PAD is tedious and complex, involving a meticulous evaluation of peripheral pulses, targeted blood pressure measurements involving brachial and tibial arteries, duplex ultrasound, as well as advanced imaging studies in some patients. Although many successful treatments frequently involve pharmaceutical and surgical procedures including arterial stents, many patients without major obstructions to blood vessels continue to be symptomatic despite conventional methodologies. Frequently, small vessel disease is present and a metabolic approach can be very supportive in reducing pain and suffering in women.

Our metabolic cardiology recommendations for women include the following targeted nutritional supplement program for PAD support:

- A high-quality multimineral/vitamin formula.
- A total of 100–300 mg of CoQ10 and 200–600 mg of magnesium, both of which help to lower blood pressure and support endothelial function.
- A total of 1–2 g of L-carnitine or 2 g of glycine propionyl L-carnitine (GPLC), a proprietary form of L-carnitine. L-carnitine helps clear our metabolic wastes that aggravate vasoconstriction in small blood vessels generated by cellular energy production. Cellular efficiency and aerobic capacity are supported when toxic by-products or the β-oxidation of fats is shuttled out of the mitochondria. GPLC does the same and also helps to improve blood flow by boosting nitric oxide, a biochemical that keeps blood vessels relaxed.
- A total of 5 g D-ribose, three times daily and prior to exercise activities.
- A total of 1–2 g omega-3 fatty acid (fish or squid oil).

Another simple and potentially therapeutic intervention for diffuse distal vessel disease is earthing. Since it was introduced years ago, and after performing cardiovascular research, it became crystal clear that earthing will be a new therapeutic strategy for PAD.[86] Please see Chapter 17 for the impressive blood viscosity effects resulting from the essence of grounding to the earth.

PAD is a widespread problem that is frequently undiagnosed and mismanaged. Arteriosclerotic CVD is a diffuse process, and when lesions show up in one area of the body, it is most likely present in other areas as well. Diagnosis of PAD should tip off the clinician that the carotid and coronary arteries are most likely involved. Although PAD has not been previously considered to be a significant issue in women, it clearly has become a major problem afflicting women, especially Black women.

SUMMARY

Women are different than men. CAD increases significantly when a women approaches peri-menopausal and menopausal years.

Risk factors are unique to women or occur disproportionately in women, including adverse pregnancy outcomes, migraine with aura and autoimmune disease. Assessing a woman's history of and risk for adverse pregnancy outcomes is an essential part of a comprehensive cardiovascular assessment in women. As a result, the AHA together with the American College of Obstetricians and Gynecologists has pleaded for obstetrician/gynecologists, cardiologists and others to perform comprehensive risk factor assessment as early as possible in women.[87]

Metabolic syndrome is another area where women need to be aggressively treated as women with type 2 diabetes or insulin resistance with higher triglyceride levels have more cardiac risk as opposed to men. DD, which is more prevalent in women with hypertension and occurring in MVP, frequently found in more women than men, is another area of marked concern given the fact that conventional medicine has very few options to offer.

Even painkillers in women can have a detrimental effect on their health. Acetaminophen has been incriminated in hundreds of cases of unexplained liver failure, while ibuprofen contributes to the high prevalence rate of hypertension in the United States which may be related to the overzealous use of these over-the-counter drugs.

CVD is the major leading cause of death in women today. Conducting appropriate gender-specific differences research and analysis of CVD trials has been difficult due to insufficient recruitment of women. Although this has contributed to a lack of understanding of gender differences in CVD, improved participation rates of women in new cardiovascular trials would yield more information concerning appropriate prevention, detection, accurate diagnosis and proper treatment of all women with heart disease. In the near future, a new subspecialty of gender-specific medicine will probably be able to stand on its own, and physicians will have a better understanding in the diagnosis and treatment of women with a wide range of cardiovascular concerns.

REFERENCES

1. Virani SS, Alonso A, Aparicio HJ, et al. 2021. American Heart Association Council on Epidemiology and Prevention Statistics Committee and Stroke Statistics Subcommittee. Heart disease and stroke statistics -2021 update: A report from the American Heart Association. *Circulation* 143(8):e254–e743.
2. Dreyer RP, Beltrame JF, Tavella R, et al. 2013. Evaluation of gender differences in door-to-balloon time in ST-elevation myocardial infarction. *Heart Lung and Circulation* 22(10):861–869.
3. Bugiardini R, Ricci B, Cenko E, et al. 2017. Delayed care and mortality among women and men with myocardial infarction. *Journal of the American Heart Association* 6(8):e005968.
4. Huded CP, Johnson M, Kravitz K, et al. 2018. 4-Step protocol for disparities in STEMI care and outcomes in women. *Journal American College of Cardiology* 71:2122–2132.
5. Hertler C, Seiler A, Gramatzki D, et al. 2020. Sex-specific and gender-specific aspects in patient-reported outcomes. *European Society for Medical Oncology Open* 5(Suppl 4):e000837.
6. Greenwood BN, Carnahan S, Huang L. 2018. Patient-physician gender concordance and increased mortality among female heart attack patients. *Proceedings of the National Academy of Sciences of the United States of America* 115(34):8569–8574.
7. Liakos M, Parikh PB. 2018. Gender disparities in presentation, management, and outcomes of acute myocardial infarction. *Current Cardiology Reports* 20(8):64–73.
8. Cushman M, Shay CM, Howard VJ, et al. 2020. Ten-year differences in women's awareness related to coronary heart disease: Results of the 2019 American Heart Association national survey: A special report from the American Heart Association. *Circulation* 143(7):e239–e248.
9. Saeed A, Kampangkaew J, Nambi V. 2017. Prevention of cardiovascular disease in women. *Methodist DeBakey Cardiovascular Journal* 13(4):185–192.
10. Reckelhoff JF. 2001. Gender differences in the regulation of blood pressure. *Hypertension* 37(5):1199–208.
11. Song JJ, Ma Z, Wang J, et al. 2019. Gender differences in hypertension. *Journal Cardiovascular Translational Research* 13(1):47–54.
12. Vaccarino V, Sullivan S, Hammadah M, et al. 2018. Mental Stress-Induced-Myocardial Ischemia in young patients with recent myocardial infarction: Sex differences and mechanisms. *Circulation* 137(8):794–805.
13. Pimple P, Hammadah M, Wilmot K, et al. 2018. Chest pain and Mental Stress-Induced Myocardial Ischemia: Sex differences. *American Journal of Medicine* 131(5):540–547.e1.
14. Thurston RC. 2011. Are vasomotor symptoms associated with alterations in hemostatic and inflammatory markers? Findings from the Study of Women's Health Across the Nation. *Menopause* 18(10):1044–1051.
15. Szmuilowicz ED, Manson JE, Rossouw JE, et al. 2011. Vasomotor symptoms and cardiovascular events in postmenopausal women. *Menopause* 18(6):603–610.
16. van den Berg MJ, Herber-Gast GC, van der Schouw YT. 2015. Is an unfavourable cardiovascular risk profile a risk factor for vasomotor menopausal symptoms? Results of a population-based cohort study. *British Journal Obstetrics and Gyneocology* 122(9):1252–1258.
17. Biglia N, Cagnacci A, Gambacciani M, et al. 2017. Vasomotor symptoms in menopause: A biomarker of cardiovascular disease risk and other chronic diseases? *Climacteric* 20(4):306–312.
18. Thurston RC. 2018. Vasomotor symptoms: Natural history, physiology, and links with cardiovascular health. *Climacteric* 21(2):96–100.
19. Houston MC. 2011. Role of mercury toxicity in hypertension, cardiovascular disease, and stroke. *Journal of Clinical Hypertension (Greenwich)* 13(8):621–627.
20. Pollard KM, Cauvi DM, Toomey CB, et al. 2019. Mercury-induced inflammation and autoimmunity. *Biochimica et Biophysica Acta General Subjects* 1863(12):129299.

21. Pelletier R, Khan NA, Cox J, et al. 2016. Sex versus gender-related characteristics: Which predicts outcome after acute coronary syndrome in the young? *Journal of American College of Cardiology* 67(2):127–135.

22. Meyer MR, Bernheim AM, Kurz DJ. 2018. Gender differences in patient and system delay for primary percutaneous coronary intervention: Current trends in a Swiss ST-segment elevation myocardial infarction population. *European Heart Journal. Acute Cardiovascular Care* 8(3):283–290.

23. Jackson EA, Ruppert K, Derby CA, et al. 2020. Is race or ethnicity associated with under-utilization of statins among women in the United States: The study of women's health across the nation. *Clinical Cardiology*. doi: 10.1002/clc.23448. Epub ahead of print. PMID: 32862481.

24. Wenger NK, Ferdinand KC, Merz CN, et al. 2016. Women, hypertension, and the systolic blood pressure intervention trial. *American Journal of Medicine* 129(10):1030–1036.

25. Rodriguez F, Foody JM, Wang Y, et al. 2015. Young Hispanic women experience higher in-hospital mortality following an acute myocardial infarction. *Journal of the American Heart Association* 4:e002089.

26. Zhang M, Wan P, Ng K, et al. 2020. Preeclampsia among African American pregnant women: An update on prevalence, complications, etiology, and biomarkers. *Obstetrical and Gynecological Survey* 75(2):111–120.

27. Deputy NP, Kim SY, Conrey EJ, et al. 2018. Prevalence and changes in preexisting diabetes and gestational diabetes among women who had a live birth–United States, 2012–2016. *MMWR Morbidity and Mortality Weekly Report* 67:1201–1207.

28. Sinatra ST. 2000. *Heart Sense for Women*. Washington, DC: Lifeline Press.

29. Mehta LS, Beckie TM, DeVon HA, et al. 2016. American Heart Association cardiovascular disease in women and special populations Committee of the Council on Clinical Cardiology, Council on epidemiology and prevention, Council on cardiovascular and stroke Nursing, and Council on quality of care and outcomes research. Acute myocardial infarction in women: A Scientific statement from the American Heart Association. *Circulation* 133(9):916–947.

30. Golomb BA, Evans MA. 2008. Statin adverse effects: A review of the literature and evidence for a mitochondrial mechanism. *American Journal of Cardiovascular Drugs* 8:373–418.

31. Hecht HS, Harman SM. 2003. Relation of aggressiveness of lipid-lowering treatment to changes in calcified plaque burden by electron beam tomography. *Journal of the American College of Cardiology* 92(3):334–336.

32. de Lorgeril M, Salen P, Abramson J, et al. 2010. Cholesterol lowering, cardiovascular diseases, and the rosuvastatin-JUPITER controversy: A critical reappraisal. *The Archives of Internal Medicine* 170(12):1032–1036.

33. Jones M, Tett S, Geeske M, et al. 2017. New-onset diabetes after statin exposure in elderly women: The Australian longitudinal study on women's health. *Drugs & Aging* 34(3):203.

34. Ma Y, Culver A, Rossouw J, et al. 2013. Statin therapy and the risk for diabetes among adult women: Do the benefits outweigh the risk? *Therapeutic Advances in Cardiovascular Disease* 7(1):41–44.

35. Raparelli V, Pannitteri G, Todisco T, et al. 2017. Treatment and response to statins: Gender-related differences. *Current Medical Chemistry* 24(24):2628–2638.

36. Ingersgaard MV, Anderson TH, Norgaard O, et al. 2020. Reasons for nonadherence to statins – a systematic review of reviews. *Patient Prefer Adherence* 14:675–691.

37. Faubion SS, Kapoor E, Moyer AM, et al. 2019. Statin therapy: Does sex matter? *Menopause* 26(12):1425–1435.

38. Sattar N, Preiss D, Murray HM, et al. 2010. Statins and risk of incident diabetes: A collaborative meta-analysis of randomized statin trials. *Lancet* 375:735–742.

39. Puri R, Nissen SE, Nicholls SJ. 2015. Statin-induced coronary artery disease regression rates differ in men and women. *Current Opinion in Lipidology*. 26(4):276–281.

40. Mitchell JD, Fergestrom N, Gage BF, et al. 2018. Impact of statins on cardiovascular outcomes following coronary artery calcium scoring. *Journal of the American College of Cardiology* 72(25):3233–3242.

41. Sinatra ST, Teter BB, Bowden J, et al. 2014. The saturated fat, cholesterol, and statin controversy a commentary. *Journal of the American College of Nutrition* 33(1):79–88.

42. Clerc Liaudat C, Vaucher P, et al. 2018. Sex/gender bias in the management of chest pain in ambulatory care. *Womens Health (London)* 14:1745506518805641.

43. Groepenhoff F, Eikendal ALM, Onland-Moret NC, et al. 2020. Coronary artery disease prediction in women and men using chest pain characteristics and risk factors: An observational study in outpatient clinics. *British Medical Journal Open* 10(4):e035928.

44. Bai MF, Wang X. 2020. Risk factors associated with coronary heart disease in women: A systemic review. *Herz* 45(Suppl 1):52–57.
45. Owan TE, Hodge DO, Herges RM, et al. 2006. Trends in prevalence and outcome of heart failure with preserved ejection fraction. *New England Journal of Medicine* 355:251–259.
46. Bhatia RS, Tu JV, Lee DS, et al. 2006. Outcome of heart failure with preserved ejection fraction in a population-based study. *New England Journal of Medicine* 355:260–269.
47. Redfield MM, Jacobsen SJ, Burnett JC, et al. 2003. Burden of systolic and diastolic ventricular dysfunction in the community: Appreciating the scope of the heart failure epidemic. *Journal of the American Medical Association* 289:194–202.
48. Hoekstra T, Lesman-Leegte I, van Veldhuisen DJ, et al. 2011. Quality of life is impaired similarly in heart failure patients with preserved and reduced ejection fraction. *European Journal of Heart Failure* 13:1013–1018.
49. Upadhya B, Kitzman DW. 2019. Heart failure with preserved ejection fraction: New approaches to diagnosis and management. *Clinical Cardiology* 43(2):145–155.
50. Ladeiras-Lopes R, Araújo M, Sampaio F, et al. 2019. The impact of diastolic dysfunction as a predictor of cardiovascular events: A systematic review and meta-analysis. *Revista Portuguesa de Cardiologis (English edition)* 38(11):789–804.
51. Nadruz W, Shah AM, Soloman SD. 2017. Diastolic dysfunction and hypertension. *Medical Clinics of North America* 101(1):7–17.
52. Stundiene L, Sarnelyte J, Norkute A, et al. 2019. Liver cirrhosis and left ventricular diastolic dysfunction: Systematic review. *World Journal of Gastroenterology* 25(32):4779–4795.
53. Roger VL, Go AS, Lloyd-Jones DM, et al. 2011. Heart disease and stroke statistics-2011 update: A report from the American Heart Association. *Circulation* 123(4):e18–e209.
54. Yancy CW, Lopatin M, Stevenson LW, et al. 2006. Clinical presentation, management, and in-hospital outcomes of patients admitted with acute decompensated heart failure with preserved systolic function: A report from the acute decompensated heart failure national registry (adhere) database. *Journal of the American College of Cardiology* 47:76–84.
55. Pfeffer MA, Shah AM, Borlaug BA. 2019. Heart failure with preserved ejection fraction in perspective. *Circulation Research* 124(11):1598–1617.
56. Tibrewala A, Yancy CW. 2019. Heart Failure with preserved ejection fraction in women. *Heart Failure Clinics* 15(1):9–18.
57. Hunt SA, Abraham WT, Chin MH, et al. 2009. Focused update incorporated into the ACC/AHA 2005 guidelines for the diagnosis and management of heart failure in adults a port of the American College of Cardiology foundation/American heart association task force on practice guidelines developed in collaboration with the international society for heart and lung transplantation. *Journal of the American College of Cardiology* 53:e1–e90
58. Paulus WJ, van Ballegoij JJ. 2010. Treatment of heart failure with normal ejection fraction: An inconvenient truth! *Journal of the American College of Cardiology* 55:526–537.
59. Loai S, Hai-Ling MC. 2020. Heart failure with preserved ejection fraction: The missing pieces in diagnostic imaging. *Heart Failure Reviews* 25(2):305–319.
60. Shah KS, Xu H, Matsouaka RA, et al. 2017. Heart failure with preserved, borderline, and reduced ejection fraction: 5-year outcomes. *Journal of American College of Cardiology* 70(20):2476–2486.
61. Gohar A, Kievit RF, Valstar GB, Hoes AW, Van Riet EE, van Mourik Y, Bertens LC, Boonman-Winter LJ, Bots ML, Den Ruijter HM, Rutten FH. Opportunistic screening models for high-risk men and women to detect diastolic dysfunction and heart failure with preserved ejection fraction in the community. *European Journal of Preventive Cardiology* 26(6):613–623. doi: 10.1177/2047487318816774. Epub 2018 Nov 27. PMID: 30482050; PMCID: PMC6431757.
62. Kim HJ, Kim MA, Kim HL, et al. 2018. Effects of multiparity on left ventricular diastolic dysfunction in women: Cross-sectional study of the KoRean wOmen'S chest pain rEgistry (KoROSE). *British Medical Journal Open* 8(12):e026968.
63. Wenger NK, Hayes SN, Pepine CJ, et al. 2013. Cardiovascular care for women: The 10-Q report and beyond. *American Journal of Cardiology* 112(4):S2.
64. Cikes M, Claggett B, Shah AM, et al. 2018. Atrial fibrillation in heart failure with preserved ejection fraction: The TOPCAT trial. *Journal of the American College of Cardiology – Heart Failure* 6(8):689–697.
65. Pitt B, Pfeffer MA, Assmann SF, et al. 2014. Spironolactone for heart failure with preserved ejection fraction. *New England Journal of Medicine* 370:1383–1392.

66. Solomon SD, Claggett B, Lewis EF. 2016. Influence of ejection fraction on outcomes and efficacy of spironolactone in patients with heart failure with preserved ejection fraction. *European Heart Journal* 37(5):455–462.

67. Alzahrani T, Tiu J, Panjrath G, et al. 2018. The effect of angiotensin-converting enzyme inhibitors on clinical outcomes in patients with ischemic cardiomyopathy and midrange ejection fraction: A pot hoc subgroup analysis from the PEACE trial. *Therapeutic Advances in Cardiovascular Diseases* 12(12):351–359.

68. Patel RB, Shah SJ, Fonarow GC, et al. 2017. Designing future clinical trials in heart failure with preserved ejection fraction: Lessons from TOPCAT. *Current Heart Failure Reports* 14(4):217–222.

69. Sinatra ST. 2009. Metabolic cardiology: An integrative strategy in the treatment of congestive heart failure. *Alternative Therapies in Health and Medicine* 15(3):44–52.

70. Bashore TM, Magorien DJ, Letterio J, et al. 1987. Histologic and biochemical correlates of left ventricular chamber dynamics in men. *Journal of the American College of Cardiology* 9(4):734–742.

71. Inwall JS, Weiss RG. 2004. Is the failing heart energy starved? On using chemical energy to support cardiac function. *Circulation Research* 95(2):135–145.

72. Dai Y, Luk T, Yiu K, et al. 2011. Reversal of mitochondrial dysfunction by coenzyme Q10 supplement improves endothelial function in patients with ischemic left ventricular systolic dysfunction: A randomized controlled trial. *Atherosclerosis* 216:395–401.

73. Raizner AE, Quiñones MA. 2021. Coenzyme Q10 for patients with cardiovascular disease: JACC focus seminar. *Journal of the American College of Cardiology* 77(5):609–619.

74. Melduni RM, Suri RM, Seward JB, et al. 2011. Diastolic dysfunction in patients undergoing cardiac surgery: A pathological mechanism underlying the initiation of new-onset post-operative atrial fibrillation. *Journal of the American College of Cardiology* 58:953–961.

75. Engberding N, Wenger NK. 2012. Management of hypertension in women. *Hypertension Research* 35:251–260.

76. Sprint Research Group, Wright JT Jr, Williamson JD, et al. 2015. A randomized trial of intensive versus standard blood-pressure control. *The New England Journal of Medicine* 373:2103–2116.

77. Forman JP, Stampfer MJ, Curhan GC. 2005. Non-narcotic analgesic dose and risk of incident hypertension in US women. *Hypertension* 46(3):500–507.

78. Kattah AG, Garovic VD. 2013. The management of hypertension in pregnancy. *Advances in Chronic Kidney Disease* 20(3):229–239.

79. Behrens I, Basit S, Melbye M, et al. 2017. Risk of post-pregnancy hypertension in women with a history of hypertensive disorders of pregnancy: Nationwide cohort study. *British Medical Journal* 358:j3078.

80. Wassertheil-Smoller S, Anderson G, Psaty BM, et al. 2000. Hypertension and its treatment in postmenopausal women: Baseline data from the Women's Health Initiative. *Hypertension* 36:780–789.

81. ZuWallack R, Sinatra S, Lahiri B, et al. 1979. Pulmonary function studies in patients with prolapse of the mitral valve. *Chest* 76(1):17–20.

82. Halley CM, Houghtaling PL, Khalil MK, et al. 2011. Mortality rate in patients with diastolic dysfunction and normal systolic function. *Archives of Internal Medicine* 171(2):1082–1087.

83. Kitlinski M, Stepniewski M, Nessler J, et al. 2004. Is magnesium deficit in lymphocytes a part of the mitral valve prolapse syndrome? *Magnesium Research* 17(1):39–45.

84. Fowkes FG, Rudan D, Rudan I, et al. 2013. Comparison of global estimates or prevalence and risk factors for peripheral artery disease in 2000 and 2010: A systematic review and analysis. *Lancet* 382(9901):1329–1340.

85. Hirsch AT, Allison MA, Gomes MS, et al. 2012. A call to action: Women and peripheral artery disease: A scientific statement from the American Heart Association. *Circulation* 125(11):1449–1472.

86. Chevalier G, Sinatra ST, Oschman JL, et al. 2013. Earthing (grounding) the human body reduces blood viscosity: A major factor in cardiovascular disease. *Journal of Alternative and Complementary Medicine* 19(2):102–110.

87. Brown HL, Warner JJ, Gianos E, et al. 2018. American Heart Association and the American College of Obstetricians and Gynecologists. Promoting risk identification and reduction of cardiovascular disease in women through collaboration with obstetricians and gynecologists: A presidential advisory from the American Heart Association and the American College of Obstetricians and Gynecologists. *Circulation* 137(24):e843–e852.

10 Hormones and Cardiovascular Disease

Sara Gottfried

Myles Spar

CONTENTS

CVD in Women...232
Estradiol and CVD..232
Low Estradiol and CVD..233
Hormones and Metabolism...234
    Effects of Menopausal Hormone Therapy...234
    How Does Hormone Therapy Affect Risk of CVD? 235
    Critical Window or "Timing" Hypothesis 236
    Is Hormone Therapy Good for Every Woman?...236
    Methods of Hormone Therapy...237
Summary: Women and CVD 237
CVD in Men...237
Low Testosterone and CVD..238
    What Causes Low T and How Prevalent Is It? 239
    What About Treating Low T with Testosterone Replacement Therapy (TRT)?.......239
    Role of DHEA 240
    Is TRT Good for Every Man with Low T? 240
    How to Treat 241
Methods of TRT...242
    Non-Pharmaceutical Approaches...243
    Exercise..243
    Natural Supplements..243
Summary: Men and CVD 243
Conclusion 244
References...244

In this chapter, we will review the hormonal drivers of cardiovascular disease (CVD) in men and women, including the epidemiology, trends, early biomarkers and warning signs with an emphasis on coronary heart disease. Based on the seminal studies, we will discuss what occurs endogenously with hypogonadism and its downstream consequences, including how it maps to a greater risk of CVD and relevant plausible mechanisms. We will highlight diagnostic testing, and our current understanding of the risk of treatment versus no treatment of reproductive aging. Overall, we will make the case to consider the full symphony of hormone signaling and how that related to CVD.

DOI: 10.1201/9781003137849-10

CVD IN WOMEN

Traditionally thought of as a man's disease, nearly as many women as men die each year of CVD.[1,2] In fact, we are witnessing an increase in mortality rates in women from 2010 to present.[3] In the United States, approximately 50 million women have CVD, which causes one in three deaths. Yet women and their physicians tend to be more concerned about breast cancer—approximately three million women have breast cancer, which causes 1 in 31 deaths.[4] Unfortunately, only about half of women realize that they are at a greater risk of CVD than any other disease.[5]

Women live longer than men but have a higher risk of age-related chronic disease. Premenopausally, women are somewhat protected against vascular dysfunction due to physiological estradiol levels, which help to relax blood vessels and reduce cardiovascular risk.[6] However, the protection depends on other factors besides endogenous estradiol that we will describe in this chapter—as indicated by rising hospitalizations of younger women with acute myocardial infarction (MI).[2] Other studies have documented a decline in hospitalization for acute MI overall in an integrated healthcare system, but that the decline is greater in men compared to women.[8] Additionally, younger women are less likely to receive guideline-based care, including lipid-lowering therapies, non-aspirin antiplatelets, beta-blockers, coronary angiography, and coronary revascularization.[2] We need to understand these trends and how they map to underlying factors to improve care of all people with acute MI, including women of all ages.

Following menopause at a mean age of 51, women's risk of disease accelerates unless there is timely intervention. Fat deposition shifts from subcutaneous to central. Downstream, the risk of cardiometabolic disease rises. Bones weaken, and sexual and cognitive function declines. Approximately 80% of women experience poor cerebral perfusion, leading to temperature dysregulation, vasomotor symptoms, sleep disruption, and cognitive decline, all of which may worsen mood and executive function.[10] These findings demonstrate progression of a hypometabolic phenotype during the menopausal transition.[10] Endogenous estradiol protects the cardiovascular system and the brain,[12] though higher levels in postmenopause are associated with a greater risk of breast cancer.[13] While genomic and environmental influences are involved, postmenopausal women with endogenous estradiol levels in the top 20% of the distribution have breast cancer risk that is two- to threefold higher than women in the bottom 20% of the distribution.[14]

Not only do women lack awareness about CVD, only 39% of primary care physicians (PCPs) rated CVD as a top concern, after weight and breast health. Further, only 22% of PCPs and 42% of cardiologists felt extremely well prepared to assess CVD risk in women.[5] The lack of awareness among both women and physicians who care for them contributes to women not getting the diagnostic testing and treatment that they may need. To improve awareness, we recommend several books to our patients for additional reading.[16,17]

Risk varies by race. Heart disease is the leading cause of death for White and Black women. For American Indian and Alaska Native women, heart disease and cancer cause the same mortality. For Latinx, Asian, and Pacific Islander women, cancer is the leading cause of death followed by heart disease.[18]

ESTRADIOL AND CVD

Estradiol protects women from CVD via a number of potential mechanisms listed below. Most of these benefits exist for women until late perimenopause when estradiol levels begin to drop as a result of gonadal senescence:

- Increases nitric oxide bioavailability, an important vasodilator[19]
- Improves plasma lipids[20]
- Anti-inflammatory[21,22]

- Anti-platelet[23]
- Anti-oxidant[24]
- Anti-apoptotic[24]
- Prevents arterial stiffening[26]
- Anti-atherogenic: inhibits monocyte adhesion to vascular endothelium via neural cell adhesion molecules[27]
- Regulates micro RNA[24]
- Favorably modulates the renin-angiotensin-aldosterone system (RAAS), involved in arterial blood pressure regulation.[29]

While more recent data show that women are experiencing risk of CVD earlier, related to the rise of multiple nontraditional risk factors such as worsening nutrition, pregnancy-related pathological changes related to vascular function, and sedentary lifestyle, most women experience increased risk beginning in their 50s with the onset of menopause owing to the loss of estradiol-related protection. Postmenopausal women demonstrate increased arterial stiffness and hypertension, as well as other biomarkers of vascular aging, compared to premenopausal women.[27] Overall, the menopausal transition is accompanied by greater vulnerability of endothelium, contributing to accelerated vascular aging and CVD risk, including a fourfold greater risk of coronary artery disease.[31,32] We now know that for the past 30 years, more men have CVD, but in absolute numbers, more women die from CVD.[33]

LOW ESTRADIOL AND CVD

What happens when women go through perimenopause and menopause without hormonal support? Heart disease rises after menopause.[34] The reduction in estradiol levels associated with the menopausal transition may cause a proatherogenic lipid profile.[35] According to the Framingham study, risk of CVD for women aged 45–54 is doubled compared to those aged 40–44.[36] Now we have an unprecedented experiment in progress since the publication of the Women's Health Initiative in 2002—more women than ever are suffering through the changes of menopause without exogenous hormone therapy. Overall, use of hormone therapy fell approximately 80% since 1999.[37]

Before menopause, ovarian production of estradiol provides partial protection to keep blood vessels relaxed and lipids in a healthier range.[6] Menopause heralds many changes. Untreated vasomotor symptoms are linked to impaired endothelial function,[39] as well as an increased risk of hypertension and CVD,[40] diminished cardiac vagal tone,[41] fracture,[42] poor or disrupted sleep,[43] depression,[44] increased white matter hyperintensities in the brain,[45] and cognitive impairment, possibly leading to a greater risk of Alzheimer's disease.[12] In fact, vasomotor symptoms are emerging as an important biomarker of future disease, not just nuisance symptoms to be managed with nonpharmacologic agents.

Multiple cardiovascular biomarkers change in women during perimenopause and menopause, including the following. Changes are accompanied by a rise in follicle-stimulating hormone:[47]

- Increased total cholesterol, low-density lipoprotein (LDL-C), and sometimes, triglycerides.[48,49]
- Higher apolipoprotein B concentrations.[50]
- Decreased high-density lipoprotein (HDL), though data are mixed.[48,49]
- Higher total cholesterol to HDL ratio.[48]
- Data on lipoprotein(a) are mixed. Most studies suggest that lipoprotein(a) is genetically determined and not affected by age,[55,56] while other studies demonstrate that lipoprotein(a) increases with age and more significantly in women, particularly over the age of 50.[57]
- Increased levels of very small very low-density lipoproteins, intermediate-density lipoproteins, low-density lipoproteins (LDLs), remnant, and reduced LDL particle size.[58]

- Lower concentrations of estradiol and sex hormone binding globulin (SHBG), and higher levels of the free androgen index (total testosterone divided by SHBG, then multiplied by 100), were associated with a more atherogenic profile of lipoprotein subclasses.[59] Note that the high androgens associated with polycystic ovary syndrome are associated with significantly increased risk of CVD.[60,61,62]
- Higher body fat and distribution in a male pattern (trunk fat mass-to-leg fat mass ratio).[63]

Given these changes associated with the menopausal change, we recommend measurement of lipoprotein subclasses and coronary artery calcium score to improve prediction of coronary artery disease in postmenopausal women—these assessments provide improved risk stratification compared to the conventional lipid panel and traditional risk factors of coronary heart disease.[64] Furthermore, frequent vasomotor symptoms were associated with smaller HDL size and higher concentrations of LDL-C and intermediate LDL-P—all linked to lower estradiol levels.[65]

When examined in aggregate, men have a more atherogenic lipid profile than women, but women catch up with regard to LDL-C after menopause.[66]

HORMONES AND METABOLISM

Estrogen is a master regulator of metabolism for women. Premenopausally, estrogen suppresses appetite and protects against insulin resistance, adiposity, and type 2 diabetes compared to age-matched men.[67] Estrogen regulates energy intake, fat storage, and energy expenditure. Estrogen modulates insulin sensitivity, glucose transport, and mitochondrial function and suppresses gluconeogenesis.[68] Loss of estrogen at menopause causes significant changes in fat distribution, insulin activity, and whole-body metabolism. Researcher Roberta Britton refers to the menopausal transition as a shift to a *metabolically compromised phenotype* characterized by the decline in circulating estrogen and diminished brain energetics.

Estrogen exerts its effects through classical endocrinology, intracrinology, and a network of estrogen receptors (estrogen receptor alpha, estrogen receptor beta, and GPER). Metabolic effects of estrogen are primarily driven through estrogen receptor alpha (ERα), though the precise mechanisms are still under investigation.[69] Imbalance in the metabolic network of estrogen receptors ERα/ERβ may promote metabolic syndrome via insulin signaling.[70]

Menopause leads to a complex metabolic disorder in many women, associated with dysregulation of cellular glucose uptake and an atherogenic serum lipid profile. Changes in the glucose and insulin pathway leading to insulin resistance cause compensatory hyperinsulinemia, which triggers increased androgen synthesis. Similar to low testosterone in men, low estradiol impacts many of the most important risk factors for CVD, including diabetes, obesity, and metabolic syndrome.

Additionally, insulin resistance seems to be riskier for women in terms of CVD.[71] Women show greater risk of downstream consequences such as coronary heart disease at lower fasting glucose relative to men.[72] Fasting insulin and the homeostasis model assessment for insulin sensitivity (HOMA-S) are associated with a combined outcome of coronary heart disease or stroke in women.[73] Diabetic women have higher risk of coronary heart disease than diabetic men.

EFFECTS OF MENOPAUSAL HORMONE THERAPY

Systemic estrogen therapy reduces total cholesterol, low-density lipoprotein (LDL-C), and lipo(a) in a dose response.[74] Oral administration induces a more significant reduction in these biomarkers and has been shown to reduce hypertriglyceridemia, but overall, the risks of oral estrogen therapy with respect to venous thromboembolic events (VTEs) outweigh the benefits.

We recommend micronized progesterone together with estrogen therapy in women with a uterus (and therefore in need of endometrial protection) due to its neutral effect on the lipid profile.

Regarding lipoprotein(a), estrogen therapy has been shown to reduce levels by up to 44%.[75]

How Does Hormone Therapy Affect Risk of CVD?

Hormone therapy was prescribed in perimenopausal and menopausal women with the promise that it would reduce the risk of CVD for approximately 59 years before a randomized trial was performed to test the hypothesis. This was based on observational data showing that most studies of hormone replacement therapy in postmenopausal women show around a 40%–50% reduction in the risk of a coronary event in women on estrogen.[6,77,78]

In 1998, the Heart and Estrogen/Progestin Replacement Study (HERS) was published—it was the first randomized trial demonstrating that in women with established CVD (mean age 67), treatment with conjugated equine estrogen and medroxyprogesterone acetate (CEE/MPA) significantly increased heart events during the first year of use.[79] This study demonstrated that conventional hormone therapy was not associated with secondary prevention of CVD.

After HERS, the race was on to settle the score about whether hormone therapy was effective at reducing chronic disease, such as CVD and osteoporosis. The problem was that the US government spent over $1 billion on the wrong study, called the Women's Health Initiative (WHI). In the 20 years since WHI was published, most clinicians have concluded that the large randomized trial enrolled the *wrong* subjects, at the *wrong* age, and randomized them to the *wrong* hormone therapy.

WHI enrolled 16,608 postmenopausal women aged 50–79 years. The subjects were supposed to be healthy postmenopausal women, but instead 36% were on medication for high blood pressure, 35% were overweight, 34% were obese, and about half were current or past smokers. They likely had vascular dysfunction at baseline. The median age was 63, so most were 10 years or more from menopause. The distribution of women by age was uneven: 10% were 50–54, whereas 70% were 60–79, an age where established CVD was likely present given the risk factors in the study population. The subjects were treated with pregnant mare's urine, or conjugated equine estrogen, and medroxyprogesterone acetate—both of which are structurally unlike the endogenous estrogen and progesterone made by the female body, and at appropriate levels for function, serve as a defense against CVD.

In 2002, after a mean of 5.2 years of follow-up, the WHI was halted "due to an increased risk of invasive breast cancer." However, the increased risk of breast cancer with conjugated equine estrogen and medroxyprogesterone acetate was not statistically significant.[80] Rossouw et al. reported that the hazard ratios (nominal 95% confidence intervals [CIs]) were as follows:

- Breast cancer 1.26 (1.00–1.59) with 290 cases
- Coronary heart disease 1.29 (1.02–1.63) with 286 cases
- Stroke 1.41 (1.07–1.85) with 212 cases
- Pulmonary embolus 2.13 (1.39–3.25) with 101 cases
- Colorectal cancer 0.63 (0.43–0.92) with 112 cases
- Endometrial cancer 0.83 (0.47–1.47) with 47 cases
- Hip fracture 0.66 (0.45–0.98) with 106 cases
- Death due to other causes 0.92 (0.74–1.14) with 331 cases
- Corresponding HRs (nominal 95% CIs) for composite outcomes were 1.22 (1.09–1.36) for total CVD (arterial and venous disease), 1.03 (0.90–1.17) for total cancer, 0.76 (0.69–0.85) for combined fractures, 0.98 (0.82–1.18) for total mortality, and 1.15 (1.03–1.28) for the global index.

Similar to HERS, the small increased relative risk of heart events—including angina, bypass, angioplasty, and death due to heart disease—occurred only in the first year of taking conventional hormone therapy with CEE/MPA.

Shortly after publication of WHI in the *Journal of the American Medical Association*, Leon Speroff, a professor of obstetrics and gynecology at Oregon Health Sciences University and director of the Women's Health Research Unit, reanalyzed the WHI data and showed that the modestly increased rate of heart events was only in women who were 20 or more years post menopause when they enrolled in the study.[81]

WHI investigators followed suit. In 2007, cardiologist Rossouw et al. changed their conclusion about WHI to indicate that when hormone therapy was initiated within 10 years of the onset of menopause, it reduces risk of coronary heart disease.[82] Multiple other randomized trials and meta-analyses concurred—including a meta-analysis of 23 randomized trials involving 39,049 women that showed a 30% decreased incidence of MI and cardiac deaths in younger postmenopausal women,[83] and a Danish randomized trial of 1,006 recently menopausal women who experienced a 50% reduction in acute cardiac events with no increased risk of cancer, venous thrombosis, or stroke.[84]

CRITICAL WINDOW OR "TIMING" HYPOTHESIS

As we continue to parse the evidence post-WHI, we believe there is a critical window during which hormone therapy, ideally with bioidentical transdermal estrogen and oral micronized progesterone, is beneficial for vascular health. This is known as the "timing" hypothesis.[85,86,87,27]

Within this critical window, estrogen causes vessels to dilate, potentially increasing blood supply to cardiac muscle.[90] In another randomized trial of 222 women aged 45 and older, the rate of progression of subclinical atherosclerosis was slower in women taking unopposed estradiol versus placebo, as measured with carotid intima-media thickness.[91]

However, at a certain point in menopause, the benefit of hormone therapy on CVD ceases.[92] In women with underlying heart disease who are 10 years or more post menopause, estrogen may trigger inflammation in existing plaques, leading to rupture or erosion. The critical window is likely 5–10 years after menopause. Beyond that window of 10 years menopausal age, risk of hormone therapy outweighs benefits.

One randomized trial tested the timing hypothesis. Hodis et al. randomized 643 postmenopausal women based on time since menopause (6 years or less versus 10 years or more). Women were treated with oral estradiol and, if they had a uterus, vaginal progesterone gel. They measured carotid intimal-medial thickness every 6 months. They found that early hormone therapy was linked to less progression when given within 6 years of menopause. No benefit was seen 10 years or more post menopause.[93]

Since 2002 when the faulty WHI trial was published, clinicians have been confused and concerned, and guidance has been controversial. However, a cogent analysis of the details of WHI—in context with the studies that pre- and postdate the trial—indicates that many women with vasomotor symptoms are candidates for the safe and responsible prescribing of hormone therapy. The details of prescription are beyond the scope of this chapter, but our general recommendation for women is a transdermal estradiol patch at a dose of 0.0375 mg together with micronized progesterone at 100 mg/day, or 200 mg for 12 days/month.

IS HORMONE THERAPY GOOD FOR EVERY WOMAN?

Not every woman is a good candidate for hormone therapy. There are several contraindications to menopausal hormone therapy, according to the Food and Drug Administration, as published by the American Association of Clinical Endocrinologists Guidelines for Clinical Practice for Menopause (shown below).[94] Trials of nonhormonal alternatives may be considered for treatment of menopausal symptoms in patients with contraindications, such as acupuncture, yoga, exercise, hypnosis, cognitive behavioral therapy, and herbal therapies.[95]

Contraindications are as follows:

• Active liver disease
• Active or recent arterial thromboembolic disease (angina, MI)

- Current, past, or suspected breast cancer
- Known hypersensitivity to the active substance of the therapy or to any of the excipients
- Known or suspected estrogen-sensitive malignant conditions
- Porphyria cutanea tarda (absolute contraindication)
- Previous idiopathic or current venous thromboembolism (deep venous thrombosis, pulmonary embolism)
- Undiagnosed genital bleeding
- Untreated endometrial hyperplasia
- Untreated hypertension.

METHODS OF HORMONE THERAPY

There are risks, benefits, and alternatives to each method of hormone therapy, and it is essential to personalize the modes of delivery, convenience, compliance, and best evidence.

- Transdermal patch
- Topical
- Oral
- Sublingual
- Injectable
- Pellets.

In addition to estrogen and progesterone, other hormones to consider include testosterone, dehydro-epiandrosterone (DHEA), and pregnenolone. Data on therapy with these other hormones regarding CVD lack evidence. For example, postmenopausal women undergoing coronary angiography for myocardial ischemia demonstrate that lower DHEA-S levels are associated with increased cardiovascular mortality and all-cause mortality.[96] However, we lack definitive trials on DHEA treatment with regard to CVD. Still, we need to consider the broader hormonal symphony in which estrogen and progesterone play.

For further information, we recommend several guidelines including the following.

- American College of Obstetrics and Gynecology[97]
- American Association of Clinical Endocrinologists and American College of Endocrinology[98]
- Endocrine Society[99]
- North American Menopause Society[100]
- US Preventive Services Task Force.[101]

SUMMARY: WOMEN AND CVD

Loss of estradiol protection in perimenopause and menopause is associated with a greater risk of CVD. Trials regarding the use of hormone therapy in women are mixed but overall show a benefit when given within 5–10 years of menopause. We recommend personalized shared decision making using the best available evidence. As we covered in the preceding sections, systemic hormone therapy is safe and effective for symptomatic women within 10 years of menopause, which is usually in women less than 60 years of age. Regular evaluation and reassessment of risks are necessary.

CVD IN MEN

While CVD is the number one killer of both men and women, its prevalence is higher in men, with nearly a quarter of deaths in men being due to this cause.[102] Part of the reason men have higher rates of mortality and morbidity from heart disease is because of lifestyle. Men "win" at all of the major lifestyle-related risk factors contributing to early mortality from heart disease:

- Men are less likely to engage in regular exercise.
- Men are more likely to be overweight.
- Men are more likely to smoke.

We can add to this list of lifestyle-related factors that men are more likely to have other risk factors for heart disease such as diabetes and hypertension. We also know that we can add to this list a biologic risk factor—low testosterone.

Just as in women, risk varies by race. While heart disease is the leading cause of death for men in most racial and ethnic groups, it is the second likeliest cause of death in Asian and Pacific Islander men, after cancer. Non-Hispanic Blacks have the highest rate of CVD in the United States and are two to three times more likely to die from heart disease. In addition, Black and Latinx men have higher rates of major risk factors for CVD such as diabetes and hypertension.[103]

LOW TESTOSTERONE AND CVD

Men with untreated low testosterone demonstrate elevated risk for heart disease. Longitudinal studies and an extensive meta-analysis of over 16,000 men showed that those with the lowest levels of testosterone had the highest risk of CVD as well as cardiovascular and all-cause mortality. A comprehensive review of the impact of testosterone on the cardiovascular system published in the *Journal of the American College of Cardiology* in 2016 reported that low levels of testosterone are associated with more atherosclerosis, coronary artery disease, and cardiovascular events.[104,105]

We know that low testosterone (T) impacts many of the strongest risk factors for heart disease, such as diabetes, obesity, and metabolic syndrome. In fact, there is a bidirectional relationship between abnormally low testosterone and the triad of high blood sugar, hypertension, and hyperlipidemia that characterize the metabolic syndrome, one of the strongest risk factors for CVD.

In a meta-analysis of cross-sectional and observational studies, Brand et al. found an inverse relationship between total T and metabolic syndrome. The longitudinal Massachusetts male aging study also found that there was an increased risk for the development of metabolic syndrome over time among men with low T, particularly for non-overweight middle-aged men—in fact men with the lowest quartile of T have double the risk for the development of metabolic syndrome and even frank diabetes.[106,107]

While low testosterone can cause insulin resistance, even in non-obese men, it appears that the converse is also true—that men with insulin resistance have a higher risk of developing low T, especially when the insulin resistance contributes to increased adipose tissue which we know is hormonally active. Adipose tissue increases the activity of the aromatase enzyme, which converts T to estradiol, thus lowering endogenous T levels. This contributes to a cycle of metabolic syndrome or hyperglycemia, higher amounts of adipose (often as belly fat), and lower male hormone levels.

In fact, treating the low T that is found in men with diabetes with exogenous testosterone has been shown to help blood sugar control among diabetics. A recent prospective study showed that testosterone replacement therapy actually reversed diabetes in one-third of men randomized to receive testosterone as compared to none of the men with low T who were not treated with exogenous testosterone.[108]

We know that CVD, specifically presenting as an MI or cerebrovascular accident, is a disease of inflammation as much as it is of atherosclerosis. It is an inflammatory reaction caused by increase in pro-inflammatory cytokines that leads to higher instability of plaque in the coronary or cerebral arteries, leading to rupture and occlusion by thrombosis. In addition to the evidence as stated above showing that abnormally low levels of testosterone contribute to atherosclerosis and the risk factors leading to it, there has also been shown to exist a relationship between low testosterone and increased inflammatory markers. This may also be mediated by adipose tissues, which increase pro-inflammatory cytokines. In fact, testosterone therapy has been shown to lower such inflammatory compounds.[109]

While low testosterone is prevalent and increases the risk for heart disease, how do clinicians identify those most at risk? Interestingly, one early warning sign of both low T and potential coronary artery disease—the canary in the coal mine—would be erectile dysfunction (ED), especially at an early age, as this could be both a symptom of low T as well as a first clue as to the presence of atherosclerosis. In fact, there is a 50-fold increase in cardiac events in 40- to 60-year-old men with ED compared with men without ED.[110]

WHAT CAUSES LOW T AND HOW PREVALENT IS IT?

By far the most common cause of low testosterone is age. Up to 40% of men over 40 have low T, as defined by total T less than 350 ng/dL. In fact, decline of T starts at age 35—up to 1% per year.[111] Chronic opioid use, hypothalamic or pituitary dysfunction, and trauma are other causes, but none of these are nearly as prevalent as age-associated hypogonadism.

Low testosterone causes many symptoms, physically, psychologically, and sexually. See Table 10.1 for a summary of such symptoms.

WHAT ABOUT TREATING LOW T WITH TESTOSTERONE REPLACEMENT THERAPY (TRT)?

Treating to normal levels has been shown to help all of the symptoms in Table 10.1, but what is the impact on CVD risk?

Most studies had shown either a favorable impact of TRT or no significant change. However, in 2013, two studies were published which purported to show a link between TRT and an increased risk of heart disease. These studies received much media attention, because at the time, the FDA was concerned that too many men were receiving TRT. In fact, these studies had important limitations and flaws, so much so that one required correction twice and was called to be retracted by 29 different medical societies.[112]

One of these studies, by Vigen et al., was a retrospective analysis of men who had undergone coronary angiography within the Veterans Administration healthcare system.[113] The authors reported that the overall rate of MI, stroke, and death in men with serum T levels less than 300 ng/dL was higher in men who received a T prescription compared with untreated men. Although no statistically significant differences were noted at years 1, 2, or 3, the overall rate of events over the course of the study was reported to be significantly higher (29%) in T-treated men. To show this, they used complicated and unconventional statistical methodologies that were refuted. In fact, the authors were found to have accidentally included women in the study and an incorrect number of men in addition to errors in their statistics, leading to two corrections. Subsequently 29 international

TABLE 10.1
Clinical Manifestations of Testosterone Deficiency

Physical	Psychological	Sexual
Decreased muscle mass	Depressed mood	Diminished libido
Increased fat mass	Diminished mental energy	Erectile dysfunction
Decreased bone mineral density	Decreased well-being	Difficulty achieving orgasm
Gynecomastia	Impaired cognition or memory	
Anemia		
Fatigue		

medical societies and more than 160 physician scientists from 32 countries petitioned *JAMA* to retract this article, citing "gross data mismanagement and contamination" that rendered the study "no longer credible."

Another study was published at the same time by Finkle et al.[114] This was a retrospective study of a health insurance database that reported rates of nonfatal MI in the period up to 90 days after a T prescription and compared these rates to MI rates in the previous 12 months. The authors reported a higher rate of adverse events in the T-treated group using something called inverse stabilized propensity weighting in which an event was counted as more than 1 event in the T-treated group and less than 1 event in the untreated group.

Because the source was an insurance claims database, available information was limited to diagnosis codes, procedure codes, and prescriptions. There was no information available regarding several standard CV risk factors, such as diabetes, hypertension, hyperlipidemia, smoking history, or obesity, and no information concerning any blood test results,

Given this fact and the unusual methodology, even the FDA concluded that "it is difficult to attribute the increased risk for non-fatal MI seen in the Finkle study to testosterone alone and not consider that the study participants might have remained hypogonadal and thus at higher risk for non-fatal MI."[115]

However, due to increased attention on the rates of TRT being prescribed and against the advice of the FDA's own advisory board which concluded, in September 2014, that with regard to the risk of CV events, "evidence linking T therapy to an increased risk of heart attack, stroke and death is inconclusive and weak signal", still in March 2015, the FDA imposed a black box warning on testosterone prescriptions, requiring that prescribers warn patients about a possible increased risk of heart attack and stroke associated with testosterone use. They called for a prospective study on the use of TRT as it relates to CVD risk.[116]

Meanwhile, over 23 studies have been published since the FDA-required label change was added in 2015 assessing TRT and CVD risk. In their review of these, Miner et al. discussed that cumulatively there have been more major adverse cardiac events in the placebo arms than the testosterone treatment arms, and TRT has been shown to improve myocardial ischemia in men with coronary artery disease. TRT has certainly been shown to decrease fat mass and insulin resistance, known risk factors for CVD.[117] Still, the prospective trail suggested by the FDA is underway, the results of which will help to resolve any concerns.

ROLE OF DHEA

Dehydroepiandrosterone, DHEA, is an androgenic hormone produced mainly in the adrenal glands. There have been numerous epidemiological studies indicating that low levels of DHEA correlate with increased risk of cardiovascular risk, morbidity, and actual coronary artery disease in men, but not in women. The impact of treatment with DHEA is not clear; however, there is some evidence that DHEA works as an antioxidant, which would imply that normalizing levels not only could attenuate any increased risk from lower-than-normal levels but could also decrease inflammation through an antioxidant effect.[118]

IS TRT GOOD FOR EVERY MAN WITH LOW T?

There are certainly contraindications to starting exogenous testosterone therapy. When looking at the primary guidelines on TRT, from the American Urological Association and the North American Endocrine Society, there are several absolute or relative contraindications to TRT.

Given the high level of concern with heart disease risk, it is recommended not to start TRT in any man with a cardiovascular event, including stroke, within the prior 6 months. While TRT has been shown not to increase risk for the development of prostate cancer, it potentially may worsen some prostate cancers; thus, TRT is not recommended for men with active prostate cancer. Lastly, as TRT can worsen poorly controlled sleep apnea, it is not recommended for men in whom sleep apnea is not well controlled.

Contraindications are as follows:

- Active prostate ca or PSA > 4 ng/mL or presence of prostate nodules on digital rectal exam
- Recent cardiovascular event (6 mos)
- Polycythemia (Hct > 54%)
- Breast cancer.

Relative contraindications are as follows:

- Hematocrit > 50%
- Severe lower urinary tract symptoms
- Uncontrolled congestive heart failure
- Untreated obstructive sleep apnea.

In addition to needing to explain the FDA black box warning regarding possible increased risk of heart disease, there is another black box warning regarding transference of topical testosterone products onto children in the home through skin contact, so it is important to document the discussion regarding ways to avoid transference if topical testosterone is being prescribed. Children and women should avoid contact with the site of application.

Lastly, men who are desiring to maintain fertility at the current time of evaluation should not be put on exogenous testosterone in any form. Testosterone therapy will lead to a decrease in hypothalamic stimulation of the pituitary hormones LH and FSH in many men, leading not only to decreased endogenous testicular production of testosterone but also to decreased sperm production. Options for therapy in such men include off-label use of Clomiphene or HCG (human chorionic gonadotropin), which both can raise endogenous T production without impairing fertility. The use of TRT generally does not cause permanent suppression of gonadal function, but should be stopped at least 6 months before fertility is desired to allow for testicular recovery.

Even with these considerations, the majority of men who have low testosterone are candidates for hormone replacement therapy and will be benefited both in terms of symptomatic improvement as well as metabolic and cardiovascular health.

How to Treat

When considering testosterone therapy, a standard work-up should include an assessment of:

- Total and bioavailable or free testosterone
- SHBG
- Estradiol
- DHEA-sulfate
- Hematocrit
- PSA
- Metabolic panel
- LH/FSH.

Free or bioavailable testosterone is important to assess, as some men may have normal levels of total testosterone, while the actual bioavailable or free levels may be low. This would still be an indication to treat. Typically, ordering total testosterone and the SHBG level will generate a calculated free level by the lab. Alternatively, salivary testing can be used, which assesses free levels, but the guidelines and most standard practice recommend blood testing.

Time of testing is also important. Especially for men under 45 years old, the diurnal fluctuations in testosterone dictate an early morning blood draw in order to best interpret the level.

Other labs that can be helpful in evaluating the risk for potential adverse cardiac events in a man being considered for TRT would include:

- Coronary artery calcium score
  - This test done by CT scan is the best non-invasive test for the true presence of athero-sclerotic plaque in the coronary artery system
- Genetic testing for genes that impact CVD, such as ApoE, ACE and genes impacting inflammation and lipid metabolism
- Advanced cardiac risk panel including cholesterol particle numbers, and ApoB as well as lipoprotein(a)
- Inflammatory markers such as hsCRP, ferritin, and/or adiponectin
- Metabolic syndrome evaluation including HOMA-IR and/or hemoglobin A1C.

METHODS OF TRT

There are advantages and disadvantages to each method of TRT, and it is important to take individual factors and preferences for particular modes of delivery into account (Table 10.2):

- Transdermal patch
- Topical T
- Injectable T
- Oral
- Pellets
- Clomiphene
- HGH.

TABLE 10.2
Methods of Testosterone Replacement

TRT Option	Dose	Advantages	Disadvantages
Transdermal patch	5 and 2 mg patches, replaced nightly	Recreation of normal circadian rhythm	Skin irritation; irregular absorption; falls off; erratic levels
Testosterone gel or cream (branded or compounded)	5–10 g/day	Skin irritation less common than with patch	Irregular absorption; concern of transfer to others
Injectable (IM or SC) testosterone: • Cypionate • Enanthate • Propionate	Cypionate or enanthate: 50–100 mg q week or BIWk Propionate: 10–25 mg 2–3x/week	Inexpensive; reliable increase in levels	Invasive, mildly painful, injection site reactions; less frequently than weekly causes uneven levels
Testosterone undecanoate IM	750 mg every 10 weeks following a 4-wk loading dose	Convenient levels; 4–5 injections/year	Painful; must be done in office; POME and anaphylaxis warnings
Testosterone undecanoate oral	237–396 mg bid	Oral	BID dosing; possible hypertension impact; black box warning MACE
Testosterone pellets	600–900 mg	Leave it in and forget it for 3–6 months; stable blood levels	Invasive in-office procedure; harder to titrate or remove

Once on treatment, it is essential to monitor the patient for response and for side effects. Typically, response varies, but it is most common to see an impact first on sexual symptoms, generally within 2–3 weeks of initiating treatment followed by an improvement in energy after 4–6 weeks and finally changes in body compositions by 2–3 months.

Side effects may include injection site reactions or skin reactions if using a topical preparation. Gynecomastia may develop in men who have an increase in estradiol. Some men may notice acne or feeling more aggressive, though these symptoms are found mainly in men being treated with doses that are higher than therapeutic level.

Any ongoing monitoring schedule should include blood testing between 6 weeks and 3 months after initiating therapy or making any changes and then every 6 months thereafter.

Such monitoring should include:

- Total testosterone
- Estradiol
- Hematocrit
- PSA (if age 40 or over)
- DHEA-s if using DHEA treatment.

In addition, prostate digital rectal exam should be done every 6 months while on therapy, with a stop in treatment and referral to urology if a nodule is palpated.

NON-PHARMACEUTICAL APPROACHES

Certainly, there are non-pharmaceutical approaches to the symptoms of low testosterone, but there are fewer options to actually raise the level of the sex hormone when it is low.

EXERCISE

One of the strongest interventions to raise testosterone is exercise to both build lean body mass and lose fat. The more muscle mass a man has, the more testosterone he produces. The more fat he has, the more testosterone gets converted into estrogen via the aromatase enzyme. Thus, resistance and cardiovascular training are both important aspects of treatment.

Furthermore, exercise has been shown to improve many of the non-physical symptoms of low testosterone, such as depressed mood and diminished cognition, and resistance training will also improve bone mineral density, which is decreased when T is low.

NATURAL SUPPLEMENTS

There are few supplements that will actually raise testosterone. Zinc is a mild aromatase inhibitor; thus, it may raise T levels somewhat in a man with high aromatase activity. Other supplements have been shown to improve the sexual symptoms of low testosterone, such as Ashwagandha, Maca Root, Asian Ginseng, and Tribulus, but these do not raise the actual level of the hormone.

SUMMARY: MEN AND CVD

In general, it is recommended to check a total and bioavailable or free testosterone level in any man over 35 with symptoms listed above. Given the prevalence of low T levels and the impact on cardiovascular health, identifying men who could benefit from normalization of their levels not only can help address symptoms, but could also reduce early mortality from cardiovascular and other causes.

Given the role sex hormone optimization has for both men and women as relates to metabolic health, it makes sense that there is also an impact on cardiovascular health.

CONCLUSION

We believe that gonadal failure is associated with greater cardiovascular risk than hormone therapy, particularly when treated early in women. In this chapter, we have reviewed the seminal studies that support hormone therapy for patients experiencing perimenopause, menopause, and low testosterone in female and male patients. Several studies were poorly designed and flawed in their conclusion, leading to substantial confusion for clinicians. While hormone therapy is not FDA approved for primary or secondary prevention of CVD, we believe that hormone therapy can be provided safely and responsibly in the right candidates.

REFERENCES

1. Virani S., Alonso A., Aparicio H. J, et al. 2021. American Heart Association Council on Epidemiology and Prevention Statistics Committee and Stroke Statistics Subcommittee. Heart disease and stroke statistics-2021 update: a report from the American Heart Association. *Circulation*. 143:e254–743.
2. Arora S., Stouffer G. A., Kucharska-Newton A. M., et al. 2019. Twenty year trends and sex differences in young adults hospitalized with acute myocardial infarction. *Circulation*. 139:1047–56.
3. Khan S.U., Yedlpati S. H., Lone A.N., et al. 2021. A comparative analysis of premature heart disease- and cancer-related mortality in women in the USA, 1999–2018. *European Heart Journal Quality of Care and Clinical Outcomes*. 2021 Feb 8 qcaa099.
4. National Cancer Institute. 2021. Cancer Stat Facts: Female Breast Cancer. https://seer.cancer.gov/statfacts/html/breast.html.
5. Bairey Merz C. N., Andersen H., Sprague E, et al. 2017. Knowledge, attitudes, and beliefs regarding cardiovascular disease in women: the Women's Heart Alliance. *Journal of the American College of Cardiology*. 70:123–32.
6. Barrett-Connor E., Bush T. L. 1991. Estrogen and coronary heart disease in women. *JAMA*. 265: 1861–7.
7. Mefford M. T., Li B. H., Qian L., et al. 2000. Sex-specific trends in acute myocardial infarction within an integrated healthcare network, 2000 through 2014. *Circulation*. 141:509–19.
8. Mosconi L., Rahman A., Diaz I., et al. 2018. Increased Alzheimer's risk during the menopause transition: a 3-year longitudinal brain imaging study. *PLoS One*. 13:e0207885.
9. Rahman A., Jackson H., Hristov H., et al. 2019. Sex and gender driven modifiers of Alzheimer's: the role for estrogenic control across age, race, medical, and lifestyle risks. *Frontiers in Aging Neuroscience*. 11:315.
10. Cummings S. R., Duong T., Kenyon E., et al. 2002. Multiple outcomes of raloxifene evaluation (MORE) trial. Serum estradiol level and risk of breast cancer during treatment with raloxifene. *JAMA*. 287:216–20.
11. Hankinson S. E. 2005. Endogenous hormones and risk of breast cancer in postmenopausal women. *Breast Disease*. 24:3–15.
12. Bluming A. and C. Tavris. 2018. *Estrogen Matters: Why Taking Hormones in Menopause Can Improve Women's Well-Being and Lengthen Their Lives—Without Raising the Risk of Breast Cancer*. New York: Little Brown.
13. Gottfried S. 2013. *The Hormone Cure*. New York: Scribner.
14. Centers for Disease Control and Prevention. 2020. Women and Heart Disease. https://www.cdc.gov/heartdisease/women.htm.
15. Somani Y. B., Pawelczyk J. A., De Souza M. J., et al. 2019. Aging women and their endothelium: probing the relative role of estrogen on vasodilator function. *American Journal of Physiology-Heart and Circulatory Physiology*. 317:H395–404.
16. Fåhraeus L. 1988. The effects of estradiol on blood lipids and lipoproteins in postmenopausal women. *Obstetrics & Gynecology*. 72:18S–22S.
17. Kovats S. 2015. Estrogen receptors regulate innate immune cells and signaling pathways. *Cellular Immunology*. 294:63–9.
18. Song C. H., Kim N., Sohn S. H., et al. 2018. Effects of 17β-estradiol on colonic permeability and inflammation in an azoxymethane/dextran sulfate sodium-induced colitis mouse model. *Gut and Liver*. 12:682–93.
19. Miller V. M., Lahr B. D., Bailey K. R., et al. 2016. Longitudinal effects of menopausal hormone treatments on platelet characteristics and cell-derived microvesicles. *Platelets*. 27:32–42.

20. Ramesh S. S., Christopher R., Indira D. B., et al. 2019. The vascular protective role of oestradiol: a focus on postmenopausal oestradiol deficiency and aneurysmal subarachnoid haemorrhage. *Biological Reviews of the Cambridge Philosophical Society.* 94:1897–917.

21. Westendorp I. C., Bots M. L., Grobbee D. E., et al. 1999. Menopausal status and distensibility of the common carotid artery. *Arteriosclerosis, Thrombosis, and Vascular Biology.* 19:713–7.

22. Naftolin F., Friedenthal J., Nachtigall R., et al. 2019. Cardiovascular health and the menopausal woman: the role of estrogen and when to begin and end hormone treatment. *F1000Research.* 8:1576.

23. O'Donnell E., Floras J. S., Harvey P. J. 2014. Estrogen status and the renin angiotensin aldosterone system. *American Journal of Physiology - Regulatory, Integrative and Comparative Physiology.* 307:R498–500.

24. Moreau K. L., Hildreth K. L., Meditz A. L., et al. 2012. Endothelial function is impaired across the stages of the menopause transition in healthy women. *The Journal of Clinical Endocrinology and Metabolism.* 97:4692–700.

25. Hildreth K. L., Kohrt W. M., Moreau K.L. 2014. Oxidative stress contributes to large elastic arterial stiffening across the stages of the menopausal transition. *Menopause.* 21:624–32.

26. Roger V. L., Go A.S., Lloyd-Jones D. M., et al. 2011. American Heart Association Statistics Committee and Stroke Statistics Subcommittee. Heart disease and stroke statistics--2011 update: a report from the American Heart Association. *Circulation.* 123:e18–e209.

27. Colditz G. A., Willett W. C., Stampfer M. J., et al. 1987. Menopause and the risk of coronary heart disease in women. *New England Journal of Medicine.* 316:1105–10.

28. El Khoudary S. R. 2017. Gaps, limitations and new insights on endogenous estrogen and follicle stimulating hormone as related to risk of cardiovascular disease in women traversing the menopause: a narrative review. *Maturitas.* 104:44–53.

29. Gordon T., Kannel W. B., Hjortland M. C., et al. 1978. Menopause and coronary heart disease. The Framingham Study. *Annals of Internal Medicine.* 89:157–61.

30. Sprague B. L., Trentham-Dietz A., Cronin K. A. 2012. A sustained decline in postmenopausal hormone use: results from the National Health and Nutrition Examination Survey, 1999–2010. *Obstetrics & Gynecology.* 120:595–603.

31. Bechlioulis A., Kalantaridou S. N., Naka K. K., et al. 2010. Endothelial function, but not carotid intima-media thickness, is affected early in menopause and is associated with severity of hot flushes. *The Journal of Clinical Endocrinology and Metabolism.* 95:1199–206.

32. Gast G. C., Grobbee D. E., Pop V. J., et al. 2008. Menopausal complaints are associated with cardiovascular risk factors. *Hypertension.* 51:1492–8.

33. Thurston R. C., Matthews K. A., Chang Y., et al. 2016. Changes in heart rate variability during vasomotor symptoms among midlife women. *Menopause.* 23:499–505.

34. Crandall C. J., Aragaki A., Cauley J. A., et al. 2015. Associations of menopausal vasomotor symptoms with fracture incidence. *The Journal of Clinical Endocrinology and Metabolism.* 100:524–34.

35. Thurston R. C., Wu M., Aizenstein H. J., et al. 2020. Sleep characteristics and white matter hyperintensities among midlife women. *Sleep.* 43:zsz298.

36. Worsley R., Bell R., Kulkarni J., et al. The association between vasomotor symptoms and depression during perimenopause: a systematic review. *Maturitas.* 77:111–7.

37. Thurston R. C., Aizenstein H. J., Derby C. A., et al. 2016. Menopausal hot flashes and white matter hyperintensities. *Menopause.* 23:27–32.

38. Cho E. J., Min Y.J., Oh M. S., et al. 2011. Effects of the transition from premenopause to postmenopause on lipids and lipoproteins: quantification and related parameters. *The Korean Journal of Internal Medicine.* 26:47–53.

39. Ambikairajah A., Walsh E., Cherbuin N. 2019. Lipid profile differences during menopause: a review with meta-analysis. *Menopause.* 26:1327–33.

40. Li H., Sun R., Chen Q., et al. 2021. Association between HDL-C levels and menopause: a meta-analysis. *Hormones* 20:49–59.

41. Schaefer E. J., Lamon-Fava S., Cohn S. D., et al. 1994. Effects of age, sex, and menopausal status on plasma low density lipoprotein cholesterol and apolipoprotein B levels in the Framingham Offspring Study. *Journal of Lipid Research.* 35:779–92.

42. Jenner J. L., Ordovas J. M., Lamon-Fava S., et al. 1993. Effects of age, sex, and menopausal status on plasma lipoprotein(a) levels. The Framingham Offspring Study. *Circulation.* 87:1135–41.

43. Tselmin S., Julius U., Müller G., et al. 2009. Cardiovascular events in patients with increased lipoprotein (a) - retrospective data analysis in an outpatient department of lipid disorders. *Atherosclerosis Supplements.* 10:79–84.

44. Yamamoto A., Horibe H., Mabuchi H., et al. 1999. Analysis of serum lipid levels in Japanese men and women according to body mass index. Increase in risk of atherosclerosis in postmenopausal women. Research Group on Serum Lipid Survey 1990 in Japan. *Atherosclerosis*. 143:55–73.
45. Wang Q., Ferreira D. L. S., Nelson S. M., et al. Metabolic characterization of menopause: cross-sectional and longitudinal evidence. *BMC Medicine*. 16:17.
46. El Khoudary S. R., Brooks M. M., Thurston R. C., et al. 2014. Lipoprotein subclasses and endogenous sex hormones in women at midlife. *Journal of Lipid Research*. 55:1498–504.
47. Christian R. C., Dumesic D. A., Behrenbeck T., et al. 2003. Prevalence and predictors of coronary artery calcification in women with polycystic ovary syndrome. *The Journal of Clinical Endocrinology and Metabolism*. 88:2562–8.
48. McCartney C. R., Marshall J. 2016. Clinical practice. Polycystic Ovary Syndrome. *New England Journal of Medicine*. 375:54–64.
49. Osibogun O., Ogunmoroti O., Michos E. D. 2020. Polycystic ovary syndrome and cardiometabolic risk: opportunities for cardiovascular disease prevention. *Trends in Cardiovascular Medicine*. 30:399–404.
50. Park J. K., Lim Y. H., Kim K. S., et al. 2013. Body fat distribution after menopause and cardiovascular disease risk factors: Korean National Health and Nutrition Examination Survey 2010. *Journal of Women's Health*. 22:587–94.
51. Mackey R. H., Kuller L. H., Sutton-Tyrrell K., et al. 2002. Lipoprotein subclasses and coronary artery calcium in postmenopausal women from the healthy women study. *The American Journal of Cardiology*. 90:71i–6i.
52. Nasr A., Matthews K. A., Brooks M. M., et al. 2020. Vasomotor symptoms and lipids/lipoprotein subclass metrics in midlife women: does level of endogenous estradiol matter? The SWAN HDL Ancillary Study. *Journal of Clinical Lipidology*. 14:685–94.
53. Anagnostis P., Stevenson J. C., Crook D., et al. 2015. Effects of menopause, gender and age on lipids and high-density lipoprotein cholesterol subfractions. *Maturitas*. 81:62–8.
54. Rettberg J. R., Yao J., Brinton R. D. 2014. Estrogen: a master regulator of bioenergetic systems in the brain and body. *Frontiers in Neuroendocrinology*. 35:8–30.
55. Yan H., Yang W., Zhou F., et al. 2019. Estrogen improves insulin sensitivity and suppresses gluconeogenesis via the transcription factor foxo1. *Diabetes*. 68:291–304.
56. Gupte A. A., Pownall H. J., Hamilton D. J. 2015. Estrogen: an emerging regulator of insulin action and mitochondrial function. *Journal of Diabetes Research*. 2015:916585.
57. Barros R. P., Gustafsson J. Å. 2011. Estrogen receptors and the metabolic network. *Cell Metabolism*. 14:289–99.
58. Emerging Risk Factors Collaboration, Sarwar N., Gao P., et al. 2010. Diabetes mellitus, fasting blood glucose concentration, and risk of vascular disease: a collaborative meta-analysis of 102 prospective studies. *Lancet*. 375:2215–22.
59. Ahn S. V., Kim H. C., Nam C. M., et al. 2018. Sex difference in the effect of the fasting serum glucose level on the risk of coronary heart disease. *Journal of Cardiology*. 71:149–54.
60. Lawlor D. A., Fraser A., Ebrahim S., et al. 2007. Independent associations of fasting insulin, glucose, and glycated haemoglobin with stroke and coronary heart disease in older women. *PLoS Medicine*. 4:e263.
61. Anagnostis P., Bitzer J., Cano A., et al. 2020. Menopause symptom management in women with dyslipidemias: an EMAS clinical guide. *Maturitas*. 135:82–8.
62. Anagnostis P., Karras S., Lambrinoudaki I., et al. 2016. Lipoprotein(a) in postmenopausal women: assessment of cardiovascular risk and therapeutic options. *International Journal of Clinical Practice*. 70:967–77.
63. Barrett-Connor E., Grady D. 1998. Hormone replacement therapy, heart disease, and other considerations. *Annual Review of Public Health*. 19:55–72.
64. Goldman L., Tosteson A. N. 1991. Uncertainty about postmenopausal estrogen. Time for action, not debate. *New England Journal of Medicine*. 325:800–2.
65. Hulley S., Grady D., Bush T., et al. 1998. Randomized trial of estrogen plus progestin for secondary prevention of coronary heart disease in postmenopausal women. Heart and Estrogen/progestin Replacement Study (HERS) Research Group. *JAMA*. 280:605–13.
66. Rossouw J. E., Anderson G. L., Prentice R. L., et al. 2002. Risks and benefits of estrogen plus progestin in healthy postmenopausal women: principal results From the Women's Health Initiative randomized controlled trial. *JAMA*. 288:321–33.

67. Speroff L. 2004. A clinician's review of the WHI-related literature. *International Journal of Fertility and Women's Medicine.* 49:252–67.
68. Rossouw J. E., Prentice R. L., Manson J. E., et al. 2007. Postmenopausal hormone therapy and risk of cardiovascular disease by age and years since menopause. *JAMA.* 297:1465–77.
69. Salpeter S. R., Walsh J. M., Greyber E., et al. Brief report: coronary heart disease events associated with hormone therapy in younger and older women. A meta-analysis. *Journal of General Internal Medicine.* 21:363–6.
70. Schierbeck L. L., Rejnmark L., Tofteng C. L., et al. 2012. Effect of hormone replacement therapy on cardiovascular events in recently postmenopausal women: randomised trial. *BMJ.* 345:e6409.
71. Hodis H. N., Mack W. J. 2014. Hormone replacement therapy and the association with coronary heart disease and overall mortality: clinical application of the timing hypothesis. *The Journal of Steroid Biochemistry and Molecular Biology.* 142:68–75.
72. Clarkson T. B., Meléndez G. C., Appt S. E. 2013. Timing hypothesis for postmenopausal hormone therapy: its origin, current status, and future. Menopause. 20:342–53.
73. Hodis H. N., Collins P., Mack W. J., et al. 2012. The timing hypothesis for coronary heart disease prevention with hormone therapy: past, present and future in perspective. *Climacteric.* 15:217–28.
74. Mikkola T. S., Clarkson T. B. 2002. Estrogen replacement therapy, atherosclerosis, and vascular function. *Cardiovascular Research.* 53:605–19.
75. Hodis H. N., Mack W. J., Lobo R. A., et al. 2001. Estrogen in the prevention of atherosclerosis. A randomized, double-blind, placebo-controlled trial. *Annals of Internal Medicine.* 135:939–53.
76. Herrington D. M., Reboussin D. M., Brosnihan K. B., et al. 2000. Effects of estrogen replacement on the progression of coronary-artery atherosclerosis. *New England Journal of Medicine.* 343:522–9.
77. Hodis H. N., Mack W. J., Henderson V. W., et al. 2016. Vascular effects of early versus late postmenopausal treatment with estradiol. *New England Journal of Medicine.* 374:1221–31.
78. Goodman N. F., Cobin R. H., Ginzburg S. B., et al. 2011. American Association of Clinical Endocrinologists medical guidelines for clinical practice for the diagnosis and treatment of menopause. *Endocrine Practice.* 6:1–25.
79. Pinkerton J. V. 2020. Hormone therapy for postmenopausal women. *New England Journal of Medicine.* 382:446–55.
80. Shufelt C., Bretsky P., Almeida C. M., et al. 2010. DHEA-S levels and cardiovascular disease mortality in postmenopausal women: results from the National Institutes of Health--National Heart, Lung, and Blood Institute (NHLBI)-sponsored Women's Ischemia Syndrome Evaluation (WISE). *The Journal of Clinical Endocrinology and Metabolism.* 95:4985–92.
81. American College of Obstetricians and Gynecologists. 2014. ACOG Practice Bulletin No. 141: management of menopausal symptoms. *Obstetrics & Gynecology.* 123:202–16.
82. Cobin R. H., Goodman N. F., AACE Reproductive Endocrinology Scientific Committee. 2017. American Association of Clinical Endocrinologists and American College of Endocrinology position statement on menopause–2017 update. *Endocrine Practice.* 23:869–81.
83. Stuenkel C. A., Davis S. R., Gompel A., et al. 2015. Treatment of symptoms of the menopause: an Endocrine Society clinical practice guideline. *The Journal of Clinical Endocrinology and Metabolism.* 100:3975–4011.
84. The NAMS 2017 Hormone Therapy Position Statement Advisory Panel. 2017. The 2017 hormone therapy position statement of The North American Menopause Society. *Menopause.* 24:728–53.
85. US Preventive Services Task Force, Grossman D. C., Curry S. J., et al. 2017. Hormone therapy for the primary prevention of chronic conditions in postmenopausal women: US Preventive Services Task Force recommendation statement. *JAMA.* 318:2224–33.
86. Centers for Disease Control and Prevention. 2020. Heart Disease Facts. https://www.cdc.gov/heartdisease/facts.htm.
87. American College of Cardiology. 2018. One Size Does Not Fit All: The Role of Sex, Gender, Race and Ethnicity in Cardiovascular Medicine. https://www.acc.org/latest-in-cardiology/articles/2018/10/14/12/42/cover-story-one-size-does-not-fit-all-sex-gender-race-and-ethnicity-in-cardiovascular-medicine.
88. Oskui P. M., French W. J., Herring M. J., et al. 2013. Testosterone and the cardiovascular system: a comprehensive review of the clinical literature. *Journal of the American Heart Association.* 2:e000272.
89. Kloner R. A., Carson C. 3rd, Dobs A., et al. 2016. Testosterone and cardiovascular disease. *Journal of the American College of Cardiology.* 67:545–57.

90. Brand J. S., Rovers M. M., Yeap B. B., et al. 2014. Testosterone, sex hormone-binding globulin and the metabolic syndrome in men: an individual participant data meta-analysis of observational studies. *PLoS One*. 9:e100409.

91. Kupelian V., Shabsigh R., Araujo A. B., et al. 2006. Erectile dysfunction as a predictor of the metabolic syndrome in aging men: results from the Massachusetts Male Aging Study. *The Journal of Urology*. 176:222–6.

92. Haider K. S., Haider A., Saad, F., et al. 2020. Remission of type 2 diabetes following long-term treatment with injectable testosterone undecanoate in patients with hypogonadism and type 2 diabetes: 11-year data from a real-world registry study. *Diabetes, Obesity and Metabolism*. 22:2055–68.

93. Mohamad N. V., Wong S. K., Wan Hasan W. N., et al. 2019. The relationship between circulating testosterone and inflammatory cytokines in men. *Aging Male*. 22(2):129–40.

94. Inman B.A., Sauver J. L., Jacobson D. J., et al. 2009. A population-based, longitudinal study of erectile dysfunction and future coronary artery disease. *Mayo Clinic Proceedings*. 84:108–13.

95. Mulligan T., Frick M. F., Zuraw Q. C., et al. Prevalence of hypogonadism in males aged at least 45 years: the HIM study. *International Journal of Clinical Practice*. 60:762–69.

96. Morgentaler A., Miner M. M., Caliber M., et al. 2015. Testosterone therapy and cardiovascular risk: advances and controversies. *Mayo Clinic Proceedings*. 90:224–51.

97. Vigen R., O'Donnell C. I., Barón A. E., et al. 2013. Association of testosterone therapy with mortality, myocardial infarction, and stroke in men with low testosterone levels. *JAMA*. 310:1829–36.

98. Finkle W. D., Greenland S., Ridgeway G. K., et al. 2014. Increased risk of non-fatal myocardial infarction following testosterone therapy prescription in men. *PLoS One*. 9:e85805.

99. US Food and Drug Administration. Citizen petition denial response from FDA CDER to Public Citizen. Regulations.gov website [Internet] Washington, D.C.: Regulationsgov; c2014. [cited 2017 Sep 9]. Available from: http://www.regulations.gov/#!documentDetail;D=FDA-2014-P-0258-0003

100. U.S. Food and Drug Administration. 2018. FDA Drug Safety Communication: FDA cautions about using testosterone products for low testosterone due to aging; requires labeling change to inform of possible increased risk of heart attack and stroke with use. https://www.fda.gov/drugs/drug-safety-and-availability/fda-drug-safety-communication-fda-cautions-about-using-testosterone-products-low-testosterone-due.

101. Miner M., Morgentaler A., Khera M., et al. 2018. The state of testosterone therapy since the FDA's 2015 labelling changes: indications and cardiovascular risk. *Clinical Endocrinology*. 89:3–10.

102. Rutkowski K., Sowa P., Rutkowska-Tulipska J., et al. 2014. Dehydroepiandrosterone (DHEA): hypes and hopes. *Drugs*. 74:1195–207.

11 The Heartbreak of Wheat-Related Disorders

Wheat, Gluten and Cardiovascular Disease

Thomas O'Bryan

CONTENTS

Frequency of a Wheat-Related Disorder 254
The Immune Response to Wheat 255
Causes of Wheats' Immunogenicity 256
Abbreviations 259
References 259

Although it is extremely unusual for an author to begin a chapter in such a text with a personal story, this will speak to the 'heartbreak' of a wheat-related disorder (WRD).

When my father died suddenly of a myocardial infarction at the age of 64, with no identified cardiovascular risk factors and a forensic pathologist's report of 'death by myocardial infarction (MI) with no known cause', questions arose. In conversation, the physician first apologized, as this was only the second time in his career he could not identify the cause of death. He reported there was no clot visible which immediately raised alarm bells. The left descending coronary, the 'widow maker', had approximately 30% blockage—not enough for an MI.[1] Toxicology screens of blood and lung biopsy (looking for inhaled toxins) were negative. Full-body scans for needle marks was negative. The doctor apologized for being unable to identify the cause of the MI. The 'heartbreak' to our family in losing our patriarch was all-encompassing (as is the case for most families when suddenly and unexpectedly losing a loved one). This author's investigation of the literature to leave no stone unturned, eventually led to Dr. Kilmer McCully. 'Dr. McCully, I know hyperhomocysteinemia can cause vasospasm. Can an elevated homocysteine (Hcy) level cause vasospasm of the left descending coronary artery at the site of a 30% blockage effectively making it 100% blockage? And after the MI and loss of life, could the blood vessel then relax and leave no evidence of the 'widow maker effect?' His response was startling. 'From our experiments, it is entirely possible such a spasm can occur at the location of a vulnerable, inflamed artery'.

By the time of this discussion, my father had long since been laid to rest—no way to check his homocysteine level. So the next best thing? I tested positive for elevated Hcy, along with my brother, my sister and 19 of my first cousins (my father had six siblings). The genetics suggested with a high degree of probability that my father had likely died of an undiagnosed elevated Hcy.

Back in the 1980s, Hcy was not a common screen performed in a cardiovascular risk profile. This simple $40 blood test could have given us many more years with my father. The 'heartbreak' to our family in losing our patriarch was all-encompassing. The goal of this chapter is to minimize the

DOI: 10.1201/9781003137849-11

'post-shock' heartbreak of a WRD, a common trigger in fueling the inflammation of cardiovascular disease (CVD), with or without celiac disease.

It is unlikely that any reader of this text has not already developed an opinion or belief on the topic of gluten- and wheat-related disorders. The topic has inundated the literature and infiltrated the minds of consumers for decades. Hundreds of studies in the past two decades have changed the paradigm of WRDs from a primary focus on celiac disease to a recognition of varied presentations in numerous systems of the body from multiple components of incompletely digested wheat.

A report from the Institute of Medicine 'Crossing the Quality Chasm' tells us that despite exponential technological advancements that have been made, the fundamental approach to medical education has not changed since 1910.[2] Patients present to our offices with CVD symptoms. We now recognize this as an acute presentation of a chronic inflammatory disease (CID). Thus, the clinician now is faced with separate, distinct, necessary lines of thought—stabilize the acute manifestations and address the underlying CID.

This chapter will address the science behind wheat consumption and its recognition as one of the two most powerful triggers of intestinal inflammation, with or without celiac disease, and give the reader a foundational understanding of the contribution of wheat to the mechanisms of pathology in CVD.

Effecting population health improvements requires understanding not only of the injuries and diseases that drive health burdens, but also the risks that drive injury and disease. The combination of increasing metabolic risks and population aging continues to drive the increasing trends in non-communicable diseases at the global level presenting an enormous public health challenge. Understanding the environmental, behavioral, and metabolic risks that drive chronic disease is the mechanism by which public health efforts can most efficiently and effectively prevent health loss.[3] This chapter addresses the role of WRD in contributing to the metabolic underpinnings of CVD.

The Global Burden of Diseases, Injuries, and Risk Factors Study (GBD 2017) cites diet as a major contributing factor behind the rise in hypertension, diabetes, obesity, and other CVD components. This study is the most comprehensive population-level comparative risk assessment across countries and risks, and offers a useful tool for synthesizing evidence on risks of morbidity, mortality, and risk–outcome associations. Quantification of the disease burden caused by different risks informs prevention by providing an account of health loss different from that provided by a disease-by-disease analysis and provides a benchmarking tool to assist the focus of local decision making.[3]

Tissue inflammation represents the 'common soil' of multifactorial diseases, such as chronic inflammatory rheumatic disease or type 2 diabetes, obesity, inflammatory bowel diseases, CVDs, neurodegenerative diseases, asthma, cancer, and accelerated aging.[4]

Originally identified in the 1870s as a lipid-storage disease of the arterial wall,[5] atherosclerosis was recognized as a CID in 1986.[6] A substantial body of evidence identifies inflammatory and immunologic mechanisms at the endothelial level as a driving force behind CVD, especially atherosclerosis and its clinical sequelae.[7,8]

Therapeutic decision making for the clinician must take into account the differentiation of cardiac inflammation from systemic inflammation. The causes of cardiac inflammation may vary depending on the part of the heart that is affected—the endocardium, the myocardium, or the pericardium.[9] However, molecular mimicry initiated by a WRD has been identified as a common mechanism initiating inflammation in cardiac tissue.[10] The inflammatory cytokines inducing cardiac remodeling and dysfunction can originate from the heart itself (cardiokines), produced by cardiomyocytes, cardiac endothelial cells, cardiac fibroblasts, cardiac tissue macrophages, and cardiac infiltrated immune cells, or can be of extra-cardiac tissue including adipose tissue, gut, and lymphoid organs. This chapter will address the gut contribution to systemic inflammation fueled by a WRD, which may impact on cardiac function.

The large diversity of inflammatory triggers further addresses the need for a tailored characterization of inflammation enabling differentiation of inflammation and subsequent target-specific strategies.[11] As you will see, the potential complications of a WRD are startling. For example, untreated CD children had larger left ventricle end diastolic dimension, reduced left ventricular ejection fraction (<55%), and a higher (>0.6) myocardial performance index as compared to controls. Re-evaluation after one year with good dietary compliance showed changes in isovolumic relaxation time and deceleration time, reflecting improved cardiac diastolic function. GFD-compliant patients had lower myocardial performance index (MPI) than non-compliant patients, reflecting improvement in load-independent echocardiographic parameters.[12]

The necessity of considering a WRD when investigating triggers of cardiovascular dysfunction is supported by the disappointing results of anti-inflammatory strategies used in heart failure (HF) patients so far.[13,14] The characterization and differentiation of inflammation will allow classification of patients into subclasses to provide appropriate treatment. For example, with 85% of acute pericarditis identified as idiopathic,[15] in the absence of an identifiable infection, searching for the trigger of inflammation may be life-saving and occasionally is as simple as eliminating a food from the diet.[16]

There are numerous mechanisms of cardiac involvement in WRDs, which may include:

- molecular mimicry activating autoimmune pathogenic mechanisms[17]
- increased intestinal permeability which leads to increased systemic absorption of various luminal antigens or infectious agents that may cause myocardial damage through immune-mediated mechanisms[18,19]
- neo-antigen formation activating a protective immune response[20]
- systemic-wide activation of metalloproteases[21]
- premature atherosclerosis from chronic systemic inflammation[22]
- myocardial injury secondary to an immune response directed against the antigen present in both the myocardium and small intestine[23,24]
- villous atrophy causing poor absorption of several nutrients such as thiamine, riboflavin, magnesium, calcium, selenium, and carnitine, which play an active role in myocardial metabolism.[25]

Such a differentiated approach identifying sources of inflammation is in line with the growing appreciation and ongoing introduction of precision medicine in cardiology.[26] Precision medicine incorporates standard clinical and health record data with advanced panomics (i.e., genomics, transcriptomics, epigenomics, proteomics, metabolomics, microbiomics) for deep phenotyping.[27] These phenotypic data can then be analyzed within the framework of molecular interaction (interactome) networks to uncover previously unrecognized disease phenotypes, relationships between comorbidities, and unique inflammatory triggers to the individual.[28] Functional medicine addresses chronic disease by delivering precision medicine with an emphasis on reducing the triggers of inflammation. The ability to deliver precision medicine relies on one's capability to not only collect data, but also organize it in a way that extracts an understanding of a patient's biological processes and then maps these processes to human disease.[29,30]

Comorbidities are the norm in CVD, rather than the exception. Patients with HF have the highest prevalence of comorbidity (92%) compared with those with other cardiovascular conditions such as stroke (81%) and CHD (80%).[31] Thus, Health-Related Quality of Life (HRQoL) protocols are recommended when addressing CVD.[32] And how do we focus on enhancing HRQoL in our busy offices?

In a first-of-its-kind analysis of the functional medicine approach to precision medicine, a retrospective cohort study was performed to compare HRQoL in 7252 patients aged 18 years or older treated in a functional medicine setting with propensity score (PS)–matched patients in a primary care setting—31.2% of these participants had a diagnostic category including CVD. Sensitivity analyses assessed improvement of patients seen at both 6 and 12 months. The study included patients who visited the Cleveland Clinic Centre for Functional Medicine or the Cleveland Clinic Family Health Centre between 1 April 2015 and 1 March 2017. Patients had a baseline Patient-Reported

Outcome Measurement Information System (PROMIS), Global Physical Health (GPH) score and at least 1 follow-up score determined within a year of their initial visit.

Although recommended, but not inherent to all functional medicine practices, the Centre for Functional Medicine at Cleveland Clinic requires that all new patients see a registered dietitian and health coach, in addition to a clinician, as part of their initial visit. Patients also have the option to meet with a behavioral health therapist as part of any visit. Dietitians and health coaches are integral because they address the nutritional, psychological, and social aspects of patients' illnesses, and support and promote long-term self-management, which are components needed for the treatment of various chronic conditions.[33] The results were startling. Patients in the Functional Medicine Centre with data at both 6 and 12 months demonstrated improvements in PROMIS GPH (mean [SD], 2.61 [6.53]) that were significantly larger compared with patients seen at the Family Health Centre (mean [SD], 0.25 [6.54]) ($p =.02$ in 91 PS-matched pairs). The Functional Medicine Model of Precision Medicine care demonstrated significantly larger beneficial and sustainable associations with patient-reported HRQoL.[34]

Thus, at a primary investigative level, the practitioner will benefit from asking the question 'how can I identify, and then reduce the multiple triggers of inflammation?' to a patient who presents with cardiovascular concerns.

A primary initiator of a systemic inflammatory response in the human body is the choice of foods consumed habitually.[7] For the past two decades, we have known that the simple addition to the diet of chocolate, wine, fish, nuts, garlic, fruit, and vegetables represented a reduction in CVD events by 76%, an increase in total life expectancy for men of 6.6 years, an increase in life expectancy free from CVD of 9.0 years, and a decrease in life expectancy having to live with CVD of 2.4 years. The corresponding differences for women were 4.8, 8.1, and 3.3 years (Figure 11.1).[35]

One of the most researched conditions diagnosed from an adverse reaction to food is celiac disease—an immune-activated response to the environmental trigger, wheat, initiating an

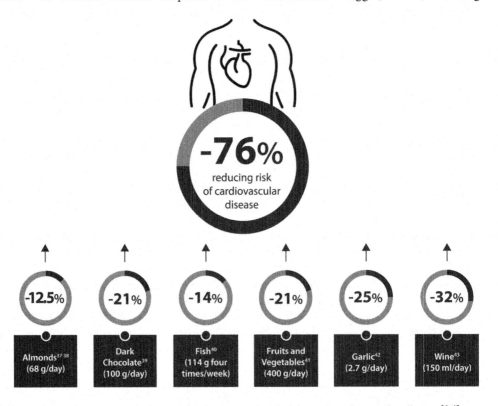

FIGURE 11.1 Effect of ingredients of the polymeal in reducing risk of cardiovascular disease.[36–42]

autoimmune attack initially on the small intestine. Celiac disease has traditionally been clinically considered and then investigated with patients presenting with gastrointestinal (GI) symptoms. However, for every adverse reaction to wheat presenting with GI symptoms, there are eight patients presenting without GI symptoms.[43] The ratio is 8:1. The classic intestinal presentation of CD of malnutrition, chronic diarrhea, a failure to thrive and nutritional deficiencies is disappearing and extraintestinal presentations are being recognized more frequently. Nowadays, we are witnessing an epidemiological shift in the disease phenotype toward a more advanced age, and increased prevalence of latent, GI hyposymptomatic or GI asymptomatic presentations.[44] Thus, requiring a GI complaint before considering a WRD will miss the vast majority of patients with a sensitivity to wheat. These patients may present with cognitive concerns,[45] cardiovascular concerns,[46] musculoskeletal concerns,[47] dermatological concerns,[48] insulin resistance,[49] anemia,[50] etc. Thus, requiring GI complaints as a prerequisite in considering an adverse reaction to wheat will allow a majority to escape diagnosis. This is a critical point of recognition for the clinician when considering an association between WRDs and cardiovascular health.

A second contributor in missing a WRD is the emphasis of considering celiac disease as its primary manifestation. This concept is a historical misconception. After referral from a primary physician with a concern of a WRD to secondary gastrointestinal care, 7% of these patients are identified as being positive for celiac disease with 93% identified as non-celiac gluten sensitivity.[51] Thus, the frequency of a WRD without CD is much more common, often less obvious to the clinician, and more challenging to identify.

The 8:1 ratio of extraintestinal versus intestinal symptoms is not limited to celiac disease. In a prospective 1-year study of suspected non-celiac gluten sensitivity (NCGS)–related disorders from 38 Italian centers (27 centers of adult gastroenterology, 5 of internal medicine, 4 of pediatrics, and 2 of allergy)—all recognized as referral centers of excellence and included in the register of the Italian Health Ministry for the diagnosis of gluten-related disorders—53% of patients presented with non-abdominal complaints. The most frequent extraintestinal manifestations were fatigue and lack of well-being, reported by 64% and 68%, respectively, of the enrolled subjects. In addition, a high prevalence of neuropsychiatric symptoms including headache (54%), anxiety (39%), 'foggy mind' (38%), and arm/leg numbness (32%) was recorded. Other extraintestinal manifestations emerging from the analysis of the survey responses were joint/muscle pain often misdiagnosed as fibromyalgia (31%), weight loss (25%), anemia (22%), due both to iron deficiency and low folic acid, depression (18%), dermatitis (18%), and skin rash (29%).[52] With its global impact in the body and lack of isolated tissue vulnerability, a high degree of suspicion is required for a clinician to investigate a presenting patient for a WRD. Any of the above comorbidities, in a presenting cardiovascular patient, may emphasize the value of screening for a WRD.

An overly active immune response to wheat increases the risk of early atherosclerosis, as suggested by the presence of chronic inflammation, vascular impairment, unfavorable biochemical patterns, and relative lack of the classical risk factors.[53] Specific cardiovascular maladies, including cardiomyopathy,[54] ischemic heart disease,[55] myocarditis,[56] arrhythmias,[57] and premature atherosclerosis,[58] are substantially more prevalent in individuals with an immune response to wheat as compared to individuals without such a response.[22,59]

With such a plethora of clinical and laboratory research on the frequency and variance of manifestations of a WRD, the obvious question arises, 'why isn't a WRD more known and looked for, with or without CD'?

Time lags in the transition from solid, reproducible research into clinical practice are startling. It is frequently stated that it takes an average of 17 years for translational research evidence to reach clinical practice.[60]

One recent study estimating the economic benefit of CVD research in the United Kingdom between 1975 and 2005, found an internal rate of return (IRR) of CVD research of 39% per annum. In other words, a £1.00 investment in public/charitable CVD research produced a stream of benefits equivalent to earning £0.39 per year in perpetuity. Varying the lag time from 10 to 25 years produced rates of return of 13% and 6%, respectively, illustrating that shortening the lag between bench and bedside improves the overall benefit of cardiovascular research.[61]

We must do better in educating our clinicians on the value of accurately screening for a WRD, and thus the true 'Heartbreak of a Wheat-Related Disorder'.

FREQUENCY OF A WHEAT-RELATED DISORDER

A 'canary in a coal mine' is an advanced warning of some danger. The metaphor originates from the times when miners used to carry caged canaries into the mines while at work; if there was any methane or carbon monoxide in the mine, the canary would die before the levels of the gas reached those hazardous to humans, and thus signal to the miners to exit the mine immediately.

The increase in the prevalence of celiac disease has been exponential in recent decades, and seroprevalence studies indicate that this is a true rise, rather than one due to increased awareness and testing.[62] If a WRD were a relatively rare occurrence, the value of this topic (and chapter) could be challenged. That, however, is not the case. The recognition of the dramatic increase in the prevalence of CD gives pause and supports the rationale of considering a WRD as a contributor to the inflammatory cascade of CVD. Numerous independent studies worldwide are identifying this continuing rise in CD (Figure 11.2):

- During the past few decades, CD prevalence increased five-fold overall in the United States since 1974. This increase was identified as due to an increasing number of subjects that lost the immunological tolerance to gluten.[63]
- A threefold increase in the incidence rate for CD in the Norwegian pediatric population during the decade of 2000–2010.[64]
- A fourfold increase in the incidence of CD in the United Kingdom over 22 years (1990–2011).[65]
- A 4.5-fold increase in the United States during 45 years of follow-up (1954–1999) with a nearly fourfold increased risk of early death (hazard ratio = 3.9; 95% CI, 2.0–7.5; $p < .001$).[66]
- 2+-fold increase in Italy between 1993 and 2016.[67]
- The prevalence of CD among children in Brazil is 5.4 times higher than that found in the present elderly group.[68]
- A 6.4-fold increase in 'Classic CD' in Scotland in the 20 years from 1990 to 2009 with an increase in non-classic presentation (children with a mono-symptomatic presentation with extraintestinal symptoms) increased by 15.66% ($p < .05$).[69]

Unfortunately, available diagnostic tools and scope of testing for a WRD beyond CD have been restricted and incomplete until the last decade.[7] Thus, comparative studies over decades for WRD outside of CD are unavailable. However, the reader is reminded that after referral from a primary

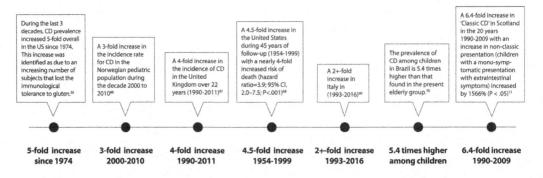

FIGURE 11.2 Increased frequency of a wheat-related disorder.

physician with a concern of a WRD to secondary gastrointestinal care, 7% of these patients are identified as being positive for celiac disease with 93% identified as non-celiac gluten sensitivity. Thus, with confirming evidence of the loss of oral tolerance and dramatic increase in CD world-wide, an assumption of likely increase to WRDs outside of CD is rational.

In summary, since the 1950s, the worldwide increase in loss of immune tolerance to wheat has exploded!

THE IMMUNE RESPONSE TO WHEAT

Because the first serology screen of a WRD identified a gluten peptide (alpha gliadin), the world has focused on gluten proteins as the exclusive toxic component of wheat. In the past few decades, gluten has been recognized as a primary, but not exclusive trigger of WRDs. Other components of incompletely digested wheat have been identified in initiating an immune response to wheat (Figure 11.2). Thus, there is increasing evidence among the scientific community that gluten is only one trigger of a WRD. Numerous studies now identify other fragments of poorly digested wheat which may activate an immune response and the onset of a WRD.[70]

Multiple components of poorly digested wheat, outside the family of gluten proteins, may have deleterious effects on cardiovascular function including fermentable oligo-, di-, and monosaccharides and polyols (FODMAPS),[71] wheat amylase trypsin inhibitors (ATIs),[72] wheat germ agglutinins (WGA),[73] and wheat exorphins[74] (Figure 11.3).

Wheat is resistant to food processing and to proteolysis in the human gastrointestinal tract and breaks into families of peptides. One family of poorly digested peptides of gluten (gliadins) are known to be the primary activating environmental trigger fueling development of the autoimmune celiac disease. However, multiple peptides of poorly digested wheat stay biologically active.[75] The final product of this partial digestion of wheat is a mix of peptides that can trigger host responses (increased intestinal permeability plus innate and/or adaptive immune response) that closely resemble those instigated by the exposure to gastrointestinal pathogens. This is a key point as to why humans have an immune reaction to wheat in the proximal part of the small intestine. Gluten (and other peptides of incompletely digested wheat) are misinterpreted as a harmful component of a microorganism.

The fact that the consumption of wheat activates an innate immune response in every human was first recognized well over a decade ago.[76] Peptides of incompletely digested wheat are able to enter the upper part of the intestine as intact proteins. Thus, they are sensed by mucosal innate immune

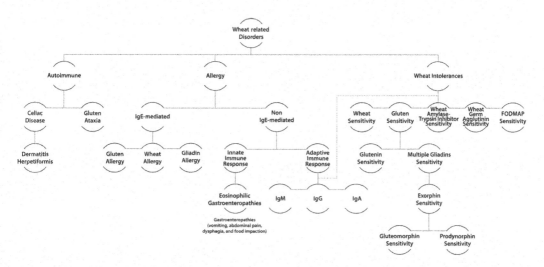

FIGURE 11.3 The diversity of wheat-related disorders.

cells and engage the toll-like receptor 4 (TLR4)-MD2-CD14 complex on monocytes, macrophages, and dendritic cells. This leads to the release of both zonulin and proinflammatory chemokines and cytokines including NFκB, IL-6, IL-8, IL-12 p(40), IL-10, IFN-α, and TNF-α, irrespective of genotype or activity of celiac disease.[77,78] This process, and the resultant transient intestinal permeability, takes place in all individuals who ingest gluten.[79] For the majority, these events do not lead to abnormal consequences. However, with the accumulative development of an inflammatory GI tract, loss of oral tolerance occurs, and these transient responses take on a pathological role.[80]

Alpha-gliadin, the most well-researched fragment of poorly digested wheat, triggers zonulin release through the CXCR3 receptor activated by its engagement to MyD88 with a subsequent increase in gut permeability,[81] suggesting that gluten is misinterpreted by the zonulin pathway as a potential harmful component of a microorganism. The critical point here for clinicians is that this occurs in all humans who consume wheat.[77] Increased proliferative activity of the epithelial cells in the crypts, enterocyte stress, activation of tissue transglutaminase 2 (TG2), induction of Ca^{2+}, IL-15, NFκB signaling, IFN-α, inhibition of CFTR, alteration of vesicular trafficking, and activation of the inflammasome platform are some of the biological effects of the gliadin peptide p31–43.[82] This process, and the resultant transient intestinal permeability, takes place in all individuals who ingest gluten.[83]

ATIs, a family of non-gluten proteins in wheat, are responsible for manifestations of mainly extraintestinal symptoms of WRDs.[84–87] In the gut, ATIs are able to stimulate immune cells residing in the lamina propria and mesenteric lymph nodes through TLR4 binding and stimulation, and the emigration of the activated myeloid cells. ATIs directly interact with TLR4 with nanomolar affinity.[88]

Cardiologist and heart surgeon Dr. Steven Gundry has impacted on millions in the last few years by revealing that the plant-based protein lectin is highly toxic to humans and its consumption may have cardiovascular consequences.[89] The lectins in wheat are the WGA. WGA induces platelet activation and aggregation.[90] WGA can pass through the blood brain barrier (BBB) through a process called 'adsorptive endocytosis'[91] and is able to travel freely among the tissues of the brain which is why it is used as a marker for tracing neural circuits.[92] At nanomolar concentrations, WGA stimulates the synthesis of proinflammatory cytokines including IL-1, IL-6, and IL-8 in intestinal and immune cells.[93] WGA has been shown to induce NADPH-oxidase in human neutrophils associated with the 'respiratory burst' that results in the release of inflammatory free radicals, reactive oxygen species.[94] WGA has been shown to play a causative role in patients with chronic thin gut inflammation possibly due to the fact that gluten itself functions as a lectin that binds to certain oligosaccharide units of glycoconjugates of the intestinal brush border initiating humoral and cellular immune processes.[95,96]

In the gluten family of protein fragments from poorly digested wheat, gliadin can be broken down into various amino acid lengths or peptides. Gliadorphin is a 7-amino acid-long peptide, Tyr-Pro-Gln-Pro-Gln-Pro-Phe, which forms from incompletely digested gliadin. When digestive enzymes are insufficient to break down gliadorphin into 2–3 amino acids length, and a compromised intestinal wall allows for the leakage of the entire 7-amino acid-long fragment into the blood, gliadorphin can pass through to the brain via circumventricular organs and activate opioid receptors resulting in disrupted brain function. In the brain, gliadorphin and other gluteomorphins can directly interfere with neuronal messaging by binding to the opioid receptors, thus inhibiting the natural binding of neurotransmitters to their receptors.[97–99] In addition, lymphocytes carry the same receptors on their own surfaces; therefore, gluteomorphins can indirectly interfere with opioid receptors through lymphocyte secretion of cytokines and cause the delivery of aberrant messages to the brain.[100] If antibodies are produced to gluteomorphins (a biomarker commonly identified in serology), these antibodies act as natural opioids on the lymphocytes and the nerve cells causing neuroimmune abnormalities.[101]

CAUSES OF WHEATS' IMMUNOGENICITY

Policies on supporting on-farm production introduced in the 1930–1960 period in the United States[102] and Europe focused on a few major crops, particularly grains (e.g., wheat, corn, rice), oilseeds (e.g., soybeans), livestock (e.g., pigs, poultry, and cattle), and critical cash crops, especially sugar cane and other sources of sugar.[103,104]

The 1960s also saw the start of significant agricultural transformation in low- and middle-income countries, with the 'Green Revolution', which focused on increasing productivity of corn, rice, and wheat. These investments and changes in production systems were designed to make calories from staples (e.g., wheat, corn, rice) cheaply available, in order to simultaneously address hunger in low- and middle-income countries and national food insecurity in high-income countries.[105]

Coupled with the breeding of wheat in the last 100+ years being focused toward increased yield and resistance, these efforts have inadvertently contributed to a higher immunostimulatory potential of modern wheat cultivars cultivated after 1950, compared to older wheat cultivars.[106,107] However, a common misconception is that the more ancient strains of wheat are not immunogenic. Numerous studies have identified that the ancient or heritage strains of wheat such as emmer, spelt, or kamut are at least as immunogenic as, and in some cases more immunogenic than, modern strains and thus are strongly recommended to be avoided in a WRD.[108–111]

Some have theorized that the increased sensitivity to wheat and CD seen in the past few decades are due to the introduction of glyphosate and other pesticides in conjunction with the development of transgenic crops (genetically modified foods).[112] Although the evidence is sound on the toxic effect of these chemicals on both human tissue and the human microbiome,[113,114] as referenced above, the increase in the prevalence of CD preceded the agricultural introduction and common use of these pesticides.

Thus, the previously held assumptions that the immunogenicity of wheat is new and due to its increased gluten content, or glyphosate content, are historical misconceptions.

Several studies have linked exposure to a variety of genetic and environmental risk factors with the onset of non-infective CID.[115] Since host genetics and environmental factors are known to influence the gut microbiota composition and function, researchers have started to explore alterations in the gut microbiota of infants at risk of autoimmune conditions such as CD, Ankylosing Spondylitis,[116] IBD,[117] and T1D.[118]

These and other studies reinforce the paradigm that the 'perfect storm' for CID development (including CVDs) includes:

- genetic vulnerabilities, activated by
- exposure to environmental triggers, activating
- TLR4 in the proximal part of the small intestine, signaling both
- zonulin release and NfK-B production, thus activating IL-1B, IL-6, IL-8, IL-12 p(40), IL-10, and TNF-α, creating
- an imbalanced inflammatory microbiome, contributing to
- excess intestinal permeability, allowing
- macromolecular transport from the intestinal lumen into the submucosa and systemic circulation, initiating
- a systemic immune response, eventually fueling
- the development of CID (Figure 11.4).

Among the numerous potential intestinal luminal stimuli that can stimulate zonulin release, thus activating an increase in intestinal permeability, small exposure to large amounts of bacteria (bacterial overgrowth) and gluten have been identified as the two most powerful triggers.[119]

With the understanding that gluten and other peptides of incompletely digested wheat activate both an innate immune response and zonulin release in every human who consumes wheat, within 5 minutes of wheat entering the proximal part of the small intestine,[120] the role of wheat as the 'most common' environmental trigger initiating an inflammatory cascade is of paramount importance. An in-depth review of the multiple studies on this topic confirms that the vast majority of time, this increase in intestinal permeability from exposure to gluten is initially asymptomatic.

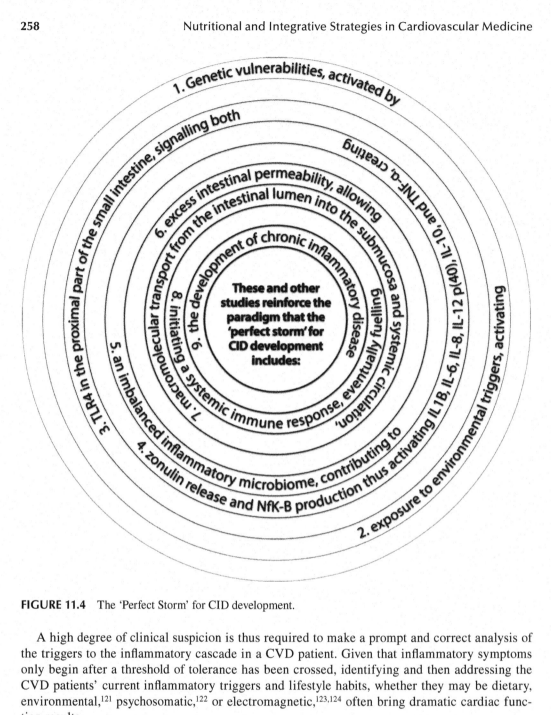

FIGURE 11.4 The 'Perfect Storm' for CID development.

A high degree of clinical suspicion is thus required to make a prompt and correct analysis of the triggers to the inflammatory cascade in a CVD patient. Given that inflammatory symptoms only begin after a threshold of tolerance has been crossed, identifying and then addressing the CVD patients' current inflammatory triggers and lifestyle habits, whether they may be dietary, environmental,[121] psychosomatic,[122] or electromagnetic,[123,124] often bring dramatic cardiac function results.

A careful medical history should be obtained to recognize inflammatory symptoms outside traditional cardiovascular risk factors. For example, in the absence of known etiologies for dilated cardiomyopathy or myocarditis, common symptoms such as iron deficiency anemia, fatigue, and neurological symptoms can alert a physician to screen for a WRD. Addressing a WRD may hold the key to arresting and/or reversing the cardiac abnormality.[125,126]

CVDs are a serious and often lethal condition. With any and every presenting cardiovascular abnormality, once acute stabilization has occurred, focused attention reducing the causes of the underlying inflammatory cascade brings the potential of arresting and/or putting the rampaging dysfunction into remission. With physician awareness and simple serology, the initiation of a gluten-free diet may bring symptomatic relief and reduction of pathology, thereby side-stepping 'the Heartbreak of a Wheat-Related Disorder'.[16,49,127]

ABBREVIATIONS

MI: myocardial infarction
HF: heart failure
WRD: wheat-related disorders
PROMIS: Patient-Reported Outcome Measurement Information System
GPH: Global Physical Health
HRQoL: Health-Related Quality of Life
MPI: myocardial performance index
NCGS: Non-Celiac Gluten Sensitivity
ATIs: amylase trypsin inhibitors
WGA: wheat germ agglutinins
TG2:   tissue transglutaminase 2
CID: chronic inflammatory diseases
CXCR3:   CXCR3 is a chemokine receptor that regulates leukocyte trafficking
MyD88:   Myeloid differentiation primary response 88 provides instructions for making a protein involved in signaling within immune cells
NFκB: nuclear factor kappa B
IFN-α: interferon alpha
CFTR: Cystic fibrosis transmembrane conductance regulator

REFERENCES

1. Holmes DR, Bell MR. Left anterior descending artery stenosis: the widow maker revisited. *Mayo Clin Proc* 2000 Nov;75(11):1113–1115.
2. Holman H. Chronic disease–the need for a new clinical education. *JAMA* 2004 Sep 1;292(9):1057–1059.
3. GBD 2017 Risk Factor Collaborators. Global, regional, and national comparative risk assessment of 84 behavioural, environmental and occupational, and metabolic risks or clusters of risks for 195 countries and territories, 1990–2017: a systematic analysis for the Global Burden of Disease Study 2017. *Lancet* 2018 Nov 10;392(10159):1923–1994.
4. Tilg H, Moschen AR. Food, immunity, and the microbiome. *Gastroenterology* 2015;148:1107–1119.
5. Virchow R. *Die cellularpathologie in ihrer begründung auf physiologische und pathologische gewebelehre.* Berlin: Hirschwald Verlag; 1871.
6. Ross R. The pathogenesis of atherosclerosis–an update. *New Engl J Med* 1986;314:488–500.
7. O'Bryan T. Food Sensitivities, Wheat-Related Disorders, and Cardiovascular Disease, Ch. 6. In *Personalized and Precision Integrative Cardiovascular Medicine.* Walters Kluwer; 2019. ISBN-13: 978-1-975115-28-9.
8. Blasi C. The autoimmune origin of atherosclerosis. *Atherosclerosis* 2008 Nov;201(1):17–32.
9. NIH. Heart inflammation. https://www.nhlbi.nih.gov/health-topics/heart-inflammation. Accessed 6-21-21.
10. Frustaci A, Cuoco L, Chimenti C, Pieroni M, Fioravanti G, Gentiloni N, Maseri A, Gasbarrini G. Celiac disease associated with autoimmune myocarditis. *Circulation* 2002 Jun 4;105(22):2611–2618.
11. Van Linthout S, Tschöpe C. Inflammation—cause or consequence of heart failure or both? *Curr Heart Fail Rep* 2017 Aug;14(4):251–265.
12. Children with untreated coeliac disease have sub-clinical cardiac dysfunction: a longitudinal observational analysis. *Scand J Gastroenterol* 2018 Jun–Jul;53(7):803–808.
13. Bozkurt B, Torre-Amione G, Warren MS, Whitmore J, Soran OZ, Feldman AM, et al. Results of targeted anti-tumor necrosis factor therapy with etanercept (ENBREL) in patients with advanced heart failure. *Circulation* 2001;103:1044–1047.
14. Anker SD, Coats AJ. How to recover from renaissance? The significance of the results of recover, renaissance, renewal and attach. *Int J Cardiol* 2002;86:123–30.

15. Andreis A, Imazio M, Casula M, Avondo S, Brucato A. Recurrent pericarditis: an update on diagnosis and management. *Intern Emerg Med* 2021 Apr;16(3):551–558.
16. Goel NK, McBane RD, Kamath PS. Cardiomyopathy associated with celiac disease. *Mayo Clin Proc* 2005;80(5):674–676.
17. Not T, Faleschini E, Tommasini A, et al. Celiac disease in patients with sporadic and inherited cardiomyopathies and in their relatives. *Eur Heart J* 2003;24:1455–1461.
18. Cosnes J, Cellier C, Viola S, et al. Incidence of autoimmune diseases in celiac disease: protective effect of the gluten-free diet. *Clin Gastroenterol Hepatol.* 2008;6:753–758.
19. van Elburg RM, Uil JJ, Mulder CJ, Heymans HS. Intestinal permeability in patients with coeliac disease and relatives of patients with coeliac disease. *Gut* 1993;34:354–357.
20. Swirski FK, Nahrendorf M. Cardioimmunology: the immune system in cardiac homeostasis and disease. *Nat Rev Immunol* 2018 Dec;18(12):733–744.
21. Daum S, Bauer U, Foss HD, Schuppan D, Stein H, Riecken EO, Ullrich R. Increased expression of mRNA for matrix metalloproteinases-1 and -3 and tissue inhibitor of metalloproteinases-1 in intestinal biopsy specimens from patients with coeliac disease. *Gut* 1999 Jan;44(1):17–25.
22. Bayar N, Çağırcı G, Üreyen ÇM, Kuş G, Küçükseymen S, Arslan Ş. The relationship between spontaneous multi-vessel coronary artery dissection and celiac disease. *Korean Circ J* 2015 May;45(3):242–244.
23. Curione M, Barbato M, Viola F, Francia P, De Biase L, Cucchiara S. Idiopathic dilated cardiomyopathy associated with coeliac disease: the effect of a gluten-free diet on cardiac performance. *Dig Liver Dis* 2002;34:866–869.
24. Chimenti C, Pieroni M, Maseri A, Frustaci A. Dilated cardiomyopathy and celiac disease [reply]. *Ital Heart J* 2002;3:385.
25. Lerner A, Gruener N, Iancu TC. Serum carnitine concentrations in coeliac disease. *Gut* 1993;34:933–935.
26. Antman EM, Loscalzo J. Precision medicine in cardiology. *Nat Rev Cardiol* 2016;13:591–602.
27. Houston, M. *Personalized and Precision Integrative Cardiovascular Medicine.* Walters Kluwer; 2019. ISBN-13: 978-1-975115-28-9.
28. Leopold JA, Loscalzo J. Emerging role of precision medicine in cardiovascular disease. *J Circ Res* 2018 Apr 27;122(9):1302–1315.
29. National Research Council. *Toward Precision Medicine: Building a Knowledge Network for Biomedical Research and a New Taxonomy of Disease.* Washington, DC: National Academies Press; 2011.
30. Collins FS, Varmus H. A new initiative on precision medicine. *N Engl J Med* 2015;372(9):793–795.
31. van Oostrom SH, Picavet HSJ, van Gelder BM, et al. Multimorbidity and comorbidity in the Dutch population—data from general practices. *BMC Public Health* 2012;12–715.
32. Buddeke J, Bots ML, van Dis I, Visseren FL, Hollander M, Schellevis FG, Vaartjes I Comorbidity in patients with cardiovascular disease in primary care: a cohort study with routine healthcare data. *Br J Gen Pract* 2019 Jun;69(683):e398–e406.
33. Lehnert T, Heider D, Leicht H, et al. Review: healthcare utilization and costs of elderly persons with multiple chronic conditions. *Med Care Res Rev* 2011;68(4):387–420.
34. Beidelschies M, Alejandro-Rodriguez M, Ji X, Lapin B, Hanaway P, Rothberg MB Association of the functional medicine model of care with patient-reported health-related quality-of-life outcomes. *JAMA Netw Open* 2019 Oct 2;2(10):e1914017.
35. Franco OH, Boneux L, de Laet C, Peeters A, Steyerberg EW, Mackenbach JP. The polymeal: a more natural, safer, and probably tastier (than the Polypill) strategy to reduce cardiovascular disease by more than 75%. *BMJ* 2004;329(7480):1447–1450.
36. DiCastelnuovo A, Rotondo S, Iacoviello L, Donati MB, DeGaetano G., Meta-analysis of wine and beer consumption in relation to vascular risk. *Circulation* 2002;105:2836–2844.
37. Whelton SP, He J, Whelton PK, Muntner P. Meta-analysis of observational studies on fish intake and coronary heart disease. *Am J Cardiol* 2004;93:1119–1123.
38. Taubert D, Berkels R, Roesen R, Klaus W. Chocolate and blood pressure in elderly individuals with isolated systolic hypertension. *JAMA* 2003;290:1029–1030.
39. John JH, Ziebland S, Yudkin P, Roe LS, Neil HA. Effects of fruit and vegetable consumption on plasma antioxidant concentrations and blood pressure: a randomised controlled trial. *Lancet* 2002;359:1969–1974.
40. Ackermann RT, Mulrow CD, Ramirez G, Gardner CD, Morbidoni L, Lawrence VA. Garlic shows promise for improving some cardiovascular risk factors. *Arch Intern Med* 2001;161:813–24.
41. Jenkins DJ, Kendall CW, Marchie A, Parker TL, Connelly PW, Qian W, et al. Dose response of almonds on coronary heart disease risk factors: blood lipids, oxidized low-density lipoproteins, lipoprotein(a), homo-cysteine, and pulmonary nitric oxide: a randomized, controlled, crossover trial. *Circulation* 2002;106:1327–1332.

42. Sabate J, Haddad E, Tanzman JS, Jambazian P, Rajaram S. Serum lipid response to the graduated enrichment of a step I diet with almonds: a randomized feeding trial. *Am J Clin Nutr* 2003;77: 1379–1384.

43. Fasano A, Catassi C. Current approaches to diagnosis and treatment of celiac disease: an evolving spectrum. *Gastroenterology* 2001;120:636–651.

44. Lerner A. Factors affecting the clinical presentation and time of diagnosis of celiac disease: the Jerusalem and the West Bank-Gaza experience. *Isr J Med Sci* 1994;30:294–295.

45. Makhlouf S, Messelmani M, Zaouali J, Mrissa R. Cognitive impairment in celiac disease and non-celiac gluten sensitivity: review of literature on the main cognitive impairments, the imaging and the effect of gluten free diet. *Acta Neurol Belg* 2018 Mar;118(1):21–27.

46. Ciaccio EJ, Lewis SK, Biviano AB, Iyer V, Garan H, Green PH. Cardiovascular involvement in celiac disease. *World J Cardiol* 2017;9(8):652–666.

47. Orbach H, Amitai N, Barzilai O, Boaz M, Ram M, Zandman-Goddard G, Shoenfeld Y. Autoantibody screen in inflammatory myopathies high prevalence of antibodies to gliadin. *Ann N Y Acad Sci* 2009 Sep;1173:174–179.

48. Bonciolini V, Bianchi B, Del Bianco E, Verdelli A, Caproni M. Cutaneous manifestations of non-celiac gluten sensitivity: clinical histological and immunopathological features. *Nutrients* 2015 Sep 15;7(9):7798–7805.

49. Soares FL, de Oliveira Matoso R, Teixeira LG, Menezes Z, Pereira SS, Alves AC, Batista NV, de Faria AM, Cara DC, Ferreira AV, Alvarez-Leite JI. Gluten-free diet reduces adiposity, inflammation and insulin resistance associated with the induction of PPAR-alpha and PPAR-gamma expression. *J Nutr Biochem* 2013 Jun;24(6):1105–1111.

50. Annibale B, Severi C, Chistolini A, Antonelli G, Lahner E, Marcheggiano A, Iannoni C, Monarca B, Delle Fave G. Efficacy of gluten-free diet alone on recovery from iron deficiency anemia in adult celiac patients. *Am J Gastroenterol* 2001 Jan;96(1):132–137.

51. Aziz I, Lewis NR, Hadjivassiliou M, Winfield SN, Rugg N, Kelsall A, Newrick L, Sanders DS. A UK study assessing the population prevalence of self-reported gluten sensitivity and referral characteristics to secondary care. *Eur J Gastroenterol Hepatol* 2014 Jan;26(1):33–39.

52. Volta U, Bardella MT, Calabrò A, Troncone R, Corazza GR, The Study Group for Non-Celiac Gluten Sensitivity. An Italian prospective multicenter survey on patients suspected of having non-celiac gluten sensitivity. *BMC Med* 2014;12:85.

53. Lebwohl B, Cao Y, Zong G, Hu FB, Green PHR, Neugut AI, Rimm EB, Sampson L, Dougherty LW, Giovannucci E, Willett WC, Sun Q, Chan AT. Long term gluten consumption in adults without celiac disease and risk of coronary heart disease: prospective cohort study. *BMJ* 2017 May 2;357:j1892.

54. Patel P, Smith F, Kilcullen N, Artis N. Dilated cardiomyopathy as the first presentation of coeliac disease: association or causation? *Clin Med (Lond)* 2018 Mar;18(2):177–179.

55. Ludvigsson JF, James S, Askling J, Stenestrand U, Ingelsson E. Nationwide cohort study of risk of ischemic heart disease in patients with celiac disease. *Circulation.* 2011 Feb 8;123(5):483–490.

56. Frustaci A, Cuoco L, Chimenti C, et al. Celiac disease associated with autoimmune myocarditis. *Circulation* 2002;105:2611–2618.

57. Emilsson L, Smith JG, West J, Melander O, Ludvigsson JF. Increased risk of atrial fibrillation in patients with coeliac disease: a nationwide cohort study. *Eur Heart J* 2011 Oct;32(19):2430—2437.

58. Rybak A, Cukrowska B, Socha J, Socha P. Long term follow up of coeliac disease—is atherosclerosis a problem? *Nutrients* 2014 Jul 21;6(7):2718–2729.

59. Wang I, Hopper I. Celiac disease and drug absorption: implications for cardiovascular therapeutics. *Cardiovasc Ther* 2014;32:253–256.

60. Morris ZS, Wooding S, Grant J. The answer is 17 years, what is the question: understanding time lags in translational research. *J R Soc Med* 2011 Dec;104(12):510–520.

61. Health Economics Research Group, Office of Health Economics, RAND Europe. *Medical Research: What's It Worth? Estimating the Economic Benefits from Medical Research in the UK.* London: UK Evaluation Forum; 2008.

62. Lebwohl B, Murray JA, Verdú EF, Crowe SE, Dennis M, Fasano A, Green PH, Guandalini S, Khosla C. Gluten introduction, breastfeeding, and celiac disease: back to the drawing board. *Am J Gastroenterol* 2016 Jan;111(1):12–14.

63. Catassi C, Kryszak D, Bhatti B, Sturgeon C, Helzlsouer K, Clipp SL, Gelfond D, Puppa E, Sferruzza A, Fasano A. Natural history of celiac disease autoimmunity in a USA cohort followed since 1974. *Ann Med* 2010 Oct;42(7):530–538.

64. Beitnes AR, Vikskjold FB, Jóhannesdóttir GB, Perminow G, Olbjørn C, Andersen SN, Bentsen BS, Rugtveit J, Størdal K. Symptoms and mucosal changes stable during rapid increase of pediatric celiac disease in Norway. *J Pediatr Gastroenterol Nutr* 2017 Apr;64(4):586–591.

65. West J, Fleming KM, Tata LJ, Card TR, Crooks CJ, Incidence and prevalence of celiac disease and dermatitis herpetiformis in the UK over two decades: population-based study. *Am J Gastroenterol* 2014 May;109(5):757–768. doi: 10.1038/ajg.2014.55.

66. Rubio-Tapia A, Kyle RA, Kaplan EL, Johnson DR, Page W, Erdtmann F, Brantner TL, Kim WR, Phelps TK, Lahr BD, Zinsmeister AR, Melton LJ 3rd, Murray JA. Increased prevalence and mortality in undiagnosed celiac disease. *Gastroenterology* 2009 Jul;137(1):88–93.

67. Gatti S, Lionetti E, Balanzoni L, Verma AK, Galeazzi T, Gesuita R, Scattolo N, Cinquetti M, Fasano A, Catassi C. Celiac screening team increased prevalence of celiac disease in school-age children in Italy. *Clin Gastroenterol Hepatol* 2020 Mar;18(3):596–603.

68. Almeida LM, Castro LC, Uenishi RH, de Almeida FC, Fritsch PM, Gandolfi L, Pratesi R, Nóbrega YK. Decreased prevalence of celiac disease among Brazilian elderly. *World J Gastroenterol* 2013 Mar 28;19(12):1930–1935.

69. White LE, Merrick VM, Bannerman E, Russell RK, Basude D, Henderson P, Wilson DC, Gillett PM. The rising incidence of celiac disease in Scotland. *Pediatrics* 2013 Oct;132(4):e924–e931.

70. Gibson PR, Muir JG, Newnham ED. Other dietary confounders: FODMAPs et al. *Dig Dis* 2015;33:269–276.

71. Wilder-Smith CH, Olesen SS, Materna A, Drewes AM. Predictors of response to a low-FODMAP diet in patients with functional gastrointestinal disorders and lactose or fructose intolerance. *Aliment Pharmacol Ther* 2017 Apr;45(8):1094–1106.

72. Ashfaq-Khan M, Aslam M, Qureshi MA, Senkowski MS, Yen-Weng S, Strand S, Kim YO, Pickert G, Schattenberg JM, Schuppan D. Dietary wheat amylase trypsin inhibitors promote features of murine non-alcoholic fatty liver disease. *Sci Rep* 2019 Nov 25;9(1):17463.

73. Ohmori T, Yatomi Y, Wu Y, Osada M, Satoh K, Ozaki Y. Wheat germ agglutinin-induced platelet activation via platelet endothelial cell adhesion molecule-1: involvement of rapid phospholipase C gamma 2 activation by Src family kinases. *Biochemistry* 2001 Oct 30;40(43):12992–3001.

74. Tanaka K, Kersten JR, Riess ML. Opioid-induced cardioprotection. *Curr Pharm Des* 2014;20(36):5696–5705.

75. Zevallos VF, Raker V, Tenzer S, Jimenez-Calvente C, Ashfaq-Khan M, Russel N, et al. Nutritional wheat amylase-trypsin inhibitors promote intestinal inflammation via activation of myeloid cells. *Gastroenterology* 2017;152:1100–13 doi: 10.1053/j.gastro.2016.12.006.

76. Drago S, El Asmar R, Di Pierro M, Grazia Clemente M, Tripathi A, Sapone A, Thakar M, Iacono G, Carroccio A, D'Agate C, Not T, Zampini L, Catassi C, Fasano A. Gliadin, zonulin and gut permeability: effects on celiac and non-celiac intestinal mucosa and intestinal cell lines. *Scand J Gastroenterol* 2006 Apr;41(4):408–419.

77. Thomas KE, Sapone A, Fasano A, Vogel SN. Gliadin stimulation of murine macrophage inflammatory gene expression and intestinal permeability are MyD88-dependent: role of the innate immune response in celiac disease. *J Immunol* 2006 Feb 15;176(4):2512–2521.

78. Rakhimova M, Esslinger B, Schulze-Krebs A, Hahn EG, Schuppan D, Dieterich W. In vitro differentiation of human monocytes into dendritic cells by peptic-tryptic digest of gliadin is independent of genetic predisposition and the presence of celiac disease. *J Clin Immunol* 2009 Jan;29(1):29–37.

79. Leonard MM, Sapone A, Catassi C, Fasano A. Celiac disease and nonceliac gluten sensitivity: a review. *JAMA* 2017 Aug 15;318(7):647–656.

80. The gut as communicator between environment and host: immunological consequences. *Eur J Pharmacol* 2011 Sep;668(Suppl 1):S16–S32.

81. Lammers KM, Lu R, Brownley J, et al. Gliadin induces an increase in intestinal permeability and zonulin release by binding to the chemokine receptor CXCR3. *Gastroenterology* 2008;135(1):194–204.

82. Chirdo FG, Auricchio S, Troncone R, Barone MV. The gliadin p31–43 peptide: inducer of multiple proinflammatory effects. *Int Rev Cell Mol Biol* 2021;358:165–205.

83. Leonard MM, Sapone A, Catassi C, Fasano A. Celiac disease and nonceliac gluten sensitivity: a review. *JAMA* 2017 Aug 15;318(7):647–656.

84. Fasano A, Sapone A, Zevallos V, Schuppan D. Nonceliac gluten sensitivity. *Gastroenterology* 2015;148:1195–204.doi: 10.1053/j.gastro.2014.12.049.

85. Schuppan D, Zevallos V. Wheat amylase trypsin inhibitors as nutritional activators of innate immunity. *Dig Dis* 2015;33:260–263. doi: 10.1159/000371476.

86. Leccioli V, Oliveri M, Romeo M, Berretta M, Rossi P. A new proposal for the pathogenic mechanism of non-coeliac/non-allergic gluten/wheat sensitivity: piecing together the puzzle of recent scientific evidence. *Nutrients* 2017;9:E1203.

87. Schuppan D, Pickert G, Shfaq-Khan M, Zevallos V. Non-celiac wheat sensitivity: differential diagnosis, triggers and implications. *Best Pract Res Clin Gastroenterol* 2015 29:469–476. doi: 10.1016/j.bpg.2015.04.002.

88. Cuccioloni M, Mozzicafreddo M, Bonfili L, Cecarini V, Giangrossi M, Falconi M, Saitoh SI, Eleuteri AM, Angeletti M. Interfering with the high-affinity interaction between wheat amylase trypsin inhibitor CM3 and toll-like receptor 4: in silico and biosensor-based studies. *Sci Rep* 2017 Oct 13; 7(1):13169.

89. Gundry S., *The Plant Paradox: The Hidden Dangers in "Healthy" Foods That Cause Disease and Weight Gain*, 1st edition. New York: Harper Wave; 2017.

90. Lebret M, Rendu F. Further characterization of wheat germ agglutinin interaction with human platelets: exposure of fibrinogen receptors. *Thromb Haemost* 1986 Dec 15;56(3):323–327.

91. Transcytotic pathway for blood-borne protein through the blood-brain barrier. *Proc Natl Acad Sci U S A* 1988 Jan;85(2):632–636. PMID:2448779.

92. Transsynaptic transport of wheat germ agglutinin expressed in a subset of type II taste cells of transgenic mice. *BMC Neurosci* 2008 Oct 2;9:96.

93. Effects of wheat germ agglutinin on human gastrointestinal epithelium: insights from an experimental model of immune/epithelial cell interaction. *Toxicol Appl Pharmacol* 2009 Jun 1;237(2):146–153. Epub 2009 Mar 28. PMID 19332085.

94. Wheat germ agglutinin induces NADPH-oxidase activity in human neutrophils by interaction with mobilizable receptors. *Infect Immun* 1999 Jul;67(7):3461–3468. PMID 10377127.

95. Guzyeyeva G. Lectin glycosylation as a marker of thin gut inflammation. *The FASEB J* 2008;22:898–893.

96. Köttgen E, Kluge F, Volk B, Gerok W. The lectin properties of gluten as the basis of the pathomechanism of gluten-sensitive enteropathy. *Klin Wochenschr.* 1983 Jan 17;61(2):111–112.

97. Cosford. PANDAS (pediatric autoimmune neuropsychiatric disease associated with Streptococcus) in autism? *Electron J Appl Psychol* 2009;5(1):39–48.

98. Vojdani A, O'Bryan T. The immunology of gluten sensitivity beyond the intestinal tract. *Eur J Inflamm* 2008;6(2):47–57.

99. Vojdani A, O'Bryan T. Immune response to dietary proteins, gliadin and cerebellar peptides in children with autism. *Nutr Neurosci* 2004;7(3):151–161.

100. Vojdani A, et al. Infections, toxic chemicals and dietary peptides binding to lymphocyte receptors and tissue enzymes are major instigators of autoimmunity in autism. *Intl J Immunopathol Pharmacol* 2003;16(3):189–199.

101. Pruimboom L, de Punder K. The opioid effects of gluten exorphins: asymptomatic celiac disease. *J Health Popul Nutr* 2015 Nov 24;33:24.

102. Gardner BL. *American Agriculture in the Twentieth Century: How It Flourished and What It Cost.* Cambridge, MA: Harvard University Press; 2002.

103. Galloway J. Sugar. In: Kiple, K.; Ornelas, K., editors. *The Cambridge World History of Food.* New York: Cambridge University Press; 2000. pp. 437–449.

104. Popkin, B. *The World Is Fat: The Fads, Trends, Policies, and Products That Are Fattening the Human Race.* New York: Avery-Penguin Group; 2008.

105. Lang T, Heasman M. *Food Wars: The Global Battle for Mouths Minds and Market.* London: Routledge; 2003.

106. Pronin D, Börner A, Weber H, Scherf KA, Wheat (*Triticum aestivum* L.) breeding from 1891 to 2010 contributed to increasing yield and glutenin contents but decreasing protein and gliadin contents. *J Agric Food Chem* 2020 Nov 18;68(46):13247–13256.

107. vanden Broeck HC, de Jong HC, Salentijn EM, Dekking L, Bosch D, Hamer RJ, Gilissen LJ, van der Meer IM, Smulders MJ. Presence of celiac disease epitopes in modern and old hexaploid wheat varieties: wheat breeding may have contributed to increased prevalence of celiac disease. *Theor Appl Genet* 2010;121:1527–1539.

108. Gregorini A, Colomba M, Ellis HJ, Ciclitira PJ. Immunogenicity characterization of two ancient wheat α-gliadin peptides related to coeliac disease. *Nutrients* 2009 Feb;1(2):276–290.

109. Ribeiro M, Rodriguez-Quijano M, Nunes FM, Carrillo JM, Branlard G, Igrejas G. New insights into wheat toxicity: breeding did not seem to contribute to a prevalence of potential celiac disease's immunostimulatory epitopes. *Food Chem* 2016 Dec 15;213:8–18.

110. Geißlitz SM. Proteins of einkorn, emmer and spelt: Influence on baking quality and role in wheat related hypersensitivities, Die Dissertation wurde am 23.05.2019 bei der Technischen Universität München eingereicht und durch die Fakultät für Chemie am 12.08.2019 angenommen, accessed 6-21-21. https://mediatum.ub.tum.de/doc/1485372/1485372.pdf.

111. Geisslitz S, Ludwig C, Scherf KA, Koehler PJ. Targeted LC-MS/MS reveals similar contents of α-amylase/trypsin-inhibitors as putative triggers of nonceliac gluten sensitivity in all wheat species except einkorn. *Agric Food Chem* 2018 Nov 21;66(46):12395–12403. doi: 10.1021/acs.jafc.8b04411. Epub 2018 Nov 6.

112. Samsel A, Seneff S. Glyphosate, pathways to modern diseases II: celiac sprue and gluten intolerance. *Interdiscip Toxicol* 2013 Dec;6(4):159–184.

113. Benachour N, Séralini GE. Glyphosate formulations induce apoptosis and necrosis in human umbilical, embryonic, and placental cells. *Chem Res Toxicol* 2009 Jan;22(1):97–105.

114. Mesnage R, Defarge N, Spiroux de Vendômois J, Séralini GE. Major pesticides are more toxic to human cells than their declared active principles. *Biomed Res Int* 2014;2014:179691.

115. Tamburini S, Shen N, Wu HC, Clemente JC. The microbiome in early life: implications for health outcomes. *Nat Med* 2016;22(7):713–22.

116. Leonard MM, Karathia H, Pujolassos M, Troisi J, Valitutti F, Subramanian P, Camhi S, Kenyon V, Colucci A, Serena G, Cucchiara S, Montuori M, Malamisura B, Francavilla R, Elli L, Fanelli B, Colwell R, Hasan N, Zomorrodi AR, Fasano A, CD-GEMM Team. Multi-omics analysis reveals the influence of genetic and environmental risk factors on developing gut microbiota in infants at risk of celiac disease. *Microbiome* 2020 Sep 11;8(1):130.

117. Torres J, Hu J, Seki A, Eisele C, Nair N, Huang R, et al. Infants born to mothers with IBD present with altered gut microbiome that transfers abnormalities of the adaptive immune system to germ-free mice. *Gut* 2020;69(1):42–51.

118. Vatanen T, Franzosa EA, Schwager R, Tripathi S, Arthur TD, Vehik K, et al. The human gut microbiome in early-onset type 1 diabetes from the TEDDY study. *Nature* 2018;562(7728):589–594.

119. Fasano A. All disease begins in the (leaky) gut: role of zonulin-mediated gut permeability in the pathogenesis of some chronic inflammatory diseases. *F1000Res* 2020 Jan 31;9:F1000 Faculty Rev-69. doi: 10.12688/f1000research.20510.1.

120. Fritscher-Ravens A, Schuppan D, Ellrichmann M, Schoch S, Röcken C, Brasch J, Bethge J, Böttner M, Klose J, Milla PJ. Confocal endomicroscopy shows food-associated changes in the intestinal mucosa of patients with irritable bowel syndrome. *Gastroenterology* 2014 Nov;147(5):1012–1020.

121. Swan SH. Environmental phthalate exposure in relation to reproductive outcomes and other health endpoints in humans. *Environ Res* 2008 Oct;108(2):177–184.

122. Rozanski A, Blumenthal JA, Davidson KW, Saab PG, Kubzansky L. The epidemiology, pathophysiology, and management of psychosocial risk factors in cardiac practice: the emerging field of behavioral cardiology. *J Am Coll Cardiol* 2005 Mar 1;45(5):637–651.

123. Levitt B, Lai H. Biological effects from exposure to electromagnetic radiation emitted by cell tower base stations and other antenna arrays. *Environ Rev* 2010;18:369–395.

124. Elmas O. Effects of electromagnetic field exposure on the heart: a systematic review. *Toxicol Ind Health* 2016 Jan;32(1):76–82.

125. Ulaş K, Kayı Eliaçık, Maşallah Baran, Ali Kanık, Nihal Özdemir, Osman Tolga İnce, Ali Rahmi Bakiler. The subclinical effect of celiac disease on the heart and the effect of gluten-free diet on cardiac functions. *Turk J Pediatr* 2016;58(3):241–245.

126. Rishi B, Anshu S, Aditya K, Surender Kumar Y, Ujjal P. Children with untreated coeliac disease have sub-clinical cardiac dysfunction: a longitudinal observational analysis. *Scand J Gastroenterol* Jun-Jul 2018;53(7):803–808.

127. Ludvigsson JF, de Faire U, Ekbom A, Montgomery SM. Vascular disease in a population-based cohort of individuals hospitalised with coeliac disease. *Heart* 2007 Sep;93(9):1111–1115.

12 The Role of the Gut Microbiome in Cardiovascular Disease

Jill C. Carnahan

CONTENTS

Pathophysiology of Cardiovascular Disease as It Relates to the Gut Microbiome.......................266
Metabolic Endotoxemia and Cardiovascular Disease..267
Hypertension and the Gut Microbiome...269
Periodontal Disease and Cardiovascular Disease 269
Specific Microbial Species and Microbiota Composition Associated with Cardiovascular
    Health Risks..270
The Effects of Certain Dietary Components on the Gut Microbiota and
    Cardiovascular Disease..271
Clinical Presentation of Cardiovascular Disease Driven by Gut Microbiology 272
Prevention and Treatment Strategies..274
Summary..277
Future Challenges 277
References..277

The intricate role of these microorganisms in human biology is so profound, and it's appropriate to consider this complex ecosystem as an organ of multiple systems, including:

The Endocrine System: The gut microbiota is arguably the largest endocrine organ[5] and capable of producing a wide range of biologically active compounds that may be carried via circulation to distant sites within the host.

The Nervous System: The gut microbiota directly influences the development, function, and activity of the enteric nervous system (ENS)[6] through neurotransmitter synthesis and the physical and chemical stimuli on intrinsic primary afferent neurons (IPANs)[7] throughout the gut lining.

The Immune System: The gut microbiota is also integral to maintaining homeostasis in the immune system[8] of the host. It plays an important metabolic role through maintaining cross-talk with the immune system.

Important metabolic functions of the gut microbiome include:

- Breakdown of dietary fiber
- Breakdown of oligosaccharides
- Gas production
- Fermentation
- Production of phenols
- Detoxification
- Mucus production
- Short-chain fatty acid (SCFA) metabolism

DOI: 10.1201/9781003137849-12

- Primary bile acid deconjugation
- Vitamin absorption
- Fats, triglycerides, and cholesterol regulation.

Similar to an ecological ecosystem, the best indicators of the overall health of the gut microbiome are richness and diversity. Richness is the number of species within the community, and diversity refers to the richness combined with how evenly distributed the species are. The gut microbiota includes bacteria, viruses, fungi, archaea, and phages. Bacteria are by far the most prominent microorganisms, comprising almost.[9]

Greater microbial diversity is associated with the body's ability to deal with stressors, such as opportunistic pathogens, dietary, and environmental perturbations. Individuals with disease are more likely[10] to have alterations in their gut microbiome compared to healthy controls. There are strong associations between reduced microbial diversity and illness.

Bacterial colonization during birth plays a major role in the formation and resilience of the gut microbiota. Babies born vaginally colonize with a gut microbiome similar to their mothers' vaginal microbiota, whereas cesarean section-born infants are colonized by bacteria found on the mothers' skin surface. It is well established that cesarean sections are associated with a higher risk of numerous diseases including asthma, food allergy, type 1 diabetes, and obesity,[11] and it appears an altered microbiota is a likely mechanism. Factors that affect diversity throughout life include:

- Genetics
- Stress
- Physiologic processes
- Anatomical structure of the digestive tract
- Diet
- Prebiotic intake
- Probiotic intake
- Antibiotic usage
- Lifestyle
- Living environment.

The importance of the gut microbiome and its various roles across human biology makes having an understanding of this "organ" essential for anyone in the medical field. Furthermore, it's critical that medical professionals remain vigilant in continuously educating themselves on the most current research.

PATHOPHYSIOLOGY OF CARDIOVASCULAR DISEASE AS IT RELATES TO THE GUT MICROBIOME

Dysbiosis is the imbalance or maladaptation of the gut microbiome. Low diversity and richness can present as dysbiosis and are associated with higher levels of inflammation,[12] higher adiposity, insulin resistance, and dyslipidemia. A 2013 study[13] published in the journal *Nature* studied participants ($n=292$) in two characterized groups, delineated by the number of gut microbial genes (gut bacterial richness) with an average 40% difference between low gene count (LGC) individuals and high gene count (HCG) individuals. Individuals with low bacterial gene richness (23% of the study population) were characterized by an increase in adiposity, insulin resistance, and dyslipidemia. Additionally, low bacterial richness individuals showed a more pronounced inflammatory phenotype when compared with high bacterial richness individuals. Various metabolic diseases, including type 2 diabetes and obesity, are associated with dysbiosis that is distinguishable by a unique microbiota profile.

Some causes of dysbiosis include:

- **Standard American Diet (SAD)**: low fiber, high in fat and simple carbs
- Broad-spectrum antibiotics
- Chronic maldigestion
- Chronic use of proton pump inhibitors
- Chronic constipation
- Suppression of *Lactobacillus*, *Bifidobacteria*, and secretory immunoglobulin A (sIgA) due to stress, for example, growth of gram-negative organisms (*Yersinia*, *Pseudomonas*) is stimulated by catecholamines
- Consumption of genetically modified foods with exposure to glyphosate.

The gut microbiota is an important player in atherogenesis.[14] Specifically, higher levels of Lactobacillales and decreased levels in *Bacteroides* have been associated with coronary artery disease.[15] Metabolism by certain intestinal flora has been linked to the deleterious association between the development of atherosclerotic plaque and egg yolk consumption, due to its choline content. Certain gut microbiota can metabolize choline, phosphatidylcholine,[16] and L-carnitine[17] to produce trimethylamine (TMA), which can be oxidized in the liver into trimethylamine N-oxide (TMAO), a proatherogenic metabolite. Inhibiting TMAO production through the gut microbiota has been found to be a promising treatment for atherosclerosis.[18] Due to the inherent complexity of the gut microbiome and its differences among individuals, this pathway is not the same for everyone. The complex ecology of the gut microbiota and its role in metabolic behavior must be considered. For example, many types of fish are still considered beneficial for cardiovascular patients[19] despite their trimethylamine content. Additionally, L-carnitine may ameliorate metabolic diseases[20] by increasing insulin sensitivity of the skeletal muscle and may reduce ischemic heart disease in some people.

METABOLIC ENDOTOXEMIA AND CARDIOVASCULAR DISEASE

Another major mechanism that causes systemic inflammation in the body and is largely modulated by the gut microbiota and gastrointestinal lining is the development of metabolic endotoxemia[21] brought on by intestinal permeability and lipopolysaccharides (LPS). There is a strong correlation between metabolic endotoxemia and an increased risk of cardiovascular disease, diabetes, and obesity. Metabolic endotoxemia is characterized by insulin resistance and low-grade inflammation.

Intestinal permeability can cause systemic inflammation through translocation of LPS. Intestinal permeability is also known as "leaky gut" and is a reinforcing process that can result in intestinal inflammation, damage to the gut lining, dysregulation of the immune system response, nutrient malabsorption (especially vitamins B12, magnesium, and iron), gastrointestinal issues, multiple food intolerances, and eventually, autoimmune disease.

The majority of microbes that reside in the digestive tract are gram-negative bacteria including *Clostridium* sp., *Enterococcus* sp., *Escherichia* sp., and *Bacteroides* sp. These trillions of bacteria in the gastrointestinal tract all contain LPS, a major component of the outer membrane of gram-negative bacteria and considered endotoxins. If they are absorbed through the gastrointestinal lining, they can elicit systemic inflammation and a strong immune system response. In addition to triggering a potent inflammatory cascade, circulating LPS can also suppress cellular anti-inflammatory protective mechanisms. This increases the effects of damaging pathological consequences.[22]

The detection of antibodies against LPS can reveal macromolecule endotoxin infiltration through the intestinal barrier into the systemic circulation. Other indicators of a compromised gastrointestinal lining include occludin, the main component of the proteins that hold together the tight junctions, and zonulin, which is a protein that regulates permeability of the intestine. Detection of antibodies for occludin and zonulin can indicate that tight junctions are breaking down or that normal regulation of tight junctions is compromised, respectively. An assessment of gut barrier damage can be done by measuring these barrier protein antibodies. This detects damage long before there is a dysregulation of the immune system response. This process can be a major driver of inflammation in the body.

Clinical indications that would warrant testing for LPS endotoxemia include:

- Cardiovascular disease
- Obesity
- Metabolic syndrome or diabetes
- Increase in food allergies or sensitivities
- History of celiac disease or other cause of villous atrophy
- Inflammatory bowel disease
- Autoimmune diseases or family history of autoimmune disease
- Neurological conditions such as Parkinson's disease or multiple sclerosis
- Mood disorders, such as bipolar, anxiety or depression
- Cognitive dysfunction, including Alzheimer's disease.

Causes of increased intestinal permeability include:

- Inflammatory bowel disease
- NSAID therapy
- Small intestinal bacterial overgrowth (SIBO)
- Small intestinal fungal overgrowth (SIFO)
- Celiac disease
- Protozoal infections
- Toxic chemical exposure
- Mold or mycotoxin exposure
- Glyphosate consumption
- Severe food allergies or lectin sensitivity
- Chronic alcoholism
- Hypochlorhydria
- Other infections
- Psychological stressors
- Surgery
- Strenuous exercise
- Advanced age
- Nutritional depletions (zinc, vitamin D, vitamin A, butyrate)
- Tobacco use.

Biomarkers of intestinal permeability include:

- **Permeability/Dysbiosis**: Bacterial endotoxin – LPS, IgG, IgM, IgA
- **Epithelial Cell Damage**: Actomyosin network – IgA
- **Tight Junction Damage**: Occludin and zonulin – IgG, IgM, IgA

Metabolic endotoxemia is characterized by:

- Insulin resistance and low-grade inflammation
- An LPS concentration of two to three times the threshold
- An increase in endotoxins during fed states and a decrease during fasting states
- An increase in the proportion of LPS containing microbiota in the gut with a high-fat diet
- Dysregulation of inflammatory processes, triggering weight gain and diabetes and cytokine production.

This mechanism suggests that lowering plasma LPS concentration is a potential strategy for controlling metabolic diseases.

HYPERTENSION AND THE GUT MICROBIOME

The gut microbiota and its metabolites have been implicated in the regulation of host physiological functions that can contribute to hypertension, a precursor to cardiovascular disease. Similar to cardiovascular disease, Firmicutes, *Bacteroides*, Actinobacteria, and Proteobacteria are the microorganisms that play a major role in the pathogenesis of hypertension. Toxic products produced by the gut microbiome like TMAO, p-Cresol sulfate, and indoxyl sulfate can contribute to salt sensitivity and affect blood pressure regulation and related epigenetic changes. SCFA receptors are expressed in the kidney and blood vessels, and have been reported to function as a regulator of blood pressure (BP).

Specific and observed gut microbiome contributors to hypertension include[23]:

- **Increased Firmicutes**: *Bacteroides* ratio lowers BP.
- Increased gut inflammation increases BP.
- Increased TMAO and phosphatidylcholine increase BP.
- **Increased Firmicutes**: *Bacteroides* ratio may trigger angiotensin II (A II)-induced hypertension.
- Norepinephrine increases virulence factors in gram-negative bacteria.

These interactions provide novel therapeutic pathways for BP regulation. The regulation of BP via SCFA receptors has provided new insights into the interactions between the gut microbiota and BP control systems. Other hypertension intervention methods via the gut microbiome worth considering include[24]:

- Angiotensin-converting enzyme inhibitory (ACEI) peptides made by the microbiome via fermentation lower BP.
- *Lactobacilli* are natural ACEI and produce biologically active peptides that inhibit ACE.
- Phenylacetylglutamine (PAG), a gut metabolite, is negatively associated with pulse-wave velocity (PWV) and systolic blood pressure (SBP).
- Probiotics with over 10^{11} CFU of multiple strains administered over 8 weeks decreased SBP and diastolic blood pressure (DBP).
- Gut-derived hormones such as gastrin, glucagon-like peptide-1 (GLP-1), and others regulate gut sodium reabsorption and renal sodium homeostasis and BP.
- Blockade of the gut Na^+/H^+ exchanger-3 (NHE3) will lower BP.
- Probiotics have been shown to lower BP.

When the brain-gut microbiome axis and the gastro-renal reflex are affected, psychological symptoms may be observed. The absence of some gut microbiota may increase anxiety and decrease dopamine in the frontal cortex, hippocampus, and striatum. There can also be alterations in renal dopamine with salt intake. Finally, changes to the gut microbiome can induce changes in microRNAs, DNA methylation, and acetylation, which can contribute to inflammatory diseases including hypertension and cardiovascular disease.

PERIODONTAL DISEASE AND CARDIOVASCULAR DISEASE

The connection between periodontal microbes and cardiovascular disease has long been observed with no definitive mechanisms identified. LPS-mediated mitochondrial dysfunction[25] is a potential origin of oxidative stress in periodontal patients, as is intestinal permeability.

Research indicates that inflammatory responses evoked by the LPS of *Porphyromonas gingivalis* are one key factor in this process. The influence of LPS on fibroblast and peripheral blood mononuclear cells appears to increase reactive oxygen species production while reducing CoQ10 levels and citrate synthase activity. Mitochondrial dysfunction promoted by the LPS of *Porphyromonas gingivalis* on these cells may also promote oxidative stress and alter cytokine homeostasis.

SPECIFIC MICROBIAL SPECIES AND MICROBIOTA COMPOSITION ASSOCIATED WITH CARDIOVASCULAR HEALTH RISKS

Certain organisms and gut microbiota composition patterns have been associated with cardiovascular disease and metabolic syndrome. Low bacterial richness is associated with a reduction in beneficial butyrate-producing bacteria. Butyrate is a SCFA with potent anti-inflammatory potential. Low bacterial richness is also associated with mucus degradation, potential gut barrier impairment, and an increase in oxidative stress.

Species and patterns associated with atherosclerosis are as follows:

- Low microbial diversity is associated with atherosclerosis.[26]
- *Chryseomonas*, *Veillonella*, and *Streptococcus* have been found in artery plaques but are believed to originate from the oral cavity and gut.
- Patients with symptomatic atherosclerosis[27] have higher levels of *Collinsella* and lower levels of *Eubacterium* and *Roseburia* in their gut.

Genus/Species	PAC Score	Previous	Reference Range	Abundance Associated With*
Collinsella	5.84··		<=6.00	
Eubacterium	5.61··		>=4.00	
Roseburia	5.80··		>=4.00	
Clostridium	3.67··		<=6.00	
Ruminococcus	1.07··		<=6.00	Atherosclerosis
Prevotella	7.80·		<=6.00	
Peptostreptococcus	5.01··		<=6.00	
Lachnospira	4.64··		>=4.00	

Species associated with cardiovascular disease:

- Increases in the abundance of the family Pseudomonadaceae
- Lower levels of Firmicutes species
- A higher ratio of Pseudomonadaceae to Firmicutes bacteria in coronary heart disease plaque.

Lactobacillus reuteri	5.26··		>=4.00	
Enterococcus faecalis	4.40··		>=4.00	High LDL-Cholesterol
Lactobacillus acidophilus	4.44··		>=4.00	
Bifidobacterium lactis	4.24··		>=4.00	
Anaerotruncus colihominis	4.02··		>=4.00	High BMI and Triglyceride levels
Lactobacillus plantarum	5.35··		>=4.00	Atherosclerosis and Triglyceride levels

Species associated with diabetes include:

- **Higher Levels Of**:
  - *Lactobacillus gasseri* and *Streptococcus mutans*
  - Certain *Clostridium* species
  - Proteobacteria.
- **Lower Prevalence of Butyrate Producers**:
  - *Roseburia intestinalis* (butyrate producer)
  - *Faecalibacterium prausnitzii*.
- Increased expression of microbial genes involved in oxidative stress leading to a proinflammatory signature.
- Reduced expression of genes involved in vitamin synthesis like riboflavin.
- Gut microbiota may increase hepatic production of triglycerides and development of insulin resistance.
- Sulfate-reducing species *Desulfovibrio* was more frequently observed in diabetic patients.
- Dietary fiber improved microbiota-related metabolic functions such as glucose tolerance, insulin sensitivity, and weight gain and reduced low-grade inflammation.

Clinically, low bacterial richness and dysbiosis are associated with:

- Inflammatory bowel disease[28]
- Obesity
- Diabetes
- Non-alcoholic fatty liver disease
- Low-grade inflammation (elevated C-reactive protein)
- Insulin resistance
  - Elevated leptin
  - Decreased adiponectin
- Dyslipidemia
- Hypertension[29]
- High BP.

THE EFFECTS OF CERTAIN DIETARY COMPONENTS ON THE GUT MICROBIOTA AND CARDIOVASCULAR DISEASE

Diet significantly affects the composition and function of the gut microbiome. Specifically, the consumption of high-fiber foods, such as fruits and vegetables high in prebiotic fibers, have been shown[30] to increase bacterial richness and improve clinical symptoms associated with obesity. Even short-term diets alter the microbial community in a predictable manner.[31] A 2010 study[32] found that switching from a low-fat, polysaccharide-rich diet to a high-fat, high-sugar Western diet changed the composition of mice with humanized microbiota within one day. Through fecal microbial transplantation, the effects of the Western diet were transferred to donor mice where increased adiposity was observed, leading researchers to conclude the effects came from the microbiota and not merely the diet. It's important to note that we need a better understanding of the extent to which the gut microbiota changes based on diet. It appears that even though changes can be seen in as little as a day, individuals have a core population that is more resilient to change. This core population has been compared to a microbial "fingerprint" because its signature can allow scientists to identify individuals based on their microbial patterns alone. This microbial pattern bears a resemblance most closely to their mother's gut or skin microbiota depending on delivery method.

Beyond diet, other factors have been associated with metabolic abnormalities through altering the gut microbiota, including:

TABLE 12.1

Summary of Diet-Induced Dysbiosis

Diet	Altered Bacteria	Effect on Bacteria	References
High-fat	*Bifidobacteria* spp.	Decreased (absent)	[45]
High-fat and high-sugar	*Clostridium innocuum, Catenibacterium mitsuokai,* and *Enterococcus* spp.	Increased	[18]
	Bacteroides spp.	Decreased	[18]
Carbohydrate-reduced	Bacteroidetes	Increased	[49]
Caloric-restricted	*Clostridium coccoides, Lactobacillus* spp., and *Bifidobacteria* spp.	Decreased (growth prevented)	[48]
Complex carbohydrates	*Mycobacterium avium* subspecies *paratuberculosis* and Enterobacteriaceae	Decreased	[49]
	B. longum subspecies *longum, B. breve* and *B. thetaiotaomicron*	Increased	[53]
Refined sugars	*C. difficile* and *C. perfringens*	Increased	[54,55]
Vegetarian	*E. coli*	Decreased	[56]
High n-6 PUFA from safflower oil	Bacteroidetes	Decreased	[59,60]
	Firmicutes, Actinobacteria, and Proteobacteria	Increased	[59,60]
	δ-Proteobacteria	Increased	[61]
Animal milk fat	δ-Proteobacteria	Increased	[62]

- **Artificial Sweeteners**[33]: Non-caloric artificial sweeteners drive the development of glucose intolerance through changing the composition and function of the gut microbiota.
- **Metformin**[34]: Metformin disrupts the bacterial folate cycle resulting in decreased levels of S-adenosylmethionine synthase (Table 12.1).

Summary of the effects of gut dysbiosis on cardiovascular disease

Balanced microbiome	Dysbiotic microbiome
High beneficial/commensal microbes vs. low opportunistic	Low beneficial/commensal microbes vs. high opportunistic
Associated lifestyle factors: high-fiber diet, prebiotics, probiotics, immune-potentiating therapeutics, nutraceuticals	**Associated lifestyle factors**: high-fat, high-caloric, high-sugar diets, sedentary lifestyle, excessive antibiotic use
Decreased gut permeability	Increased gut permeability
Decreased toxemia and sepsis	Increased toxemia and sepsis
Decreased proinflammation	Increased proinflammation
Increased insulin sensitivity	Decreased insulin sensitivity
Better gut, metabolic, cardiovascular health	Poorer gut, metabolic, cardiovascular health

CLINICAL PRESENTATION OF CARDIOVASCULAR DISEASE DRIVEN BY GUT MICROBIOLOGY

A well-functioning gut microbiome is essential to modulating inflammation, suggesting initial symptoms of dysregulation or dysbiosis could potentially be preclinical symptoms of cardiovascular disease. Gastrointestinal issues could be an early indicator of mechanisms that can contribute to and drive cardiovascular disease, creating a unique opportunity for intervention. Should gastroenterologists check for cardiovascular disease markers? Research suggests so.

Clinical presentation of cardiovascular disease driven by gut microbiology include the following:

- **Exocrine Pancreatic Insufficiency** (EPI)[35]: EPI should be ruled out in all patients with cardiovascular disease in the presence of overt malnutrition or in the case of persistent gastrointestinal symptoms despite a gluten-free diet.
- **Inflammatory Bowel Disease**
- **Small Intestinal Bacterial Overgrowth (SIBO)**: Symptoms of SIBO include excessive gas, abdominal bloating, distention, diarrhea, and abdominal pain. Few patients with SIBO have chronic constipation over diarrhea. If overgrowth is severe and prolonged, it can interfere with digestion and absorption of food and may result in nutrient deficiencies.
- **Celiac Disease**
- **Protozoal Infections**
- **Food Allergy**
- **Low Stomach Acid**
- **Diarrhea**
- **Nutritional Depletion.**

In addition to these indicators of dysbiosis and/or a compromised intestinal lining, additional testing can be done to measure the influence of the gut on systemic inflammation which is potentially contributing to or driving cardiovascular disease.

Current testing to assess gut microbiome-modulated inflammation in cardiovascular patients breaks down into three categories:

1. Digestion and absorption
2. Inflammation and Immunology
3. Gastrointestinal microbiota and metabolic markers.

- **Digestion and Absorption**:
  - **Pancreatic elastase 1 (PE1)** – PE1 is a proteolytic enzyme exclusively secreted by the human pancreas and serves as a noninvasive fecal biomarker of pancreatic exocrine function (producing amylase, lipase, and protease). This test is used for initial determination of pancreatic exocrine insufficiency and monitoring of pancreatic exocrine function in patients.[36,37] Replacement of pancreatic enzymes is warranted until PE1 levels rebound (i.e., when underlying etiology can be corrected). Prescription and non-prescription formulations are available.
  - **Products of protein break down into putrefactive SCFAs** – These SCFAs (isovalerate, valerate, and isobutyrate) are produced by bacterial fermentation of proteinaceous material (polypeptides and amino acids) in the distal colon. Elevated levels suggest increased protein material in the distal colon which may be due to underlying gastrointestinal conditions such as hypochlorhydria and exocrine pancreatic insufficiency (maldigestion), bacterial overgrowth of the small intestine (SIBO), or gastrointestinal irritation. Levels may also be elevated with increased protein intakes.

    Potential causes of inadequate protein digestion and bacterial fermentation and their corresponding tests include the following:
    - **Low hydrochloric (HCl) acid** – Symptoms include bloating/belching after meals, intolerance for protein, rectal itching, weak, peeling, or cracked fingernails/vertical ridges, adult acne, and undigested food in stool. Potential causes include advanced age (30% of elderly), use of proton pump inhibitors, autoimmunity, fasting, and chronic medical conditions. Consequences include SIBO, dysbiosis, chronic candida infections, unexplained low ferritin or anemia, and deficiency of minerals such as Ca, Mg, Zn, Fe, Cr, Mo, Mn, Cu, and B_{12}.

- **Protease insufficiency** – Majority of protein digestion is due to the pancreatic proteases. Trypsin and chymotrypsin are two primary pancreatic proteases, which are synthesized and packaged into secretory vesicles as the inactive proenzymes trypsinogen and chymotrypsinogen.
    - **Small intestinal bacterial overgrowth (SIBO)** – Breath test for SIBO.
    - **Intolerance to fructose** – Can be counterbalanced with a low FODMAP diet.
  - **Fecal fat** – Fecal fat measurement is an extraction method that provides a quantitative result for the amount of fat in the stool. Excess fecal fat may be due to a lack of bile acids (caused by liver damage, hyperlipidemia drugs, or impaired gallbladder function), disorders that impact pancreatic exocrine function (such as chronic pancreatitis or cystic fibrosis), celiac disease, small bowel bacterial overgrowth, or other conditions and medications.
- **Inflammation and Immunology**:
  - Calprotectin[38] and EPX primary markers of inflammation – elevated in:
    - Inflammatory bowel disease
    - Post-infectious irritable bowel syndrome
    - Irritable bowel syndrome
    - Gastrointestinal cancers
    - Certain gastrointestinal infections
    - NSAID enteropathy
    - Food allergy
    - Chronic pancreatitis.
  - **Eosinophilic protein X (EPX)** – Benefits of EPX as an inflammation biomarker and test include its release in eosinophil degranulation, sensitivity as a marker of gastrointestinal inflammation and low-level inflammation, possible predictor of relapse in inflammatory bowel disease (IBD), and stability of transport up to 7 days.[39–42] EPX can be elevated in inflammatory bowel disease, celiac disease, parasitic infection, and allergic reaction. It is less common in GERD, chronic diarrhea, chronic alcoholism, and protein-losing enteropathy.[43–47]
- **Gastrointestinal Metabolic Markers**:
  - **Beneficial SCFAs** – Includes acetate, n-butyrate, and propionate, which are produced by anaerobic bacterial fermentation of indigestible carbohydrate (fiber). The role of SCFAs includes providing nutrients for the colonic epithelium, modulating colonic and intracellular pH, cell volume, and other functions associated with ion transport, and regulating proliferation, differentiation, and gene expression.[48] SCFAs may enter the systemic circulation and directly affect metabolism or the function of peripheral tissues. SCFAs can beneficially modulate adipose tissue, skeletal muscle, and liver tissue function. SCFAs may contribute to improved glucose homeostasis and insulin sensitivity.[49]

PREVENTION AND TREATMENT STRATEGIES

A diet consisting of whole foods high in vegetables and sufficient exercise are common recommendations for those with cardiovascular disease. However, gut microbiome science provides new insights into the various mechanisms behind why these recommendations are beneficial. A diet high in fermentable fibers and plant polyphenols[50] appears to regulate microbial activities within the gut and increase beneficial SCFA[51] production. New insights into microbiota activity support the increased consumption of whole plant foods and provide a scientific rationale for the use of efficacious prebiotics.

Furthermore, the gut microbiota plays a major role in inflammation mediation throughout the body and offers novel treatment strategies through nutrition, nutritional supplements, and lifestyle changes. Targeting the gut microbiota or related metabolic pathways may offer potential therapeutic benefits to cardiovascular disease patients.

I. **Select Interventions for Reducing LPS Levels**:
   - **Quercetin**[52]: Quercetin, a naturally occurring flavonoid, has been shown to down-regulate inflammatory responses and provide cardioprotection by inhibiting LPS-induced phosphorylation of stress-activated protein kinases (JNK/SAPK) and p38 MAP kinases.
   - **Curcumin**[53]: Studies indicate that curcumin attenuates LPS-induced cardiac hypertrophy in vivo.
   - **Sulforaphane**[54]: Sulforaphane is a biologically active compound often found in cruciferous vegetables, such as broccoli. Sulforaphane is both anti-inflammatory and has anti-cancer properties. It is been shown to significantly suppress LPS-induced COX-2 protein and mRNA expression in a dose-dependent manner. In animal studies, sulforaphane activated the nuclear factor-E2-related factor 2 (Nrf2)/antioxidant response element (ARE) pathway in mice with LPS-induced injury.
   - **Resveratrol**[55]: Resveratrol is naturally occurring stilbenoid phenol with free radical scavenging activity.
   - **EPA/DHA**[56]: EPA and DHA have been shown to down-regulate LPS-induced activation of NF-kappaB.
   - **Bifidobacteria**[57]: *Bifidobacterium* is effective in inhibiting LPS-induced intestinal inflammation and could be an intervention for chronic intestinal inflammation. Byproducts associated with fermentation of prebiotics by *Bifidobacterium*, such as SCFAs (butyrate, propionate, and lactate), positively affect leaky gut and improve tight junctions.

II. **Dietary Interventions to Decrease Endotoxemia Include**:
   - Increase whole plant food.
   - Increase low-mercury fish consumption.
   - Avoid sugar and processed foods.
   - Incorporate intermittent fasting.
   - Increase dietary fiber and prebiotic consumption (especially foods high in oligofructose, inulin, and galactooligosaccharide).
     - Soluble fibers are digested by enzymes into SCFAs.
     - SCFAs constitute approximately 5%–10% of the energy source in healthy people.
     - Fiber-enriched diets improve insulin sensitivity[58] in lean and obese diabetic subjects.

III. **Pancreatic Elastase Treatment**:
   - Smoking cessation
   - Reduced alcohol consumption
   - Small frequent meals
   - Replacement of fat-soluble vitamins
   - Supplemental lipase or pancreatic enzymes (plant-based digestive enzymes may not be strong enough for EPI)
   - Prescription strength enzymes: CREON®, ZENPEP®, and others.

IV. **Recommendations for Adequate Protein Digestion and Fermentation by Anaerobic Bacteria Include**:
   - A low FODMAP diet if intolerance to fructose is suspected.

V. **To Increase Beneficial SCFAs**:
   - Increase dietary fiber.
   - Use prebiotics and probiotics.
   - Take *Saccharomyces boulardii*.

VI. **To Reduce High Levels of Beta-Glucuronidase**:
- Decrease meat intake and increase insoluble fiber.
- Take probiotics.
- Consider *Silybum marianum* for liver support.
- Take calcium-D-glucarate.

VII. **Pre- and Probiotics are Essential**.

VIII. **Probiotics**: An animal study[59] that examined the effects of probiotics on circulating cytokine levels and severity of ischemia/reperfusion injury in the heart, found that the leptin-suppressing bacteria, *Lactobacillus plantarum 299v*, resulted in decreased circulating leptin levels by 41%, smaller myocardial infarcts by 29%, and greater recovery of post-ischemic mechanical function by 35%, when compared to its untreated controls. Finally, a pretreatment with leptin abolished the protective properties of the probiotic. This demonstrated the mechanistic link between microbiota composition and myocardial infarction, and demonstrated that probiotic supplementation can have a beneficial effect on those with cardiovascular disease.

IX. **Spore-Forming Probiotics**: While over-the-counter probiotics (like *Lactobacillus* and *Bifidobacterium*) have proven to address some symptoms associated with digestive abnormalities, the concern is that these strains of probiotics are unable to deliver fully viable bacteria to the small intestine. However, spore-forming probiotic strains of the bacillus species are encapsulated by endospores, allowing them to endure the hostile environment of the upper gastrointestinal tract and deliver more viable probiotics to the gut. While spore-forming bacilli are typically considered soil organisms, they are able to adapt and sporulate within the human digestive tract. The introduction and amplification of these species have been found to have a number of beneficial therapeutic effects, including:
- The amelioration of dysbiosis by supporting the growth of beneficial microbiota in the gastrointestinal tract. Supplementation with spore-forming probiotics has been found to increase populations of beneficial SCFA-producing microbes including *Lactococcus*, *Prevotella*, and *Akkermansia*.
- Increased repair of intestinal mucosa and improved intestinal permeability.
- Potent antilipemic effects – reducing triglycerides, total serum cholesterol, LDL, and VLDL47, while simultaneously promoting HDL cholesterol.[60]
- The reduction of biomarkers (like blood glucose and troponin) associated with metabolic disorders and cardiovascular disease.
- Demonstrated to have immunomodulatory effects as well as remarkable pathogen exclusion, and antimicrobial effects.
- A significant reduction in the biomarkers associated with metabolic endotoxemia. One study found an incredible 42% reduction in LPS and serum endotoxin levels.[61]
- Impressive hepatoprotective and antioxidant activities due to their ability to produce carotenoids – highly potent and bioavailable antioxidants that the human body is unable to synthesize on its own.[62]

X. **Polyphenol-rich foods** are extensively metabolized[63] by gut bacteria into anti-inflammatory end products. One study found that foods such as coffee and cocoa support a significant effect on the functional ecology of symbiotic partners that can affect the host physiology.

Cacao is a prebiotic for beneficial microbes including *Bifidobacterium* and lactic acid bacteria. These bacteria ferment the cacao and produce anti-inflammatory compounds.[64]

Coffee consumption attenuated an increase in Firmicutes to Bacteroidetes to ratios normally associated with high-fat eating. Coffee also increases levels of SCFAs while lowering branched-chain amino acid.

XI. **Mediterranean-Style Diet Recommended** – Lean protein (fish, poultry), nuts, vegetables, and fruit, and extra virgin olive oil (EVOO) together with regular physical activity, are recommended to maintain cardiovascular health.

SUMMARY

- The products of the microbiome can have a dramatic effect on risk of developing cardiovascular disease.
- The microbiome may contribute to obesity, insulin resistance, diabetes, hypertension, dyslipidemia, congestive heart failure, myocardial infarction, and coronary artery disease.
- Always check the microbiome and intestinal integrity in a patient who presents with cardiovascular disease.
- It is critical to rule out LPS endotoxemia as a contributing factor in diabetes and cardiovascular disease.
- Assume that intestinal permeability is likely present in patients presenting with cardiovascular or metabolic disorders.
- TMAO can come from choline, phosphatidylcholine, and carnitine and increases heart disease risk. The microbiome metabolism of these compounds is what determines the actual risk.
- Beneficial SCFAs include butyrate, propionate, and acetate and are critical to cardiovascular health.
- Check bile acid metabolism in cardiovascular disease patients with gut-related symptoms.
- Test for metabolic switches for FXR, PRP, TGR5, glucose metabolism, lipid metabolism, and thermogenesis in BAT.
- **Key Treatment Options**: Mediterranean diet, added soluble and insoluble fiber, fasting mimicking diet or intermittent fasting, prebiotics, probiotics, butyrate, extra virgin olive oil (EVOO) and DMB (dimethyl butanol).

FUTURE CHALLENGES

As the cost of metatranscriptomic or RNA sequencing continues to come down, research of the gut microbiome will continue to improve. Currently, metatranscriptomic technology is the best means we have of analyzing the gut microbiome because of its ability to see function and pathways of the gut microbiome. Defining what a healthy gut microbiome looks like and its variations among diseases is a meticulous and arduous process that requires a high input of data for accurate statistical analysis.

REFERENCES

1. Qin J, Li R, Raes J, et al. 2010. A human gut microbial gene catalogue established by metagenomic sequencing. *Nature.* 464(7285):59–65. http://dx.doi.org/10.1038/nature08821.
2. Ursell L, Metcalf J, Parfrey LW, et al. 2013. Defining the human microbiome. *Nutr Rev.* 70(Suppl 1):S38–44. https://doi.org/10.1111/j.1753-4887.2012.00493.x.
3. Lozupone CA, Stombaugh JI, Gordon JI, et al. 2012. Diversity, stability and resilience of the human gut microbiota. *Nature.* 489(7415):220–30. http://dx.doi.org/10.1038/nature11550.
4. Blaser MJ. 2014. *Missing Microbes: How the Overuse of Antibiotics Is Fueling Our Modern Plagues.* New York: Henry Holt & Company.
5. Ahlman H, Nilsson O. 2001. The gut as the largest endocrine organ in the body. *Ann Oncol.* 12(Suppl 2):S63–8. http://dx.doi.org/10.1093/annonc/12.suppl_2.S63.
6. Hyland NP, Cryan JF. 2016. Microbe-host interactions: influence of the gut microbiota on the enteric nervous system. *Dev Biol.* 417(2):182–7. http://dx.doi.org/10.1016/j.ydbio.2016.06.027.
7. Furness JB, Jones C, Nurgali K, et al. 2004. Intrinsic primary afferent neurons and nerve circuits within the intestine. *Prog Neurobiol.* 72(2):143–64. http://dx.doi.org/10.1016/j.pneurobio.2003.12.004.
8. Wu H, Wu E. 2012. The role of gut microbiota in immune homeostasis and autoimmunity. *Gut Microbes.* 3(1):4–14. http://dx.doi.org/10.4161/gmic.19320.
9. Clemente J, Ursell L, Parfrey L, et al. 2012. The impact of the gut microbiota on human health: an integrative view. *Cell.* 148(6):1258–70. http://dx.doi.org/10.1016/j.cell.2012.01.035.

10. Shreiner AB, Kao JY, Young VB. 2015. The gut microbiome in health and disease. *Cur Opin Gastroenterol.* 31(1):69–75. http://dx.doi.org/10.1097/MOG.0000000000000139.

11. Magne F, Silva AP, Carvajal B, et al. 2017. The elevated rate of cesarean section and its contribution to non-communicable chronic diseases in Latin America: the growing involvement of the microbiota. *Front Pediatr.* 5:192. http://dx.doi.org/10.3389/fped.2017.00192.

12. Fang S, Evans R. 2013. Wealth management in the gut. *Nature.* 500:538–9. http://dx.doi.org/10.1038/500538a.

13. Le Chatelier E, Neilsen T, Qin J, et al. 2013. Richness of human gut microbiome correlates with metabolic markers. *Nature.* 500(7464):541–6. http://dx.doi.org/10.1038/nature12506.

14. Jie Z, Xia H, et al. 2017. The gut microbiome in atherosclerotic cardiovascular disease. *Nat Commun.* 8(1):845. http://dx.doi.org/10.1038/s41467-017-00900-1.

15. Yamashita T. 2017. Intestinal immunity and gut microbiota in atherogenesis. *J Atheroscler Thromb.* 24(2):110–9. http://dx.doi.org/10.5551/jat.38265.

16. Wang Z, Klipfell E, Bennett B, et al. 2011. Gut flora metabolism of phosphatidylcholine promotes cardiovascular disease. *Nature.* 472(7341):57–63. http://dx.doi.org/10.1038/nature09922.

17. Koeth RA, Wang Z, Levinson BS, et al. 2013. Intestinal microbiota metabolism of *L*-carnitine, a nutrient in red meat, promotes atherosclerosis. *Nat Med.* 19(5):576–85. http://dx.doi.org/10.1038/nm.3145.

18. Wang Z, Roberts AB, Buffa JA, et al. 2015. Non-lethal inhibition of gut microbial trimethylamine production for the treatment of atherosclerosis. *Cell.* 163(7):1585–95. http://dx.doi.org/10.1016/j.cell.2015.11.055.

19. Morris MC, Manson JE, Rosner B, et al. 1995. Fish consumption and cardiovascular disease in the physicians' health study: a prospective study. *Am J Epidemiol.* 142(2):166–75. http://dx.doi.org/10.1093/oxfordjournals.aje.a117615.

20. Ruggenenti P, Cattaneo D, Loriga G, et al. 2009. Ameliorating hypertension and insulin resistance in subjects at increased cardiovascular risk: effects of acetyl-L-carnitine therapy. *Hypertension.* 54(3):567–74. http://dx.doi.org/10.1161/HYPERTENSIONAHA.109.132522.

21. Cani PD, Amar J, Iglesias MA, et al. 2007. Metabolic endotoxemia initiates obesity and insulin resistance. *Diabetes.* 56(7):1761–72. http://dx.doi.org/10.2337/db06-1491.

22. Krishnan, K. 2017. Metabolic endotoxemia: a driving force behind chronic illness. *AAPI'S Nutrition Guide to Optimal Health Using Principles of Functional Medicine & Nutritional Genomics* Part 3:265–86. https://www.aapiusa.org/wp-content/uploads/2020/04/Functional-Medicine-and-Nutritional-Genomics.pdf.

23. Jose PA, Raj D. 2015. Gut microbiota in hypertension. *Curr Opin Nephrol Hypertens.* 24(5):403–9. http://dx.doi.org/10.1097/MNH.0000000000000149.

24. Afsar B, Vaziri ND, Aslan G, et al. 2016. Gut hormones and gut microbiota: implications for kidney function and hypertension. *J Am Soc Hypertens.* 10(12):954–61. http://dx.doi.org/10.1016/j.jash.2016.10.007.

25. Bullon P, Cordero MD, Quiles JL, et al. 2011. Mitochondrial dysfunction promoted by Porphyromonas gingivalis lipopolysaccharide as a possible link between cardiovascular disease and periodontitis. *Free Radic Biol Med.* 50(10):1336–43. http://dx.doi.org/10.1016/j.freeradbiomed.2011.02.018.

26. Menni C, Lin C, Cecelja M, et al. 2018. Gut microbial diversity is associated with lower arterial stiffness in women. *Eur Heart J.* 39(25):2390–97. http://dx.doi.org/10.1093/eurheartj/ehy226.

27. Karlsson F, Fak F, Nookaew I, et al. 2012. Symptomatic atherosclerosis is associated with an altered gut metagenome. *Nat Commun.* 3:1245. http://dx.doi.org/10.1038/ncomms2266.

28. Machiels K, Joossens M, Sabino J, et al. 2014. A decrease of the butyrate-producing species Roseburia hominis and Faecalibacterium prausnitzii defines dysbiosis in patients with ulcerative colitis. *Gut.* 63(8):1275–83. https://www.ncbi.nlm.nih.gov/pubmed/24021287. Accessed October 21, 2018.

29. Yang T, Santisteban MM, Rodriguez V. 2015. Gut dysbiosis is linked to hypertension. *Hypertension.* 65(6):1331–40. http://dx.doi.org/10.1161/HYPERTENSIONAHA.115.05315.

30. Cotillard A, Kennedy SP, Kong LC, et al. 2013. Dietary intervention impact on gut microbial gene richness. *Nature.* 500(7464):585–88. http://dx.doi.org/10.1038/nature12480.

31. David LA, Maurice CF, Carmody RN, et al. 2014. Diet rapidly and reproducibly alters the human gut microbiome. *Nature.* 505(7484):559–53. http://dx.doi.org/10.1038/nature12820.

32. Turnbaugh PJ, Ridaura VK, Faith JJ, et al. 2009. The effect of diet on the human gut microbiome: a metagenomic analysis in humanized gnotobiotic mice. *Sci Transl Med.* 1(6):6ra14. http://dx.doi.org/10.1126/scitranslmed.3000322.

33. Suez J, Korem T, Zeevi D, et al. 2014. Artificial sweeteners induce glucose intolerance by altering the gut microbiota. *Nature.* 514(7521):181–6. http://dx.doi.org/10.1038/nature13793.

34. Cabreiro F, Au C, Leung K. 2013. Metformin retards aging in C. elegans by altering microbial folate and methionine metabolism. *Cell.* 153(1):228–39. http://dx.doi.org/10.1016/j.cell.2013.02.035.

35. Vujasinovic M, Tepes B, Volfrand J, et al. 2015. Exocrine pancreatic insufficiency, MRI of the pancreas and serum nutritional markers in patients with coeliac disease. *Postgrad Med J.* 91(1079):497–500. http://dx.doi.org/10.1136/postgradmedj-2015-133262.

36. Stein J, Jung M, Sziegoleit A, et al. 1996. Immunoreactive elastase I: clinical evaluation of a new noninvasive test of pancreatic function. *Clin Chem.* 42(2):222–6. https://www.ncbi.nlm.nih.gov/pubmed/8595714. Accessed October, 2018.

37. Loser C, Mollgaard A, Folsch UR. 1996. Faecal elastase 1: a novel, highly sensitive, and specific tubeless pancreatic function test. *Gut.* 39(4):580–6. http://dx.doi.org/10.1136/gut.39.4.580.

38. Pouillis A, Foster R, Mendall MA, et al. 2003. Emerging role of calprotectin in gastroenterology. *J Gastroenterol Hepatol.* 18(7):756–62. http://dx.doi.org/10.1046/j.1440-1746.2003.03014.x.

39. Carlson M, Raab Y, Peterson C, et al. 1999. Increased intraluminal release of eosinophil granule proteins EPO, ECP, EPX, and cytokines in ulcerative colitis and proctitis in segmental perfusion. *Am J Gastroenterol.* 94(7):1876–83. http://dx.doi.org/10.1111/j.1572-0241.1999.01223.x.

40. Bischoff SC, Mayer J, Nguyen QT, et al. 1999. Immunohistological assessment of intestinal eosinophil activation in patients with eosinophilic gastroenteritis and inflammatory bowel disease. *Am J Gastroenterol.* 94(12):3521–9. http://dx.doi.org/10.1111/j.1572-0241.1999.01641.x.

41. Hau J, Andersson E, Carlsson HE. 2001. Development and validation of a sensitive ELISA for quantification of secretory IgA in rat saliva and faeces. *Lab Anim.* 35(4):301–6. http://dx.doi.org/10.1258/0023677011911822.

42. Choi SW, Park CH, Silva TM, et al. 1996. To culture or not to culture: fecal lactoferrin screening for inflammatory bacterial diarrhea. *J Clin Microbiol.* 34(4):928–32. https://www.ncbi.nlm.nih.gov/pubmed/8815110. Accessed October 21, 2018.

43. Saitoh O, Kojima K, Sugi K, et al. 1999. Fecal eosinophil granule-derived proteins reflect disease activity in inflammatory bowel disease. *Am J Gastroenterol.* 94(12):3513–20. http://dx.doi.org/10.1111/j.1572-0241.1999.01640.x.

44. Liu LX, Chi J, Upton MP, et al. 1995. Eosinophilic colitis associated with larvae of the pinworm Enterobius vermicularis. *Lancet.* 346(8972):410–12. http://dx.doi.org/10.1016/S0140-6736(95)92782-4.

45. Bischoff SC, Grabowsky J, Manns MP. 1997. Quantification of inflammatory mediators in stool samples of patients with inflammatory bowel disorders and controls. *Dig Dis Sci.* 42(2):394–403. https://www.ncbi.nlm.nih.gov/pubmed/9052525. Accessed October 21, 2018.

46. Rothenberg ME, Mishra A, Brandt EB, et al. 2001. Gastrointestinal eosinophils. *Immunol Rev.* 179:139–55. http://dx.doi.org/10.1034/j.1398-9995.2001.00905.x.

47. Clouse RE, Alpers DH, Hockenbery DM, et al. 1992. Pericrypt eosinophilic enterocolitis and chronic diarrhea. *Gastroenterology.* 103(1):168–76. http://dx.doi.org/10.1016/0016-5085(92)91110-P.

48. Hijova E, Chmelaravo A. 2007. Short chain fatty acids and colonic health. *Bratisl Lek Listy.* 108(-8):354–8. https://www.ncbi.nlm.nih.gov/pubmed/18203540. Accessed October 21, 2018.

49. Canfora EE, Jocken JW, Blaak EE. 2015. Short-chain fatty acids in control of body weight and insulin sensitivity. *Nat Rev Endocrinol.* 11(10):577–91. http://dx.doi.org/10.1038/nrendo.2015.128.

50. Tuohy KM, Fava F, Viola R. 2014. "The way to a man's heart is through his gut microbiota" – dietary pro- and prebiotics for the management of cardiovascular risk. *Proc Nutr Soc.* 73(2):172–85. http://dx.doi.org/10.1017/S0029665113003911.

51. Ohira H, Tsutsui W, Fujioka Y. 2017. Are short chain fatty acids in gut microbiota defensive players for inflammation and atherosclerosis? *J Atheroscler Thromb.* 24(7):660–72. http://dx.doi.org/10.5551/jat.RV17006.

52. Angeloni C, Hrelia S. 2012. Quercetin reduces inflammatory responses in LPS-stimulated cardiomyoblasts. *Oxid Med Cell Longev.* http://dx.doi.org/10.1155/2012/837104.

53. Chowdhury R, Nimmanapalli R, Graham T, et al. 2013. Curcumin attenuation of lipopolysaccharide induced cardiac hypertrophy in rodents. *ISPN Inflamm.* 2013:539305. http://dx.doi.org/10.1155/2013/539305.

54. Qi T, Xu F, Yan X, et al. 2016. Sulforaphane exerts anti-inflammatory effects against lipopolysaccharide-induced acute lung injury in mice through the Nrf2/ARE pathway. *Int J Mol Med.* 37(1):182–8. http://dx.doi.org/10.3892/ijmm.2015.2396.

55. Sharafkhaneh A, Velamuri S, Badmaev V, et al. 2007. The potential role of natural agents in treatment of airway inflammation. *Ther Adv Respir Dis.* 1(2):105–20. http://dx.doi.org/10.1177/1753465807086096.

56. Li H, Ruan XZ, Powis SH, et al. 2005. EPA and DHA reduce LPS-induced inflammation responses in HK-2 cells: evidence for a PPAR-gamma-dependent mechanism. *Kidney Int.* 67(3):867–74. http://dx.doi.org/10.1111/j.1523-1755.2005.00151.x.

57. Riedel CU, Foata F, Philippe D, et al. 2006. Anti-inflammatory effects of bifidobacteria by inhibition of LPS-induced NF-kappaB activation. *World J Gastroenterol*. 12(23):3729–35. https://www.ncbi.nlm.nih.gov/pubmed/16773690. Accessed October, 2018.
58. Morenga LT, Docherty P, Williams S. 2017. The effect of a diet moderately high in protein and fiber on insulin sensitivity measured using the dynamic insulin sensitivity and secretion test (DISST). *Nutrients*. 9(12):1291. http://dx.doi.org/10.3390/nu9121291.
59. Lam V, Su J, Koprowski S, et al. 2012. Intestinal microbiota determine severity of myocardial infarction in rats. *FASEB J*. 26(4):1727–35. http://dx.doi.org/10.1096/fj.11-197921.
60. Campbell AW, Sinatra D, Zhang Z, Sinatra ST. 2020. Efficacy of spore forming bacilli supplementation in patients with mild to moderate elevation of triglycerides: A 12 week, randomized, double-blind, placebo controlled trial. *Integr Med (Encinitas)*. 19(2):22–7.
61. McFarlin BK, Henning AL, Bowman EM, Gary MA, Carbajal KM. 2017. Oral spore-based probiotic supplementation was associated with reduced incidence of post-prandial dietary endotoxin, triglycerides, and disease risk biomarkers. *World J Gastrointest Pathophysiol*. 8(3):117–26. http://dx.doi.org/10.4291/wjgp.v8.i3.117.
62. Neag MA, Catinean A, Muntean DM, Pop MR, Bocsan CI, Botan EC, Buzoianu AD. 2020. Probiotic bacillus spores protect against acetaminophen induced acute liver injury in rats. *Nutrients*. 12(3):632. http://dx.doi.org/10.3390/nu12030632.
63. Moco S, Martin FP, Rezzi S. 2012. Metabolomics view on gut microbiome modulation by polyphenol-rich foods. *J Proteome Res*. 11(10):4781–90. http://dx.doi.org/10.1021/pr300581s.
64. *The Precise Reason for the Health Benefits of Dark Chocolate: Mystery Solved* [news release]. Dallas, TX: American Chemical Society; March 18, 2014. https://www.acs.org/content/acs/en/pressroom/newsreleases/2014/march/the-precise-reason-for-the-health-benefits-of-dark-chocolate-mystery-solved.html. Accessed October, 2018.

13 Environmental Toxins and Cardiovascular Disease

Joseph Pizzorno

CONTENTS

Introduction 281
Lead 283
    Sources 284
    Primary Measure 284
    Primary Intervention 284
Air Pollution 285
    Sources 285
    Primary Measure 285
    Primary Intervention 285
Persistent Organic Pollutants (POPs) 286
    Sources 287
    Primary Measure 287
    Primary Intervention 287
Bisphenols 287
    Sources 287
    Primary Measure 288
    Primary Intervention 288
Systemic Approaches 288
    GGTP (Gamma Glutamyl Transferase) 288
    Sauna 289
Conclusion 289
References 290

INTRODUCTION

Environmental toxins damage cardiovascular tissues in many ways.[1] While this chapter focuses on specific toxins, total toxic load is equally important. As the body load of toxic chemicals and metals increases, so do oxidative stress and depletion of antioxidants, especially glutathione. This increased oxidative stress not only systemically increases virtually all the mechanisms of cardiovascular damage but also depletes physiological resources for detoxification and protection from toxins.

The several tables for toxin load come from an extensive, regularly updated CDC database made available to researchers, clinicians, and the public through a large two-volume book titled *Fourth National Report on Human Exposure to Environmental Chemicals.* (While the date says 2019, tables are regularly updated (Figure 13.1).)

This chapter covers the toxins causing the most cardiovascular damage, where they come from, how to access body load, and methods to increase detoxification or excretion. It is not meant to be a

DOI: 10.1201/9781003137849-13

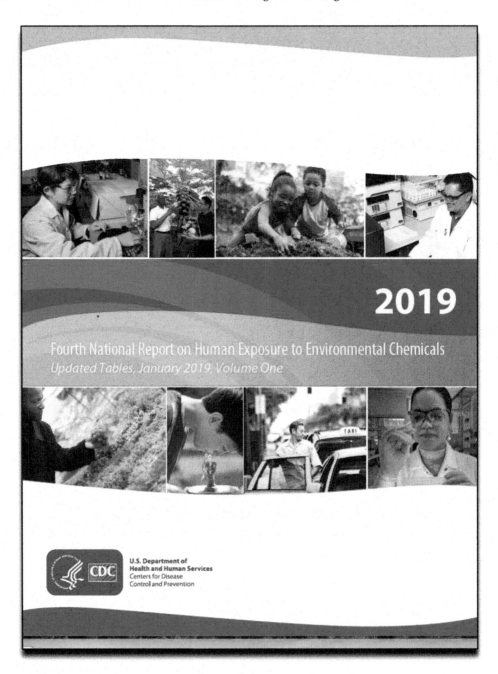

FIGURE 13.1 Fourth National Report on human exposure to environmental chemicals.

comprehensive treatise, but rather a focused guide for busy clinicians. Obviously, many other toxins also cause cardiovascular damage, and the hope of the author is that all clinicians will systematically increase their skills in environmental medicine since every person on the earth is being damaged by environmental pollution. Those interested in delving more deeply into this important area of medicine will find the textbook *Clinical Environmental Medicine* (Elsevier 2019, I coauthored with Dr. Walter Crinnnion) useful.

LEAD

As one of the earliest metals mined and refined by humans, its health consequences were probably the first recognition of an environmental toxin. Study of the history of the evolution of the standards of "safe" levels reveals an important story: In general, the threshold for toxicity was defined by population norms. Those in the top 5% are considered toxic, while the rest of the population is considered normal. This thinking resulted in a toxic threshold level for lead of 60 ug/dL in 1965. Then decade by decade as research evolved, the "safe" levels dropped: 40 ug/dL in 1970, 30 ug/dL in 1975 to 10 ug/dL in 1990. Now the CDC is recommending <3.5 ug/dL for children.[2] There is no safe level of lead. For example, one study showed that those with a supposedly safe level of 5.0–9.0 ug/dL of lead had increased risk of all-cause mortality, cancer, and cardiovascular disease.[3]

The good news is that the public health work to reduce lead release into the environment has been hugely successful. As can be seen in Table 13.1 from the CDC, average population-wide blood levels have been decreasing significantly.

The primary dysfunctions/diseases caused by lead are cognitive decline, mood disorders, Parkinsonism, cardiovascular disease, renal disease, and respiratory and reproductive issues.

A huge number of studies have reported on the role of lead in chronic disease, especially cardiovascular disease. They also show a simple linear relationship between virtually every measure of lead and cardiovascular disease. A comprehensive systematic review and metanalysis comparing top versus bottom thirds of body load found relative risks for lead of 1.43 (1.16–1.76) for cardiovascular disease, 1.85 (1.27–2.69) for coronary heart disease, and 1.63 (1.14–2.34) for stroke.[5]

TABLE 13.1
Blood Lead Levels over Time[4]

Categories (Survey Years)	Geometric Mean (95% Conf. Interval)	50th Percentile (95% Conf. Interval)	75th Percentile (95% Conf. Interval)	90th Percentile (95% Conf. Interval)	95th Percentile (95% Conf. Interval)	Sample Size
Total population (1999–2000)	1.66 (1.60–1.72)	1.60 (1.60–1.70)	2.50 (2.40–2.60)	3.80 (3.60–4.00)	5.00 (4.70–5.50)	7,970
Total population (2001–2002)	1.45 (1.39–1.51)	1.40 (1.40–1.50)	2.20 (2.10–2.30)	3.40 (3.20–3.60)	4.50 (4.20–4.70)	8,945
Total population (2003–2004)	1.43 (1.36–1.50)	1.40 (1.30–1.50)	2.10 (2.10–2.20)	3.20 (3.10–3.30)	4.20 (3.90–4.40)	8,373
Total population (2005–2006)	1.29 (1.23–1.36)	1.27 (1.20–1.34)	2.01 (1.91–2.11)	3.05 (2.86–3.22)	3.91 (3.64–4.18)	8,407
Total population (2007–2008)	1.27 (1.21–1.34)	1.22 (1.18–1.30)	1.90 (1.80–2.00)	2.80 (2.67–2.96)	3.70 (3.50–3.90)	8,266
Total population (2009–2010)	1.12 (1.08–1.16)	1.07 (1.03–1.12)	1.70 (1.62–1.77)	2.58 (2.45–2.71)	3.34 (3.14–3.57)	8,793
Total population (2011–2012)	0.973 (0.916–1.06)	0.930 (0.880–0.980)	1.52 (1.41–1.61)	2.38 (2.17–2.61)	3.16 (2.77–3.68)	7,920
Total population (2013–2014)	0.858 (0.813–0.906)	0.830 (0.780–0.870)	1.32 (1.24–1.42)	2.10 (1.96–2.30)	2.81 (2.49–3.14)	5,215
Total population (2015–2016)	0.820 (0.722–0.872)	0.780 (0.740–0.840)	1.32 (1.21–1.42)	2.14 (2.02–2.24)	2.75 (2.50–2.98)	4,988

Blood Lead (1999–2010).

CAS Number 7439-92-1.

Geometric mean and selected percentiles of blood concentrations (in μg/dL) for the U.S. population from the National Health and Nutrition Examination Survey.

An especially relevant and worrisome large study determined that lead accounted for 18.0% of all-cause mortality, 28.7% of cardiovascular disease mortality, and 37.4% of ischemic heart disease mortality.[6]

Lead is currently the worst toxin damaging the cardiovascular system. Lead is such a serious problem that I recommend every patient, regardless of apparent disease burden, be tested for blood level.[7]

SOURCES

In adults, diet is the source of most low-level environmental exposure to lead. Unfortunately, a surprising number of public water supplies are contaminated with lead. Worse, if water pH and corrosiveness are not properly controlled, lead can be leached from old water supply pipes and from copper pipes installed before 1987 when lead was banned from solder. While the Flint lead fiasco received a lot of media attention, it is only one of hundreds of cities with too much lead in their water supply. Older adults formed the majority of their bones when environmental lead levels were much higher. Therefore, those losing bone have substantially higher blood levels leading to more disease.[8] Other potential sources of lead include contaminated herbal medicines,[9] cosmetics, and ceramic and metal cookware. Industrial exposure can occur in smelting and battery manufacturing. Sources of lead for children are somewhat different. They can be exposed to lead from crawling and hand-to-mouth activities which increase exposure to the contaminated dust and soil around older homes that contain lead-based paint or from eating paint chips that contain lead.

PRIMARY MEASURE

Assessing body load of lead is controversial. While most research looking at the correlation between disease and lead use blood measures, blood measures only modestly correlate with bone levels. Challenge testing is more accurate at assessing total body load. However, this methodology is controversial and not needed by the clinician. Blood lead is a good measure of disease risk and useful for monitoring efficacy of intervention. This author recommends active intervention for anyone with a blood lead above 5.0 ug/dL.

PRIMARY INTERVENTION

As with all toxins, avoidance of exposure is always the foundational approach. In addition, since most older adults have high levels of lead in their bones, preventing bone loss is very important. If living in a house built before 1987, water in the house must be tested.

Since excretion of lead is slow by normal metabolic processes, intervention is usually required. This means both minimizing damage as well as increasing excretion. Calcium, vitamin C, and NAC (N-acetyl cysteine) help prevent damage, while chelating agents such as EDTA and DMSA increase excretion.[10–12] While the vast majority of research on chelating agents is on high dose and/or IV administration, this author suggests lower dosages over longer periods of time to decrease the risk of adverse events and redistribution.

Supplements:
Calcium: 500 bid
Vitamin C: 500 bid
NAC: 500 mg bid
If high blood lead and symptoms:
DMSA: oral, 250 mg/3 day
EDTA: oral, 5 g/day

IV (if especially high and should only be performed by those who are expert in environmental medicine).

Rarely, a patient may indicate signs of sulfur overload (such as GERD, IBS, and allergic rhinitis). All sulfur supplements should be stopped. Some patient can improve their sulfur metabolism by taking 300 ug/day of molybdenum—the trace mineral required by the sulfur-manipulating enzymes.

AIR POLLUTION

While no individual toxin in this group is a primary cause of cardiovascular disease, as a group they appear the second worst environmental causes of cardiovascular disease. Since the mitigation strategy is similar for all, they are addressed together for efficiency. Indoor and outdoor air contains many classes of toxins especially damaging to the cardiovascular system. These include mycotoxins, ozone, sulfur oxides, nitrogen oxides, polycyclic aromatic hydrocarbons (PAHs), and particulate matter (PM). The effects of ozone and sulfur and nitrogen oxides have been known for decades and have been substantially reduced by various public health measures. The good news is that PM has been decreased as well. The bad news is that a substantial amount of research shows that PM, especially $PM_{2.5}$, continues to be a huge problem. The focus here is on PM and PAHs since they appear to currently account for most of the cardiovascular damage from air pollutants. The reason this particle size is worse than the others is that not only do these small particles adsorb PAHs, but they also facilitate their penetration deeply into the tissues by bypassing the cilia of the respiratory tract. Covering all these toxins is far beyond the scope of this chapter.

There is a direct, linear correlation between air toxin exposure and virtually every cardiovascular disease and measures of inflammation. For example, urinary levels of urinary pyrenes—a measure of PAH exposure—directly correlate with all-cause mortality, MI, malondialdehyde, high-sensitivity C-reactive protein, and many other measures of inflammation.[13] Living in a city or within 100 yards of a highway substantially increases exposure and risk of cardiovascular disease. Each increase of 10 μg/m³ $PM_{2.5}$ in the air is associated with a 16% increase in mortality from ischemic heart disease and a 14% increase in mortality from stroke.[14]

SOURCES

PAHs and PM are produced whenever organic materials like wood, tobacco, gasoline, and diesel are burned. Typical sources are cigarette smoke, barbeque smoke, moving vehicles, burning coal for energy, etc. The worst source—accounting for about 90% of air pollution—is diesel trucks. Yes, that blue/black smoke coming out of their exhaust stacks is as bad as it looks.

PRIMARY MEASURE

Research has shown a correlation between several measures of inflammation (e.g., hsCRP) and coagulation (e.g., plasminogen activator inhibitor-10 with exposure to PM).[15] Since these measures are non-specific as they respond to many other factors as well, they are not reliable for measuring exposure to PM. However, they are useful for assessing efficacy of air pollution reduction measures.

Reasonably priced devices to measure air toxins are becoming available for home use. Their reliability is unclear at this time, but accurate and sophisticated devices are under development.[16] Most convenient and accurate is to monitor local reports by public health agencies. These reports are now available to a radius of a few blocks.

PRIMARY INTERVENTION

Good-quality air filters are extremely effective at clearing out PM and their associated PAHs. Optimal is a whole-house air filter with a rating of at least MERV-8, preferably MERV-12. As can

TABLE 13.2

Improvement in Cardiovascular Measures after 48 Hours with a MERV-12 Filter Unit[17]

Measure	After 48 Hours
Clinical Measures	
Systolic pressure	2.7 mmHg decrease
Diastolic pressure	3.0 mmHg decrease
Lung function	No change
Laboratory Measures	
MCP-1, pg/mL	11% reduction
IL-1β, pg	67% reduction
MPO, ng/mL	20% reduction
sCD40L, ng/mL	64% reduction

TABLE 13.3

Improvement in Cardiovascular Measures after 72 Hours with Unit High-Efficiency HEPA-Filtered Air in Bedroom and Living Room

Measure	After 72 Hours
Clinical Measures	
Systolic pressure	2.9 mmHg decrease
Diastolic pressure	0.8 mmHg decrease

be seen in Table 13.2, just 48 hours in a clean room dramatically decreased physical and laboratory measures of cardiovascular damage.

If a whole-house air filter is not possible, then every room the patient spends significant time in should include a HEPA filter. As can be seen in Table 13.3, these are also effective.

All patients who live in a city or within 100 yards of a highway, whether or not suffering from cardiovascular or respiratory disease, should be advised to limit direct exposure to air toxins from the sources listed above and to install air filters in their home or place of work.

PERSISTENT ORGANIC POLLUTANTS (POPS)

Persistent organic pollutants are manmade, new to nature molecules that are very difficult to break down by physical and biological processes. They are a large class of organic molecules with one or more halogen substitutes. These include many of the chemicals used in industry and agriculture. Serum levels of dioxins, furans, polychlorinated biphenyls [PCBs], and chlorinated pesticides directly correlate with risk of virtually every type of cardiovascular disease.

Perhaps worst are the polychlorinated biphenyls (PCBs) which have very long half-lives (measured in years to decades), body load which increases with age, and are strongly associated with cardiovascular disease in both men and women. Example clinical correlations are as follows:

- Cholesterol and triglycerides: directly proportional to total PCBs[18]
- Hypertension: OR 1.70 highest to lowest quartiles (meta-analysis)[19]

- Myocardial infarction: OR 1.74 highest to lowest quintiles (12-year prospective)[20]
- Stroke: OR 3.0 highest to lowest TEQ (composite measure).[21]

SOURCES

Even though banned in the 1970s, exposure to PCBs continues every day due to the general contamination of the environment and eating animal foods which concentrate these fat-soluble toxins, especially farmed fish.[22]

PRIMARY MEASURE

Serum levels of several PCBs are commercially available. They are reported as absolute levels (PPB) or as lipid-adjusted values (ng/g lipid). In general, lipid adjusted is preferred since they correlate better with levels in fat stores. No level of PCBs is considered safe. These measures are best used to access efficacy of intervention.

PRIMARY INTERVENTION

Due to the great difficulty removing these toxins, avoidance is extremely important. This basically means avoiding farmed fish and land animals fed with the feed contaminated with PCBs.

Most any fiber should help excretion, but few have been studied. Rice bran fiber increases excretion by binding to the PCBs as they are released into the gut.[23] The typical dosage is at least 5 g bid. Chlorophyll and chlorophyll-rich foods also facilitate excretion through the stools.[24] The higher the dosage, the more rapid the excretion. In general, 500–1.000 mg/day is an effective dosage with little risk of adverse events (other than stool possibly turning green).

The rate of excretion can be substantially increased with bile sequestrants.[25] While the rate of excretion increases with dosage, so does the risk of the typical ADRs (adverse drug reactions) for these agents, such as smelly, oily diarrhea. The recommendation is to use the highest dosage (typically 5–10 g/day) which does not produce side effects. Be aware this may also decrease absorption of fat-soluble vitamins.

BISPHENOLS

Bisphenols are synthesized chemicals with two phenol groups and one acetone molecule. They were first researched for their estrogenic effects and later came into widespread use in the manufacturing and stabilization of plastic polymers. As the public became aware of the toxicity of BPA, manufacturers substituted it with other bisphenols like BPS, BPA, and BPZ. Unfortunately, these appear as toxic as BPA.

A recent comprehensive meta-analysis of NHANEs data on over 10,000 adults found that risk of cardiovascular disease using urinary BPA/Cr as the measure was 1.13.[26] Another recent large meta-analysis similarly found an OR of 1.19 for CVD.[27]

Very worrisome is the research showing that maternal exposure increases risk of cardiovascular disease in their children. One study that measured urinary levels of BPA at week 20 of gestation found that if the mothers' urinary level exceeded 4.5 ug/g cr, their children at age 4 had a 7.9 mm of Hg increase in diastolic blood pressure.[28] Approximately 10% of the population exceeds these BPA levels. The epigenetic and transgenerational effects of environmental toxins are distorting the "normal" baselines and likely resulting in an underappreciation of the devastating effects of the progressively higher body load of toxins.

SOURCES

Exposure is ubiquitous. The main sources include food, food packaging (especially cans), dust, dental materials, healthcare equipment, thermal paper, toys, and products for children and infants.

Although there are many sources, food, especially canned food, is the primary source for most people. Since BPA has a short half-life, it is technically a non-persistent toxin. However, since exposure is so continuous, some classify them as semi-persistent.

While the statistic above may not sound as alarming as the other toxins covered here, the problem is that the whole population has substantial exposure throughout their entire life.

PRIMARY MEASURE

While total bisphenols is the preferred measure, at this time the only commercially available tests are for urinary and blood BPA. Obviously, the less the better.

PRIMARY INTERVENTION

Since these are non-persistent toxins, avoidance is very effective. However, they are so ubiquitous in food, clothing, packaging, plastics, etc. that total avoidance is almost impossible. Key is to avoid all food stored in plastic or cans and to remove all plastic food storage containers from the home.

The oxidative stress from BPA can be decreased by 1,000 mg/day of NAC (N-acetylcysteine).[29] Curcumin and melatonin have also been shown to decrease the toxicity of BPA.[30,31]

SYSTEMIC APPROACHES

Most of the common environmental metal and chemical pollutants increase risk for cardiovascular disease. While important to understand the worst cardiovascular system damaging toxins, total toxin load is equally important. In addition, while toxin-specific interventions are required, equally important are systemic therapies that indiscriminately increase excretion of all toxins. In this last section, I will cover clinical application of a key measure of total toxic load and saunas for systemic detoxification.

GGTP (GAMMA GLUTAMYL TRANSFERASE)

Measuring body load of every toxin is not only prohibitively expensive, but many are not currently measurable through commercial laboratories. Fortunately, there is a readily available and inexpensive test to monitor total body load of toxins: GGTP. While blood levels of this liver enzyme were measured in the past to diagnose liver inflammation, its better use is in environmental medicine. The role of this enzyme in the liver is to recycle glutathione which plays a key role in both increasing the detoxification and excretion of many toxins as well as protecting normal tissues from the oxidative stress the toxins induce. Within the normal range, GGTP increases in proportion to toxic load—including alcohol consumption—and oxidative stress. (A small percentage of the population does not increase GGTP in response to toxic load. In the author's experience, these people are usually more sensitive to chemicals. They also will not show an increase in GGTP after alcohol consumption.)

As a measure of toxicity and oxidative stress, the fact GGTP levels correlate with many chronic diseases and all-cause mortality is not surprising.[32] The correlation with cardiovascular disease is especially strong. Several review articles documented direct correlation of GGTP with risk of arrhythmias, arterial hypertension, atherosclerosis, congestive heart failure, coronary heart disease, embolic disease, stroke, and sudden cardiac death.[33,34] In general, the many studies show that the GGTP threshold for increased disease risk is at about 24 IU. This author uses 20 IU as the threshold for likely toxin exposure unless the patient is drinking regularly or suffering from oxidative stress from another source.

SAUNA

Sweating is very effective at eliminating many toxins. Research clearly demonstrates high levels of virtually all toxic metals and chemicals in sweat taken from people in saunas.[35] While we cannot say the cardiovascular benefits from sauna are due to detoxification, the results are extremely impressive. Compared to once a week (so not a true control), saunas two to three times a week decreased sudden cardiac death by 29% and fatal cardiovascular disease by 32%. Increasing saunas to four to seven times a week dropped those numbers to a remarkable 51% and 45%, respectively. The protocol I recommend:

- Temperature: high enough to start sweating freely in 15–20 minutes
- Type not critical—all that counts is frequency and length of sweating
- Fluids:
  - Take weight before and after (empty bladder)
  - Drink enough fluids to maintain weight
  - Typically need about 1 pint/20 min heavy sweating
  - Improved detoxification by mildly alkalinizing with trace minerals such as magnesium and potassium citrates
- 20–40 minutes of heavy sweating
- Leave earlier if not feeling well
- Every 2–4 days—listen to body.

All should be aware of the need for careful control of core body temperature in pregnant women. While some simply recommend against pregnant women using sauna, hot tubs, heavy exercise, etc. (i.e., anything that raises body temperature), careful research has shown that the teratogenic effects don't start until her core body temperature exceeds 39°C.[36] This helps explain why pregnant women in Finland who sauna regularly have the lowest rates of anencephaly in the world, while women who sauna infrequently suffer elevated risk for neural tube disorders.[37]

CONCLUSION

Applying environmental medicine concepts to the practice is straightforward and can provide huge benefits to our patients suffering cardiovascular disease. A doctor does not need to be an expert in environmental medicine to help their patient decrease their toxic load. The following are the key priorities:

1. Advise all patients to only eat organically grown foods and if eating fish, only wild caught. If eating land animal products, only eat those raised in a low-toxin environment.
2. Measure the blood lead level of every patient. If above 5.0 ug/dL (3.0 in children), determine and eliminate source and implement methods discussed above to decrease body burden as quickly and safely as possible.
3. Measure the serum GGTP in every patient. If above 20 IU, determine and eliminate sources of chemical or metal toxins and implement methods discussed above to decrease body burden as quickly and safely as possible.
4. If the patient is living in a city or near a major highway, advise them to install as effective air filters as they can afford in their homes and places of work.
5. All patients should be advised to increase dietary fiber, which increases excretion of essentially all toxins.
6. Provide guidance to patients to systematically replace all plastic containers, cooking utensils with non-stick coatings, etc. with less toxic alternatives.
7. Advise patients to sauna two to four times a week until toxic load has substantially declined and then once a week as a health-promoting practice.

REFERENCES

1. Crinnion W, Pizzorno J. (2019) *Clinical Environmental Medicine*. Elsevier, Amsterdam.
2. Blood Lead Reference Value l Lead l CDC (Accessed 01/10/2022).
3. Schober SE, Mirel LB, Graubard BI, Brody DJ, Flegal KM. (2006) Blood lead levels and death from all causes, cardiovascular disease, and cancer: results from the NHANES III mortality study. *Environ Health Perspect*. Oct;114(10):1538–41. PMID: 17035139.
4. Fourth National Report on human exposure to environmental chemicals. Updated tables, January 2019, Volume One.
5. Chowdhury R, Ramond A, O'Keeffe LM, Shahzad S, Kunutsor SK, Muka T, Gregson J, Willeit P, Warnakula S, Khan H, Chowdhury S, Gobin R, Franco OH, Di Angelantonio E. (2018) Environmental toxic metal contaminants and risk of cardiovascular disease: systematic review and meta-analysis. *BMJ*. Aug 29;362:k3310. doi: 10.1136/bmj.k3310. PMID: 30158148; PMCID: PMC6113772.
6. Lanphear BP, Rauch S, Auinger P, et al. (2018) Low-level lead exposure and mortality in US adults: a population-based cohort study. *Lancet Public Health*. Apr;3(4):e177–e184. PMID: 29544878.
7. Pizzorno J. (2019) Time to change standard of care to include screening for common disease-inducing toxicants. *Integr Med (Encinitas)*. Oct;18(5):8–13. PMID: 32549838; PMCID: PMC7219443.
8. Mendola P, Brett K, Dibari JN, Pollack AZ, Tandon R, Shenassa ED. (2013) Menopause and lead body burden among US women aged 45–55, NHANES 1999–2010. *Environ Res*. Feb;121:110–3. doi: 10.1016/j.envres.2012.12.009. Epub 2013 Jan 24. PMID: 23352036; PMCID: PMC3578085.
9. Mathee A, Naicker N, Teare J. (2015). Retrospective investigation of a lead poisoning outbreak from the consumption of an ayurvedic medicine: Durban, South Africa. *Int J Environ Res Public Health*. 12(-7):7804–13. PubMed PMID: 26184256.
10. Flora SJ, Pande M, Mehta A. (2003) Beneficial effect of combined administration of some naturally occurring antioxidants (vitamins) and thiol chelators in the treatment of chronic lead intoxication. *Chem Biol Interact*. Jun 15;145(3):267–80. doi: 10.1016/s0009-2797(03)00025-5. PMID: 12732454.
11. Patrick L. (2006) Lead toxicity part II: the role of free radical damage and the use of antioxidants in the pathology and treatment of lead toxicity. *Altern Med Rev*. Jun;11(2):114–27. PMID: 16813461.
12. Čabarkapa A, Borozan S, Živković L, Stojanović S, Milanović-Čabarkapa M, Bajić V, et al. (2015) CaNa2EDTA chelation attenuates cell damage in workers exposed to lead—a pilot study. *Chem Biol Interact*. 242:171–8. PubMed PMID: 26460059.
13. Brucker N, Moro AM, Charão MF, Durgante J, Freitas F, Baierle M, et al. (2013). Biomarkers of occupational exposure to air pollution, inflammation and oxidative damage in taxi drivers. *Sci Total Environ*. 463–464:884–93. PubMed PMID: 23872245.
14. Hayes RB, Lim C, Zhang Y, Cromar K, Shao Y, Reynolds HR, Silverman DT, Jones RR, Park Y, Jerrett M, Ahn J, Thurston GD. (2020) PM2.5 air pollution and cause-specific cardiovascular disease mortality. *Int J Epidemiol*. Feb 1;49(1):25–35. doi: 10.1093/ije/dyz114. PMID: 31289812; PMCID: PMC7124502.
15. Davis E, Malig B, Broadwin R, Ebisu K, Basu R, Gold EB, Qi L, Derby CA, Park SK, Wu XM. (2020) Association between coarse particulate matter and inflammatory and hemostatic markers in a cohort of midlife women. *Environ Health*. Nov 5;19(1):111. doi: 10.1186/s12940-020-00663-1. PMID: 33153486; PMCID: PMC7643259.
16. Gillooly SE, Zhou Y, Vallarino J, Chu MT, Michanowicz DR, Levy JI, Adamkiewicz G. (2019) Development of an in-home, real-time air pollutant sensor platform and implications for community use. *Environ Pollut*. Jan;244:440–50. doi: 10.1016/j.envpol.2018.10.064. Epub 2018 Oct 15. PMID: 30359926; PMCID: PMC6250577.
17. Chen R, Zhao A, Chen H, Zhao Z, Cai J, Wang C, Yang C, Li H, Xu X, Ha S, Li T, Kan H. (2015) Cardiopulmonary benefits of reducing indoor particles of outdoor origin: a randomized, double-blind crossover trial of air purifiers. *J Am Coll Cardiol*. Jun 2;65(21):2279–87. doi: 10.1016/j.jacc.2015.03.553. PMID: 26022815; PMCID: PMC5360574.
18. Goncharov A, Haase RF, Santiago-Rivera A, Morse G; Akwesasne Task Force on the Environment, McCaffrey RJ, Rej R, Carpenter DO. (2008) High serum PCBs are associated with elevation of serum lipids and cardiovascular disease in a Native American population. *Environ Res*. Feb;106(2):226–39. doi: 10.1016/j.envres.2007.10.006. Epub 2007 Dec 4. PMID: 18054906; PMCID: PMC2258089.
19. Raffetti E, Donat-Vargas C, Mentasti S, Chinotti A, Donato F. (2020) Association between exposure to polychlorinated biphenyls and risk of hypertension: a systematic review and meta-analysis. *Chemosphere*. Sep;255:126984. doi: 10.1016/j.chemosphere.2020.126984. Epub 2020 May 8. PMID: 32679627.

20. Bergkvist C, Berglund M, Glynn A, Julin B, Wolk A, Åkesson A. (2016) Dietary exposure to polychlori-nated biphenyls and risk of myocardial infarction in men—a population-based prospective cohort study. *Environ Int.* Mar;88:9–14. doi: 10.1016/j.envint.2015.11.020. Epub 2015 Dec 12. PMID: 26690540.

21. Lim JE, Lee S, Lee S, Jee SH. (2018) Serum persistent organic pollutants levels and stroke risk. *Environ Pollut.* Feb;233:855–61. doi: 10.1016/j.envpol.2017.12.031. Epub 2017 Dec 15. PMID: 29248762.

22. Rodríguez-Hernández Á, Camacho M, Henríquez-Hernández LA, Boada LD, Valerón PF, Zaccaroni A, Zumbado M, Almeida-González M, Rial-Berriel C, Luzardo OP. (2017) Comparative study of the intake of toxic persistent and semi persistent pollutants through the consumption of fish and seafood from two modes of production (wild-caught and farmed). *Sci Total Environ.* Jan 1;575:919–31. doi: 10.1016/j.scitotenv.2016.09.142. Epub 2016 Sep 23. PMID: 27670595.

23. Morita K, Hamamura K, Iida T. (1995) Binding of PCB by several types of dietary fiber in vivo and in vitro. *Fukuoka Igaku Zasshi.* May;86(5):212–7. Japanese. PMID: 7628811.

24. Morita K, Ogata M, Hasegawa T. (2001) Chlorophyll derived from Chlorella inhibits dioxin absorp-tion from the gastrointestinal tract and accelerates dioxin excretion in rats. *Environ Health Perspect.* Mar;109(3):289–94. doi: 10.1289/ehp.01109289. PMID: 11333191; PMCID: PMC1240248.

25. Mochida Y, Fukata H, Matsuno Y, Mori C. (2007) Reduction of dioxins and polychlorinated biphenyls (PCBs) in human body. *Fukuoka Igaku Zasshi.* Apr;98(4):106–13. PMID: 17533984.

26. Moon S, Yu SH, Lee CB, Park YJ, Yoo HJ, Kim DS. (2021) Effects of bisphenol A on cardiovascular disease: an epidemiological study using National Health and Nutrition Examination Survey 2003–2016 and meta-analysis. *Sci Total Environ.* Apr 1;763:142941. doi: 10.1016/j.scitotenv.2020.142941. Epub 2020 Oct 14. PMID: 33158523.

27. Fu X, Xu J, Zhang R, Yu J. (2020) The association between environmental endocrine disruptors and cardiovascular diseases: a systematic review and meta-analysis. *Environ Res.* Aug;187:109464. doi: 10.1016/j.envres.2020.109464. Epub 2020 Apr 9. PMID: 32438096.

28. Bae S, Lim YH, Lee YA, Shin CH, Oh SY, Hong YC. (2017) Maternal urinary bisphenol a concentration during midterm pregnancy and children's blood pressure at age 4. *Hypertension.* Feb;69(2):367–74. doi: 10.1161/HYPERTENSIONAHA.116.08281. Epub 2016 Dec 5. PMID: 27920131.

29. Jain S, Kumar CH, Suranagi UD, Mediratta PK. (2011) Protective effect of N-acetylcysteine on bisphe-nol A-induced cognitive dysfunction and oxidative stress in rats. *Food Chem Toxicol.* Jun;49(6):1404–9. doi: 10.1016/j.fct.2011.03.032. Epub 2011 Mar 31. PMID: 21440025.

30. Aslanturk A, Uzunhisarcikli M. (2020) Protective potential of curcumin or taurine on nephrotoxicity caused by bisphenol A. *Environ Sci Pollut Res Int.* Jul;27(19):23994–24003. doi: 10.1007/s11356-020-08716-1. Epub 2020 Apr 17. PMID: 32304054.

31. Kobroob A, Peerapanyasut W, Chattipakorn N, Wongmekiat O. (2018) Damaging effects of bisphenol a on the kidney and the protection by melatonin: emerging evidences from in vivo and in vitro studies. *Oxid Med Cell Longev.* Feb 18;2018:3082438. doi: 10.1155/2018/3082438. PMID: 29670679; PMCID: PMC5835250.

32. Yang P, Wu P, Liu X, Feng J, Zheng S, Wang Y, Fan Z. (2019) Association between γ-glutamyltransferase level and cardiovascular or all-cause mortality in patients with coronary artery disease: a systematic review and meta-analysis. *Angiology.* Oct;70(9):844–52. doi: 10.1177/0003319719850058. Epub 2019 May 23. PMID: 31122026.

33. Ndrepepa G, Colleran R, Kastrati A. (2018) Gamma-glutamyl transferase and the risk of atherosclerosis and coronary heart disease. *Clin Chim Acta.* Jan;476:130–8. doi: 10.1016/j.cca.2017.11.026. Epub 2017 Nov 23. PMID: 29175647.

34. Bulusu S, Sharma M. (2011) What does serum γ-glutamyltransferase tell us as a cardiometabolic risk marker? *Ann Clin Biochem.* 2016 May;53(Pt 3):312–32. doi: 10.1177/0004563215597010. Epub 2015 Jul 2. PMID: 26139450.

35. Genuis SJ, Birkholz D, Rodushkin I, Beesoon S. (2010) Blood, urine, and sweat (BUS) study: monitor-ing and elimination of bioaccumulated toxic elements. *Arch Environ Contam Toxicol.* Aug;61(2):344–57. doi: 10.1007/s00244-010-9611-5. Epub 2010 Nov 6. PMID: 21057782.

36. Ravanelli N, Casasola W, English T, et al. (2019) Heat stress and fetal risk. Environmental limits for exercise and passive heat stress during pregnancy: a systematic review with best evidence synthesis. *Br J Sports Med.* Jul;53(13):799–805.

37. Waldenström U. (1994) Warm tub bath and sauna in early pregnancy: risk of malformation uncertain. *Acta Obstet Gynecol Scand.* Jul;73(6):449–51.

14 Dental Disease, Inflammation, Cardiovascular Disease, Nutrition and Nutritional Supplements

Douglas G. Thompson

Gregori M. Kurtzman

Chelsea Q. Watkins

CONTENTS

Introduction 294
Periodontal Disease, Caries, Periapical Infections, Inflammatory Infiltrates and the
    Inflammatory Cascade 294
    What Is Periodontal Disease and What Causes It? 294
The Guilty Bugs: Oral Biofilm in Periodontal Disease, Caries and Periapical Disease –
    Effects on Cardiovascular Disease...295
    What We Know about the Systemic Connection 296
The Dynamic Duo: How Does Blood Glucose Control and Diabetes Impact Periodontal and
    Cardiovascular Diseases 296
    Cardiovascular Disease (CVD)..297
    Periodontal Disease and Atherosclerosis as an Inflammatory Process 298
    Diagnosing Periodontal Disease 299
    Periodontal Disease: Treatment and Maintenance 303
    Host Modulation 305
    How Can We Better Manage Oral Biofilms? 306
    Host Modulation Using Nutrition 309
    Biofilm Elimination over the Long Term 312
    Collaboration between the Physician and Dentist 315
    Collaborative Inflammation and Biofilm Treatment: Dentistry and Medicine 316
References 322

DOI: 10.1201/9781003137849-14

INTRODUCTION

Periodontal (gum) disease, dental caries and periapical infections are some of the most common dental diseases affecting humans. They all are inflammatory diseases that affect either the gingival tissue, bone supporting the teeth, structure of the teeth or the root end of an infected tooth.

Periodontal disease, when left untreated, can lead to tooth loss from the destruction of the bone supporting the teeth. Recent studies suggest that in adults over the age of 30, 42%–47% have some form of periodontal disease. In those aged 65 and above, that incidence increases to 70.1% affecting 64.7 million Americans.[1–3] Prevalence is highest in Hispanics (63.5%) and non-Hispanic blacks (59.1%), followed by non-Hispanic Asian Americans (50.0%) and lowest in non-Hispanic whites (40.8%).[4] With respect to gender, this condition is more common in men than women (56.4% vs 38.4%). Additionally, this disease is more prevalent in those living below the federal poverty level (65.4%), in individuals with less than a high school education (66.9%) and in current smokers (64.2%). This data was confirmed with the 2017–2018 NHANES report, and its updated data was reported in May 2021.[5] Research has demonstrated that periodontal disease is associated with multiple systemic health conditions, including cardiovascular disease, diabetes, osteoporosis, pulmonary disorders, renal issues and Alzheimer's to name a few. It is currently being studied and cross-referenced to 57 other systemic diseases.[6,7]

Dental caries is the disease process causing cavities that structurally compromise the tooth structure (enamel and dentin). Caries is a very prevalent disease affecting or having affected 92% of adults aged 20–64 in their permanent teeth, with 26% of adults aged 20–64 having untreated decay.[8] Caries is also the most common chronic disease among youth aged 6–19 years.[9] Among children aged 5–19 years, 13.2%[10] have been reported as having untreated caries. Caries is especially prevalent in children and older adults with specific bacteria responsible for the caries infection. It is clearly a biofilm disease modulated by host susceptibility, and not all children are victims of it. Interestingly, those bacteria associated with the caries disease are also associated with changes in vascular biology which subsequently contribute to the cardiovascular disease process.

Periapical infections (infections at the root end of the teeth) can be of pulpal (nerve) or periodontal (gum) origin. Bacterial invasion of the pulpal tissue related to caries of the overlying tooth structure is the most common cause of devitalization of the tooth's pulp. During this devitalization process, the body responds with a foreign body reaction at the root end (apex) of the tooth. This may result in suppuration, pain and/or swelling in addition to bacterial accumulation in the area surrounding the tooth's apex. *Streptococcus viridans*, a facultative anaerobe, is typically the putative pathogen in this infection; however,[11] *Staphylococcus aureus* has been frequently reported from acute dental abscesses, ranging from 0.7% to 15%.[12] It has been reported that 41%–59% of individuals have had at least one endodontic treatment (root canal), and 24%–65% of these endodontically treated teeth remain associated with secondary apical periodontitis (SAP).[13] Both primary and secondary periapical periodontitis have a direct effect on inflammation and generalized inflammatory biomarkers. These streptococci have systemic implications in various systemic diseases, such as infective endocarditis, purulent infections, brain hemorrhage, intestinal inflammation and autoimmune diseases, as well as generalized bacteremia.[14]

PERIODONTAL DISEASE, CARIES, PERIAPICAL INFECTIONS, INFLAMMATORY INFILTRATES AND THE INFLAMMATORY CASCADE

WHAT IS PERIODONTAL DISEASE AND WHAT CAUSES IT?

Periodontal disease, a chronic inflammatory process, is initiated by oral bacteria, yeast, viruses and their byproducts that stimulate a unique host immunoinflammatory response to them. Although the microbial community stimulates a response that initiates the periodontal inflammation, over-activation of the host immune response directly activates osteoclastic activity leading to alveolar bone loss.[15] The inflammatory response can become chronic, producing continual inflammation and ultimately a dysregulation of bone metabolism that leads to bone loss, tooth mobility and eventual tooth loss if left untreated. Severe periodontitis affects more than 700 million people (11% of the world's population), making it one of the most prevalent chronic inflammatory diseases worldwide.[16]

Each patient has a unique host response to the oral biofilm generated from their combined innate (genetic) and acquired (environmental) risk factors. Innate (genetic) risk factors are things you cannot change like ethnicity, gender assigned at birth and age. Acquired (environmental) risk factors are alterable things such as smoking, nutrition, stress management and sleep quantity/quality to name a few. This polymicrobial disease can be slowly progressing or quite aggressive depending on an individual's host response. It may also be episodic in nature, based on the varying health and strength of the immune system. Thus, periodontal disease is oral biofilm induced but host modulated. Dentistry's traditional focus has been on controlling this disease to prevent bone loss and ultimately tooth loss; yet, in recent years, additional concerns to systemic health have come to light.

Plaque is a community of microorganisms found on the tooth surface or within the gingival sulcus (periodontal pocket), which are embedded in a matrix of polymers of host and bacterial origin. This is much more of a complex bio-environment than previously recognized and has been re-termed a community called oral biofilm as a result.[17,18] Between 700 and 1,500 different species of bacteria naturally reside in the mouth.[19-22] Most of those oral bacteria are considered innocuous, but some of these microorganisms have been identified as pathogenic. This aggregation of bacteria work symbiotically together as a community, producing specific proteins and enzymes utilizing oral fluids as the vector for transmission and the source of nutrients.[23] It has been long demonstrated that those microbial communities can display enhanced pathogenicity (pathogenic synergism) compared to bacteria that are planktonic (free floating). Additionally, unlike planktonic bacteria, those in biofilms are protected by the surrounding slime layer which restricts the host's ability to remove them via an immunological action or from the penetration of antimicrobial agents. This means that biofilm infections are less susceptible to antimicrobials applied locally or administered systemically.[24,25] To summarize, bacteria in these complex biofilms act and react differently than bacteria that are planktonic in nature which complicates management and treatment, and makes them potentially more harmful. In addition to oral bacteria, yeast and viruses are also found in the biofilm of some patients with periodontal disease. The composition of the biofilm in periodontal and periapical disease has long been ignored for any affects outside the oral cavity because the connection to systemic health had been poorly understood. Research has now linked pathogenic biofilm to the vascular disease process and negative effects on the biology of the blood vessels.[26]

THE GUILTY BUGS: ORAL BIOFILM IN PERIODONTAL DISEASE, CARIES AND PERIAPICAL DISEASE – EFFECTS ON CARDIOVASCULAR DISEASE

The bacterial community's composition in the pathogenic biofilm is very diverse. Variations in the many species may be different from site to site in the same patient.[27] With biofilm maturation and disease progression, the microbial composition changes from one that is primarily gram-positive and streptococcus-rich to a structure filled with gram-negative anaerobes.[28-31]

Formation of the biofilm includes a series of steps that begins with the initial colonization of the pellicle through adsorption of bacterial molecules creating an adhesive layer on the tooth surface. This leads to other diverse bacterial species' co-adhesion using bacterial receptors to create diversity. There are both synergistic and antagonistic biochemical interactions among the inhabitants of the pellicle. Those bacteria continue to divide until a three-dimensional mixed-culture biofilm forms that is specially and functionally organized with polymer production leading to development of an extracellular matrix. This matrix is a key structural aspect of the biofilm offering the inhabitants protection from external factors. As the biofilm matrix thickens and microbiome becomes more mature, anaerobic bacteria are able to live deeper within the biofilm, and with the biofilm and aerobic bacteria further protecting them from the oxygen-rich environment within the oral cavity they survive in. The early biofilm is able to withstand frequent mechanisms of oral bacterial removal such as chewing, swallowing and salivary fluid flow. Early biofilm colonizers are also able to survive in the high oxygen concentrations present in the oral cavity. This initial biofilm is always present orally, forming immediately after oral cleansing (toothbrushing) by the patient.

The understanding of how complex oral biofilm, and the dentists' management of it, has evolved as science has demonstrated that "plaque" is not as innocuous as previously thought. The current understanding is what is contained in the oral biofilm, and how its components interact, has far-reaching (systemic) actions that have an effect on multiple systems and conditions of the body including cardiac, pulmonary, renal, diabetes, colon, arthritis, Alzheimer's and a variety of other areas of the body. In fact, periodontal pockets and atheromatous plaques associated with cardiovascular disease can present similarities in microbial composition, indicating possible bacterial translocation between periodontal pockets and coronary arteries.[32–34] Pathogenic organisms in the biofilm associated with dental caries can also be found in atheromatous plaques far distant from the site of the infection.[35] This has been reported in older patients and may be a contributor to coronary artery disease in the aging population.[36] Similar results can be said for periapical infections, and this biofilm can now be taught of as "traveling oral microbiome" having vascular and systemic health effects far from oral infectious sites of the teeth, gingiva and bone. For the purposes of this chapter, those organisms in all three of these dental infections (caries, periapical abscess and periodontal disease) will be grouped together and referred to as disease-producing biofilm components.

WHAT WE KNOW ABOUT THE SYSTEMIC CONNECTION

Harmful strains of bacteria and their byproducts in the oral biofilm can enter the bloodstream during the inflammatory response and travel to other areas of the body.[37,38] Increasing evidence indicates that patients with periodontal disease have a much higher risk of developing cardiovascular and other systemic issues than those individuals who take preventive measures to eliminate and control the biofilm in their mouths.[39]

THE DYNAMIC DUO: HOW DOES BLOOD GLUCOSE CONTROL AND DIABETES IMPACT PERIODONTAL AND CARDIOVASCULAR DISEASES

Diabetes is a significant public health problem globally, specifically in the United States.[40] Current statistics report that 34.2 million people, or 10.5% of the US population, have diabetes, with 7.3 million (21.4%) of those people being undiagnosed.[41,42] Additionally, 88 million people above the age of 17 have been reported as prediabetic (34.5% of the adult US population).

Patients with diabetes have twice the risk for periodontal disease than those without the metabolic disorder.[43] In addition, periodontal disease progresses more rapidly and is often more severe in patients with type I or type II diabetes.[44–46] Periodontal disease has been classified as the sixth most common complication of diabetes and is a strong, well-established risk factor for severe periodontal disease. Patients with periodontal infections have worse glycemic control over time and thus have greater difficulty managing their diabetes. Treatment of periodontitis appears to improve glycemic control.[47,48] Diabetic patients who are having difficulty controlling their blood sugar following medication recommendations and prescriptions from their physician, may be affected negatively by the oral biofilm microbiome. Ultimate control of their oral condition by the dentist may aid in controlling their blood sugar since the relationship with oral pathogens is bidirectional. Diabetes provides a collaborative opportunity between dentists in coordination with their physicians. Therefore, control of the periodontal infection and associated biofilm should be part of the standard treatment for the diabetic patient.

Cardiovascular Disease (CVD)

The connection between periodontal and cardiovascular diseases and the impact of the oral biofilm is the most apparent. Unfortunately, this connection has been ignored or misunderstood by dentists and physicians alike until recent literature has provided evidence of that connection.

CVD, an umbrella term for cardiac and blood vessel conditions, such as atherosclerosis, coronary heart disease, stroke and myocardial infarction, is the result of a complex set of genetic and environmental factors.[49,50] It is commonly accepted that genetic factors including age, lipid metabolism, obesity, hypertension and diabetes have a direct connection to CVD and its severity. Environmental risk factors also play a key role and include socioeconomic status, exercise, stress, diet, smoking and chronic infections. Classic risk factors such as hypertension, hypercholesterolemia and cigarette smoking may only account for one-half to two-thirds of the incidence of CVD.[32] Increasing evidence has been reported linking chronic infection and its associated inflammation to CVD with biofilm as a predisposing factor.[51–56] The connection between oral bacteria and cardiac disease is not a recent development. Connections have been reported for over more than two decades and are well supported in the literature. Oral bacteria, specifically *Porphyromonas gingivalis* (periodontitis), *Streptococcus mutans* (cariogenic) and *Streptococcus viridians* (periapical infections), induce platelet aggregation, which leads to thrombus formation.[57,58] Research shows that these microorganisms have a negative effect on vascular elasticity, endothelial function, HDL efflux, lipids, the atheromatous process, and various inflammatory biomarkers and mediators. Schenkein reported "increased systemic levels of inflammatory mediators stimulated by bacteria and their products at sites distant from the oral cavity, elevated thrombotic and hemostatic markers that promote a prothrombotic state and inflammation, cross-reactive systemic antibodies that promote inflammation and interact with the atheroma, promotion of dyslipidemia with consequent increases in proinflammatory lipid classes and subclasses, and common genetic susceptibility factors present in both diseases leading to increased inflammatory responses."[59] Such mechanisms may increase systemic inflammation in periodontal disease, promoting or exacerbating atherogenesis. Those patients with acute myocardial infarction were reported to have worse periodontal status compared to patients who were without CVD. Additionally, greater severity of the periodontitis, plaque accumulation and bleeding on probing are associated with acute myocardial infarction. Therefore, periodontal disease as a risk factor for myocardial infarction affects the degree of post-infarction damage, providing an inflammatory link between these two diseases.[60]

One or more periodontal pathogens as reported in the literature are found in 42% of atheroma in patients with severe periodontal disease.[61] It has been reported that *P. gingivalis* actively can adhere to and invade fetal bovine heart endothelial cells and aortic endothelial cells.[62] Additionally, *P. gingivalis* has been reported to impair endothelial integrity by inhibiting cell proliferation, which induces endothelial mesenchymal transformation and apoptosis of endothelial cells. This reduces cell levels causing the endothelium to lose its ability to repair itself.[63] Research also supports similar findings for *Fusobacterium nucleatum* and endothelial permeability. A 14-year study found that patients with periodontal disease had a 25% higher risk to develop CVD than their healthy counterparts.[64] Men younger than 50 years with periodontal disease demonstrate 72% more risk to develop CVD, with a twofold increased risk for both fatal and non-fatal strokes.[65] Despite the strong evidence of an association between periodontal disease and CVD, it is unknown if it is a direct or causal relationship. It has been reported that the occurrence of periodontitis leads to an increase in blood pressure, suggesting that the presence of periodontitis may increase the risk of arterial hypertension and lead to ineffectiveness of antihypertensive treatment.[66,67] Patients with higher levels of bacteria in their mouths tend to have thicker carotid arteries, which is an indicator of CVD.[68] Bacteria associated with diseased gingiva appear to induce platelet clumping, which may then cause clotting and blockages that can lead to heart attacks or strokes.

The body's response to periodontal infection includes production of inflammatory mediators, which travel through the circulatory system and may cause harmful effects on the heart and blood vessels. Inflammatory mediators such as lipoprotein and triglycerides are significantly higher in patients with periodontitis than in control groups.[69] Increased levels of C-reactive protein (CRP), a biomarker for inflammation, is associated with periodontitis.[70] Periodontal disease releases bacteria which may enter the circulation, invading the heart and vascular tissue, causing harmful effects. Clinical evidence suggests that periodontal disease is associated with a systemic host response and a low-grade inflammatory state that can affect serum levels of CRP and endothelial dysfunction. The overall effect of periodontal therapy was associated with a reduction in CRP and improvement in endothelial dysfunction.[71]

Emergence of periodontal disease as a potential risk factor for CVD is leading to a convergence in oral and medical care. Proper management of oral health may very well be key to prevention of cardiac disease, and when the oral factors are not properly managed, existing heart conditions may worsen. Proper management requires coordination by the patient's physician and dentist, in addition to improved homecare by the patients themselves.

PERIODONTAL DISEASE AND ATHEROSCLEROSIS AS AN INFLAMMATORY PROCESS

The major pathological component of cardiovascular disease, particularly atherosclerosis, involves an inflammatory response to the multiple components of the adaptive immune system.[72] Links between atherosclerosis and periodontal disease can be predicted based on the bacteria-initiated inflammatory mechanisms created by periodontal disease both locally and systemically.[73] This has an influence on the initiation and propagation of atherosclerotic lesions which may be initiated by local or systemic inflammation.

Inflammation produces cytokines and chemotactic agents causing endothelial changes which include up-regulation of adhesion molecules.[59] The role of inflammation in CVD offers the possibility that other disorders characterized by inflammation, such as periodontal disease, may have an indirect role influencing risk, manifestation and progression of vascular events.[74] Those endothelial changes promote interactions with leucocytes (monocytes) promoting leucocyte migration into the interior layer of the arteries, resulting in lipid streaks. Up-regulation of the endothelium releases chemotactic cytokines (monocyte chemotactic protein-1 (MCP-1)), which further attract cells that can transport bacteria into the lesion. Resident dendritic cells (DCs) and monocytes attracted by those cytokines become foam cells following ingestion of LDLs releasing inflammatory cytokines and matrix metalloproteinases (MMPs), which further enhances the localized inflammatory response.[75,76] Thus, initiation and propagation of early atherosclerotic lesions may be enhanced by periodontal disease when periodontal bacteria or their effects on the host immune response, such as t-cell responses, contribute to endothelial dysfunction. Additionally, attraction of monocytes with enhanced lipid uptake by the cells leads to plaque formation in the vessel wall (Figure 14.1).

Excess inflammation mediated by those inflammatory cells may lead to plaque cap instability, which can lead to rupture or erosion of the vessel walls resulting in myocardial infarction or a stroke.[77,78]

Periodontal disease is generated by microorganisms which may enter the general circulation causing a bacteremia. Some species of these microorganism have been identified as high-risk pathogens. Those high-risk pathogens are currently understood as *Aggregatibacter actinomycetemcomitans* (Aa), *Porphyromonas gingivalis* (Pg), *Tannerella forsythia* (Tf), *Treponema denticola* (Td) and *Fusobacterium nucleatum* (Fn). High-risk pathogens may adversely influence the atherosclerosis pathogenesis triad in three distinct ways. High-risk periodontal pathogens affect serum lipoprotein concentration, endothelial permeability and lipoprotein binding in the intima. Strong evidence also supports that periodontal bacteria affect vascular elasticity, lipid concentration, vascular biomarkers, HDL efflux and endothelial function. Therefore, the dental community has a substantial opportunity to assist in mitigating the number one cause of morbidity and mortality, namely cardiovascular disease, by effective management of periodontal disease and reduction or elimination of those high-risk pathogens.[79–81]

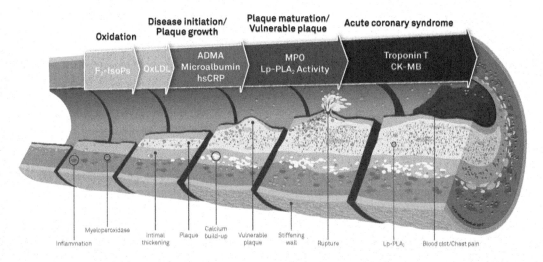

FIGURE 14.1 Cutaway of an artery at various disease stages with related biomarkers. Initiation and propagation of endothelial inflammation leading to plaque formation may be initiated by periodontal inflammation and other risk factors. (Photo courtesy Cleveland Heart Lab.)

DIAGNOSING PERIODONTAL DISEASE

Periodontal disease is not strictly a bacterial issue. It has been demonstrated that yeast and viruses play a role in periodontal disease progression and are part of the complex biofilm. This biofilm initiates an individualized patient immunoinflammatory process that is host dependent on genetics and environmental influence. It is this unique host response that ultimately determines the individual's sensitivity and reaction to the initiating insult.[82] Lifestyle and multiple risk factors can modulate the disease expression. For example, chronic stress has been shown to increase the severity of the pathologic progression of periodontal disease. It has been shown that lifestyle modification may not only improve oral health status, but also its systemic connections.[83,84] As with systemic inflammation, response will vary from patient to patient to the same insult. Periodontally, some patients will exhibit high degrees of inflammation with minimal insult from the biofilm present, whereas other patients will present with high biofilm levels but exhibit minimal or no gingival inflammation. Recognizing the etiology and the inflammatory nature of periodontal disease opens new opportunities for diagnosis, treatment and long-term management of the disease. Managing the disease can prevent tooth loss as well as reduce cardiovascular and other systemic involvement or complications to systemic diseases already present.

Traditionally, periodontal disease has been diagnosed by increases in pocket depth, bleeding gums and bone loss around the teeth leading to clinical attachment loss. Today, the same information is utilized to determine if the disease is and has been present; however, dentists are using the presence of gingival bleeding (bleeding on probing) to determine if the disease is active or stable. The presence of a periodontal pocket (4 mm or greater) is not indicative of active disease, especially when bleeding is not identified on probing. Radiographic evidence of bone loss associated with the teeth indicates prior disease, but it is the presence of bleeding on probing that determines disease activity and the presence of inflammation or in the case of zero bleeding on probing disease stability. When inflammation is identified, it signifies that there has been a histological alteration and bleeding on probing is a result of that change. Dental practitioners recognize that bleeding on probing and gingival inflammation can also be initiated by other systemic issues as well such as caries, failing restorative dentistry, herbals taken in supplement form and other factors. These other initiators of bleeding on probing need to be taken into consideration during the formulation of the diagnosis.

For the purposes of this chapter, we are referring to inflammation of the gingival complex that is biofilm mediated and host modulated due to periodontal disease pathogens. When periodontal disease is biofilm related, treatment traditionally consists of mechanical debridement of the supra- and subgingival tooth surfaces (scaling and root planing) to remove any hard deposits (calculus) present and disrupt the oral biofilm.[85] Following a healing period, traditionally of 6 weeks, a favorable host response is expected as evidenced by the elimination of bleeding on probing. Observing zero bleeding on probing becomes a surrogate endpoint and a sign that the periodontal disease, and its associated inflammation, has been arrested. Studies show that zero bleeding on probing has a 98%–99% negative predictive value for further bone breakdown. The absence of bleeding on probing can therefore be used as a sign of periodontal stability.[86,87]

Numerous studies have demonstrated that in addition to the bacteria in the biofilm, periodontal disease severity in adults is intricately linked with increases in local inflammatory mediators due to genetic mutations of genes regulating the production of inflammatory cytokines. One commonly recognized inflammatory cytokine is interleukin-1. A mutation of the interleukin-1 (IL-1) gene can cause overexpression of IL-1 making it a key player in the inflammatory process and a prime candidate for a genetic association with periodontal disease.[88–90] Thirty percent of the population can be identified with IL-1 polymorphisms.[91,92] The presence of the IL-1 genotype does not confer an expected periodontal disease diagnosis. However, this gene mutation has been implicated as a contributory factor to the host's immunoinflammatory response contributing to the severity of adult periodontitis.[93] The IL-1 gene has also been connected to atherothrombosis.[94]

Saliva consists of the fluid excreted from the major and minor salivary glands, containing proteins, enzymes and buffers that are designed to provide protection, buffering, digestion and aid in swallowing. Saliva also contains a serum exudate known as gingival crevicular fluid. In inflamed tissues, this serum exudate serves as a protective mechanism to cleanse the "pocket" of the bacteria and debris that reside within the sites. Gingival crevicular fluid contains bacteria, yeast, viruses, serum, white blood cells, inflammatory mediators and matrix metalloproteinases. Thus, saliva is an excellent source for bacterial and human cell DNA. Both kinds of DNA can be extracted and analyzed through a laboratory process called polymerase chain reaction (PCR). In molecular biology, PCR is a technique for detection and elongation of DNA strands, an indispensable technique for duplicating DNA so that it can be analyzed for the identification of hereditary diseases, as well as the detection and diagnosis of infectious disease. DNA-PCR also permits identification of mycobacteria, anaerobic bacteria or viruses from the saliva sample sent for testing. Several unique salivary tests are now available to dentists that are reliable, affordable and easy – requiring only minutes to collect. These tests evaluate bacteria, yeast, viruses and genetic variations in genes that express inflammatory mediators. Within 4–5 days of receipt of the sample, a comprehensive interpretation of the periodontal pathogens detected and their concentrations present in the saliva are sent to the clinician.

Utilizing modern salivary diagnostic tests or a combination of them can significantly enhance the practitioner's knowledge about the initiators of the periodontal disease process. Just like the tests for oral pathogens, tests also exist for genetic mutations that may affect the disease process. These tests identify potential genetic mutations that may increase the risk of acquiring periodontal disease or reacting more severely to the disease if the patient already has it. Examples of some of the genes significant to this and other inflammatory disease processes are beta-defensin 1, CD14, toll-like receptor 4, tumor necrosis factor-alpha, interleukin-1, interleukin-6, interleukin-17A and matrix metallopeptidase 3. The Celsus One™ (OralDNA® Labs, Eden Prairie, MN) test evaluates for mutations in eight gene markers related to a potential exaggerated inflammatory response: IL-1 composite genotype, IL-6, IL-17 A, beta-defensin 1, CD14, tumor necrosis factor-alpha, toll-like receptor 4 composite genotype and matrix metalloproteinase 3. These gene mutations are associated with an increased risk for more severe periodontal infections, as well as increased risk for periimplantitis (periodontal disease associated with dental implants), diabetes and cardiovascular disease (Figure 14.2).[95,96]

Reason for Testing: Patient assessment/post treatment, Diabetes, Cardiovascular disease

CELSUS ONE: GENETIC ANALYSIS FOR MARKERS OF ORAL AND SYSTEMIC INFLAMMATION

Type of Immunity	Gene Marker	Genotype	Inflammation Index
Innate	Beta-defensin 1 (DEFB1)	G/A	Low Risk
	CD14 (CD14)	T/T	
	Toll-like receptor 4 (TLR4)	AA/CC	
Acquired	Tumor necrosis factor alpha (TNF-alpha)	C/C	Intermediate Risk
	Interleukin 1 (IL1)	TT/CT	
	Interleukin 6 (IL6)	C/C	
	Interleukin 17A (IL17A)	G/G	
	Matrix Metallopeptidase 3 (MMP3)	5A/5A	

Interpretation:

The genotypes for markers DEFB1, CD14 and TLR4 for this individual collectively predict a normal phenotype for the innate immune system and a low risk for chronic systemic inflammation. Specifically, the expected level of gene expression, and/or levels of these proteins, is normal in response to environmental and disease-causing bacteria and other effectors of inflammation. See comment.

The genotypes for markers TNF-alpha, IL1, IL6, IL17A, and MMP3 predict a slightly enhanced immune response to specific pathogens and an intermediate risk for chronic systemic inflammation. Based on this, gene expression and the corresponding protein levels, in response to disease causing bacteria and the other effectors of the acquired immune system, are predicted to be increased. See comment.

Disclaimer: The reported genotypes are a subset of the group of genes that comprise the complete immune system. This genetic analysis may not detect specific immunologic diseases or predict the health and effectiveness of a person's immunity for specific diseases. Such an evaluation may require genetic counseling and testing directed to characterize those genetic conditions.

Comments:

The innate immune system is the body's first line of defense against pathogenic organisms and a major cause of oral and systemic inflammation. The innate immunity functions to create a physical and chemical barrier to bacteria, the recruitment of inflammatory cells to the site of infection, the release of cytokines and the activation of the complement cascade to localize and eliminate bacteria and recruit antigen-recognizing lymphocytes. The acquired immune system involves the production of specialized cells that eliminate or prevent pathogen growth and is the basis for immunologic memory.

- **Periodontitis:** The genotype for the innate immune system marker, DEFB1, predicts an inability to maintain a balance of commensal oral bacteria. Thus, there is a predisposition to periodontal pathogenic bacterial infection. The acquired immune system IL1 and MMP3 genotypes predict an accentuated inflammatory response to specific periodontal bacteria. The cytokine IL1 acts in concert with TNF-alpha to stimulate bone resorption by osteoclasts and to promote the release of matrix metalloproteinases. Further, the presence of a 'T' allele in both the IL1 alpha and beta polymorphic loci is associated with an increased severity of chronic periodontitis. Individuals with the MMP3 5A/5A genotype have elevated levels of gene transcription and an increased local expression of MMP3, and are 3 times more likely to develop chronic periodontitis.
- **Cardiovascular:** Chronic inflammation is implicated in the etiology of cardiovascular disease (CVD). There is also strong evidence to support that polymorphisms within the promoter regions of the cytokine genes for IL1, IL6 and MMP3 are linked to levels of gene expression which are associated with chronic inflammation. The cytokine IL1 beta upregulates the recruitment of inflammatory cells and the levels of matrix metalloproteinase to the site of cholesterol deposition at sites of atherosclerosis. Matrix metalloproteinases function to remove extracellular matrix products which is considered a risk factor to destabilize arterial plaque. Specifically, the 5A/5A genotype is associated with a higher risk of myocardial infarction (MI) at young age (males < 60 years) which increases to a 10-fold risk in those who smoke.
- **Type II Diabetes:** The 'T' allele of the IL1 beta gene is correlated with elevated serum glucose and altered glucose homeostasis. Further, it has been shown that insulin producing beta cells in the pancreas in persons with type 2 diabetes mellitus (T2DM) also have increased levels of the cytokine IL1 beta. Consequently, clinical studies conclude that the IL1 SNPs are associated with development of diabetic nephropathy through interactions with other pro- and anti-inflammatory mediators.

FIGURE 14.2 An example of a Celsus One™ report indicating the genes present in the patient via saliva testing to identify the factors that can influence inflammation.

One of the most common bacterial tests is the MyPerioPath test (OralDNA® Labs), which is utilized to determine both the quality (type) and quantity (bacterial inflammatory burden) of specific pathogenic microorganisms associated with periodontal infections.[97,98] Both tests are intended as supportive adjuncts to conventional diagnostic methods of recording probing depths, recession, bleeding, mobility, as well as radiographic examination and a personal/family history of periodontal disease and its associated risk factors. Depending on the test results, the practitioner can make informed decisions on what type of treatment enhancers may be necessary to manage the disease. These reports are also invaluable for patient education.

These clinical lab reports, as in medicine, serve to help further define risk for disease and/or disease progression allowing management decisions to be made based on objective biological information. Test reports also serve as a persuasive means to instill the need for periodontal therapy and patient compliance in order to achieve the best possible treatment outcome. Furthermore, a "control analysis" post therapy using microbial, yeast or viral testing also serves to confirm the efficacy of the treatment.

A hallmark of periodontal disease management is biofilm control involving mechanical debridement and pharmacotherapeutics which include oral rinses, systemic antibiotics and other biofilm reduction strategies based on disease severity. Pathogens identified by the most common microbial tests are classified in two taxa: facultative and anaerobic. This data plus data about their concentration can help determine if antibiotic antimicrobial therapy should be used to help stabilize the disease. Antimicrobial therapy may be used systemically or locally with use of antiseptics and topically applied medications. However, without knowing the virulence and pathogenic properties of the bacteria, there is no organized way to determine which patients are best suited for which antimicrobials. Salivary tests help identify the bacteria present to guide the use and selection of medicaments and antimicrobials. The graphical portion of the report shows the types of pathogens present, and the pathogen load (Figure 14.3).

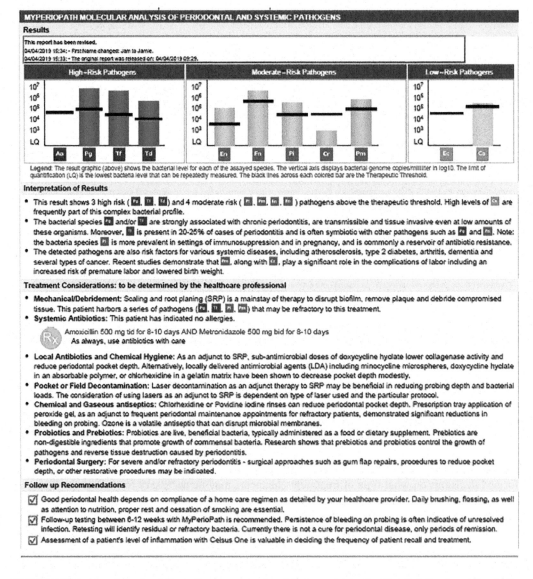

FIGURE 14.3   An example of the pathogens present and their concentration (load) following saliva testing with the MyPerioPath test.

The report section discusses the risk of each pathogen based on virulence factors. Longitudinal studies have shown the potential risk for each of these pathogens. This gives the clinician information to "target" pathogens with the goal of elimination, suppression or alteration in the composition of pathogens associated with disease. Knowing which pathogens are present and their concentrations yields a suggestion of a specific antibiotic regimen that most effectively targets the taxa of the pathogens detected. This allows selection of antibiotics based on the actual causative agent(s) rather than the indiscriminate use without objective data.

Without salivary diagnostics, dental practitioners have been unable to determine if bacterial levels have changed, pathogenic species have been eliminated or a microbial shift has taken place. Elimination of bleeding does not confirm an absence of bacteria or the offending biofilm.

Figure 14.4 is from an actual patient who presented with isolated bleeding on probing during periodontal examination, a history of periodontal disease confirmed by prior bone loss and increased periodontal pocketing. Salivary testing was performed to learn the microbial makeup prior to disinfection treatment. Based on the data from the testing, treatment consisted of traditional scaling and root planing and the recommendation to rinse for 2 weeks with chlorhexidine (a common periodontal disease treatment approach taught in most dental schools). (Figure 14.4 left) At the 6-week periodontal recall to evaluate the gingival healing, probing identified less bleeding and the periodontal chart showed improving pocket depths. Salivary testing was performed to check type and levels of pathogenic bacteria post-treatment. Although clinical evidence of periodontal disease and the associated inflammation had improved, the retest report demonstrated no significant changes in the pathogenic bacteria load. (Figure 14.4 right) The retest results confirmed that traditional nonsurgical periodontal treatment methods were not effective in shifting the oral biofilm to levels that would encourage long-term periodontal stability. The goals of periodontal treatment are eliminating or reducing the pathogenic biofilm to levels that do not initiate a host immunoinflammatory response. Squelching the host immunoinflammatory response prevents the release of cytokines that break down connective tissue, supporting bone and induces inflammation and ultimately a dysregulation of bone metabolism resulting in more destruction. Additionally, this patient will continue to have systemic changes in vascular biology with continued exposure to the high-risk periodontal pathogens that are still present after failed conventional therapy.

PERIODONTAL DISEASE: TREATMENT AND MAINTENANCE

The goals of periodontal treatment are twofold. Clinically the goal is to eliminate deep pockets, gingival bleeding and inflammation/infection, in addition to educating the patient so that they can attain and maintain adequate plaque control at home. Microbially the goal of treatment is to shift the biofilm, so the makeup is less than 5% pathogenic organisms and the balance are health- or core-related species that do not initiate an immune response.[99] Periodontal disease is a complex disease that, when left untreated, ultimately results in significant hard and soft tissue damage with possible subsequent tooth loss. Contemporary periodontal treatment goals should be based on recognizing the multifactorial nature of the disease and the individual variability in how patients manifest that disease. Ultimately, the goal is to have the patient free of pathogenic microorganisms and inflammation, and undertake personalized homecare regimes based on their ability to control the biofilm. An innovative approach takes into account individual differences in people's genes, environments, and lifestyles or behaviors.[100,101] Nutrition is an example of a lifestyle behavior under patient control that has an effect on biofilm diseases, such as periodontal disease and caries.[102] Nutrition will be discussed later in this chapter.

As outlined, periodontal disease is identified by the presence of gingival bleeding, increased probing depth, evidence of bone loss on radiographs and potential tooth mobility during routine examination. Once identified, goal of treatment is the mechanical debridement (scaling and root planing) of the periodontal pockets and the associated teeth to remove hard formations (calculus), and disrupt and remove the soft sulcular biofilm (plaque) to levels that do not provoke a host response.

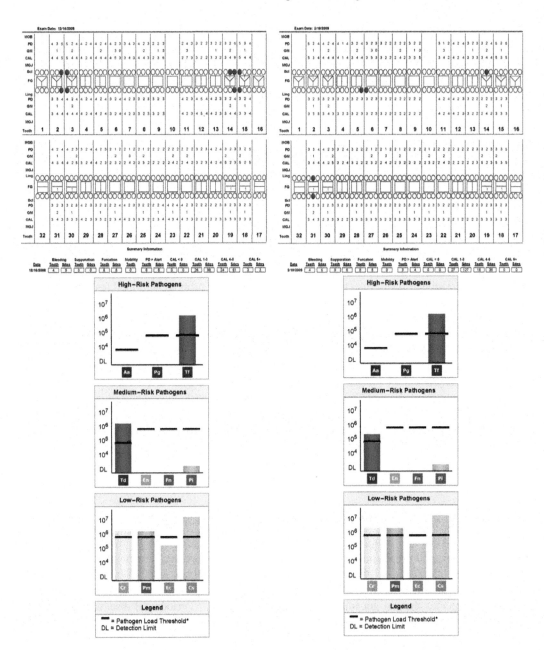

FIGURE 14.4 Pre- and post-treatment results of patient with pretreatment clinical signs of active periodontal disease. Testing produced objective information showing unaltered microbial flora after traditional mechanical debridement methods. This revelation resulted in developing the Thompson Disinfection Protocol.

Additionally, other host modulatory strategies, for example better nutrition, may be employed to alter the host response and to strengthen the autoimmune system. Salivary testing is performed prior to treatment to identify those patients who are at higher risk based on pathogenicity of the bacteria present and their concentrations. This information serves as a pretreatment baseline to compare to a post-treatment report confirming if the flora has been altered and if additional care is required. Genetic testing can also be obtained to learn information about the possible severity of the innate and acquired host response.

Host Modulation

When we recognize the importance of modulating the inflammatory response, new treatment opportunities arise that may be adjunctive to mechanical debridement. In the future, various methods to modulate the host response will offer a significant opportunity to guard against disease progression. These will focus on controlling or resolving inflammation either during the dental appointment or with homecare.[103,104]

As the individual patient's host response consists of a person's genetics and their acquired risk factors, several opportunities present.[105] Depending on the innate genetic makeup and lifestyle factors that increase the risk of disease severity like smoking, stress, nutrition, etc., several options are available. One method of host modulation that has been available clinically for many years is the administration of a sub-antimicrobial dose of doxycycline that acts as a collagenase inhibitor.[106] This has the benefit of limiting breakdown within the soft tissue that may allow bacterial invasion of that tissue and help reduce exposure to inflammatory cytokines that contribute to systemic issues.

Although doxycycline has been used as an antibacterial agent, its use in lower doses has proven to help modulate the activities of some host-derived matrix metalloproteinases responsible for tissue breakdown.[107,108] Additionally, it has an inhibitory effect on collagenase. During the inflammatory responses observed in periodontal and cardiovascular diseases, proinflammatory mediators are up-regulated not only in affected tissues, but also in the secreted, disease-affected oral fluids (saliva) as well as in serum and plasma. Therefore, inhibiting collagenase activity not only has a benefit orally with those hard and soft tissues, but also cadiovascularly.[109] Studies show the use of a sub-antimicrobial dose of doxycycline 20 mg (Periostat® (doxycycline hyclate)) prescribed BID daily as an adjunct following scaling and root planing (SRP) provided significantly greater clinical benefits than SRP alone in the treatment of moderate to severe periodontal disease.[110,111] It can be prescribed for up to 9 months followed by a 3-month drug holiday and then repeated. Usage beyond 9 months has not been well reported, so continued benefits may be present, but further studies are needed to confirm.

Anti-cytokine therapy is another promising host modulation therapy that targets interleukin-1 and tumor necrosis factor.[112,113] Cytokines play a primary role in tissue homeostasis, recruitment of immune cells to control pathogenic impact and regulation of osteoclastic activity.[5] Thus, they are modulating the intensity and duration of the immune response. They also play a critical regulatory role in the inflammatory process and immune cell response that underlies the bone destruction associated with periodontal disease.[114] Etanercept, a tumor necrosis factor-alpha receptor antagonist, has been reported in animal models studying periodontitis to assist in the reduction of inflammation by way of decreased neutrophil infiltration, increased nitric oxide levels and apoptosis.[115] Unfortunately, reports in human patients found a negligible influence on the periodontal condition.[116] One of the major problems with anticytokine therapy is that a functional redundancy of cytokines can enable the host to activate alternative pathways of inflammation if only one specific cytokine is targeted.[117]

Biological resolution of inflammation is driven largely by resolvins, lipoxins, maresins and protectins. Collectively coined specialized pro-resolving mediators (SPMs), these endogenous molecules are oxygenated polyunsaturated fatty acids biosynthesized by enzymes lipoxygenases and cyclooxygenases. These chemically sensitive molecules produced in nano- to pico-gram amounts in vivo exhibit potent anti-inflammatory and pro-resolving bioactions. They help clear bacterial infections, while reducing pain and displaying bioactivities toward host defense, organ protection and tissue remodeling.[118] Statins, like aspirin, have demonstrated anti-inflammatory and bone-preserving actions by upregulating production of SPMs. Emerging evidence from novel drugs, including SPMs and complement inhibitors, suggests future availability of adjunctive therapeutic strategies for the management of periodontal disease.[119]

Two areas of considerable interest are utilizing diet and resolvins (synthetic and natural) as adjuncts to periodontal therapy. Omega-3 polyunsaturated fatty acids (resolvin precursor) have well-documented anti-inflammatory properties and are utilized in the treatment of periodontal disease.[120,121] There is emerging evidence that dietary supplementation with fish oil may be of some benefit.[122] A cost-effective adjunctive therapy to the management of periodontal disease could be dietary supplementation with fish oil.[123–125] Several studies report the clinical benefit is enhanced when combined with low-dose aspirin.[126–128] The addition of aspirin to the treatment regime is based on its ability to significantly increase the production of stable resolvins.[129] This has been shown to be of significant benefit in patients with type 2 diabetes, providing clinical and immunological benefits.[130] In this context, resolvin E1 has been shown to regulate inflammation at the tissue and cellular levels. It has been demonstrated that by resolving experimentally induced inflammation and periodontitis, damaged bone is able to regenerate in the absence of any adjunctive antimicrobial or regenerative therapies.[71]

Statins modulate the host response activated by a bacterial challenge and prevent inflammation-mediated bone resorption, while promoting bone formation. Furthermore, this class of drugs reduce bacterial growth, disrupt bacterial membrane stability and increase bacterial clearance, which leads to a decrease in the infection. Local statin delivery may be considered as an adjunct to both nonsurgical and surgical periodontal therapy resulting in better periodontal treatment.[131,132]

How Can We Better Manage Oral Biofilms?

Professional mechanical debridement, no matter the method or the amount of time spent, has been shown to leave some residual biofilm within the gingival sulcus and on the teeth. Complete removal of biofilm is impossible using mechanical methods alone.[133] Despite our best mechanical attempts and the patient's homecare approaches of brushing, flossing or other plaque management modalities, we are learning that biofilm is hard to manipulate or eliminate completely. Additionally, biofilm is present in other areas of the mouth that mechanical debridement does not target such as the cheeks, tongue and pharyngeal spaces.[134] Additionally, there has been detection of periodontal pathogens (A. actinomycetemcomitans and P. gingivalis) in edentulous patients, as these species were thought to disappear after removal of all-natural teeth and in the absence of dental implants.[135] This becomes an issue in senior patients wearing removable prosthetics (full and partial dentures) as these can be coated in biofilm especially where they contact the underlying gingiva, becoming a source of biofilm that may be aspirated leading to pulmonary infections.[136] Thus, keeping the dentures clean either by the patient or their caretakers can decrease potential aspiration of oral biofilm and improve the patient's health. It is very well supported that pathogenic biofilm can exist even in the edentulous patient.

It has become clear that to achieve success in the management of oral health, and consequently systemic health, mechanical methods of plaque removal in both the dental office and at home are necessary. Additionally, the patient also needs chemotherapeutic methods of plaque disruption in both the dental office and at home for the areas of the mouth that are not accessible to mechanical methods. Nonsurgical periodontal disease management must begin with debridement of the teeth and follow with methods to target the biofilm in the rest of the mouth. Following biofilm manipulation in the dental office, disease minimalization and elimination must be maintained with meticulous homecare by the patient if therapy is to succeed. Since we cannot mechanically manipulate the other soft tissues of the mouth, use of antimicrobial rinses and other chemotherapeutics are indicated to improve overall health by controlling oral biofilm. Various oral rinses are available for oral biofilm maintenance. When biofilm is being rebalanced, a rinse that is virucidal, fungicidal and bactericidal is desired. When maintaining a healthy biofilm balance, rinses that suppress pathogenic biofilm are rinses of choice.

Due to limitations with mechanical homecare methods used alone, the addition of select antimicrobial rinses is critical for long-term biofilm management in patients with periodontal disease. An ideal adjunctive rinse would be one with antibacterial, antiviral and antifungal properties with no side effects. It would also be accessible and inexpensive if it is to be used in therapy or maintenance of the disease. We will outline some of the most popular adjunctive rinses.

Chlorhexidine has been the gold standard in periodontal disease and caries management for many years. It is a broad-spectrum antiseptic oral rinse that acts against Gram-positive and Gram-negative bacteria, aerobes, facultative anaerobes and fungi by increasing bacterial cell wall permeability causing cell wall lysis.[137] It has a long history in dentistry to reduce dental plaque and to augment biofilm management when treating periodontal disease.[138] Numerous studies have confirmed the antiplaque and anti-gingivitis effects of chlorhexidine.[139] Chlorhexidine has the ability to adhere to the dental pellicle and oral mucosa extending its antiplaque effect and is used in dentistry as a 0.12%–0.2% mouthwash used twice daily. The cationic chlorhexidine is incompatible with anionic surfactant compounds in toothpastes, which neutralize its antimicrobial action. Therefore, chlorhexidine should not be used in conjunction with tooth brushing.[140] Chlorhexidine has poor taste, and allergic reactions have been reported. Chlorhexidine has been reported to affect gingival fibroblasts, periodontal ligament cells and osteoblast cells which can impair periodontal healing in both soft and hard tissues.[141] As oral biofilm can be thought of like an onion, with many layers, chlorhexidine has been shown to break through oral biofilm breaking up the exterior layers allowing access to deeper bacteria being protected by the biofilm's structure.[142] Patient daily use may have a negative effect on healing following nonsurgical and surgical periodontal treatments. On the other hand, chlorine dioxide has no reported effect on those cells, and no negative effects have been reported with its use as an oral rinse or daily home use.[143] Chlorhexidine has been reported to have an effect on young biofilms, but the bacteria in mature biofilms and nutrient-limited biofilms have been shown to be more resistant to its affects.[144,145] Today, there are other options to chlorhexidine that are better.

Another oral rinse that has well-documented action on oral biofilm is chlorine dioxide (ClO_2). Chlorine dioxide acts as an oxidizing agent, reacting with several cellular constituents including the cell membrane of microbes. Oxidation of proteins and lipids in the cell membrane leads to the death of the organism. The rinse is available in a stabilized or activated formulation. Chlorine dioxide has been reported in the literature to reduce both plaque and gingival indices and bacterial counts in the oral cavity, similar to other routinely used oral rinses.[146] The solution has shown a high safety and efficacy with concentrations of up to 40 ppm in drinking water reported to not show any toxicity in sub-chronic oral toxicity tests.[147] The lack of cytotoxicity to human cells and its selective toxicity to bacteria appear to be related to the cell membrane structure. Microbial cells are killed extremely fast, with kill times for bacteria occurring in seconds of contact time with chlorine dioxide. Thus, contact time with oral rinsing is sufficient to kill all bacteria, but short enough to keep chlorine dioxide from penetrating into the living tissues of the patient, minimizing cytotoxic effects when applying it as an antiseptic such as an oral rinse. Most importantly, bacteria are not able to develop resistance against chlorine dioxide.[148] Chlorine dioxide has an effective antiplaque action as well as oral bacterial load reduction that have been found to be comparable to chlorhexidine.[149] No significant difference has been reported between chlorine dioxide and chlorhexidine with respect to mean reduction in plaque and gingival scores.[150]

Sodium hypochlorite (NaOCl) is a highly active cytotoxic oxidant recognized as a potent antiseptic and disinfectant agent against bacteria, fungi and viruses. Sodium hypochlorite reacts with proteins, nucleic acids and lipids, and inactivates enzymes essential in the energy-yielding metabolism of microorganisms. Hydrolysis occurs when NaOCl contacts water-forming hypochlorous acid (HOCl) and the less active hypochlorite ion (OCl). Hypochlorous acid then splits into hydrochloric acid (HCl) and the oxygen atom (O), a strong oxidator, which diffuses through the microbial cell wall, changing the oxidation–reduction potential of the cell. As NaOCl is naturally occurring in human neutrophils, monocytes and macrophages, an allergic reaction does not occur, is not mutagenic or carcinogenic, and it has a century-long safety record of use.[151,152] For periodontal disease management, studies have shown that a very dilute solution 0.2% is highly effective as an antiseptic. NaOCl, at concentrations of 5%–6% as found in common household bleach, can cause irritation to the skin, mucous membranes and the eyes, and although the irritant effect is reversible, NaOCl at these concentrations should never be used for oral rinsing.

NaOCl has been used as an antiseptic agent in dentistry for more than a century and remains a widely used root canal irrigant at concentrations of 1.0%–5.25%.[153] NaOCl rinsing at lower concentrations (0.01%–0.05%) exerts broad antimicrobial activity against oral biofilms, with an 80-fold decrease in biofilm endotoxin when compared to water.[154–156] One study reported that patients who abstained from oral hygiene for 21 days but performed supervised twice-daily 0.05% sodium hypochlorite oral rinses, had a 48% reduction in Plaque Index score, 52% reduction in Gingival Index score and 39% reduction in bleeding on probing sites compared with water rinse alone.[157] In another study in college students abstaining from oral hygiene, the clinical effect of rinsing with 0.5% NaOCl (Carrel-Dakin solution) reported similar results and produced a 47% greater reduction in dental plaque amount compared with water-rinsing. Low pretreatment gingivitis scores were maintained around teeth receiving the sodium hypochlorite rinse, whereas the gingivitis score increased by 50% in water-treated sites.[158] Zou et al. reported that NaOCl can also penetrate into and potentially kill cariogenic bacteria within dentinal tubules decreasing potential for dental caries.[159] Histologically, it was found that concentrated NaOCl solution applied subgingivally exhibited no detrimental effect on periodontal healing and dilute NaOCl has no contraindications.[160]

NaOCl in low concentrations has a basic pH and does not pose a risk of tooth erosion and does not corrode titanium implant surfaces.[161] The lowest concentration of NaOCl solution found to reliably inactivate bacteria in vitro is 0.01%.[162] However, a suitable concentration of NaOCl for periodontal pocket irrigation is up to 0.5%. Following are Dr. Jorgen Slots' recommendations to make this effective rinse using regular household bleach. Proper concentrations can be obtained by mixing 10 ml (two teaspoonful) of 6.0% household bleach in 125 mL (one-half glass) of water. Patients are advised to rinse 2–3 times weekly for 30 seconds with 8 mL of the solution for continual biofilm management when disease stability is present. This solution may also be used in an oral irrigator (Waterpik) at a low-pressure setting for patients with deeper periodontal pockets to aid in contact with subgingival biofilm. For an adjunctive rinse to be used to treat disease and to help shift the oral biofilm, other commercially prepared 0.2% NaOCl preparations are available (CariFree CTx4Rinse is an example).

Hydrogen peroxide solution has little effect on periodontal pathogens; however, hydrogen peroxide gel (H_2O_2) has been documented as a very effective means of both eliminating the biofilm as well as preventing its reformation without bacterial resistance issues found with other site-specific treatment modalities. H_2O_2 has been documented with daily use for up to 6 years with no adverse effects or carcinogenic activity, while showing a decrease in biofilm (plaque), enhanced wound healing and improved gingival bleeding.[163] Further, no allergic reactions have been reported, and bacterial strains demonstrate no resistance. Functionally it debrides the biofilm slime matrix and bacterial cell walls, essentially peeling the biofilm back layer by layer. This causes irreversible cleaving of the amino acids in the protein chains of the bacteria in the biofilm, which breaks down the protein pellicle attaching the biofilm to the tooth surface and decreases localized inflammation in the pocket by inhibiting IL-8mRNA.[164]

Oxygen is required for successful wound healing due to increased demand of the reparative processes such as cell proliferation, bacterial defense, angiogenesis and collagen synthesis.[165]

New cell growth requires oxygen, which induces the growth of new blood vessels. This increases flow of oxygenated blood to the wound beginning the healing process. As healing progresses, new granulation tissue that is exposed to oxygen is better vascularized, leading to higher tensile strength collagen being formed during wound healing. Hyperbaric oxygen has been well documented to be bactericidal for anaerobic bacteria.[166] Hydrogen peroxide gel delivered to the teeth and gums in a specialized tray delivery system (PerioProtect) oxygenates the pocket changing the environment from anaerobic to aerobic creating a hyperbaric oxygen chamber in the sulcus to destroy the biofilms occupants. Published studies have documented that the ideal concentration of hydrogen peroxide gel is 1.7% as this is effective in breaking down the biofilm and virtually eliminates any irritation issues reported with higher concentrations. It has been determined that a 10-minute exposure to a 1.7% hydrogen peroxide gel penetrates the biofilm slime matrix, debriding the bacterial cell walls within. Maintaining the peroxide in the periodontal pocket releases oxygen and changes the subgingival micro-environment, making survival of the anaerobic bacteria more difficult.[167,168] Biofilm can be quick to redevelop, so to be effective, the 1.7% hydrogen peroxide application needs to be part of the daily homecare routine. Additionally, neutrophils in the presence of hydrogen peroxide and chloride will produce ozone through the cholesterol ozonolysis process.[169]

Ozone has antimicrobial activity by oxidation of biomolecule precursors and microbial toxins that have been implicated in periodontal diseases causing healing and tissue regeneration.[96] Ozone therapy has been reported to significantly improve clinical parameters in smokers and nonsmokers when applied in addition to periodontal therapy.[170,171] When compared to chlorhexidine, topical application of ozone to patients as part of their daily homecare routine have shown similar results and may be considered an alternative in those patients who object to the taste or staining associated with chlorhexidine, or if the practitioner is concerned about the fibroblast issues reported with its use.[171]

A study examining the antibacterial properties of various oral rinses, including sodium hypochlorite (NaOCl), chlorhexidine, Listerine and chlorine dioxide on selected common oral pathogens and on oral biofilm, demonstrated that chlorine dioxide was most effective against aerobic bacteria and *Candida* (yeast). Evaluating chlorine dioxide's efficacy against anaerobes showed it is similar to chlorhexidine. Chlorine dioxide was found to be superior at dissolving the biofilm when compared to chlorhexidine and Listerine. Therefore, it was concluded that chlorine dioxide is a potent disinfectant with high efficacy on oral pathogenic microorganisms and a powerful biofilm-dissolving effect compared to the other antiseptic oral rinses.[172]

Since maintenance in the dental office is of such limited time, two to four appointments annually depending on the degree of periodontal disease present, homecare becomes a critical component of overall care. Despite great diligence, homecare can be compromised by limitations of our cleaning devices. For example, toothbrush bristles are unable to extend more then 3–4 mm into the pocket and is unable to mechanically contact the biofilm located at deeper depths. A similar problem presents with oral irrigators not allowing irrigation to the bottom of the pockets. Compliance with regular daily use can also be a challenge. The sulcular environment is difficult for most patients to reach with brushing and flossing, making it impossible to control oral biofilms by mechanical means alone as the bacteria grow and replicate so rapidly. Post-cleaning biofilm redevelopment is more rapid and complex, and without great care can exceed pre-cleaning levels within 2 days.[24,173,174] Bacteria embedded in the biofilm are up to 1,000-fold more resistant to antibiotics compared to planktonic bacteria. Therefore, the use of antibiotics either systemically or in oral rinses is often unable to eliminate or manage the biofilm bacteria adequately.[175,176] This has implications both with natural teeth and with dental implants.[177] As a consequence, homecare must be consistent to keep biofilm levels down that were removed during dental periodontal treatment.

HOST MODULATION USING NUTRITION

Nutrition plays a key role in overall health and can help the host moderate genetic factors and improve health when systemic issues are present. Nutrients also have a major impact on periodontal health.[178–180] The influence of the traditional diet on the formation of oxidative stress caused by bacterial biofilm in the oral cavity has a direct causative action on inflammation intraorally and systemically. Diets that contain high sugar, high saturated fat, low fiber and low polyunsaturated fat causes an increased risk of periodontal diseases. This is classically found in the Western diet, a diet that is considered an 'unhealthy' diet contributing to the cause/exacerbation of cardiovascular diseases, diabetes and other health issues. Conversely, diets that contain low sugar, high fiber and high omega-6-to-omega-3 fatty acid ratio reduce the risk of periodontal diseases. These include the Mediterranean and vegetarian diets. These diets are considered "healthy" diets and have been found to reduce the risk of cardiovascular diseases, diabetes and cancer.

Increasing evidence presents that a diet inspired by the Mediterranean diet is associated with numerous health benefits.[181,182] This type of diet has been demonstrated to exert a preventive effect on cardiovascular diseases with a positive action on the cardiometabolic risk.[183,184] Additionally, it has the added benefit of decreasing the risk of diabetes and metabolic-related conditions,[185] and lower risk of cancer mortality.[186] Recent research has also demonstrated that adherence to the Mediterranean diet is associated with a lower risk of mental disorders, including cognitive decline and depression.[187] With regard to periodontal health, in patients following the Mediterranean diet, there was a reported decrease in periodontal pathogenic bacteria in the saliva. Specifically, a significant decrease in the relative abundances of *P. gingivalis*, *Prevotella intermedia* and *T. denticola* which are considered associated with periodontal disease.[188] Alternatively, an inflammatory diet that is high in carbohydrates and fats but deficient in necessary nutrients elevates leukocyte counts and systemic inflammation with periodontal disease.[189]

There is an association between periodontal pockets and patients who are type 2 diabetics and/or obese. These patients also present with increased inflammation related to periodontal disease and its associated biofilm formation.[190] Intermittent fasting has reported a decrease in inflammation in those patients with metabolic disorders such as diabetes. One study reported that clinically supervised periodic fasting in female patients with diabetes facilitated a reduction in periodontal inflammation.[191] Patients who are diabetic or obese with periodontal disease may wish to coordinate with their physician on a program of intermittent fasting to help with their physical/systemic issues as well as the added benefit of decreasing periodontal inflammation which will have a positive effect systemically.

High carbohydrate intake has been implicated in periodontal disease and dental caries. The relationship of nutrition and oral health is well known.[192,193] High carbohydrate intake is especially prevalent in adolescents, and those dietary habits become lifelong habits affecting oral health and consequently systemic health as well.[194] This is especially true for those patients consuming soft drinks, as those are high in carbohydrates.[195] A diet high in sugar encourages plaque formation, with bacterial breakdown of those sugars leading to an acid attack of the tooth structure with the onset or worsening of dental decay in reaction to poor oral hygiene. Dentists need to counsel patients on nutritional strategy and to avoid eating a high carbohydrate diet.[196]

The role of micronutrients (such as vitamins D, E and K and magnesium) and others (such as vitamins A, B and C, calcium, zinc and polyphenols) has some relationship to periodontal disease. Some have a bigger influence on the disease than others. Studies show that B-vitamin supplementation results in higher clinical periodontal attachment following periodontal surgery, and many studies support that vitamin D deficiency contributes to negative outcomes following periodontal surgery.[197,198] Vitamins play a vital role in cell metabolism, but also have potent antioxidant properties.

The human diet contains several antioxidants in the form of micronutrients. Antioxidant micronutrients include vitamin A (carotenoids and carotene),[199] vitamin C (ascorbic acid),[200] vitamin E,[201] and melatonin.[202] Studies have suggested that antioxidants may help overcome the mediated inflammation of periodontal tissues.[203] Vitamins A, C and E have all been observed to modulate the antioxidant defense system, with vitamins C and E having a potential role in reducing oxidative stress in the periodontium. A lower intake of vitamin A has been associated with decreased oral epithelial development and periodontitis.[204] A diet deficient in vitamin A can increase susceptibility to pathogenic periodontal bacteria and may trigger or aggravate an immune-inflammatory response.[205] Supplementation with vitamin C in patients undergoing non-surgical periodontal therapy increased the total antioxidant capacity (TAOC). Additionally, vitamin C has been found to act as anti-senescence allowing periodontal ligament stem cell (PDLSCs) proliferation, which are potential "seed cells" for periodontal tissue repair and regeneration.[206,207] Another study noted a significant reduction in gingival inflammation with increased vitamin E supplementation.[208] Additionally, when combined with SRP, vitamin E has demonstrated to be effective in controlling the levels of inflammatory mediators and pain in patients with periodontitis.[209] Intake of these important vitamins, whether through the diet or supplementation, has demonstrated to decrease the severity of periodontal disease. These micronutrients may also be able to aid in prevention of the initiation of periodontal disease in minor cases.[210] A recent study reported that increased intake of foods high in vitamins A, C and E has decreased the severity of periodontitis in non-smokers; however, the same effects could not be replicated in smokers.[211]

Vitamin D has gained much attention as an important nutrient, and in the United States, 50% of the population is deficient in this critical vitamin.[212] That number increases in elderly patients and has been reported to be 61% of that population.[213] Vitamin D plays an important role in bone maintenance, and patients who are deficient have lower bone density, which may allow more rapid progression of periodontal disease. This is also important in those patients with dental implants, as higher failure rates of implants have been reported in those who are vitamin D deficient.[214] As the gingival tissue is supported by the underlying bone, bone of lower density is affected earlier and more profoundly when periodontal inflammation presents. Supplementation with vitamin D aids in bone health and provides resistance to resorption resulting from periodontal disease and inflammation from the adjacent biofilm. The vitamin D receptor binds zinc, and the ability of vitamin D to work within the cells is influenced by intracellular zinc concentrations.[215] Zinc acts as a cofactor in many enzyme-controlled processes, modulating the processes of auto-debridement and keratinocyte migration during wound repair.[216] Additionally, it exerts an antioxidative effect by scavenging reactive oxygen species (ROS) in addition to neutralizing bacterial toxins while providing anti-inflammatory actions.[217] Thus, dietary zinc plays an important role in maintaining periodontal health, and a lack of dietary zinc leads to worsening of periodontal disease in patients with type 2 diabetes mellitus.[218] Zinc supplementation may have the potential to augment the therapeutic effects of periodontal therapy.[219,220]

Lycopene, a red pigment present in vegetables such as tomatoes and carrots, may prevent cancer and cardiac diseases due to its antioxidant effects.[221] Some studies have investigated lycopene as an adjunct to non-surgical periodontal therapy and suggest its supplementation may enhance periodontal health.[222] Later studies have reported a possible therapeutic role of lycopene in the management of periodontitis.[223,224] As increased oxidative stress has emerged as one of the prime factors in the pathogenesis of periodontitis, antioxidant therapy may become a promising tool in the treatment of periodontal disease. Lycopene with green tea extract may prove to be an adjunctive therapeutic modality in the treatment of patients with gingival inflammation.[225]

Green tea is an important source of polyphenol antioxidants. The most interesting polyphenol components with proven health benefits are the catechins.[226] Green tea catechins possessed antibacterial and anti-inflammatory effects on periodontal disease and have the potential to improve the outcome of periodontal nonsurgical treatment.[227]

Melatonin, a potent antioxidant, is secreted by various organs of the human body and also found in plants and cereal sources. Recently, research has focused on possible therapeutic supplementation in the oral cavity and, in particular, the periodontal tissues.[228] Melatonin supplementation, either topical or systemic, in patients with periodontitis made an improvement in key periodontal parameters including reduction in pocket depth and decreased clinical attachment loss.[229] Melatonin, additionally, may aid in the prevention of periodontitis by decreasing inflammation.[230] Melatonin has shown to reduce inflammation, inhibit cell proliferation and regulate differentiation with increased odontoblast activities and seems to have beneficial effects in periodontitis by promoting wound healing.[231] Additionally, combination of nonsurgical periodontal treatment and systemic treatment with melatonin supplementation provided additional improvements to severe periodontitis, and the glycemic control of patients with diabetes type 2, when compared to nonsurgical periodontal treatment alone.[232]

Magnesium is required for cell metabolism for maintenance and bone formation. Deficiencies have been shown to interfere with the parathyroid hormone and directly affect bone metabolism resulting in osteoporosis and harm to the bone supporting the teeth.[233] An association between magnesium and periodontitis has been reported, and nutritional magnesium supplementation may improve periodontal health.[234,235] One study has suggested a positive effect of magnesium-rich diets on nonsurgical periodontal therapy.[236] Further research is needed to ascertain the effect of dietary magnesium on periodontal health.

Iron is required for the synthesis of proteins, including hemoglobin and enzymes. Foods such as red meat, spinach, fish (tuna and salmon), and beans are rich sources of iron. Iron deficiency leads to anemia, which is associated with many oral manifestations including recurrent ulceration, pale mucosa and oral burning sensation. Iron-deficiency anemia leads to a reduction in antioxidant enzymes, leading to an increased oxidative stress and a worsening of periodontal diseases.[237] Iron supplements should be considered in those patients who have iron anemia and conditions such as Crohn's disease as this deficiency can complicate periodontal disease due to an increase in inflammation.[238]

Coenzyme Q10 (CoQ10) is an antioxidant the body produces naturally that cells use for growth and maintenance. Levels of CoQ10 decrease with age and are reported to be lower in patients with certain conditions, such as heart disease, and in those who take cholesterol-lowering drugs (statins). CoQ10 is found in meat, fish and nuts, although the amount found in those dietary sources is not enough to significantly increase CoQ10 levels in your body. Supplementation with CoQ10 could counteract the negative effects of polyunsaturated fatty acid on alveolar bone loss, which is a major feature of periodontitis associated with age.[239] Coenzyme Q10 has a beneficial effect on smokers with periodontitis when used as an adjunct to SRP and can be used in nonsmokers as a treatment adjunct.[240] The majority of the population has poor dietary habits, which include intake of too many carbohydrates, fats and insufficient levels of vitamins, and other necessary nutrients. This has direct and indirect effects on systemic health. Directly as other chapters in this textbook have addressed, cardiac and other systemic issues are associated with insufficient or poor nutrition. Indirectly, as outlined in this chapter, the periodontal tissue is affected, and oral biofilm is able to increase inflammation dependent on the host immunomodulatory response to the bacteria and its byproducts within that biofilm. Improving the diet by decreasing carbohydrates and supplementing with vitamins A, C, D and E and essential components such as CoQ10, lycopene, magnesium and melatonin can aid the host in decreasing inflammation and allow better localized management of the biofilm's effects on the adjacent tissues. Those patients who are iron deficient should also be supplemented with iron supplements to improve both systemic health as well as oral health.

BIOFILM ELIMINATION OVER THE LONG TERM

The key to elimination of oral inflammation and long-term alteration of the bacteria in the biofilm relies on treatment in the dental office as well as daily patient homecare. With strict homecare compliance and following a thorough in-office disinfection program, long-term alteration of the bacteria with a shift to non-pathogenic species can be accomplished. Elimination of bleeding on probing is a positive clinical sign yet does not guarantee a change in the pathogenicity of the bacteria intraorally. As an example, a patient presented with pathogenic bacteria as documented by the MyPerioPath saliva test prior to traditional periodontal treatment. (Figure 14.4 left) Traditional treatment consisted of SRP (mechanical debridement with specialized instruments) and the use of chlorhexidine for 3 weeks and reevaluation at 6 weeks. The microbial test was repeated at 6 weeks post periodontal treatment with surprising results demonstrating no alteration in the pathogenic bacteria (Figure 14.4 right). This highlighted a need for a more comprehensive approach to disease treatment. A very comprehensive protocol was developed that has a multipronged approach to biofilm management and employs a Total Mouth Disinfection methodology developed by Dr. Doug Thompson of Integrative Oral Medicine a Bloomfield Hills, MI general dental practice. This Total Mouth Disinfection approach employed a much more robust treatment protocol including the use of systemic antibiotics in conjunction with professional debridement and utilizes chemotherapeutics and some host modulatory methods. When this protocol was used, a follow-up microbial test from OralDNA showed a significant shift in the biofilm as evidenced in Figure 14.5 (right).

Total Mouth Disinfection method developed by Dr. Thompson addresses the following areas:

1. Occlusal analysis to identify and remove any fremitus (vibration or movement of a tooth when teeth come into contact together) in chewing.
2. Mechanical removal of the bacteria and biofilm in the pockets using SRP.

Initial (pretreatment)	6 weeks after conventional scaling and root planing	4 months post Total Mouth Disinfection Protocol
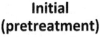		

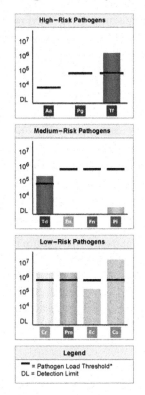

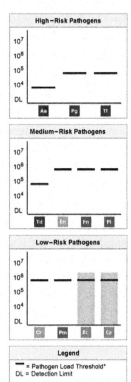

FIGURE 14.5 Biofilm management demonstrating microflora prior to conventional treatment (left), after conventional treatment that did not alter the microbial profile (middle), and after Dr. Thompson's Total Mouth Disinfection protocol (far right) that altered the microbial profile significantly.

3. Chemically attack the bacteria in the pockets by irrigating with a 0.2% dilute NaOCl rinse (CariFree Treatment Rinse, www.carifree.com), and depositing a locally applied timed release antibiotic (Arestin® OraPharma, Inc., www.orapharma.com) in all pockets equal to or greater than 5 mm.
4. Manage the systemic bacteria in the bloodstream and gingival crevicular fluid with the antibiotic regimen suggested on the microbial report (OralDNA MyPerioPath).
5. Treat the bacteria in the oral cavity with 0.2% NaOCl rinse (CariFree Treatment Rinse), to control microbial load. Use this rinse for one minute twice daily until zero bleeding on probing during periodontal charting is achieved.
6. Prescribe homecare adjuncts such as an electric toothbrush, water flosser such as a Waterpik® (Water Pik, Inc., www.waterpik.com) or Hydroflosser (Shazzam Tsunami™, Bling Dental Products, www.blingdentalproducts.com) and interproximal aids, etc., for enhanced bacteria load control.
7. Maintain regular 2-month reevaluation appointments until zero bleeding on probing during periodontal charting has been achieved. Zero bleeding on probing is a clinical goal of therapy and can be used to represent periodontal stability from a clinical standpoint.
8. Retest using the same testing method that was used pretreatment to re-evaluate the microbial profile. Microbial endpoints of therapy require elimination, suppression or an alteration of the pathogenic profile that does not evoke a negative host immune response.

The patient in the example (Figure 14.5) was kept on a regular 2-month (8-week) reevaluation schedule until zero bleeding was established. Retesting was performed using MyPerioPath (Figure 14.5 right). With the use of a Total Mouth Disinfection approach and utilizing oral rinses with the highest microbial killing efficiency (CTx4 Treatment from CariFree.com), the microbial profile was significantly altered. The goal was to eradicate, suppress, or alter the bacterial load to a point where it does not provoke an immune-inflammatory response. Finally, in this case, these goals have been achieved. It is important to note that this profile was measured when there was zero bleeding, a clinical sign to suggest periodontal stability. Many cases have been treated by Dr. Thompson this way, and it has been learned that a rapid and sudden "shift" of the biofilm is possible only when a multipronged approach is employed that targets the biofilm in several ways. Following an enhanced disinfection protocol addressing the teeth, sulcus around the teeth, and the rest of the mouth, in addition to placing the patient on a biofilm altering rinse for up to 4 months following SRP and then a therapeutic maintenance rinse plus meticulous home care, the 26–51 months (2–4 years) follow-up bacterial tests (Figure 14.6) show a sustained significant biofilm shift from original disease levels. As the science unfolds about the significance of pathogen exposure to systemic health risks, it is only a guess what may have been prevented from eliminating exposure to this type of pathogen presence for over 10 years in a person in his fifth decade of life. If periodontal disease is diagnosed and treated with success, it would mean that pathogen exposure is reduced or eliminated in younger individuals and it would make sense that the overall health impact would be even greater.

The next logical question to ask is: How much longer can the practitioner and the patient working together maintain periodontal stability? Looking further at Figure 14.7, you can see subsequent reports for up to 11 years. This 11-year follow-up demonstrates that continuation of the recommended homecare plus routine in office supportive periodontal maintenance appointments maintained the elimination of the high-risk pathogenic bacteria and reduction of moderate risk pathogenic bacteria.

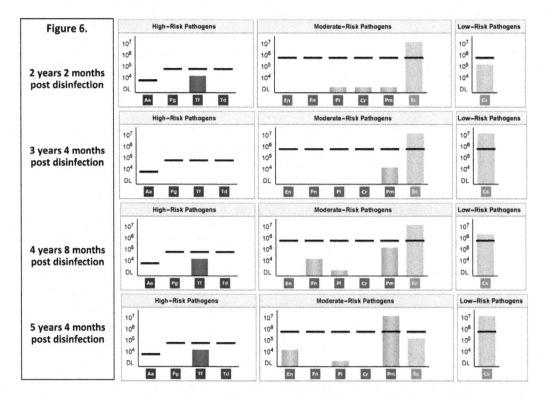

FIGURE 14.6 Microbiological stability is monitored with the MyPerioPath test to check success of the patient's homecare and allow alterations when needed.

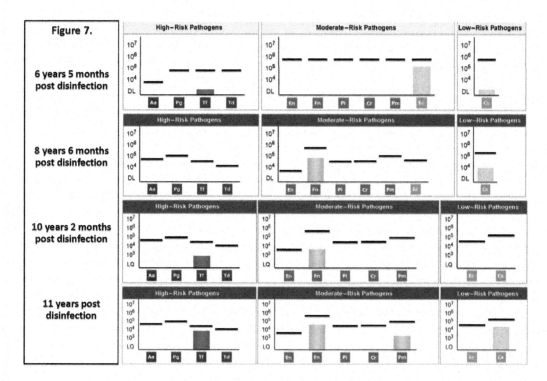

FIGURE 14.7 Long-term stability as monitored with the MyPerioPath test verifying subsequent elimination or suppression of high-risk pathogens over an 11-year plus period without reactivation of the disease. Even though the presence of some occasional high-risk pathogens is a reality over the 11 plus years, the overall exposure during this time is significantly less than it would be without treatment and maintenance. Figure 14.5 (left) is original disease presentation and a reference to initial pathogen exposure.

With modification and maintenance of the oral bacteria associated with the biofilm, inflammation can be controlled, and its effect systemically becomes much less of an overall health risk factor and the ultimate result is the patient is healthier.

COLLABORATION BETWEEN THE PHYSICIAN AND DENTIST

Current research has connected the mouth with the whole body, and total body healthcare connects these areas by bacteria, yeast, and viruses and ultimately inflammation that they stimulate. As has been suggested, oral biofilm represented by high- and moderate-risk periodontal pathogens and the host response results in chronic inflammation that when identified and managed have a positive outcome on systemic issues, especially cardiac and vascular diseases. Considering the 55 plus other associative systemic disease conditions related to periodontal biofilm, dentists will help their patients best by personalizing treatment strategies to eliminate or suppress a pathogenic biofilm load. They will also better serve their patients by providing options to modulate the host response to the biofilm, ultimately reducing exposure to inflammatory by products that slowly degrade health. Host modulation will come in the form of products, medicines, or supplements as well as lifestyle factors that alter the immune response. It is becoming clearer and clearer that periodontal disease is a medical condition harbored in the mouth and has been left to dentists to diagnose and treat. Since this disease is polymicrobial, multifactorial and episodic with a bidirectional relationship to other systemic diseases (e.g. diabetes), dentists cannot best treat the disease alone. Dentists and physicians need to collaborate to help their patients be as successful as they can be. The result is improvement in total healthcare for our mutual patients.

Physicians can screen for some obvious clinical signs of periodontal disease. When the physician is examining a patient, some simple questions may aid in coordination of care. Those include "When was the last time you saw a dentist for a cleaning and exam?", "Do your gums bleed when you brush and floss?", "Do you floss?", "Do you have bad breath?", and "Have you noticed any teeth shifting or getting loose or sensitive?". Those patients with diagnosed cardiac or vascular issues should be encouraged to see a dentist on a routine basis to help manage the oral biofilm and associated bacteria. Taking it a step further, physicians practicing preventative cardiology would like to know the biofilm makeup utilizing a metric to see the level of high- and moderate-risk pathogens that have research behind them implicating them in the vascular disease process. Ultimately, controlling this biofilm may help improve vascular and other systemic issues being treated and managed.

COLLABORATIVE INFLAMMATION AND BIOFILM TREATMENT: DENTISTRY AND MEDICINE

A collaborative effort with coordination between dentistry and medicine is the best approach to management of biofilm and its systemic affects. In the next example of an actual patient, he was referred for an oral inflammatory illness evaluation due to an elevation in myeloperoxidase (MPO). This MPO elevation was discovered during an initial vascular disease evaluation by his physician and did not have an obvious systemic cause.

On dental examination, the patient presented with active periodontal disease represented by prior radiographic bone loss, 50 sites of line bleeding on probing (Figure 14.8) and high levels of pathogenic biofilm as evidenced by the salivary diagnostic tests from two independent companies: OralDNA labs (Eden Prairie, MN) (Figure 14.9) and FidaLab (Seattle, WA) (Figure 14.10).

Exam Date: 6/5/2019

Upper arch (buccal PD/CAL):

Tooth	1	2	3	4	5	6	7	8	9	10	11	12	13	14	15	16
PD	3 3 5		4 3 3	3 2 3	3 1 3	3 1 3	3 1 4	4 3 3	3 2 3	3 1 3	4 3 4	6 1 5	5 2 5	6 3 5		6 3 4
CAL	3 3 5		4 3 3	3 2 3	3 1 3	3 1 3	3 1 4	4 3 3	3 2 3	3 1 3	4 3 4	6 1 5	5 2 5	6 3 5		6 3 4

Upper arch (lingual PD/CAL):

Tooth	1	2	3	4	5	6	7	8	9	10	11	12	13	14	15	16
PD	4 3 4		4 1 3	3 1 3	3 1 3	3 1 3	3 2 3	3 2 3	3 3 3	3 3 4	3 2 3	3 2 3	3 2 3	3 2 3		3 3 3
CAL	4 3 4		4 1 3	3 1 3	3 1 3	3 1 3	3 2 3	3 2 3	3 3 3	3 3 4	3 2 3	3 2 3	3 2 3	3 2 3		3 3 3

Lower arch (buccal PD/CAL):

Tooth	32	31	30	29	28	27	26	25	24	23	22	21	20	19	18	17
PD	5 4 6		6 3 5	5 3 4	3 3 4	4 3 3	3 2 3	3 2 3	3 2 3	3 2 3	3 2 3	4 3 4	3 2 3	3 3 4		5 3 5
CAL	5 4 6		6 3 5	5 3 4	3 3 4	4 3 3	3 2 3	3 2 3	3 2 3	3 2 3	3 2 3	4 3 4	3 2 3	3 3 4		5 3 5

Lower arch (lingual PD/CAL):

Tooth	32	31	30	29	28	27	26	25	24	23	22	21	20	19	18	17
PD	3 2 3		3 2 3	3 2 3	3 3 3	3 2 3	3 2 3	3 2 1	3 3 1	3 3 1	3 1 3	2 2 3	3 2 3	3 3 4		4 4 3
CAL	3 2 3		3 2 3	3 2 3	3 3 3	3 2 3	3 2 3	3 2 1	3 3 1	3 3 1	3 1 3	2 2 3	3 2 3	3 3 4		4 4 3

FIGURE 14.8 Initial periodontal charting demonstrating 50 areas of bleeding on probing (red).

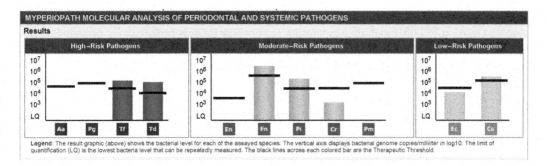

FIGURE 14.9 Initial MyPerioPath test demonstrating pathologic bacteria with high and moderate risks.

Type	Bacteria	Copies/oral rinse sample (x10^5)	10^5	10^6	10^7	10^8	10^9	10^{10}
A	Porphyromonas gingivalis (PG)	0.099 ✱						
	Tannerella forsythia (TF)	1112.903						
	Treponema denticola (TD)	294.132						
B	Prevotella nigrescens (PN)	5066.026						
	Porphyromonas endodontalis (PE)	441.076						
	Prevotella intermedia (PI)	N/A						
	Eubacterium nodatum (EN)	N/A						
	Filifactor alocis (FA)	N/A						
	Fretibacterium sp. HOT360 (Fr)	34.678						
	Treponema socranskii (TS)	63.533						
C	Bacteroidales [G-2] sp. HOT274 (Ba)	165.354						
	Campylobacter rectus (CR)	156.396						
	Parvimonas micra (PM)	230.025						
	Desulfobulbus sp. HOT041 (De)	N/A						
	Eikenella corrodens (EC)	11118.619						
	Selenomonas sputigena (SS)	2241.958						
	Eubacterium saphenum (ES)	0.006 ✱						
	TM7 [G1] sp. HOT349 (TM7)	4681.516						
	Fretibacterium fastidiosum (FF)	9.345						
	Treponema lecithinolyticum (TL)	27.717						
	Treponema maltophilum (TM)	7.950						
	Fusobacterium nucleatum ss animalis (FNa)	1113.589						
	Fusobacterium nucleatum ss polymorphum (FNp)	14762.175						
	Treponema sp. HT237 (Tr)	142.579						
	Fusobacterium nucleatum ss vincenti (FNv)	3292.834						
D	Capnocytophaga gingivalis (CG)	1602.330						
	Capnocytophaga ochracea (CO)	612.957						
	Capnocytophaga sputigena (CS)	259.171						
E	Aggregatibacter actinomycetemcomitans (AA)	N/A						

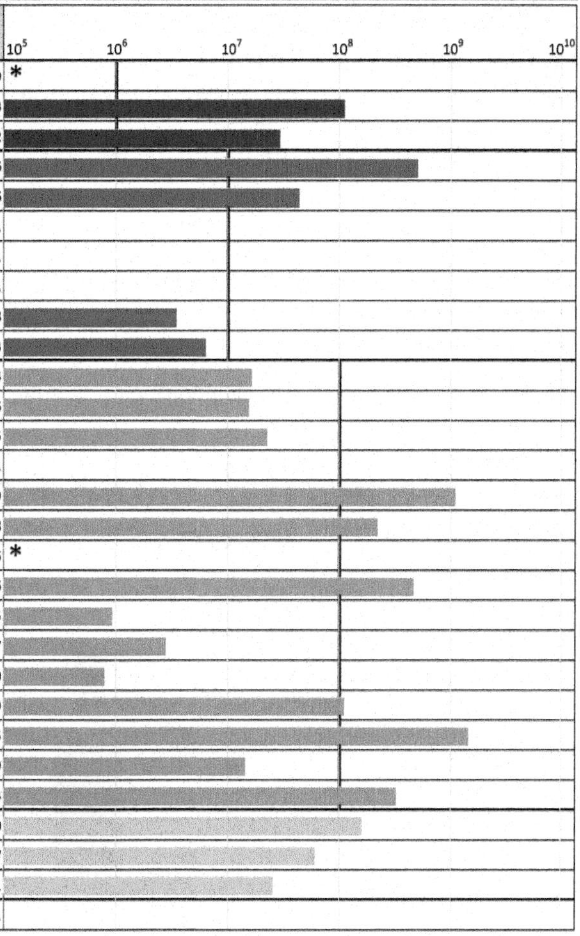

N/A   Below detection limit   **Periodontal Pathogen Composite Score: 881.65**

✱ $<10^5$ copies / sample

FIGURE 14.10 Initial Disease Diagnosis (FidaLab).

The FidaLab report presents a pathogen composite score rating scale, and the patient's initial score was rated at 881.65. FidaLab uses a rating scale where 0–20 is Low Risk for periodontal disease, 20–150 is Moderate Risk and Over 150 is High Risk for periodontal disease. The patient also had elevated MPO represented by his medical lab report (Figure 14.11).

The carotid intima-media thickness test (CIMT) is a measure used to diagnose the extent of carotid atherosclerotic vascular disease, and an abnormal CIMT was evidenced by the report for the patient (Figure 14.12).

After completion of comprehensive Total Mouth Disinfection protocol developed by Dr. Thompson (TMD) as presented in this chapter, the patient's 2-month periodontal chart demonstrated zero bleeding on probing (Figure 14.13).

This represents achievement of our clinical goals of therapy. His OralDNA Report showed a significant reduction in periodontal pathogens (Figure 14.14), which was confirmed by the FidaLab post-treatment report as well with a reduction of a pathogen composite score of 881.64 down to 4.0 (Figure 14.15).

This microbial change represents achievement of our microbial goals of therapy. Post-treatment also yielded a favorable reduction in MPO down from 527 pretreatment to 474. (Figure 14.16) This case represents successful collaborative care for a patient treated by a physician who understands and manages vascular inflammation to reduce heart attack and stroke risk. Figure 14.5 shows that in this 11-year case study both microbial and clinical goals of therapy were achieved with good

Patient Name: Scott ▓▓▓▓ | **Date of Birth:** 07/26/1968

MYELOPEROXIDASE (MPO) 05/02/2019 (#248146, Final, 04/25/2019 12:01am)

Report	Result	Ref. Range	Units		Status		Lab
MYELOPEROXIDASE	527	<470	pmol/L	High	Final		CHL

Based on a high risk sub-population (N=920) defined as ambulatory stable patients without acute coronary syndrome who underwent elective diagnostic coronary angiography (1) and a reference range study of apparently healthy donors, we have defined the following cut-offs for MPO: A cut-off of <470 pmol/L defines an 'apparently healthy' population at lower risk for a cardiovascular event, 470-539 pmol/L defines a population at intermediate risk for a cardiovascular event (2-fold increased risk of MACE at 3 years), and > = 540 pmol/L defines a population with an increased risk for a cardiovascular event. (Reference: 1. Tang et al. Am J Cardiol. 2013; 111:465-470 and personal communication with Tang et al). This test is performed by a turbidimetric immunoassay method. This test was developed and its performance characteristics determined by the Cleveland HeartLab, Inc. It has not been cleared or approved by the U.S. FDA. The Cleveland HeartLab, Inc. is regulated under Clinical Laboratory Improvement Amendments (CLIA) as qualified to perform high-complexity testing. This test is used for clinical purposes. It should not be regarded as investigational or for research.

FIGURE 14.11   Abnormal MPO lab information as reported.

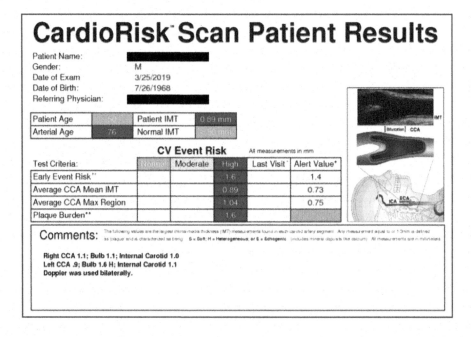

FIGURE 14.12   Abnormal CIMT results as evidenced in the lab report.

Exam Date: 9/23/2019

Maxillary arch (Teeth 1–16)

Row	1	2	3	4	5	6	7	8	9	10	11	12	13	14	15	16
MOB																
PD (Bcl)	3 2 4		4 2 3	3 2 3	3 2 3	3 2 3	3 2 3	3 2 2	2 2 2	2 2 3	3 2 3	3 2 3	3 2 3	3 2 3		3 2 3
GM																
CAL (Bcl)	3 2 4		4 2 3	3 2 3	3 2 3	3 2 3	3 2 3	3 2 2	2 2 2	2 2 3	3 2 3	3 2 3	3 2 3	3 2 3		3 2 3
MGJ																
PD (Ling)	3 2 3		3 2 3	3 2 3	3 2 3	3 2 3	3 2 2	2 2 2	2 2 2	2 2 2	2 2 2	2 2 2	2 2 3	3 2 3		3 2 3
GM																
CAL (Ling)	3 2 3		3 2 3	3 2 3	3 2 3	3 2 3	3 2 2	2 2 2	2 2 2	2 2 2	2 2 2	2 2 2	2 2 3	3 2 3		3 2 3
MGJ																

Mandibular arch (Teeth 32–17)

Row	32	31	30	29	28	27	26	25	24	23	22	21	20	19	18	17
MOB																
PD	3 2 4		4 2 3	3 2 3	3 2 2	2 2 2	2 2 2	2 2 2	2 2 2	2 2 2	2 2 3	3 2 3	3 2 3	3 2 3		3 2 4
GM																
CAL	3 2 4		4 2 3	3 2 3	3 2 2	2 2 2	2 2 2	2 2 2	2 2 2	2 2 2	2 2 3	3 2 3	3 2 3	3 2 3		3 2 4
MGJ																
PD (Bcl)	3 2 3		3 2 3	3 2 3	3 2 3	3 2 3	3 2 2	2 2 2	2 2 2	2 2 2	2 2 2	2 2 3	3 2 3	3 2 3		4 2 4
GM																
CAL (Bcl)	3 2 3		3 2 3	3 2 3	3 2 3	3 2 3	3 2 2	2 2 2	2 2 2	2 2 2	2 2 2	2 2 3	3 2 3	3 2 3		4 2 4
MGJ																

FIGURE 14.13 Periodontal disease stability as evidenced in follow-up periodontal probing with resolution of all bleeding on probing.

homecare by the patient and routine maintenance visits. This gives dentists new found hope of managing this complex disease for best health outcomes. Salivary diagnostics has shed new light on a disease that has traditionally reactivated often and continually progressed.

Physicians are now taking a much broader "root cause" approach to disease management. Finding disease when it is subclinical and providing treatment to stabilize or reverse the disease process is the goal of this application. This idea parallels the dentists' goal of identifying oral diseases early and treating them to stability for not only dental health but for systemic implications. Traditional symptom management or late-stage disease management carries a high expense burden of unnecessary hospital experiences, and less than favorable disease outcomes. One example of a medical model with a disease-inflammation approach (the BaleDoneen Method) has been found to be effective in preventing heart attack, stroke and diabetes. An 8-year outcome study using sequential CIMT reports suggests that following a vascular disease management method such as this has positive outcomes on lipids and CIMT thickness.[101] The BaleDoneen Method is effective in generating a positive effect on the atherosclerotic disease process by achieving regression of disease in the carotid arteries. A large part of the BaleDoneen Method is stressing the importance of oral health in the reduction of inflammation and bacterial burden causing vascular changes.[241,242] This model challenges the current standard of health care, utilizing a preventative, comprehensive, holistic approach focused on a disease/inflammatory treatment paradigm to achieve optimum health.

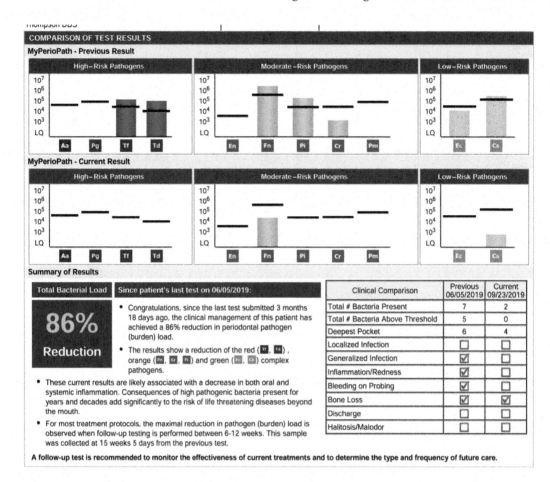

FIGURE 14.14 MyPerioPath test results following periodontal treatment and improved homecare by the patient demonstrating elimination of high-risk pathogens and significant reduction in both moderate- and low-risk pathogens.

The BaleDoneen Method is comprised of six basic elements that should be considered in any vascular disease management program. This includes the following:

1. **Education**: Each patient is educated about the disease state of atherosclerosis and understands how myocardial infarctions and ischemic strokes occur.
2. **Disease**: Each patient is evaluated for the presence of atherosclerosis, using noninvasive office-based techniques, to find asymptomatic vascular disease, and is monitored annually with a carotid intima-media thickness test (CIMT) test to follow the individual trajectory of atherosclerotic disease. In addition, all patients are monitored annually with a CIMT test to follow the atherosclerotic disease over time in the individual patient.
3. **Inflammation**: Biomarkers are used to routinely determine the inflammatory state of the vascular system. Endothelial markers include hs-CRP, microalbumin/creatinine urine ratio and fibrinogen. Lipoprotein-associated phospholipase A2 is evaluated for intima activity. Patients are instructed to have these assessed at least biannually.
4. **Root Causes**: The root cause or causes of the atherosclerotic process are determined and managed for each patient. Root causes of atherosclerosis can include insulin resistance, lipoprotein(a), familial hyperlipidemia, potentially myeloperoxidase and vitamin D deficiency. Appropriate follow-up testing for effective management of a root cause is done on average quarterly to semiannually.

Periodontal Pathogen Composite Score: 04.00

Type	Organism	Copies/oral rinse sample (x10^5)	10^5	10^6	10^7	10^8	10^9	10^{10}
A	Porphyromonas gingivalis (PG)	N/A						
	Tannerella forsythia (TF)	N/A						
	Treponema denticola (TD)	N/A						
B	Prevotella nigrescens (PN)	34.767						
	Porphyromonas endodontalis (PE)	N/A						
	Prevotella intermedia (PI)	N/A						
	Eubacterium nodatum (EN)	N/A						
	Filifactor alocis (FA)	N/A						
	Fretibacterium sp. HOT360 (Fr)	N/A						
	Treponema socranskii (TS)	N/A						
C	Bacteroidales [G-2] sp. HOT274 (Ba)	N/A						
	Campylobacter rectus (CR)	00.072	*					
	Parvimonas micra (PM)	N/A						
	Desulfobulbus sp. HOT041 (De)	N/A						
	Eikenella corrodens (EC)	1160.061						
	Selenomonas sputigena (SS)	554.768						
	Eubacterium saphenum (ES)	N/A						
	TM7 [G1] sp. HOT349 (TM7)	612.037						
	Fretibacterium fastidiosum (FF)	N/A						
	Treponema lecithinolyticum (TL)	N/A						
	Treponema maltophilum (TM)	00.032	*					
	Fusobacterium nucleatum ss animalis (FNa)	N/A						
	Fusobacterium nucleatum ss polymorphum (FNp)	801.406						
	Treponema sp. HT237 (Tr)	N/A						
	Fusobacterium nucleatum ss vincenti (FNv)	N/A						
D	Capnocytophaga gingivalis (CG)	322.524						
	Capnocytophaga ochracea (CO)	N/A						
	Capnocytophaga sputigena (CS)	26.115						
E	Aggregatibacter actinomycetemcomitans (AA)	N/A						

N/A   Below Detection Limit
*   < 10^5 Copies/sample

FIGURE 14.15 FidaLab post-treatment report demonstrated a reduction of the pathogen composite score of 881.64 down to 4.0.

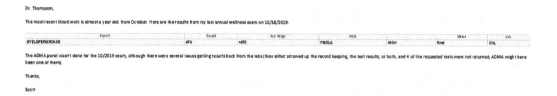

Dr. Thompson,

The most recent blood work is almost a year old: from October. Here are the results from my last annual wellness exam on 10/16/2019.

	Report	Result	Ref Range	WLb		Ftus	Lab
MYELOPEROXIDASE		474	<470	PMOLL	HIGH	final	CHL

The ADMA panel wasn't done for the 10/2019 exam, although there were several issues getting results back from the labs (they either screwed up the record keeping, the test results, or both, and 4 of the requested tests were not returned; ADMA might have been one of them).

Thanks,

Scott

FIGURE 14.16 Post-treatment yielded a favorable reduction in MPO down from 527 pretreatment to 474 post-treatment.

5. **Optimal Goals**: Goals of therapy are set based on peer-reviewed, reliable research and guidelines, with optimal targets to minimize risk and often going beyond the values set for the standard of care. Attainments of goals are evaluated, on average, every 3–6 months.
6. **Genetics**: Genetic information is obtained on patients to aid in the assessment of their cardiovascular risk and to help guide therapy. These tests are never repeated. Their clinical utility never expires, unlike other biomarkers. This makes them arguably the least expensive tests performed.

This method is mentioned and outlined here because a significant source of inflammation can be from the mouth in both periodontal and endodontic diseases. Therefore, oral health is a major root factor, and anyone practicing preventative cardiology needs a competent oral healthcare provider to evaluate the mouth for any contributing pathology.

These basic elements of the disease prevention strategy presented need to be reinforced with abundant patient education. A huge part of this education is on lifestyle modification, the number one way to prevent cardiovascular disease and a contributor to oral disease. Lifestyle skills need to be taught in physical activity, proper diet, adequate sleep, anxiety management, weight control, nicotine cessation, and mindfulness and connectedness. Of course, oral health maintenance is critical for success. Many of these are all host modulation issues that affect cardiovascular disease and oral disease, and are modifiable by the patient. Many similarities exist between cardiovascular disease and the lifestyle issues that affect periodontal disease. Because of this, there is great opportunity to collaborate on patient education reinforcement between the medical and dental disciplines. The future is bright for medical/dental collaboration for the best overall oral and systemic disease management.

REFERENCES

1. Eke PI, Thornton-Evans GO, Wei L, Borgnakke WS, Dye BA, Genco RJ. 2018 Periodontitis in US adults: National health and nutrition examination survey 2009–2014. *J Am Dent Assoc.* 149(7):576–588. e6. doi: 10.1016/j.adaj.2018.04.023. PMID: 29957185; PMCID: PMC8094373.
2. Eke PI, Dye BA, Wei L, et al. 2012 Prevalence of periodontitis in adults in the United States: 2009 and 2010. *J Dent Res.* 91(10):914–20. Epub 2012 Aug 30. doi: 10.1177/0022034512457373.
3. https://www.perio.org/newsroom/periodontal-disease-fact-sheet.
4. https://wwwn.cdc.gov/Nchs/Nhanes/2017–2018/OHXDEN_J.htm.
5. https://www.cdc.gov/oralhealth/conditions/periodontal-disease.html#:~:text=A%20recent%20CDC%20report1,and%20older%20have%20periodontal%20disease.
6. Monsarrat P, Blaizot A, Kémoun P, Ravaud P, Nabet C, Sixou M, Vergnes JN. 2016 Clinical research activity in periodontal medicine: A systematic mapping of trial registers. *J Clin Periodontol.* 43(5):390–400. doi: 10.1111/jcpe.12534. Epub 2016 Apr 13. PMID: 26881700.
7. Cecoro G, Annunziata M, Iuorio MT, Nastri L, Guida L. 2020 Periodontitis, Low-Grade Inflammation and Systemic Health: A Scoping Review. *Medicina (Kaunas).* 56(6):272. doi: 10.3390/medicina56060272. PMID: 32486269; PMCID: PMC7353850.
8. https://www.nidcr.nih.gov/research/data-statistics/dental-caries/adults#:~:text=92%25%20of%20adults%2020%20to,education%20have%20had%20more%20decay.
9. Fleming E, Afful J. 2018 Prevalence of total and untreated dental caries among youth: United States, 2015–2016. NCHS Data Brief, no 307. Hyattsville, MD: National Center for Health Statistics.
10. https://www.cdc.gov/nchs/data/hus/2019/028-508.pdf.
11. Fowell C, Igbokwe B, MacBean A. 2012 The clinical relevance of microbiology specimens in orofacial abscesses of dental origin. *Ann R Coll Surg Engl.* 94(7):490–2. doi: 10.1308/003588412X13373405385539. PMID: 23031767; PMCID: PMC3954244.
12. Shweta S. 2013 Dental abscess: A microbiological review. *Dent Res J (Isfahan).* 10(5):585–91. PMID: 24348613; PMCID: PMC3858730.
13. Manoil D, Al-Manei K, Belibasakis GN. 2020 A systematic review of the root canal microbiota associated with apical periodontitis: Lessons from next-generation sequencing. *Proteomics Clin Appl.* 14(-3):e1900060. doi: 10.1002/prca.201900060. Epub 2020 Jan 24. PMID: 31950679.
14. Yumoto H, Hirota K, Hirao K, Ninomiya M, Murakami K, Fujii H, Miyake Y. 2019 The pathogenic factors from oral streptococci for systemic diseases. *Int J Mol Sci.* 20(18):4571. doi: 10.3390/ijms20184571. PMID: 31540175; PMCID: PMC6770522.
15. Pan W, Wang Q, Chen Q. 2019 The cytokine network involved in the host immune response to periodontitis. *Int J Oral Sci.* 11:30.
16. Eke PI, Dye BA, Wei L, Slade GD, Thornton-Evans GO, Borgnakke WS, Taylor GW, Page RC, Beck JD, Genco RJ. 2015 Update on Prevalence of Periodontitis in Adults in the United States: NHANES 2009 to 2012. *J Periodontol.* 86(5):611–22. doi: 10.1902/jop.2015.140520. Epub Feb 17. PMID: 25688694; PMCID: PMC4460825.
17. Marsh PD. 2004 Dental plaque as a microbial biofilm. *Caries Res.* 38(3):204–11.
18. Socransky SS, Haffajee AD. 2002 Dental biofilms: Difficult therapeutic targets. *Periodontology.* 28:12–55.

19. Mehrotra N, Singh S. 2021 Periodontitis. In: StatPearls [Internet]. Treasure Island (FL): StatPearls Publishing; PMID: 31082170.

20. Thurnheer T, Paqué PN. 2021 Biofilm models to study the etiology and pathogenesis of oral diseases. *Monogr Oral Sci.* 29:30–7. doi: 10.1159/000510197. Epub 2020 Dec 21. PMID: 33427216.

21. Minarovits J. 2021 Anaerobic bacterial communities associated with oral carcinoma: Intratumoral, surface-biofilm and salivary microbiota. *Anaerobe.* 68:102300. doi: 10.1016/j.anaerobe.2020.102300. Epub 2020 Nov 24. PMID: 33246097.

22. Sharma D, Sharma S, Pal V, Lal R, Patil P, Grover V, Korpole S. 2020 Bacterial populations in subgingival plaque under healthy and diseased conditions: Genomic insights into oral adaptation strategies by Lactobacillus sp. Strain DISK7. *Indian J Microbiol.* 60(1):78–86. doi: 10.1007/s12088-019-00828-8. Epub 2019 Oct 8. PMID: 32089577; PMCID: PMC7000561.

23. Hojo K, Nagaoka S, Ohshima T, Maeda N. 2009 Bacterial interactions in dental biofilm development. *J Dent Res.* 88(11):982–90. doi: 10.1177/0022034509346811.

24. Kanwar IL, Sah AK, Suresh PK. 2017 Biofilm-mediated antibiotic-resistant oral bacterial infections: Mechanism and combat strategies. *Curr Pharm Des.* 23(14):2084–95.

25. van Steenbergen TJ, van Winkelhoff AJ, de Graaff J. 1984 Pathogenic synergy: Mixed infections in the oral cavity. *Antonie Van Leeuwenhoek.* 50(5–6):789–98.

26. Schenkein HA, Papapanou PN, Genco R, Sanz M. 2020 Mechanisms underlying the association between periodontitis and atherosclerotic disease. *Periodontology 2000.* 83(1):90–106. doi: 10.1111/prd.12304. PMID: 32385879.

27. Seidel CL, Gerlach RG, Wiedemann P, Weider M, Rodrian G, Hader M, Frey B, Gaipl US, Bozec A, Cieplik F, Kirschneck C, Bogdan C, Gölz L. 2020 Defining metaniches in the oral cavity according to their microbial composition and cytokine profile. *Int J Mol Sci.* 21(21):8218. doi: 10.3390/ijms21218218. PMID: 33153049; PMCID: PMC7663680.

28. Hua, X, Cook, GS, Costerton, JW, et al. 2000 Intergeneric communication in dental plaque biofilms. *J Bacteriol.* 182:7067–9.

29. Pöllänen MT, Laine MA, Ihalin R, Uitto VJ. 2012 Host-bacteria crosstalk at the dentogingival junction. *Int J Dent.* 2012:821383. doi: 10.1155/2012/821383. Epub 2012 Jul 26. PMID: 22899931; PMCID: PMC3412119.

30. Lovegrove JM. 2004 Dental plaque revisited: Bacteria associated with periodontal disease. *J N Z Soc Periodontol.* 87:7–21. PMID: 15143484.

31. Al-Ahmad A, Muzafferiy F, Anderson AC, Wölber JP, Ratka-Krüger P, Fretwurst T, Nelson K, Vach K, Hellwig E. 2018 Shift of microbial composition of peri-implantitis-associated oral biofilm as revealed by 16S rRNA gene cloning. *J Med Microbiol.* 67(3):332–40. doi: 10.1099/jmm.0.000682. Epub 2018 Jan 24. PMID: 29458668.

32. Serra e Silva Filho W, Casarin RC, Nicolela EL Jr, Passos HM, Sallum AW, Gonçalves RB. 2014 Microbial diversity similarities in periodontal pockets and atheromatous plaques of cardiovascular disease patients. *PLoS One.* 9(10):e109761. doi: 10.1371/journal.pone.0109761. eCollection 2014.

33. Zardawi F, Gul S, Abdulkareem A, Sha A, Yates J. 2021 Association between periodontal disease and atherosclerotic cardiovascular diseases: Revisited. *Front Cardiovasc Med.* 7:625579. doi: 10.3389/fcvm.2020.625579. PMID: 33521070; PMCID: PMC7843501.

34. Herrera D, Molina A, Buhlin K, Klinge B. 2020 Periodontal diseases and association with atherosclerotic disease. *Periodontology 2000.* 83(1):66–89. doi: 10.1111/prd.12302. PMID: 32385870.

35. Menon T, Gopalakrishnan SN, Balasubramanian R, Justin SR. 2017 Characterization of the human oral microbiome in patients with coronary artery disease using next-generation sequencing of 16SrRNA amplicons. *Indian J Med Microbiol.* 35(1):101–4. doi: 10.4103/ijmm.IJMM_16_370. PMID: 28303827.

36. Jiang Q, Liu J, Chen L, Gan N, Yang D. 2019 The oral microbiome in the elderly with dental caries and health. *Front Cell Infect Microbiol.* 8:442. doi: 10.3389/fcimb.2018.00442. PMID: 30662876; PMCID: PMC6328972.

37. https://www.aegisdentalnetwork.com/id/2016/03/oral-biofilms-and-the-systemic-connection.

38. https://cdeworld.com/ebooks/biofilms-the-oral-systemic-connection.

39. Párkányi L, Vályi P, Nagy K, Fráter M. 2018 Odontogenic foci and systemic diseases. A review. *Orv Hetil.* 159(11):415–22. doi: 10.1556/650.2018.31008.

40. National Diabetes Statistics Report, 2014. Centers for Disease Control and Prevention website. www.cdc.gov/diabetes/pubs/statsreport14/national-diabetes-report-web.pdf.

41. https://www.diabetesresearch.org/diabetes-statistics#:~:text=34.2%20million%20people%2C%20or%2010.5,yet%20been%20diagnosed%20(2018).

42. https://www.cdc.gov/diabetes/data/statistics-report/index.html.

43. Polak D, Sanui T, Nishimura F, Shapira L. 2020 Diabetes as a risk factor for periodontal disease-plausible mechanisms. *Periodontology 2000.* 83(1):46–58. doi: 10.1111/prd.12298. PMID: 32385872.
44. Kim EK, Lee SG, et al. 2013 Association between diabetes-related factors and clinical periodontal parameters in type-2 diabetes mellitus. *BMC Oral Health.* 13:64. doi: 10.1186/1472-6831-13-64.
45. Stanko P, Izakovicova Holla L. 2014 Bidirectional association between diabetes mellitus and inflammatory periodontal disease. A review. *Biomed Pap Med Fac Univ Palacky Olomouc Czech Repub.* 158(1):35–8. doi: 10.5507/bp.2014.005. Epub 2014 Jan 27.
46. Zheng M, Wang C, Ali A, Shih YA, Xie Q, Guo C. 2021 Prevalence of periodontitis in people clinically diagnosed with diabetes mellitus: A meta-analysis of epidemiologic studies. *Acta Diabetol.* doi: 10.1007/s00592-021-01738-2. Epub ahead of print. PMID: 34028620.
47. Taylor GW, Burt BA, Becker MP, et al. 1996 Severe periodontitis and risk for poor glycemic control in patients with non-insulin-dependent diabetes mellitus. *J Periodontol.* 67(10 suppl):1085–93.
48 Stoicescu M, Calniceanu H, Ţig I, Nemeth S, Tent A, Popa A, Brisc C, Ignat-Romanul I. 2021 Significant aspects and correlation between glycemic control and generalized chronic periodontitis in type 2 diabetes mellitus patients. *Exp Ther Med.* 22(1):671. doi: 10.3892/etm.2021.10103. Epub 2021 Apr 23. PMID: 33986836; PMCID: PMC8112123.
49. Herzberg MC, Weyer MW. 1998 Dental plaque, platelets, and cardiovascular diseases. *Ann Periodontol.* 3(1):151–60.
50. Çakmak HA, Bayoğlu B, Durmaz E, Can G, Karadağ B, Cengiz M, Vural VA, Yüksel H. 2015 Evaluation of association between common genetic variants on chromosome 9p21 and coronary artery disease in Turkish population. *Anatol J Cardiol.* 15(3):196–203. doi: 10.5152/akd.2014.5285. Epub 2014 Apr 8. PMID: 25333979; PMCID: PMC5337054.
51. Scannapieco FA. 1998 Position paper of The American Academy of Periodontology: Periodontal disease as a potential risk factor for systemic diseases. *J Periodontol.* 69(7):841–850.
52. Syrjänen J. 1990 Vascular diseases and oral infections. *J Clin Periodontol.* 17(7 pt 2):497–500.
53. Valtonen VV. 1991 Infection as a risk factor for infarction and atherosclerosis. *Ann Med.* 23(5):539–43.
54. Cotti E, Dessì C, Piras A, Mercuro G. 2011 Can a chronic dental infection be considered a cause of cardiovascular disease? A review of the literature. *Int J Cardiol.* 148(1):4–10. doi: 10.1016/j.ijcard.2010.08.011. Epub 2010 Sep 18. PMID: 20851474.
55. Humagain M, Nayak DG, Uppoor AS. 2006 Periodontal infections and cardiovascular disease: Is it a mere association? *Kathmandu Univ Med J (KUMJ).* 4(3):379–82. PMID: 18603938.
56. Zoellner H. 2011 Dental infection and vascular disease. *Semin Thromb Hemost.* 37(3):181–92. doi: 10.1055/s-0031-1273082. Epub 2011 Mar 31. PMID: 21455852.
57. Nomura R, Otsugu M, Naka S, et al. 2014 Contribution of the interaction of Streptococcus mutans serotype k strains with fibrinogen to the pathogenicity of infective endocarditis. *Infect Immun.* 82(12):5223–34.
58. Otsugu M, Nomura R, Matayoshi S, Teramoto N, Nakano K. 2017 Contribution of streptococcus mutans strains with collagen-binding proteins in the presence of serum to the pathogenesis of infective endocarditis. *Infect Immun.* 85(12):e00401-17. doi: 10.1128/IAI.00401-17. PMID: 28947650; PMCID: PMC5695098.
59. Schenkein HA, Loos BG. 2013 Inflammatory mechanisms linking periodontal diseases to cardiovascular diseases. *J Periodontol.* 84(4 Suppl):S51–69.
60. Wojtkowska A, Zapolski T, Wysokińska-Miszczuk J, Wysokiński AP. 2021 The inflammation link between periodontal disease and coronary atherosclerosis in patients with acute coronary syndromes: Case-control study. *BMC Oral Health.* 21(1):5. doi: 10.1186/s12903-020-01356-4. PMID: 33407375; PMCID: PMC7789370.
61. Haraszthy VI, Zambon JJ, Trevisan M, et al. 1998 Identification of pathogens in atheromatous plaques [abstract 273]. *Dent Res.* 77(spec. iss. B):666.
62. Deshpande RG, Khan MB, Genco CA. 1998 Invasion of aortic and heart endothelial cells by *Porphyromonas gingivalis. Infect Immun.* 66(11):5337–43.
63. Xie M, Tang Q, Yu S, Sun J, Mei F, Zhao J, Chen L. 2020 *Porphyromonas gingivalis* disrupts vascular endothelial homeostasis in a TLR-NF-κB axis dependent manner. *Int J Oral Sci.* 12(1):28. doi: 10.1038/s41368-020-00096-z. PMID: 32999278; PMCID: PMC7527479.
64. Dhadse P, Gattani D, Mishra R. 2010 The link between periodontal disease and cardiovascular disease: How far we have come in last two decades? *J Indian Soc Periodontol.* 14(3): 148–54. doi: 10.4103/0972-124X.75908. PMCID: PMC3100856
65. Persson GR, Imfeld T. 2008 Periodontitis and cardiovascular disease. *Ther Umsch.* 65(2):121–6.

66. Surma S, Romańczyk M, Witalińska-Łabuzek J, Czerniuk MR, Łabuzek K, Filipiak KJ. 2021 Periodontitis, blood pressure, and the risk and control of arterial hypertension: Epidemiological, clinical, and pathophysiological aspects-review of the literature and clinical trials. *Curr Hypertens Rep.* 23(-5):27. doi: 10.1007/s11906-021-01140-x. PMID: 33961166; PMCID: PMC8105217.

67. Pietropaoli D, Del Pinto R, Ferri C, Wright JT Jr, Giannoni M, Ortu E, Monaco A. 2018 Poor oral health and blood pressure control among us hypertensive adults. *Hypertension.* 72(6):1365–73. doi: 10.1161/HYPERTENSIONAHA.118.11528. PMID: 30540406.

68. Desvarieux M, Demmer RT, Rundek T, et al. 2005 Periodontal microbiota and carotid intima-media thickness: The Oral Infections and Vascular Disease Epidemiology Study (INVEST). *Circulation.* 111(5):576–82.

69. Loesche WJ, Schork A, Terpenning MS, et al. 1998 The relationship between dental disease and cerebral vascular accident in elderly United States veterans. *Ann Periodontol.* 3(1):161–74.

70. Wu T, Trevisan M, Genco RJ, Falkner KL, Dorn JP, Sempos CT. 2000 Examination of the relation between periodontal health status and cardiovascular risk factors: Serum total and high density lipoprotein cholesterol, C-reactive protein, and plasma fibrinogen. *Am J Epidemiol.* 151(3):273–82.

71. Moura Foz A, Alexandre Romito G, Manoel Bispo C, Luciancencov Petrillo C, Patel K, Suvan J, D'Aiuto F. 2010 Periodontal therapy and biomarkers related to cardiovascular risk. *Minerva Stomatol.* 59(5):271–83. PMID: 20502435.

72. Libby P, Ridker PM, Hansson GK. 2009 Inflammation in atherosclerosis: From pathophysiology to practice. *J Am Coll Cardiol.* 54(23):2129–38. doi: 10.1016/j.jacc.2009.09.009.

73. Paul O, Arora P, Mayer M, Chatterjee S. 2021 Inflammation in periodontal disease: Possible link to vascular disease. *Front Physiol.* 11:609614. doi: 10.3389/fphys.2020.609614. PMID: 33519515; PMCID: PMC7841426.

74. Ridker PM, Silvertown JD. 2008 Inflammation, C-reactive protein, and atherothrombosis. *J Periodontol.* 79(8 Suppl):1544–51. doi: 10.1902/jop.2008.080249. PMID: 18673009.

75. Cybulsky MI, Jongstra-Bilen J. 2010 Resident intimal dendritic cells and the initiation of atherosclerosis. *Curr Opin Lipidol.* 21(5):397–403. doi:10.1097/MOL.0b013e32833ded96.

76. Allahverdian S, Pannu PS, Francis GA. 2012 Contribution of monocyte-derived macrophages and smooth muscle cells to arterial foam cell formation. *Cardiovasc Res.* 95(2):165–72. doi: 10.1093/cvr/cvs094. Epub 2012 Feb 15. PMID: 22345306.

77. Imanishi T, Akasaka T. 2012 Biomarkers associated with vulnerable atheromatous plaque. *Curr Med Chem.* 19(16):2588–96.

78. Shah PK. 2014 Biomarkers of plaque instability. *Curr Cardiol Rep.* 16(12):547. doi: 10.1007/s11886-014-0547-7. PMID: 25326730.

79. Bale, B., Doneen, A., Vigerust, D. 2016 High-risk periodontal pathogens contribute to the pathogenesis of atherosclerosis. *Postgrad Med J* 0:1–6. Online 11–29–2016.

80. Kozarov EV, Dorn BR, Shelburne CE, Dunn WA Jr, Progulske-Fox A. 2005 Human atherosclerotic plaque contains viable invasive *Actinobacillus actinomycetemcomitans* and *Porphyromonas gingivalis.* *Arterioscler Thromb Vasc Biol.* 25(3):e17–8. Epub 2005 Jan 20.

81. Doneen AL, Bale BF, Vigerust DJ, Leimgruber PP. 2020 Cardiovascular prevention: Migrating from a binary to a ternary classification. *Front Cardiovasc Med.* 7:92. doi: 10.3389/fcvm.2020.00092. PMID: 32528979; PMCID: PMC7256212.

82. Socransky SS, Haffajee AD. 1992 The bacterial etiology of destructive periodontal disease: Current concepts. *J Periodontol.* 63(Suppl 4):322–31.

83. Lu H, Xu M, Wang F, Liu S, Gu J, Lin S. 2014 Chronic stress enhances progression of periodontitis via α1-adrenergic signaling: A potential target for periodontal disease therapy. *Exp Mol Med.* 46:e118. doi:10.1038/emm.2014.65.

84. A Tanveer S, Afaq A, Alqutub MN, Aldahiyan N, AlMubarak AM, Shaikh AC, Naseem M, Vohra F, Abduljabbar T. 2021 Association of self-perceived psychological stress with the periodontal health of socially deprived women in shelter homes. *Int J Environ Res Public Health.* 18(10):5160. doi: 10.3390/ijerph18105160. PMID: 34068018.

85. Apatzidou DA. 2012 Modern approaches to non-surgical biofilm management. *Front Oral Biol.* 15:99–116. doi: 10.1159/000329674. Epub 2011 Nov 11. PMID: 22142959.

86. Lang NP, Bartold PM. 2018 Periodontal health. *J Periodontol.* 89(Suppl 1):S9–16. doi: 10.1002/JPER.16-0517. PMID: 29926938.

87. Mariotti A, Hefti AF. 2015 Defining periodontal health. *BMC Oral Health.* 15(Suppl 1):S6. doi: 10.1186/1472-6831-15-S1-S6. Epub 2015 Sep 15. PMID: 26390888; PMCID: PMC4580771.

88. Ferreira SB Jr, Trombone AP, Repeke CE, et al. 2008 An interleukin-1beta (IL-1beta) single-nucleotide polymorphism at position 3954 and red complex periodontopathogens independently and additively modulate the levels of IL-1beta in diseased periodontal tissues. *Infect Immun.* 76:3725–3734.

89. Socransky SS, Haffajee AD, Smith C, et al. 2000 Microbiological parameters associated with IL-1 gene polymorphisms in periodontitis patients. *J Clin Periodontol.* 27:810–8; Parkhill JM, Hennig BJ, Chapple IL, et al. Association of interleukin-1 gene polymorphisms with early-onset periodontitis. *J Clin Periodontol.* 2000;27:682–689.

90. Havemose-Poulsen A, Sørensen LK, Bendtzen K, et al. 2007 Polymorphisms within the IL-1 gene cluster: Effects on cytokine profiles in peripheral blood and whole blood cell cultures of patients with aggressive periodontitis, juvenile idiopathic arthritis, and rheumatoid arthritis. *J Periodontol.* 78:475–92.

91. Caffesse RG, de la Rosa MR, de la Rosa MG. 2002 Interleukin-1 gene polymorphism in a well-maintained periodontal patient population. *Braz J Oral Sci.* 1:1–6.

92. Caffesse RG, De LaRosa MR, De LaRosa MG, Mota LF. 2002 Prevalence of interleukin 1 periodontal genotype in a Hispanic dental population. *Quintessence Int.* 33(3):190–4. PMID: 11921766.

93. Laine ML, Leonhardt A, Roos-Jansåker AM, et al. 2006 IL-1RN gene polymorphism is associated with periimplantitis. *Clin Oral Implants Res.* 17:380–5.

94. Bugueno IM, Benkirane-Jessel N, Huck O. 2021 Implication of Toll/IL-1 receptor domain containing adapters in *Porphyromonas gingivalis*-induced inflammation. *Innate Immun*:17534259211013087. doi: 10.1177/17534259211013087. Epub ahead of print. PMID: 34018827.

95. Nabors TW, McGlennen RC, Thompson D. 2010 Salivary testing for periodontal disease diagnosis and treatment. *Dent Today.* 29(6):53–4, 56, 58–60; quiz 61. PMID: 20565019.

96. Zhang Y, Kang N, Xue F, Qiao J, Duan J, Chen F, Cai Y. 2021 Evaluation of salivary biomarkers for the diagnosis of periodontitis. *BMC Oral Health.* 21(1):266. doi: 10.1186/s12903-021-01600-5. PMID: 34001101; PMCID: PMC8130171.

97. Kinane DF. 2000 Periodontal diagnostics. *Ann R Australas Coll Dent Surg.* 15:34–41. PMID: 11709970.

98. Baima G, Iaderosa G, Citterio F, Grossi S, Romano F, Berta GN, Buduneli N, Aimetti M. 2021 Salivary metabolomics for the diagnosis of periodontal diseases: A systematic review with methodological quality assessment. *Metabolomics.* 17(1):1. doi: 10.1007/s11306-020-01754-3. PMID: 33387070.

99. Diaz PI, Hoare A, Hong BY. 2016 Subgingival microbiome shifts and community dynamics in periodontal diseases. *J Calif Dent Assoc.* 44(7):421–35. PMID: 27514154.

100. Lang NP, Tonetti MS. 2003 Periodontal risk assessment (PRA) for patients in supportive periodontal therapy (SPT). *Oral Health Prev Dent.* 1: 7–16.

101. Kinane DF, Hart TC. 2003 Genes and gene polymorphisms associated with periodontal disease. *Crit Rev Oral Biol Med.* 14(6):430–49. doi: 10.1177/154411130301400605. PMID: 14656898.

102. Anderson AC, Rothballer M, Altenburger MJ, Woelber JP, Karygianni L, Vach K, Hellwig E, Al-Ahmad A. 2020 Long-term fluctuation of oral biofilm microbiota following different dietary phases. *Appl Environ Microbiol.* 86(20):e01421–20. doi: 10.1128/AEM.01421-20. PMID: 32801176; PMCID: PMC7531951.

103. Bartold PM, Van Dyke TE. 2017 Host modulation: Controlling the inflammation to control the infection. *Periodontology 2000.* 75(1):317–29. doi: 10.1111/prd.12169.

104. Curtis MA, Diaz PI, Van Dyke TE. 2020 The role of the microbiota in periodontal disease. *Periodontol 2000.* 83(1):14–25. doi: 10.1111/prd.12296. PMID: 32385883.

105. Ebersole JL, Al-Sabbagh M, Dawson DR 3rd. 2019 Heterogeneity of human serum antibody responses to *P. gingivalis* in periodontitis: Effects of age, race/ethnicity, and sex. *Immunol Lett.* 218:11–21. doi: 10.1016/j.imlet.2019.12.004. Epub 2019 Dec 18. PMID: 31863783; PMCID: PMC6956649.

106. Golub LM, Lee HM, Ryan ME, Giannobile WV, Payne J, Sorsa T. 1998 Tetracyclines inhibit connective tissue breakdown by multiple non-antimicrobial mechanisms. *Adv Dent Res.* 12(2):12–26. doi: 10.1177/08959374980120010501. PMID: 9972117.

107. Ashley RA. 1999 Clinical trials of a matrix metalloproteinase inhibitor in human periodontal disease. SDD Clinical Research Team. *Ann N Y Acad Sci.* 878:335–46. doi: 10.1111/j.1749-6632.1999.tb07693.x. PMID: 10415739.

108. Lee HM, Ciancio SG, Tüter G, Ryan ME, Komaroff E, Golub LM. 2004 Subantimicrobial dose doxycycline efficacy as a matrix metalloproteinase inhibitor in chronic periodontitis patients is enhanced when combined with a non-steroidal anti-inflammatory drug. *J Periodontol.* 75(3):453–63. doi: 10.1902/jop.2004.75.3.453. PMID: 15088884.

109. Sorsa T, Tervahartiala T, Leppilahti J, Hernandez M, Gamonal J, Tuomainen AM, Lauhio A, Pussinen PJ, Mäntylä P. 2011 Collagenase-2 (MMP-8) as a point-of-care biomarker in periodontitis and cardiovascular diseases. Therapeutic response to non-antimicrobial properties of tetracyclines. *Pharmacol Res.* 63(2):108–13. doi: 10.1016/j.phrs.2010.10.005. Epub 2010 Oct 16. PMID: 20937384.

110. Novak MJ, Dawson DR 3rd, Magnusson I, Karpinia K, Polson A, Polson A, Ryan ME, Ciancio S, Drisko CH, Kinane D, Powala C, Bradshaw M. 2008 Combining host modulation and topical antimicrobial therapy in the management of moderate to severe periodontitis: A randomized multicenter trial. *J Periodontol.* 79(1):33–41. doi: 10.1902/jop.2008.070237.

111. Preshaw PM, Novak MJ, Mellonig J, Magnusson I, Polson A, Giannobile WV, Rowland RW, Thomas J, Walker C, Dawson DR, Sharkey D, Bradshaw MH. 2008 Modified-release subantimicrobial dose doxycycline enhances scaling and root planing in subjects with periodontal disease. *J Periodontol.* 79(-3):440–52. doi: 10.1902/jop.2008.070375. PMID: 18315426.

112. Gokhale SR, Padhye AM. 2013 Future prospects of systemic host modulatory agents in periodontal therapy. *Br Dent J.* 214:467–71.

113. Deo V, Bhongade ML. 2010 Pathogenesis of periodontitis: Role of cytokines in host response. *Dent Today.* 29(9):60–2, 64–6; quiz 68–9. PMID: 20973418.

114. Plemmenos G, Evangeliou E, Polizogopoulos N, Chalazias A, Deligianni M, Piperi C. 2020 Central regulatory role of cytokines in periodontitis and targeting options. *Curr Med Chem.* doi: 10.2174/0929867327666200824112732. Epub ahead of print. PMID: 32838709.

115. Di Paola R, Mazzon E, Muia C, Crisafulli C, Terrana D, Greco S, Britti D, Santori D, Oteri G, Cordasco G, Cuzzocrea S. 2007 Effects of etanercept, a tumour necrosis factor-alpha antagonist, in an experimental model of periodontitis in rats. *Br J Pharmacol.* 150:286–97.

116. de Smit MJ, Westra J, Posthumus MD, Springer G, van Winkelhoff AJ, Vissink A, Brouwer E, Bijl M. 2021 Effect of anti-rheumatic treatment on the periodontal condition of rheumatoid arthritis patients. Int J *Environ Res Public Health.* 18(5):2529. doi: 10.3390/ijerph18052529. PMID: 33806304; PMCID: PMC7967392.

117. Han JY, Reynolds MA. 2012 Effect of anti-rheumatic agents on periodontal parameters and biomarkers of inflammation: A systematic review and meta-analysis. *J Periodontal Implant Sci.* 42:3–12.

118. Vik A, Hansen TV. 2021 Stereoselective syntheses and biological activities of E-series resolvins. *Org Biomol Chem.* 19(4):705–21. doi: 10.1039/d0ob02218g. Epub 2021 Jan 7. PMID: 33410452.

119. Balta MG, Papathanasiou E, Blix IJ, Van Dyke TE. 2021 Host modulation and treatment of periodontal disease. *J Dent Res:*22034521995157. doi: 10.1177/0022034521995157. Epub ahead of print. PMID: 33655803.

120. Stańdo M, Piatek P, Namiecinska M, Lewkowicz P, Lewkowicz N. 2020 Omega-3 polyunsaturated fatty acids EPA and DHA as an adjunct to non-surgical treatment of periodontitis: A randomized clinical trial. *Nutrients.* 12(9):2614. doi: 10.3390/nu12092614. PMID: 32867199; PMCID: PMC7551834.

121. Nicolai E, Sinibaldi F, Sannino G, Laganà G, Basoli F, Licoccia S, Cozza P, Santucci R, Piro MC. 2017 Omega-3 and omega-6 fatty acids act as inhibitors of the matrix metalloproteinase-2 and matrix metalloproteinase-9 activity. *Protein J.* 36(4):278–85. doi: 10.1007/s10930-017-9727-9. PMID: 28646265.

122. Chee B, Park B, Fitzsimmons T, Coates AM, Bartold PM. 2016 Omega-3 fatty acids as an adjunct for periodontal therapy – a review. *Clin Oral Investig.* 20:879–94.

123. El-Sharkawy H, Aboelsaad N, Eliwa M, Darweesh M, Alshahat M, Kantarci A, Hasturk H, Van Dyke TE. 2010 Adjunctive treatment of chronic periodontitis with daily dietary supplementation with omega-3 fatty acids and low-doseaspirin. *J Periodontol.* 81:1635–43.

124. Rajaram SS, Nisha S, Ali NM, Shashikumar P, Karmakar S, Pandey V. 2021 Influence of a low-carbohydrate and rich in omega-3 fatty acids, ascorbic acid, antioxidants, and fiber diet on clinical outcomes in patients with chronic gingivitis: A randomized controlled trial. *J Int Soc Prev Community Dent.* 11(-1):58–67. doi: 10.4103/jispcd.JISPCD_365_20. PMID: 33688474; PMCID: PMC7934824.

125. Kujur SK, Goswami V, Nikunj AM, Singh G, Bandhe S, Ghritlahre H. 2020 Efficacy of omega 3 fatty acid as an adjunct in the management of chronic periodontitis: A randomized controlled trial. *Indian J Dent Res.* 31(2):229–35. doi: 10.4103/ijdr.IJDR_647_18. PMID: 32436902.

126. Elkhouli AM. 2011 The efficacy of host response modulation therapy (omega-3 plus low-dose aspirin) as an adjunctive treatment of chronic periodontitis (clinical and biochemical study). *J Periodontal Res.* 46:261–8.

127. Naqvi AZ, Hasturk H, Mu L, Phillips RS, Davis RB, Halem S, Campos H, Goodson JM, Van Dyke TE, Mukamal KJ. 2014 Docosahexaenoic acid and periodontitis in adults: A randomized controlled trial. *J Dent Res.* 93:767–73.

128. Dos Santos NC, Araujo CF, Andere NMRB, Miguel MMV, Westphal MRA, Van Dyke T, Santamaria MP. 2020 Omega-3 fatty acids and low-dose aspirin in the treatment of periodontitis and metabolic syndrome: Case report. *J Int Acad Periodontol.* 22(4):223–30. PMID: 32980834.

129. Serhan CN, Chiang N, Van Dyke TE. 2008 Resolving inflammation: Dual anti-inflammatory and pro-resolution lipid mediators. *Nat Rev Immunol.* 8:349–61.

130. Castro Dos Santos NC, Andere NMRB, Araujo CF, de Marco AC, Kantarci A, Van Dyke TE, Santamaria MP. 2020 Omega-3 PUFA and aspirin as adjuncts to periodontal debridement in patients with periodontitis and type 2 diabetes mellitus: Randomized clinical trial. *J Periodontol.* 91(10):1318–27. doi: 10.1002/JPER.19-0613. Epub 2020 Jun 21. PMID: 32103495; PMCID: PMC7483813.

131. Petit C, Batool F, Bugueno IM, Schwinté P, Benkirane-Jessel N, Huck O. 2019 Contribution of statins towards periodontal treatment: A review. *Mediators Inflamm.* 2019:6367402. doi: 10.1155/2019/6367402. PMID: 30936777; PMCID: PMC6415285.

132. Bertl K, Steiner I, Pandis N, Buhlin K, Klinge B, Stavropoulos A. 2017 Statins in nonsurgical and surgical periodontal therapy. A systematic review and meta-analysis of preclinical in vivo trials. *J Periodontal Res.* 53(3):267–87. doi: 10.1111/jre.12514. Epub 2017 Dec 6. PMID: 29211309.

133. Bastendorf KD, Strafela-Bastendorf N, Lussi A. 2021 Mechanical removal of the biofilm: Is the curette still the gold standard? *Monogr Oral Sci.* 29:105–18. doi: 10.1159/000510187. Epub 2020 Dec 21. PMID: 33427229.

134. Cortelli JR, Aquino DR, Cortelli SC, Nobre Franco GC, Fernandes CB, Roman-Torres CV, Costa FO. 2008 Detection of periodontal pathogens in oral mucous membranes of edentulous individuals. *J Periodontol.* 79(10):1962–5. doi: 10.1902/jop.2008.080092. PMID: 18834252.

135. Sachdeo A, Haffajee AD, Socransky SS. 2008 Biofilms in the edentulous oral cavity. *J Prosthodont.* 17(5):348–56. doi: 10.1111/j.1532-849X.2008.00301.x. PMID: 18355168.

136. Przybyłowska D, Mierzwińska-Nastalska E, Swoboda-Kopeć E, Rubinsztajn R, Chazan R. 2016 Potential respiratory pathogens colonisation of the denture plaque of patients with chronic obstructive pulmonary disease. *Gerodontology.* 33(3):322–7. doi: 10.1111/ger.12156. Epub 2014 Nov 12. PMID: 25393518.

137. Milstone AM, Passaretti CL, Perl TM. 2008 Chlorhexidine: Expanding the armamentarium for infection control and prevention. *Clin Infect Dis.* 46(2):274–81. doi: 10.1086/524736. PMID: 18171263.

138. da Costa LFNP, Amaral CDSF, Barbirato DDS, Leão ATT, Fogacci MF. 2017 Chlorhexidine mouthwash as an adjunct to mechanical therapy in chronic periodontitis: A meta-analysis. *J Am Dent Assoc.* 148(5):308–18. doi: 10.1016/j.adaj.2017.01.021. Epub 2017 Mar 9. PMID: 28284417.

139. Addy M, Moran JM. 1997 Clinical indications for the use of chemical adjuncts to plaque control: Chlorhexidine formulations. *Periodontology 2000.* 15:52–4.

140. Jones CG. 1997 Chlorhexidine: Is it still the gold standard? *Periodontology 2000.* 15:55–62.

141. Wirthlin MR, Ahn BJ, Enriquez B, Hussain MZ. 2006 Effects of stabilized chlorine dioxide and chlorhexidine mouth rinses in vitro on cells involved in periodontal healing. *J West Soc Periodontol Periodontal Abstr.* 54(3):67–71.

142. Vitkov L, Hermann A, Krautgartner WD, Herrmann M, Fuchs K, Klappacher M, Hannig M. 2005 Chlorhexidine-induced ultrastructural alterations in oral biofilm. *Microsc Res Tech.* 68(2):85–9. doi: 10.1002/jemt.20238. PMID: 16228984.

143. Coelho AS, Laranjo M, Gonçalves AC, et al. 2020 Cytotoxic effects of a chlorhexidine mouthwash and of an enzymatic mouthwash on human gingival fibroblasts. *Odontology.* 108(2):260–70. doi: 10.1007/s10266-019-00465-z.

144. Shen Y, Stojicic S, Haapasalo M. 2011 Antimicrobial efficacy of chlorhexidine against bacteria in biofilms at different stages of development. *J Endod.* 37(5):657–61. doi: 10.1016/j.joen.2011.02.007. Epub 2011 Mar 23.

145. Guggenheim B, Meier A. 2011 In vitro effect of chlorhexidine mouth rinses on polyspecies biofilms. *Schweiz Monatsschr Zahnmed.* 121(5):432–41.

146. Kerémi B, Márta K, Farkas K, et al. 2020 Effects of chlorine dioxide on oral hygiene–A systematic review and meta-analysis. *Curr Pharm Des.* 26(25):3015–25. doi: 10.2174/1381612826666200515134450.

147. Ma JW, Huang BS, Hsu CW, et al. 2017 Efficacy and safety evaluation of a chlorine dioxide solution. *Int J Environ Res Public Health.* 14(3):329. doi:10.3390/ijerph14030329.

148. Nosticzius Z, Wittmann M, Kály-Kullai K, et al. 2013 Chlorine dioxide is a size-selective antimicrobial agent. *PLoS One.* 8(11):e79157. doi: 10.1371/journal.pone.0079157.

149. Yadav SR, Kini VV, Padhye A. 2015 Inhibition of tongue coat and dental plaque formation by stabilized chlorine dioxide vs chlorhexidine mouthrinse: A randomized, triple blinded study. *J Clin Diagn Res.* 9(9):ZC69–74. doi: 10.7860/JCDR/2015/14587.6510.

150. Yeturu SK, Acharya S, Urala AS, Pentapati KC. 2016 Effect of aloe vera, chlorine dioxide, and chlorhexidine mouth rinses on plaque and gingivitis: A randomized controlled trial. *J Oral Biol Craniofac Res.* 6(1):54–8. doi: 10.1016/j.jobcr.2015.08.008.

151. Bruch MK. 2007 Toxicity and safety of topical sodium hypochlorite. *Contrib Nephrol.* 154:24–38.

152. Hussain AM, van der Weijden GA, Slot DE. 2021 Effect of a sodium hypochlorite mouthwash on plaque and clinical parameters of periodontal disease. *Int J Dent Hyg.* doi: 10.1111/idh.12510. Epub ahead of print. PMID: 33971082.
153. Zehnder M. 2006 Root canal irrigants. *J Endod.* 32:389–98.
154. Gosau M, Hahnel S, Schwarz F, Gerlach T, Reichert TE, Burgers R. 2010 Effect of six different peri-implantitis disinfection methods on in vivo human oral biofilm. *Clin Oral Implants Res.* 21:866–72.
155. Sarbinoff JA, O_Leary TJ, Miller CH. 1983 The comparative effectiveness of various agents in detoxi-fying diseased root surfaces. *J Periodontol.* 54:77–80.
156. Spratt DA, Pratten J, Wilson M, Gulabivala K. 2001 An in vitro evaluation of the antimicrobial efficacy of irrigants on biofilms of root canal isolates. *Int Endod J.* 34:300–7.
157. De Nardo R, Chiappe V, Go´mez M, Romanelli H, Slots J. 2012 Effect of 0.05% sodium hypochlorite oral rinse on supragingival biofilm and gingival inflammation. *Int Dent J.* 62:208–12.
158. Lobene RR, Soparkar PM, Hein JW, Quigley GA. 1972 A study of the effects of antiseptic agents and a pulsating irrigating device on plaque and gingivitis. *J Periodontol.* 43:564–8.
159. Zou L, Shen Y, Li W, Haapasalo M. 2010 Penetration of sodium hypochlorite into dentin. *J Endod* 36:793–6.
160. Kalkwarf KL, Tussing GJ, Davis MJ. 1982 Histologic evaluation of gingival curettage facilitated by sodium hypochlorite solution. *J Periodontol.* 53:63–70.
161. Slots J. 2012 Low-cost periodontal therapy. *Periodontology 2000.* 60(1):110–37. doi: 10.1111/j.1600-075 7.2011.00429.x.
162. Rutala WA, Cole EC, Thomann CA, Weber DJ. 1998 Stability and bactericidal activity of chlorine solu-tions. *Infect Control Hosp Epidemiol.* 19:323–7.
163. Marshall MV, Cancro LP, Fischman SL. 1995 Hydrogen peroxide: A review of its use in dentistry. J Periodontol. 66(9):786–96.
164. Lekstrom-Himes JA, Kuhns DB, Alvord WG, Gallin JI. 2005 Inhibition of human neutrophil IL-8 production by hydrogen peroxide and dysregulation in chronic granulomatous disease. *J Immunol.* 174(1):411–7.
165. Schreml S, Szeimies RM, et al.: 2010 Oxygen in acute and chronic wound healing. *Br J Dermatol.* 163(-2):257–68. doi: 10.1111/j.1365-2133.2010.09804.x. Epub 2010 Apr 15.
166. Phillips J. 1996 The Wound Care Institute, Inc. for the Advancement of Wound Healing & Diabetic Footcare. Wound Care Institute Newsletter, Fall 1996.
167. Dunlap T, Keller DC, Marshall MV, Coserton JW, Schaudinn C, Sindelar B, Cotton JR. 2011 Subgingival delivery of oral debriding agents: A proof of concept. *J Clin Dent.* 22:149–58.
168. Schaudinn C, et al. 2010 Manipulation of the microbial ecology of the periodontal pocket. *World Dental.* 2(1):14–8.
169. Tomono S, Miyoshi N, et al. 2009 Formation of cholesterol ozonolysis products through an ozone-free mechanism mediated by themyeloperoxidase-H_2O_2-chloride system. *Biochem Biophys Res Commun.* 383(2):222–7. doi: 10.1016/j.bbrc.2009.03.155. Epub 2009 Apr 5.
170. Talmaç AC, Çalişir M. 2021 Efficacy of gaseous ozone in smoking and non-smoking gingivitis patients. *Ir J Med Sci.* 190(1):325–33. doi: 10.1007/s11845-020-02271-x. Epub 2020 Jul 1. PMID: 32613563.
171. Gandhi KK, Cappetta EG, Pavaskar R. 2019 Effectiveness of the adjunctive use of ozone and chlorhexi-dine in patients with chronic periodontitis. *BDJ Open.* 5:17. doi: 10.1038/s41405-019-0025-9. PMID: 31814999; PMCID: PMC6882833.
172. Herczegh A, Gyurkovics M, Agababyan H, et al. 2013 Comparing the efficacy of hyper-pure chlorine-dioxide with other oral antiseptics on oral pathogen microorganisms and biofilm in vitro. *Acta Microbiol Immunol Hung.* 60(3):359–73. doi:10.1556/AMicr.60.2013.3.10.
173. Teles FR, Teles RP, Sachdeo A. 2012 Comparison of microbial changes in early redeveloping biofilms on natural teeth and dentures. *J Periodontol.* 83(9):1139–48. doi: 10.1902/jop.2012.110506. Epub 2012 Mar 23.
174. Teles FR, Teles RP, Uzel NG, et al.: 2011 Early microbial succession in redeveloping dental biofilms in periodontal health and disease. *J Periodontal Res.* 47(1):95–104. doi: 10.1111/j.1600-0765.2011.01409.x. Epub 2011 Sep 5.
175. Kouidhi B, Al Qurashi YM, Chaieb K. 2015 Drug resistance of bacterial dental biofilm and the potential use of natural compounds as alternative for prevention and treatment. *Microb Pathog.* 80:39–49. doi: 10.1016/j.micpath.2015.02.007. Epub 2015 Feb 21.
176. Rams TE, Degener JE, van Winkelhoff AJ. 2014 Antibiotic resistance in human chronic periodontitis microbiota. *J Periodontol.* 85(1):160–9. doi: 10.1902/jop.2013.130142. Epub 2013 May 20.

177. Rams TE, Degener JE, van Winkelhoff AJ. 2014 Antibiotic resistance in human peri-implantitis micro-biota. *Clin Oral Implants Res.* 25(1):82–90. doi: 10.1111/clr.12160. Epub 2013 Apr 2.

178. Rowińska I, Szyperska-Ślaska A, Zariczny P, Pasławski R, Kramkowski K, Kowalczyk P. 2021 The influence of diet on oxidative stress and inflammation induced by bacterial biofilms in the human oral cavity. *Materials (Basel).* 14(6):1444. doi: 10.3390/ma14061444. PMID: 33809616; PMCID: PMC8001659.

179. Martinon P, Fraticelli L, Giboreau A, Dussart C, Bourgeois D, Carrouel F. 2021 Nutrition as a key modifiable factor for periodontitis and main chronic diseases. *J Clin Med.* 10(2):197. doi: 10.3390/jcm10020197. PMID: 33430519; PMCID: PMC7827391. [33–35].

180. Najeeb S, Zafar MS, Khurshid Z, Zohaib S, Almas K. 2016 The role of nutrition in periodontal health: An update. *Nutrients.* 8(9):530. doi: 10.3390/nu8090530. PMID: 27589794; PMCID: PMC5037517.

181. Galbete C, Schwingshackl L, Schwedhelm C, Boeing H, Schulze MB. 2018 Evaluating Mediterranean diet and risk of chronic disease in cohort studies: An umbrella review of meta-analyses. *Eur J Epidemiol.* 33:909–31.

182. D'Alessandro A, De Pergola G. 2018 The Mediterranean Diet: Its definition and evaluation of a priori dietary indexes in primary cardiovascular prevention. *Int J Food Sci Nutr.* 69:647–59.

183. Dinu M, Pagliai G, Casini A, Sofi F. 2018 Mediterranean diet and multiple health outcomes: An umbrella review of meta-analyses of observational studies and randomised trials. *Eur J Clin Nutr.* 72:30–43.

184. Rosato V, Temple NJ, La Vecchia C, Castellan G, Tavani A, Guercio V. 2019 Mediterranean diet and cardiovascular disease: A systematic review and meta-analysis of observational studies. *Eur J Nutr.* 58:173–91.

185. Becerra-Tomás N, Blanco Mejía S, Viguiliouk E, Khan T, Kendall CWC, Kahleova H, Raheli'c D, Sievenpiper JL, Salas-Salvadó J. 2019 Mediterranean diet, cardiovascular disease and mortality in diabetes: A systematic review and meta-analysis of prospective cohort studies and randomized clinical trials. *Crit. Rev Food Sci Nutr.* 1–21.

186. Morze J, Danielewicz A, Przybyłowicz K, Zeng H, Hoffmann G, Schwingshackl L. 2021 An updated systematic review and meta-analysis on adherence to mediterranean diet and risk of cancer. *Eur J Nutr.* 60(3):1561–86. doi: 10.1007/s00394-020-02346-6. Epub 2020 Aug 8. PMID: 32770356; PMCID: PMC7987633.

187. Shafiei F, Salari-Moghaddam A, Larijani B, Esmaillzadeh A. 2019 Adherence to the Mediterranean diet and risk of depression: A systematic review and updated meta-analysis of observational studies. *Nutr Rev.* 77:230–9.

188. Laiola M, De Filippis F, Vitaglione P, Ercolini D. 2020 A Mediterranean Diet intervention reduces the levels of salivary periodontopathogenic bacteria in overweight and obese subjects. *Appl Environ Microbiol.* 86(12):e00777–20. doi: 10.1128/AEM.00777-20. PMID: 32276980; PMCID: PMC7267188

189. Machado V, Botelho J, Viana J, Pereira P, Lopes LB, Proença L, Delgado AS, Mendes JJ. 2021 Association between dietary inflammatory index and periodontitis: A cross-sectional and mediation analysis. *Nutrients.* 13(4):1194. doi: 10.3390/nu13041194. PMID: 33916342; PMCID: PMC8066166.

190. Takeda K, Mizutani K, Minami I, Kido D, Mikami R, Konuma K, Saito N, Kominato H, Takemura S, Nakagawa K, Izumi Y, Ogawa Y, Iwata T. 2021 Association of periodontal pocket area with type 2 diabetes and obesity: A cross-sectional study. *BMJ Open Diabetes Res Care.* 9(1):e002139. doi: 10.1136/bmjdrc-2021-002139. PMID: 33879517; PMCID: PMC8061845.

191. Pappe CL, Steckhan N, Hoedke D, Jepsen S, Rauch G, Keller T, Michalsen A, Dommisch H. 2021 Prolonged multimodal fasting modulates periodontal inflammation in female patients with metabolic syndrome: A prospective cohort study. *J Clin Periodontol.* 48(4):492–502. doi: 10.1111/jcpe.13419. Epub 2021 Feb 2. PMID: 33393121.

192. Palmer, CA, Burnett DJ, Dean B. 2010 It's more than just candy: Important relationships between nutrition and oral health. *Nutr Today.* 45:154–64.

193. O'Connor JP, Milledge KL, O'Leary F, Cumming R, Eberhard J, Hirani V. 2020 Poor dietary intake of nutrients and food groups are associated with increased risk of periodontal disease among community-dwelling older adults: A systematic literature review. *Nutr Rev.* 78(2):175–88. doi: 10.1093/nutrit/nuz035. PMID: 31397482.

194. Moreira ARO, Batista RFL, Ladeira LLC, Thomaz EBAF, Alves CMC, Saraiva MC, Silva AAM, Brondani MA, Ribeiro CCC. 2021 Higher sugar intake is associated with periodontal disease in adolescents. *Clin Oral Investig.* 25(3):983–91. doi: 10.1007/s00784-020-03387-1. Epub 2020 Jun 9. PMID: 32519237.

195. Hong SJ, Kwon B, Yang BE, Choi HG, Byun SH. 2021 Evaluation of the relationship between drink intake and periodontitis using KoGES data. *Biomed Res Int.* 2021:5545620. doi: 10.1155/2021/5545620. PMID: 33816614; PMCID: PMC7990540.

196. Valenzuela MJ, Waterhouse B, Aggarwal VR, Bloor K, Doran T. 2021 Effect of sugar-sweetened beverages on oral health: A systematic review and meta-analysis. *Eur J Public Health.* 31(1):122–9. doi: 10.1093/eurpub/ckaa147. PMID: 32830237.

197. Neiva RF, Al-Shammari K, Nociti FH, Jr., Soehren S, Wang H. 2005 Effects of vitamin-B complex supplementation on periodontal wound healing. *J Periodontol.* 76:1084–91.

198. Bashutski JD, Eber RM, Kinney JS, Benavides E, Maitra S, Braun TM, Giannobile WV, McCauley LK. 2011 The impact of vitamin D status on periodontal surgery outcomes. *J Dent Res.* 90:1007–12.

199. Pérez-Gálvez A, Viera I, Roca M. 2020 Carotenoids and chlorophylls as antioxidants. *Antioxidants (Basel).* 9(6):505. doi: 10.3390/antiox9060505. PMID: 32526968; PMCID: PMC7346216.

200. Van der Velden U. 2020 Vitamin c and its role in periodontal diseases - The past and the present: A narrative review. *Oral Health Prev Dent.* 18(1):115–24. doi: 10.3290/j.ohpd.a44306. PMID: 32238982.

201. Shadisvaaran S, Chin KY, Shahida MS, Ima-Nirwana S, Leong XF. 2021 Effect of vitamin E on periodontitis: Evidence and proposed mechanisms of action. *J Oral Biosci.* S1349-0079(21)00053-0. doi: 10.1016/j.job.2021.04.001. Epub ahead of print. PMID: 33864905.

202. Najeeb S, Khurshid Z, Zohaib S, Zafar MS. 2016 Therapeutic potential of melatonin in oral medicine and periodontology. *Kaohsiung J Med Sci.* 32:391–6.

203. Muniz FW, Nogueira SB, Mendes FLV, Rösing CK, Moreira MMSM, de Andrade GM, de Sousa RC 2015 The impact of antioxidant agents complimentary to periodontal therapy on oxidative stress and periodontal outcomes: A systematic review. *Arch Oral Biol.* 60:1203–14.

204. Gutierrez Gossweiler A, Martinez-Mier EA. 2019 Chapter 6: Vitamins and oral health. *Monogr Oral Sci.* 28:59–67. doi: 10.1159/000455372. Epub 2019 Nov 7. PMID: 31940621.

205. Lin XP, Zhou XJ, Liu HL, DU LL, Toshihisa K. 2010 [Effect of vitamine A on mice immune response induced by specific periodontal pathogenic bacteria-immunization]. *Shanghai Kou Qiang Yi Xue.* 19(6):630–4. Chinese. PMID: 21431265.

206. Yang Y, Wang T, Zhang S, Jia S, Chen H, Duan Y, Wang S, Chen G, Tian W. 2021 Vitamin C alleviates the senescence of periodontal ligament stem cells through inhibition of Notch3 during long-term culture. *J Cell Physiol.* 236(2):1237–51. doi: 10.1002/jcp.29930. Epub 2020 Jul 13. PMID: 32662081.

207. Gauthier P, Yu Z, Tran QT, Bhatti FU, Zhu X, Huang GT. 2017 Cementogenic genes in human periodontal ligament stem cells are downregulated in response to osteogenic stimulation while upregulated by vitamin C treatment. *Cell Tissue Res.* 368(1):79–92. doi: 10.1007/s00441-016-2513-8. Epub 2016 Oct 18. Erratum in: Cell Tissue Res. 2017 Apr;368(1):227. PMID: 27757536; PMCID: PMC5366101.

208. Hong JY, Lee JS, Choi SH, Shin HS, Park JC, Shin SI, Chung JH. 2019 A randomized, double-blind, placebo-controlled multicenter study for evaluating the effects of fixed-dose combinations of vitamin C, vitamin E, lysozyme, and carbazochrome on gingival inflammation in chronic periodontitis patients. *BMC Oral Health.* 19(1):40. doi: 10.1186/s12903-019-0728-2. PMID: 30845920; PMCID: PMC6407240.

209. Isola G, Polizzi A, Iorio-Siciliano V, Alibrandi A, Ramaglia L, Leonardi R. 2021 Effectiveness of a nutraceutical agent in the non-surgical periodontal therapy: A randomized, controlled clinical trial. *Clin Oral Investig.* 25(3):1035–45. doi: 10.1007/s00784-020-03397-z. Epub 2020 Jun 17. PMID: 32556659.

210. Luo PP, Xu HS, Chen YW, Wu SP. 2018 Periodontal disease severity is associated with micronutrient intake. *Aust Dent J.* 63(2):193–201. doi: 10.1111/adj.12606. Epub 2018 Apr 23. PMID: 29509277.

211. Dodington DW, Fritz PC, Sullivan PJ, Ward WE. 2015 Higher intakes of fruits and vegetables, beta-carotene, Vitamin C, α-tocopherol, EPA, and DHA are positively associated with periodontal healing after nonsurgical periodontal therapy in nonsmokers but not in smokers. *J Nutr.* 145:2512–9.

212. Nair R, Maseeh A. 2012 Vitamin D: The "sunshine" vitamin. *J Pharmacol Pharmacother.* 3(2):118–26. doi: 10.4103/0976-500X.95506. PMID: 22629085; PMCID: PMC3356951.

213. Palacios C, Gonzalez L. 2014 Is vitamin D deficiency a major global public health problem? *J Steroid Biochem Mol Biol.* 144 Pt A:138–45. doi: 10.1016/j.jsbmb.2013.11.003. Epub 2013 Nov 12. PMID: 24239505; PMCID: PMC4018438.

214. Nastri L, Moretti A, Migliaccio S, Paoletta M, Annunziata M, Liguori S, Toro G, Bianco M, Cecoro G, Guida L, Iolascon G. 2020 Do dietary supplements and nutraceuticals have effects on dental implant osseointegration? A scoping review. *Nutrients.* 12(1):268. doi: 10.3390/nu12010268. PMID: 31968626; PMCID: PMC7019951.

215. Shams B, Afshari E, Tajadini M, Keikha M, Qorbani M, Heshmat R, Motlagh ME, Kelishadi R. 2016 The relationship of serum vitamin D and Zinc in a nationally representative sample of Iranian children and adolescents: The CASPIAN-III study. *Med J Islam Repub Iran.* 30:430. PMID: 28210595; PMCID: PMC5307609.

216. Mirastschijski U, Haaksma CJ, Tomasek JJ, Ågren, MS. 2004 Matrix metalloproteinase inhibitor GM 6001 attenuates keratinocyte migration, contraction and myofibroblast formation in skin wounds. *Exp Cell Res.* 299:465–75.

217. Jarosz M, Olbert M, Wyszogrodzka G, Młyniec K, Librowski T. 2017 Antioxidant and anti-inflammatory effects of zinc. Zinc-dependent NF-κB signaling. *Inflammopharmacology.* 25(1):11–24. doi: 10.1007/s10787-017-0309-4. Epub 2017 Jan 12. PMID: 28083748; PMCID: PMC5306179.

218. Pushparani, D.S. 2015 Serum zinc, and d glucuronidase enzyme level in type 2 diabetes mellitus with periodontitis. *Curr Diabetes Rev.* 12(4):449–53.

219. Varela-López A, Navarro-Hortal MD, Giampieri F, Bullón P, Battino M, Quiles JL. 2018 Nutraceuticals in periodontal health: A systematic review on the role of vitamins in periodontal health maintenance. *Molecules.* 23(5):1226. doi: 10.3390/molecules23051226. PMID: 29783781; PMCID: PMC6099579.

220. Kulkarni V, Bhatavadekar NB, Uttamani JR. 2014 The effect of nutrition on periodontal disease: A systematic review. *J Calif Dent Assoc.* 42(5):302–11. PMID: 25087348.

221. Rao AV, Agarwal S. 2000 Role of antioxidant lycopene in cancer and heart disease. *J Am Coll Nutr.* 2000 Oct;19(5):563–9. doi: 10.1080/07315724.2000.10718953. PMID: 11022869.

222. Chandra RV, Prabhuji M, Roopa DA, Ravirajan S, Kishore HC. 2007 Efficacy of lycopene in the treatment of gingivitis: A randomised, placebo-controlled clinical trial. *Oral Health Prev Dent.* 5:327.

223. Arora N, Avula H, Kumar Avula J. 2013 The adjunctive use of systemic antioxidant therapy (lycopene) in nonsurgical treatment of chronic periodontitis: A short-term evaluation. *Quintessence Int.* 44:395–405.

224. Belludi SA, Verma S, Banthia R, Bhusari P, Parwani S, Kedia S, Saiprasad S. 2013 Effect of lycopene in the treatment of periodontal disease: A clinical study. *J Contemp Dent Pract.* 14:1054.

225. Tripathi P, Blaggana V, Upadhyay P, Jindal M, Gupta S, Nishat S. 2019 Antioxidant therapy (lycopene and green tea extract) in periodontal disease: A promising paradigm. *J Indian Soc Periodontol.* 23(-1):25–30. doi: 10.4103/jisp.jisp_277_18. PMID: 30692739; PMCID: PMC6334550.

226. Forouzanfar A, Mohammadipour HS, Forouzanfar F. 2021 The potential role of tea in periodontal therapy: An updated review. *Curr Drug Discov Technol.* 18(1):1–7. doi: 10.2174/1389200221666200127114119. PMID: 31985382.

227. Wang Y, Zeng J, Yuan Q, Luan Q. 2021 Efficacy of (-)-epigallocatechin gallate delivered by a new-type scaler tip during scaling and root planing on chronic periodontitis: A split-mouth, randomized clinical trial. *BMC Oral Health.* 21(1):79. doi: 10.1186/s12903-021-01418-1. PMID: 33602197; PMCID: PMC7890979.

228. Reiter R, Rosales-Corral S, Liu X, Acuna-Castroviejo D, Escames G, Tan D. 2015 Melatonin in the oral cavity: Physiological and pathological implications. *J Periodont Res.* 50:9–17.

229. Balaji TM, Varadarajan S, Jagannathan R, Mahendra J, Fageeh HI, Fageeh HN, Mushtaq S, Baeshen HA, Bhandi S, Gupta AA, Raj AT, Reda R, Patil S, Testarelli L. 2021 Melatonin as a topical/systemic formulation for the management of periodontitis: A systematic review. *Materials (Basel).* 14(9):2417. doi: 10.3390/ma14092417. PMID: 34066498; PMCID: PMC8124881.

230. Şehirli AÖ, Aksoy U, Koca-Ünsal RB, Sayıner S. 2021 Role of NLRP3 inflammasome in COVID-19 and periodontitis: Possible protective effect of melatonin. *Med Hypotheses.* 151:110588. doi: 10.1016/j.mehy.2021.110588. Epub 2021 Mar 30. PMID: 33848919; PMCID: PMC8007534.

231. Vaseenon S, Chattipakorn N, Chattipakorn SC. 2021 Effects of melatonin in wound healing of dental pulp and periodontium: Evidence from in vitro, in vivo and clinical studies. *Arch Oral Biol.* 123:105037. doi: 10.1016/j.archoralbio.2020.105037. Epub 2021 Jan 6. PMID: 33440268.

232. Anton DM, Martu MA, Maris M, Maftei GA, Sufaru IG, Tatarciuc D, Luchian I, Ioanid N, Martu S. 2021 Study on the effects of melatonin on glycemic control and periodontal parameters in patients with type ii diabetes mellitus and periodontal disease. *Medicina (Kaunas).* 57(2):140. doi: 10.3390/medicina57020140. PMID: 33562452; PMCID: PMC7915328.

233. Castiglioni S, Cazzaniga A, Albisetti W, Maier JA. 2013 Magnesium and osteoporosis: Current state of knowledge and future research directions. *Nutrients.* 5:3022–33.

234. Meisel P, Schwahn C, Luedemann J, John U, Kroemer HK, Kocher T. 2005 Magnesium deficiency is associated with periodontal disease. *J Dent Res.* 84(10):937–41. doi: 10.1177/154405910508401012. PMID: 16183794.

235. Merchant AT. 2006 Higher serum magnesium: Calcium ratio may lower periodontitis risk. *J Evid Based Dent Pract.* 6(4):285–6. doi: 10.1016/j.jebdp.2006.09.007. PMID: 17174255.

236. Staudte H, Kranz S, Völpel A, Schütze J, Sigusch BW. 2012 Comparison of nutrient intake between patients with periodontitis and healthy subjects. *Quintessence Int.* 43(10):907–16. PMID: 23115770.

237. Chakraborty S, Tewari S, Sharma RK, Narula SC, Ghalaut PS, Ghalaut V. 2014 Impact of iron deficiency anemia on chronic periodontitis and superoxide dismutase activity: A cross-sectional study. *J Periodontal Implant Sci.* 44:57–64.

238. Nagpal S, Acharya AB, Thakur SL. 2012 Periodontal disease and anemias associated with Crohn's disease. A case report. *N Y State Dent J.* 78(2):47–50. PMID: 22685916.
239. Varela-Lopez A, Bullon P, Battino M, Ramirez-Tortosa MC, Ochoa JJ, Cordero MD, Ramirez-Tortosa CL, Rubini C, Zizzi A, Quiles JL. 2016 Coenzyme Q protects against age-related alveolar bone loss associated to n-6 polyunsaturated fatty acid rich-diets by modulating mitochondrial mechanisms. *J Gerontol A Biol Sci Med Sci.* 71(5):593–600. doi: 10.1093/gerona/glv063. Epub 2015 Jul 28. PMID: 26219851.
240. Raut CP, Sethi KS, Kohale B, Mamajiwala A, Warang A. 2019 Subgingivally delivered coenzyme Q10 in the treatment of chronic periodontitis among smokers: A randomized, controlled clinical study. *J Oral Biol Craniofac Res.* 9(2):204–8. doi: 10.1016/j.jobcr.2018.05.005. Epub 2018 May 9. PMID: 31211037; PMCID: PMC6562101.
241. Bale B, Doneen A, Collier L. 2014 *Beat the Heart Attack Gene: The Revolutionary Plan to Prevent Heart Disease, Stroke, and Diabetes.* New York, NY: Wiley Gen. Trade, Turner Publishing, pp. 135–137.
242. Doneen AL, Bale BF. 2018 The BaleDoneen Method (BDM): A disease-inflammation approach to achieve arterial wellness. *Cranio.* 36(4):209–10. doi: 10.1080/08869634.2018.1479491.

15 COVID-19

An Evidence-Based Integrative Approach to Disease Management

Douglas S. Harrington

CONTENTS

What Is COVID-19 (Virology)?...335
What Are COVID-19 Variants?..336
Pathophysiology of COVID-19..337
Why Is the Endothelium a Prime Target Organ in COVID-19? 337
How Is COVID-19 Transmitted? 338
How Is Testing Impacted by Viral Replication and Immune Responses? 339
    Incubation Periods and Impact on PCR Testing Strategies 339
    Period of Infectivity...339
    Serology and B-Cell Immunity..339
    T-Cell Responses to COVID-19 340
    Antigen Tests and Limitations 341
Tests to Define Prognosis and Status 341
    PULS Cardiac Test...341
    D-Dimer..342
    Other Tests Useful in COVID-19...342
How to Apply an Integrative Approach to Preventing and Caring for COVID-19 Patients..........342
Strategies to Boost Immunity...343
Summary..345
References..345

WHAT IS COVID-19 (VIROLOGY)?

COVID-19 is a corona virus also known as SARS-CoV-2 that causes an infectious disease characterized by intense respiratory symptoms, fever, cough, headache, fatigue, and loss of taste and smell.[1] While initial studies suggested that the first known case occurred in Wuhan, China in December 2019, later analyses of data suggest it actually occurred in October of 2019.[2] The disease subsequently spread worldwide resulting in the pandemic that we are still dealing with today. The official name of the virus is severe acute respiratory syndrome coronavirus 2 (SARS-CoV-2) virus strain.[3] This virus strain is closely related to the original SARS-CoV-1 that occurred in Foshan, China in 2002–2004, but significantly less related to the 2012 Middle East respiratory syndrome virus (MERS-CoV).[4] The COVID-19 virus is very similar to the MERS and SARS-CoV-1 viruses. The

DOI: 10.1201/9781003137849-15

components of the virus include a membrane glycoprotein (M), envelope protein (E), nucleocapsid protein (N), and the spikeprotein (S) (Figure 15.1).[5]

WHAT ARE COVID-19 VARIANTS?

COVID-19 variants are mutated forms of the original virus. All viruses constantly change as they pass through the population. Most do not persist at significant levels or completely disappear. When they confer characteristics that impact transmission, severity, test detection, treatment, or resistance to vaccines, they become a public health concern.[5] The current variants of concern that could have significant clinical impact are as follows:

- B.1.1.7 (Alpha) variants are associated with approximately 50% increased transmission, and likely with increased disease severity and risk of death. Appears to have minimal impact on the effectiveness of treatments with antibodies.
- B.1.351 (Beta) variants are associated with approximately 50% increased transmission. May have moderately decreased response to antibody treatments.
- P.1 (Gamma) variants may have moderately decreased response to some antibody treatments.
- B.1.617.2 (Delta) variants are associated with increased transmission. May have moderately decreased response to antibody treatments (Delta totals include Delta sublineages AY.1 and AY.2) (Table 15.1).

Variants of interest which have not shown significant clinical impact yet are as follows:

- B.1.526 (Iota) is associated with significantly reduced efficacy of some antibody treatments.
- B.1.525 (Eta) and P.2 (Zeta) variants may have moderately decreased response to some antibody treatments.

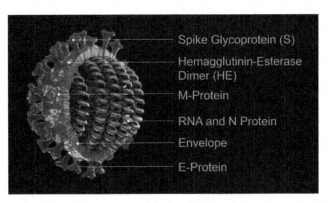

Spike Glycoprotein (S)

Hemagglutinin-Esterase Dimer (HE)

M-Protein

RNA and N Protein

Envelope

E-Protein

FIGURE 15.1　COVID-19 Structural Components.

TABLE 15.1
Data from California Department of Health

Variant as of August 5, 2021	WHO Label	Number of Cases Caused by Variant
B.1.1.7	Alpha	14,019
B.1.351	Beta	163
P.1	Gamma	2,520
B.1.617.2[a]	Delta	4,808

[a] Includes sublineages B.1.617.2.1 (AY.1), B.1.617.2.2 (AY.2), and B.1.617.2.3 (AY.3).

TABLE 15.2

Data from California Department of Health

Variant as of August 5, 2021	WHO Label	Number of Cases Caused by Variant
B.1.427 and B.1.429	Epsilon	29,509
P.2	Zeta	107
B.1.525	Eta	63
B.1.526	Iota	2,092
B.1.617.1	Kappa	67
B.1.617.3	Not available	1

- B.1.617.1 (Kappa) and B.1.617.3 may have moderately decreased response to some antibody treatments.
- B.1.427 and B.1.429 (Epsilon) are associated with approximately 20% increased transmission. There is significantly reduced efficacy of some antibody treatments.

Currently, the Delta variant is of great public health concern due to its higher transmission rate, but luckily, not a higher virulence (Table 15.2).[6,7]

PATHOPHYSIOLOGY OF COVID-19

SARS-CoV-2 binds to the human ACE2 (hACE2) receptor. ACE-2 has homology to ACE, an enzyme long known to be a key player in the Renin-Angiotensin System (RAS) and a target for the treatment of hypertension. ACE-2 is mainly expressed in arterial and venous vascular endothelial cells and arterial smooth muscle cells in all organs, renal tubular epithelium, Leydig cells in the testes, oral and nasal mucosa, nasopharynx, lung, stomach, small intestine, colon, skin, lymph nodes, thymus, bone marrow, spleen, liver, kidney, and brain.[8] The ACE-2 receptor is also highly expressed on lung alveolar epithelial cells and enteric epithelial cells.[8]

While the main target of COVID-19 is the upper respiratory tract with the resultant fever, dry cough, fatigue, and dyspnea, recent evidence has emerged that the endothelial system is the key to many of the more detrimental symptoms.[9] The virus enters the alveolar epithelial cells via the ACE-2 receptor and disrupts the cells causing intense inflammation with damage to the significant vascular element of the lungs.[9] One of the severe consequences of this unchecked process is a "cytokine storm" resulting in a propagating hyper-inflammatory process that causes extensive ongoing tissue damage.[10] A second process that has been identified as a "bradykinin storm" may be equally or more significant.[11] The cytokine storm creates extensive damage, while the bradykinin storm induces extensive vascular leakage which allows the virus to get into the circulation and extends the damage throughout the circulatory tree resulting in a series of unusual consequences: blood clots, heart attacks, and strokes (especially in individuals under 50 years of age).[12]

This pathologic process is an endotheliopathy.[13,14] The unusual feature of the COVID-19 virus when compared to the earlier SARS-CoV-1 is that it is a vasculotropic respiratory virus which is very rare.[14] Each of the viruses requires an extra protein to activate and insert their genetic material into a cell to propagate and spread in addition to the ACE-2 receptor.[14] The SARS-CoV-1 virus requires an additional protein that is only found in lung tissue restricting its spectrum of infection, whereas SARS-CoV-2 uses a protein (furin) that is found in all tissues (especially endothelial cells) allowing it to infect the vascular tree and multiple organs.[14]

WHY IS THE ENDOTHELIUM A PRIME TARGET ORGAN IN COVID-19?

The **endothelium** is the inner cell lining of all blood vessels and is the largest organ in the human body.[15] The endothelium weighs about 1 kg in the average patient and has a total surface area of

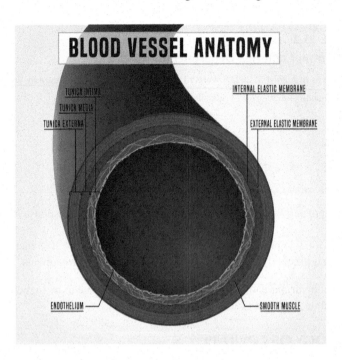

FIGURE 15.2　Artery Endothelium.

4,000–7,000 m², whereas the epidermis is only about 2 m² in the average adult.[15] The length of the circulatory system is about 60,000 miles, and the disease process is inflammation—the body's response to injury or infection.[13,15]

The COVID-19 virus has had a disproportionate impact on certain individuals such as those with diabetes, obesity, metabolic syndrome, sickle cell disease, COPD, heart disease (especially CHF), autoimmune diseases, kidney or liver disease, cancer, blood disorders, immune disorders, and increasing age.[16] These conditions all have a common intersection in that they have increased susceptibility to endothelial injury.[16,17] Many of these conditions, such as T2 diabetes, have attenuated glycocalyx, a layer of highly glycosylated proteins that coats the endothelium forming a barrier between the endothelial cells and the blood to protect it from injury and infection.[18] In certain conditions like diabetes, the thickness of the glycocalyx is markedly reduced increasing the susceptibility of the endothelium to injury and infection.[18] The endothelial cell layer is responsible for modulating the body's clotting processes.[13] Infection and inflammation of endothelial cells result in vascular damage and a disruption of the clot protection function of the endothelium resulting in the observed heart attacks, strokes, and blood clots in individuals with COVID-19 infection, especially those less than 50 years old.[13–18] In fact, in a study examining the pathology of COVID-19 patients versus H1N1 patients who died of pulmonary complications, COVID-19 patients had nine times the alveolar microthrombi as H1N1 patients (Figure 15.2).[19]

HOW IS COVID-19 TRANSMITTED?

There are four main ways that COVID-19 is transmitted:[20,21]

1. **Droplets or Aerosols**: This most commonly occurs when people are close to each other for an extended period such as in a car where an infected person coughs, sneezes, or talks sending out a spray of droplets that can carry the virus to another individual who inhales it.

2. **Airborne Transmission**: Varying studies indicate that the virus can survive up to 3 hours in an aerosol droplet. These droplets can be inhaled resulting in infection long after the infected individual has left.
3. **Surface Transmission**: This type of transmission is rare. The virus has variable survival rates depending on the surface, and the amount of virus decreases with time making it less infectious:
   - Glass—5 days
   - Wood—4 days
   - Plastic and stainless steel—3 days
   - Cardboard—24 hours
   - Copper surfaces—4 hours.
4. **Fecal-Oral Transmission**: This is one of the most ignored routes of infection during the early days of the pandemic. However, many cities have multi-generational families living in a single household who share one or two bathrooms, and aerosols can be present for several hours after a flush.[22,23] The virus sheds in urine and feces which is why sewage is tested to find outbreaks present in certain areas.[24]

HOW IS TESTING IMPACTED BY VIRAL REPLICATION AND IMMUNE RESPONSES?

INCUBATION PERIODS AND IMPACT ON PCR TESTING STRATEGIES

PCR-swab tests are primarily meant for symptomatic patients. In a large meta-analysis, the mean incubation period ranged from 5.2 to 6.5 days, but periods up to 14 days have been observed.[25] In the first 4 days after infection, the swab test (PCR) false negative rate is 67% in asymptomatic patients.[26] In symptomatic patients, 38% will have a false negative result.[26,27] Data indicates that the optimum time to test an individual is on day 8 after infection or 3 days after symptom onset but still has a false negative rate of 20%. In other words, 1 in 5 patients with the virus will test negative. This data is the reason repeat and frequent testing is recommended for symptomatic patients. Collection skill impacts clinical sensitivity and specificity.

PERIOD OF INFECTIVITY

The Singapore Academy of Medicine did an extensive review of infectivity.[28] One of the challenges of tracking infectivity is the fact that between 18% and 78% (depending on the study population) of individuals are asymptomatic or have minimal symptoms. For symptomatic cases of COVID-19, about 80% will be mild, 15% will develop more severe disease (mainly pneumonia), and about 5% may require critical care.[28] The period of infectivity relates to exposure and host response. In symptomatic individuals, the period of infectivity begins 2 days before symptoms and continues for 7–10 days after symptom onset.[28] Reports of virus shedding for months after resolution of symptoms have been shown to have detected non-viable virus (PCR-swab cannot tell the difference between living and dead virus).[28] Viable virus is not found after the second week post symptom onset.

SEROLOGY AND B-CELL IMMUNITY

Since most COVID-19 infections are asymptomatic or have minimal symptoms, serology has evolved into an important tool to determine the true prevalence of COVID-19 infections in the population from a public health perspective. Additionally, there is a push to do antibody testing post-vaccination or confirmed COVID-19 infection to determine immune status. Antibodies can appear as early as a few days in COVID-19 patients.[28] Serology tests have an analytical sensitivity of 100% and a specificity of 99.6%. Unlike most infections where IgM precedes IgG, in COVID-19, they can appear simultaneously and then IgM wanes over time. The half-life of antibodies is approximately 73 days.[29,30] Even if antibodies fall below detectable levels after an immune response, memory B-cells can respond to new exposure within minutes.

Patients with any detectable antibodies (IgM, IgG, or both) have significantly lower levels of virus in the upper respiratory tract and are much less likely to infect someone else. True prevalence with Ab+ has resulted in a significant decrease in the reported death rate statistics. In Table 15.3, data from Crenshaw-Baldwin Hills in Los Angeles, the seropositivity data for asymptomatic individuals, is outlined.[31] Of note is the fact that the Hispanic/Latino, Native Hawaiian, Native American, and under 18 years had the highest seropositive rates (17%–19%), while the African American group and Asian were the lowest (4% and 6%, respectively). The African American seropositivity was significantly lower than nationally reported numbers which were closer to 18%; this was attributed to an aggressive community prevention program.

T-Cell Responses to COVID-19

Immunity involves a partnership of memory B- and T-cells. B-cells are responsible for humoral immunity which produces specific antibodies to the virus. However, T-cells are an important component to the immune system. T-cells respond directly to the virus in a form of cell-mediated immunity.[31] CD4+ and CD8+ T-cells show a response to COVID-19 in 100% and 70% of convalescent COVID patients, respectively. T-cell responses target the spike, M, N, and other ORFs.[31] T-cell reactivity to SARS-CoV-2 epitopes is also detected in approximately 50% of non-exposed individuals.[31] Tests to measure T-cell reactivity are not routinely available. However, both the B-cell and T-cell arms of the immune system contain memory cells which activate within minutes of exposure to the virus, even after detectable levels are not evident. Mild COVID-19 may elicit strong T-cell responses in the absence of detectable virus-specific antibodies. Scientists see signs of lasting immunity to COVID-19, even after mild infections. Approximately 50% of patients who have had colds (coronavirus) have T-cells active against COVID-19.[31] 100% of patients who recover have T-cells active against COVID-19.[31] The T-cell arm of the immune system contributes to herd immunity (Figure 15.3).

TABLE 15.3
Racial/Ethnic Variation in COVID-19 Antibody Levels in Los Angeles

Ethnic/Racial Variation in Antibody Positivity Rates for COVID					
Race/Ethnicity	Patient #	% IgG	IgG+IgM %	Tot Positives %	Tot Negative %
White	257	3%	2%	5%	95%
Hispanic Latino	817	6%	13%	19%	81%
Not Disclosed	101	7%	5%	12%	88%
Native Hawaiian	12	0%	17%	17%	83%
African American	674	1%	3%	4%	96%
Asian	149	1%	5%	6%	94%
Native American	65	3%	14%	17%	83%
Total	2,075	4%	7%	11%	89%
Male	922			12%	88%
Female	1,153			10%	90%
18 y/o or younger	122			19%	81%

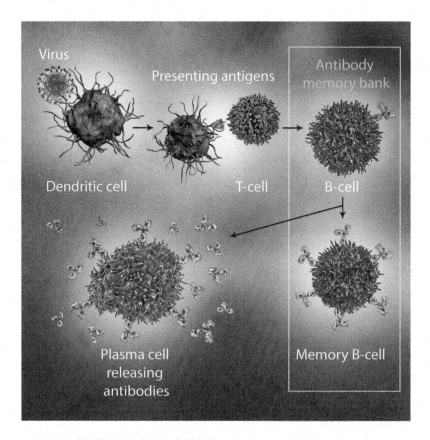

FIGURE 15.3 Interpreting Tests for SARS-CoV-2.

ANTIGEN TESTS AND LIMITATIONS

Abbott BinaxNow sensitivity is 95%–100% if samples are collected within a week of the onset of symptoms. Detection sensitivity dropped to 75% for samples taken a week after symptoms onset.[32] Specificity is 100%. Sensitivity and specificity of other Ag tests are similar. Sensitivity ranges from 84% to 98% if tested in the week after showing symptoms and specificity is 100%.[32]

TESTS TO DEFINE PROGNOSIS AND STATUS[33]

PULS CARDIAC TEST

The PULS Cardiac test is an algorithmic serum test that directly measures endothelial injury and inflammation caused by free radicals such as oxidized LDL or infectious agents like COVID-19.[34] PULS is normally used to identify the "vulnerable" patient who is at risk of having a heart attack but does not know it. PULS stands for Protein Unstable Lesion Signal and contains 13 components: age, sex, diabetes, family history, and nine biomarkers (IL-16, FAS, FASLigand, HGF, CTACK, EOTAXIN, MCP-3, HDL, and HbA1c). One of the biomarkers, MCP-3, has been shown to be a strong independent predictor of disease progression in COVID-19 patients.[35] Because PULS quantifies inflammation and injury to endothelium, studies have shown that within a month of COVID-19 infection, the integrated score increases by as much as 40% over pre-infection scores. Two patients are illustrated in Figure 15.4 who show the rise after infection.

PULS can quantify risk associated with COVID-19 injury to the endothelium and serial samples can document clinical progress. In fact, all vaccines induce biologically active spike proteins which

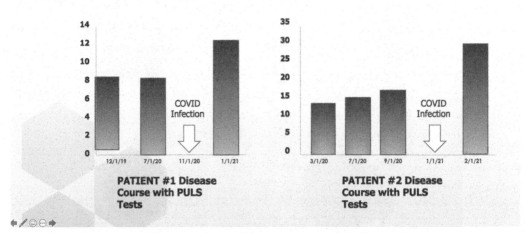

FIGURE 15.4 Memory B and T cells in COVID-19 Immunity.

bind to the ACE-2 receptor and create a transient inflammatory response, especially in the endothelium. It is not surprising, therefore, that a recent study of 566 vaccinated patients who had pre and post-vaccination PULS tests performed showed a significant increases in both specific biomarkers of the PULS test but also in the overall PULS score (11%–25%).[36]

D-Dimer

D-dimer can predict hospital mortality.[33] Patients with D-dimer levels ≥ 2.0 μg/mL had a higher incidence of mortality when compared to those with D-dimer levels < 2.0 μg/mL (12/67 vs 1/267, $P < 0.001$, HR: 51.5, 95%CI: 12.9–206.7).[33]

Other Tests Useful in COVID-19[33]

- Von Willebrand Factor Antigen (565% ICU Patients vs 278% non-ICU)
- Soluble P-Selectin (15.9 ICU vs 11.2 ng/mL non-ICU)
- Soluble thrombomodulin levels > 3.26 ng/mL lower discharge rates and HR 5.9
- HsCRP
- IL-6.

HOW TO APPLY AN INTEGRATIVE APPROACH TO PREVENTING AND CARING FOR COVID-19 PATIENTS

There are numerous articles and scientific debates directed at pharmaceutical agents like Hydroxychloroquine, Ivermectin, Remdesivir, etc., but the fact remains that the overall survival in this disease is as follows and many non-pharmacologic interventions are effective:

- CDC COVID-19 Survival Rates
- Age 0–19—99.997%
- Age 20–49—99.98%

- Age 50–69—99.5%
- Age 70+—94.6%.

However, seemingly healthy people with no comorbidities can become deathly ill. A hidden immune defect has been identified in 14% of severely ill COVID-19 patients resulting in a genetically flawed interferon response to COVID-19 infection.[36] An additional group of patients developed rogue antibodies that attack interferon resulting in severe infections (94% male).[37] The following is a list of some of the more common COVID-19 disease manifestations and the targeted therapies:[38,39]

- Bradykinin storm
  - Hereditary angioedema medication
    - Icatibant
    - Ecallantide
  - Antihistamines
  - Corticosteroids (dexamethasone)
  - PnfC1-INH
  - Fresh frozen plasma
- Cytokine storm
  - Dexamethasone
  - SP16 (AAT fragment)
  - Extracorporeal selective cytopheresis (an immunomodulatory therapy that's been evaluated in several FDA-approved clinical trials in patients with excessive inflammation)
- Antivirals
  - HCQ (conflicting data—most other countries use it)
  - Ivermectin (conflicting data—most other countries use it)
  - Remdesivir (high liver toxicity—WHO against its use)
  - Favipiravir (antiviral)
  - Molnupiravir (antiviral)
- Respiratory treatments
  - Budesonide (inhaled corticosteroid)
- Immunomodulatory monoclonal antibodies
  - Tocilizumab—IL-6 receptor antagonist
  - Sarilumab—IL-6 receptor antagonist
  - Anakinra—IL-1
  - Baricitinib—inhibits JAKs 1&2
- Monoclonal antibodies directly targeting COVID-19
  - Bamlanivimab (LY-CoV555)
  - VIR-7831
  - REGN-COV2-Neutralizing Antibody Cocktail

STRATEGIES TO BOOST IMMUNITY

The immune status of an individual determines their ability to resist infections and to quickly respond once infected. Malnutrition has a profound effect on immune response and should be corrected to the maximum degree for patients with comorbidities like obesity and diabetes.[39] Examples of specific micronutrients which impact the immune system include arginine which is essential for generation of nitric oxide by macrophages and endothelial cells, vitamin A, and zinc, which regulate cell division and are therefore critical to the B and T-cell proliferative responses to COVID-19 when infected.[39] In certain situations, some micronutrients can be detrimental such as supplemental iron in malaria endemic areas which is associated with an increase in morbidity and mortality.[40] COVID-19 patients who experienced severe illness manifest elevated serum ferritin levels, and iron chelation is being explored as a way to prevent "cytokine storm" which is associated with increased ferritin levels and as a prophylactic in conditions associated with increased ferritin levels such as diabetics.[42] Some supplements have multiple functions; vitamin E can be an antioxidant and inhibitor of protein kinase C activity, and interacts with enzymes and transport proteins.[42]

Another often overlooked component to the immune system is the GALT (Gut-Associated Lymphoid Tissue) which actually contains the majority of immune cells in the body and is heavily influenced by the microbiome.[42] The gut contains ACE-2 receptors in the epithelial cells and, as such, should be kept as healthy as possible by not only good nutritional practices, but also by care and feeding of the microbiome.[42] Probiotics can foster microbiome diversity along with prebiotics, which are usually non-digestible oligosaccharides like inulin, that feed the microbiome.[42] In addition to the pre- and probiotics, vitamin D is critical to gut health and avoiding "leaky gut" which increases susceptibility to systemic infections. The probiotics actually reduce inflammation, while prebiotics appear to maintain barrier function of the gut.[42] Developed countries have a surprisingly high rate of what is referred to as "micronutrient malnutrition" in the elderly.[44] The elderly do not always maintain a healthy diet and are at increased risk from COVID-19 infection. Common lacking nutrients include zinc, selenium, iron, copper, folic acid, and vitamins A, B6, C, D, and E.[43] The vitamin D receptor is involved in the RAS and bradykinin pathways. COVID-19 infection has two detrimental effects: (1) reduced expression of vitamin D receptors and (2) increased vitamin D degradation enzymes. This suggests that increased vitamin D requirements exist in COVID-19 patients, and this is observed clinically.

Mushrooms have been associated with immune boosting capacity as have other plant-based foods and supplements.[44] Mushrooms (medicinal varieties like Lion's Mane, Chaga, Reishi, and Cordyceps) are being used to counter the cognitive defects from COVID-19 infection and boost immunity.[44] They have a number of benefits including immune support, antioxidant activity, anti-inflammatory activity, blood sugar homeostasis, brain health and cognition support, nervous system health, and providing increased energy and stamina.

Fruits and vegetables contain a wealth of phytochemicals like carotenes, polyphenols, flavonoids, and anthocyanidins. Bitter greens are also of great value in countering COVID-19. Bitter greens such as dandelion and arugula fortify the liver and enhance natural killer and T-cell production.[44] The inclusion of whole grains and legumes in the diet provides fiber, and prebiotics along with B vitamins and zinc promote gut health and interaction of the GALT with the complete immune system. Flax seed is a source of anti-inflammatory omega-3s, but fish oil is a better source, as plant-based omega-3s are predominantly in the form of ALA (alpha-linolenic acid) which must be converted to EPA (eicosapentaenoic acid) and DHA (docosahexaenoic acid) to have an effect.[45] Less than 1% is converted to EPA and DHA indicating that fish-sourced omega-3s are the only effective form. One complication of COVID-19 is coagulation defects including microthrombi. Natural products, besides omega-3s which are evidence-based blood thinners, include turmeric, cayenne pepper, cinnamon, ginger, and garlic. Other supplements and treatments which have shown benefit include high-dose vitamin C, vitamin K2, magnesium, and hydrotherapy including saunas and whirlpool baths. Finally, spirulina has been shown using in vitro studies to have antiviral activity and also positive immune modulation.[46]

Finally, one of the key contributing factors to disease severity and death in COVID-19 patients is an endogenous deficiency of glutathione.[47] The various consequences of this deficiency are illustrated in Figure 15.5. There are a number of strategies to increase glutathione: L-cysteine-rich foods like whey protein, N-acetylcysteine (prodrug for glutathione), ALA which is chemically similar to glutathione and promotes intracellular conversion of L-cystine (by reduction) to two molecules of L-cysteine upregulating glutathione synthetase, L-citrulline which acts as a glutathione enhancer and increases L-arginine through the arginine-citrulline cycle increasing nitric oxide more than L-arginine alone (mostly broken down in liver), liposomic glutathione, nano-glutathione, and Swish30.

Endogenous Deficiency of Glutathione is a Contributing Factor to Serious Manifestations and Death in COVID-19 Patients

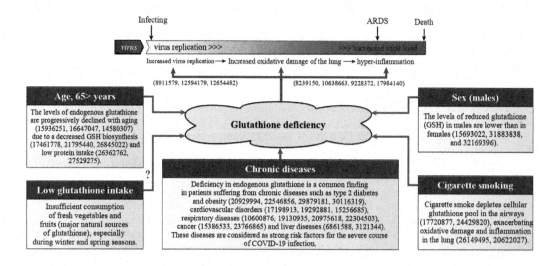

https://dx.doi.org/10.1021/acsinfecdis
.0c00288

FIGURE 15.5 Consequences of Glutathione Deficiency.

SUMMARY

COVID-19 can manifest multiple pathologies: endothelial dysfunction and increased plaque fragility, hemorrhagic damage to the endothelium and epithelium of numerous organs, thrombotic microangiopathy, and direct toxicity and inducement of autoimmunity. Awareness of this pathophysiology can enhance the differential diagnosis and improve patient care by guiding nutrition, supplementation, and other therapies. Death rates have continued to fall, and treatment regimens are more effective, both from an integrative and allopathic perspective.

REFERENCES

1. "Symptoms of Coronavirus". *U.S. Centers for Disease Control and Prevention (CDC)*. 13 May 2020. (https://www.cdc.gov/coronavirus/2019-ncov/symptoms-testing/symptoms.html)
2. Pekar J, Worobey M, Moshiri N, et al. 2021. Timing the SARS-CoV-2 index case in Hubei province. *Science*. 372:412–417. doi: 10.1126/science.abf8003.
3. Hu B, Guo H, Zhou Pe, et al. 2020. Characteristics of SARS-CoV-2and COVID-19. *Nature Reviews Microbiology*. 19(3):141–154. (https://www.ncbi.nlm.nih.gov/pmc/articles/PMC7537588).
4. Balkhy HH, Alenazi TH, Alshamrani MM, et al. 2016. Description of a hospital outbreak of middle east respiratory syndrome in a large tertiary care hospital in Saudi Arabia. *Infection Control & Hospital Epidemiology*. 37(10):1147–1155.
5. Andersen KG, Rambaut A, Lipkin WI, et al. 2020. The proximal origin ofSARS-CoV-2. *Nature Medicine*. 26(4):450–452.
6. California Department of Public Health: Tracking Variants, 8/5/2021.
7. Li B, Deng A, Li K, et al. 2021. Viral Infection and Transmission in a Large Well-Traced Outbreak Caused by the Delta SARS-CoV-2 Variant. *medRxiv*, July 12.

8. Hamming I, Timens W, Bulthuis MLC, et al. 2004. Tissue distribution of ACE2 protein, the functional receptor for SARS coronavirus. A first step in understanding SARS pathogenesis. *Journal of Pathology*. 203(2):631–637.

9. Lake MA. 2020. What we know so far: COVID-19 current clinical knowledge and research. *Clinical Medicine (London)*. 20:124–127.

10. Merad M, Martin JC. 2020. Pathological inflammation in patients with COVID-19: A key role for monocytes and macrophages. *Nature Reviews | Immunology*. doi: 10.1038/s41577-020-0331-4.

11. Rocheleau J. 2020. The Bradykinin Hypothesis: What It Is and What It Can Tell Us. https://www. forbes.com/sites/jackierocheleau/2020/10/02/the-bradykinin-hypothesis-what-it-is-and-what-it-can-tell-us/#3aed1d27204e.

12. Terry M. 2020. Unexpected Cause of Death in Younger COVID-19 Patients is Related to Blood Clotting. *BioSpace*, April 28.

13. Smith DG. 2020. Covid-19 May Be a Blood Vessel Disease, Which Explains Everything. *Elemental*, May 28.

14. Varga Z, Flammer AJ, Steiger P, et al. 2020. Endothelial cell infection and endothelitis in COVID-19. *Lancet*. 395(10234):1401–1460, e75–e82.

15. "Coronary Artery Calcification, Epidemiology, Imaging Methods, and Clinical Implications" the American Heart Association Science Advisory and Coordinating Committee on June 20, 1996.

16. CDC updates, expands list of people at risk of severe COVID-19 illness. June 25, 2020.

17. Pons S, Fodil S, Azoulay E, et al. 2020. The vascular endothelium: The cornerstone of organ dysfunction in severe SARS-CoV-2 infection. *Critical Care*. 24:Article Number 353.

18. Lemkes BA, Nieuwdorp M, Hoekstra JB, et al. 2012. The glycocalyx and cardiovascular disease in diabetes: Should we judge the endothelium by its cover? *Diabetes Technology & Therapeutics*. 14(Suppl 1):S3–S10.

19. Ackermann M, Verleden SE, Kuehnel M, et al. 2020. Pulmonary vascular endothelialitis, thrombosis, and angiogenesis in Covid-19. *New England Journal of Medicine*. 383:120–128.

20. How COVID-19 Spreads. *CDC Updates*-July 14th, 2021.

21. How Does Coronavirus Spread? *WebMD*-8/13/2021.

22. Johnson D, Lynch R, Marshall C, et al. 2013. Aerosol generation by modern flush toilets. *Aerosol Science and Technology*. 47(9):1047–1057.

23. Knowlton SD, Boles CL, Perencevich EN, et al. 2018. Bioaerosol concentrations generated from toilet flushing in a hospital-based patient care setting. *Antimicrobial Resistance & Infection Control*. 7:Article Number 16.

24. Kang M, Jianjian Wei J, Jun Yuan J, et al. Probable evidence of fecal aerosol transmission of SARS-CoV-2 in a high-rise building. *Annals of Internal Medicine*. doi: 10.7326/M20-0928.

25. Dhouib W, Maatoug J, Ayouni I, et al. 2021. The incubation period during the pandemic of COVID-19: A systematic review and meta-analysis. *Systematic Reviews*. 10:101.

26. Kucirka LM, Lauer SA, Laeyendecker O, et al. 2020. Variation in false-negative rate of RT-PCR–Based SARS-CoV-2 tests by time since exposure. *Annals of Internal Medicine*. 173(4):262–267.

27. How Accurate Are COVID-19 PCR Tests? https://www.biotechniques. com/coronavirus-news/false-negatives-how-accurate-are-pcr-tests-for-covid-19/.

28. Position Statement from the National Centre for Infectious Diseases and the Chapter of Infectious Disease Physicians, Academy of Medicine, Singapore –23 May 2020.

29. Hou H, Wang T, Zhang B, et al. 2020. Detection of IgM and IgG antibodies in patients with coronavirus disease. *Clinical & Translational Immunology*. 9:e1136.

30. Gudbjartsson DF, Norddahl GL, Melsted P, et al. 2020. Humoral immune response to SARS-CoV-2 in Iceland. *New England Journal of Medicine*. 383(18):1724–1734.

31. Crenshaw-Baldwin Hills seropositivity data in multi-ethnic asymptomatic individuals. Courtesy of GuardaHeart Foundation, 2020.

31. Grifoni A, et al. 2020. Targets of T cell responses to SARS-CoV-2 coronavirus in humans with COVID-19 disease and unexposed individuals. *Cell*. 181:1–13.

32. Interim Guidance for Rapid Antigen Testing for SARS-CoV-2. Updated September 4, 2020.

33. Conners JM. 2020. Thromboinflammation and the hypercoagulability of COVID-19. *Journal of Thrombosis and Haemostasis*. 18(7):1559–1561.

34. Cross DS, McCarty CA, Hytopoulos E, et al. 2012. Improved coronary risk assessment among intermediate risk patients using a clinical and biomarker based algorithm developed and validated in two population cohorts. *Current Medical Research & Opinion*. 28(11):1819–1830.

35. Yang Y, Shen C, Li J, et al. 2020. Plasma IP-10 and MCP-3 levels are highly associated with disease severity and predict the progression of COVID-19. *Journal of Allergy and Clinical Immunology.* 146(1):119–127.
36. Gundry SN. 2021. Abstract 10712: MRNA COVID vaccines dramatically increase endothelial inflammatory markers and ACS risk as measured by the PULS cardiac test: A warning. *Circulation.* 144(1).
37. Wadman M. 2020. Hidden immune weakness found in 14% of gravely ill COVID-19 patients. *Science.* doi: 10.1126/science.abe9395.
38. European Centre for Disease Prevention and Control. 5 May 2021.
39. Weinreich DM, Sivapalasingam S, Norton T, et al. 2021. REGN-COV2, a neutralizing antibody cocktail, in outpatients with Covid-19. *New England Journal of Medicine.* 384:238–251.
40. Childs CE, Calder PC, Miles EA. 2019. Diet and immune function. *Nutrients.* 11:1993.
41. Vargas-Vargas M, Cortés-Rojo C. 2020. Ferritin levels and COVID-19. *Revista Panamericana de Salud Publica.* 44:e72.
42. Lee GY, Han SN. 2018. The role of vitamin E in immunity. *Nutrients.* 10:1614.
43. How to boost your immune system. 2021. *Harvard Health.* February 15.
44. Houghton TS. 2020. How Does Nutrition Affect the Immune System? - Center for Nutrition Studies. March 20.
45. Omega-3 Fatty Acids. *NIH Fact Sheet for Consumers.* National Institute of Health Office of Dietary Supplements.
46. Karkos PD, Leong SC, Karkos CD, et al. 2011. Spirulina in clinical practice: Evidence-based human applications. *Evidence-Based Complementary and Alternative Medicine.* 2011:Article ID 531053.
47. Polonikov A. 2020. Endogenous deficiency of glutathione as the most likely cause of serious manifestations and death in COVID-19 patients. *CS Infectious Diseases.* 6(7):1558–1562.

16 Lymphstasis, Inflammation and Atherogenesis – Connecting the Dots

Gerald M. Lemole

CONTENTS

Inflammation and Covid 353
Lymph and Chronic Inflammation 354
Lifestyle Plus Epigenetics... 354
References.. 355

In the 1960s, technology gave us jaw-dropping advances in space exploration and a milestone moment when mankind landed on the moon. Our race to get into space also delivered cutting-edge technology and synthetic material that could be used in health care.

I spent 2 years (1967–1969) training in the cardiac surgical program of pioneers Dr. Michael DeBakey and Dr. Denton Cooley. Not only was it an honor and a privilege, but it also a time of great excitement.

Since NASA was headquartered in Houston and because doctors Cooley and DeBakey were well connected with local and governmental scientists and executives, we were the beta test site for equipment, like wireless patient monitoring and more durable materials like Teflon, titanium and Pyrolite for medical devices.

We were working in the laboratory with artificial heart models, testing new valve designs in the Calf Lab and entering the new field of cardiac transplantation after the successful operation performed by Dr. Christian Bernard in South Africa. Because of these advances, new specialties were even being created; there was no such thing as an immunologist nor a specialty of immunology until the need arose for immunosuppression in organ transplantation.

And in May 1968, we reached a moon of our own—a year before Neil Armstrong reached the literal one: We performed the first successful cardiac transplant in the United States.

That, for me, was a world-changing event.

In all, I was involved in five cardiac transplants, and all of the patients did well. I spent a further 14 months in Houston, during which time I closely followed the progress of our patients, who became our newfound friends.

Upon the completion of my residency, I accepted the position of chief of cardiac surgery at Temple University Medical Center. It was an exciting new phase of my career, and with the help of Dr. Richard Geis, a fellow surgeon from Houston who came with us to Philadelphia, we got the program up and running.

However, during this period, a very disconcerting event occurred. In the first few years, all of the cardiac-transplant patients I was involved with (and many of the patients around the world) died.

The diagnosis: "galloping atherosclerosis."

DOI: 10.1201/9781003137849-16

What did that mean? These healthy hearts that were transplanted from young individuals with smooth clean arteries had now become 90-year-old vessels filled with cholesterol. These deaths were not only a professional failure, but a personal loss. These patients stayed with us for several months after the surgery. We became friends, met their families, went to the baseball games, ate meals and had good times together.

Over the years, I not only remembered these people, but I also remembered what happened—the rapid progression of the coronary disease in these transplanted hearts.

Our practice grew to several hundred open heart patients per year, and being in a university surrounding, we had an active research program doing cardiac and aortic procedures to further scientific advancement.

During this time, a professor of pathology, Dr. Elizabeth Lausche, approached me with some questions about the cardiac-transplant procedure.

Her interest?
The function of the foam cell.

At the time, there was little known about it. Today, we know it as a cell that develops from a type of white cell named monocyte, which migrates into the inner layer of the artery (intima) and morphs into a macrophage to then collect cholesterol to take away and prevent atherosclerosis. It's a trash collector of sorts, removing the cholesterol and clearing the artery.

Back then, we didn't know much about foam cells,[1] but Dr. Lausche made that one of her major endeavors.

Her question that prompted it all: Did we sew the lymph vessels of the transplanted heart back to the patient's lymph system?

I laughed. We couldn't even see those vessels, because they were so small and transparent—how would we sew them back?

But the question was a good one, because it got at the root of the purpose of our lymph system, which was to help clear waste from our bodies.

Over the next several months, we developed a research project. Here's how it worked:

We identified the cardiac lymphatics: I operated on six rhesus monkeys and injected a charcoal solution into the cardiac area, followed the uptake into the lymphatics, and ligated them away from the heart. This was a simple operation that could easily identify the cardiac lymphatics and interrupt them.

We created atherosclerosis: We placed the monkeys on a high-cholesterol diet and sacrificed them after 8–12 weeks. All the monkeys had developing signs of early atherosclerosis. I conjectured that if we could create early atherosclerosis with acute interruption of the lymphatics of the heart, why wouldn't chronic obstruction over a long period of time create what we see now in coronary disease in our population? So we measured the composition of the pericardial fluid, which surrounds the heart, and found that this fluid, which is very similar to lymphatic fluid, has more of the cholesterol-laden HDL than the patient's blood had at that same time. Also, patients with arterial sclerosis had a higher LDL/HDL ratio in the blood than those patients with normal vessels. We also observed that patients with coronary artery disease had fine, sclerotic, scarred, shrunken, narrow lymphatic vessels following the vascular bed.[2]

We made correlations: Now we had strong circumstantial evidence that lymphatic dysfunction was related to cardiovascular disease. Lymph drainage from the tissue primarily is carried by the thoracic duct, which is dependent on deep breathing, diaphragmatic massage and upward drainage of the lymph fluid. Certainly, stress, lack of exercise and poor diet containing few vegetables that produce polyphenols and flavonoids, which encourage lymph flow, correlated closely with heart disease. While massage encourages flow, cigarette smoking constricts the lymphatic vessels. Our practice grew to 1,500 open heart cases a year, mostly coronary bypass procedures. The surgical team had ample opportunity to observe firsthand the real-time consequences of this process, and of which they all agreed made sense.

As the years progressed, case after case substantiated the postulation:

Lymphatic flow was necessary for clearance of cholesterol from the arterial wall.

Although not named as such at that time, it described "reverse cholesterol transport".[3,4] However, at that time, clearing the arteries through lymph vessels situated in the arterial connective tissue (adventitia) was not included in what was described as "reverse cholesterol transport" but only the relationship of cholesterol to HDL and liver clearance. In 1979, I decided to write the paper describing our work and I wanted it to be published in the finest journal in my field, *The Annals of Thoracic Surgery*. It took almost 2 years to get published in 1981[2] after multiple back-and-forth communication from the editorial board of cardiac surgeons (who didn't seem to be interested in a lymphatic based postulation), although it was received with some interest—generating requests for reprints from 12 countries.

Between 1981 and 2013, only 30 papers were produced in the medical literature on this topic, some with significant advances in the understanding of this process. Some examples are as follows:

- In 1984, Rudra and associates[5] showed that there was a greater percentage of cholesterol-laden HDL in the lymph fluid than there was in the blood—implying that the cholesterol is cleared through the lymphatics.
- In 1990, doctors Nordestgaard and Hjelms[6] from Denmark showed that 95% of the cholesterol in the innermost intima is carried through the strong, restrictive internal lamina of the intima to the lymphatics.
- In 2013, interest in the lymphatic clearance of the arterial wall was stimulated by the work done in Mount Sinai New York.

With the work done since 2014 by multiple centers,[7–9] it is possible to outline a theoretical process of lymphatic clearance of the arteries. With that in mind, here are some take-home messages about the processes from an article that I wrote in the journal *Lymphology* in 2016.[10]

Role of Cholesterol: Cholesterol is normally delivered to the tissue through the capillaries, to be utilized to create cell membrane, bile acids, hormones, vitamins and other necessary metabolites.[11] Coincidently, because of aging,[12] inflammation, turbulence, hypertension[13] and metabolic disorders,[14] the arterial endothelium becomes dysfunctional[15,16] and loses its integrity.

That permits LDL cholesterol (especially the small dense particles) to pass into the intima. The LDL rapidly becomes oxidized initiating an endothelial inflammatory process.[17] Monocytes are attracted, and they become macrophages in the intima. They then enhance inflammation.[18]

Macrophages engulf the cholesterol, subsequently transforming into foam cells and, unless they can transfer the cholesterol or migrate through the arterial wall, create further inflammation and deposition of the cholesterol. The development of arteriosclerosis depends on how efficiently the cholesterol can be cleared from the sub-intimal space.[19]

Clearing of Cholesterol: In the smallest arteries, this can occur with little difficulty, but in the large and mid sized arteries, the high-density lipoprotein and foam cells must pass from the intima through many layers before coming into contact with lymphatic vessels.[19]

In the past, passage of cholesterol through the arterial wall was not considered to be involved in reverse cholesterol transport because of the thickness of the arterial wall, the integrity of the internal elastic lamina, and the distance to the lymphatic vessels. The inflamed, hypertrophied arterial wall and foam cells manufacture enzymes creating oxidative stress[15–17] which immobilizes the macrophages and increases the fibroblasts and collagen, further slowing down the cholesterol's progression to the lymphatics.[20–22]

Various inflammatory processes prevent cholesterol from being transported from the arteries. Foam cells can facilitate clearance by removing significant amounts of cholesterol when unimpeded,[23,24] and research shows that the lymph system is a major transport venue for egress of cholesterol. And perhaps most importantly, the lymphatic system is not just a passive conduit, but essential for moving lipids and proteins.

Role of Lymphatics: Lymph channels contain contractile smooth muscle fibers and autonomic nerve endings.[25,26] The lymphatic system is the immune domain, warehousing lymphocytes and providing a conduit for them. It is intimately connected with the nervous and endocrine systems.

There are many causes for slowing of lymphatic clearance, such as inflammation, absence or diminished lymph channels, viscosity of lymph liquid, tissue pressure gradient, gravity, sclerosis of the lymphatic vessels, radiation, poor muscle pumping action, sluggish lymph peristalsis, shallow breathing, and/or a diet poor in flavonoids and polyphenols. Increasing lymphatic flow can diminish the oxidative stress, increasing cholesterol clearance and potentially decreasing atherosclerotic deposition. Recognizing the involvement of the lymphatic system in atherogenesis helps shed new light on the process.[27]

Lymphatic involvement in atherogenesis permits us to formulate an overarching, unifying concept in the development of arteriosclerosis and helps explain the inverse relationship between cardiovascular disease and exercise and deep breathing, high-vegetable diet, stress modification, and the direct relationship to sedentary lifestyle, stress, a pro-inflammatory diet and reactive oxygen species. In addition, establishing the involvement of lymphatic with atherogenesis underscores, explains and encourages a lifestyle of exercise, healthy diet and stress modification, to prevent cardiovascular disease. The conclusions are as follows:

- A diet high in vegetables and fruits has much scientific evidence that it is cardiovascular protective. All plants contain flavonoids and polyphenols, which are lymph stimulating.[24,28–30]
- Vitamin D has been shown to slow the ingress of monocytes and immune message transporting, dendritic cells into the intima and, in addition, downregulates the inflammation of the macrophages and monocytes.[31,32]
- Exercise is considered part of an optimum lifestyle for cardiovascular health. Besides positively affecting anti-inflammatory markers and reducing pro-inflammatory ones, exercise considerably increases lymphatic circulation.[33,34]
- Since it is necessary for the lymph to egress through the chest cavity to the subclavian vein, where it returns into the bloodstream and ultimately reaches the liver, its circulation is affected by increased deep breathing. Such respiration creates larger diaphragmatic excursions and increases negative intrathoracic pressure, and thus will stimulate lymphatic flow maximizing lipid clearance. The complete cycle of lymphatic circulation is about 2 days. The life of an HDL particle is 4 days, while a macrophage lifespan is several weeks to months.[35] This means that, with exercise, by tripling the lymphatic flow, we can significantly increase cholesterol clearance.[33,34]
- Both physical and mental stresses play an important role in the development of inflammation and atherosclerosis. Stress has been documented to increase cortisol and epinephrine, thus creating an immune suppression and a subsequent decrease in lymphatic function. Increases in long-term cortisol levels create lymphatic atrophy, which can then decrease reverse cholesterol transport.[36–39]
- Smoking induces oxidative injury, promotes altered eicosanoid production and contributes to the dysfunction of lymphatics under normal conditions, as well as a variety of clinical disorders.[40]

Chronic inflammation sounds like it could be a buzzword because it's used so often to describe medical problems, but it's very much a real issue—and one that has inspired a whole new area of therapy for chronic disease. And that is extremely promising.

To get to understand it, we must first look at the acute inflammatory process that occurs and sometimes goes on to chronic inflammation.

As the name implies, acute inflammation is a short-term process that works to help protect the body. It's one that destroys toxins, whether from the outside as a virus or a bacteria, or from within.

This is accomplished by strong chemicals, e.g., cytokines, peroxides and antibodies, and immune cells that engulf or destroy alien substances. While the destruction of the unwelcome molecules is progressing, there is collateral damage to the normal tissue in the area.[41–48]

Think of a twist of an ankle or a cut of the skin; an acute inflammatory process develops when there's been some type of insult to the body, and the system works to repair the area.

The ideal scenario? The inflammatory activity stops when the offending organism or toxins are removed. At that point, healing should begin with resolution and repair of the local tissue. In the normal course of events, this is accomplished by a recently identified group of fats called the Special Pro-Resolving Mediators (SPM). Lipoxin, Resolvin, Protectin and Maresin are these SPMs that are derived from the omega 3s and importantly, from the omega 6s that also create the "pro-inflammatory" substances – arachidonic acid and PGE2.[49,50]

The standard therapy is to treat acute inflammation with anti-inflammatories, like ibuprofen and Aleve. These Cox 2 inhibitors block the "pro-inflammatory" arachidonic acid and prostaglandin 2 series, which are also necessary to create several of the SPM substances.

This usage could contribute to the prolongation of the acute inflammation and the possible development of a chronic inflammatory condition, like heart disease, diabetes or cancer. This prevention of SPM production may be the cause of some side effects of these medications. Current research implies that certain supplements such as EPA and DHA along with fractionated marine lipid concentrates from sardines, anchovy and mackerel, and especially a concentrate from the seaweed known as krill, may be extremely helpful in resolving inflammation in the tissue.

With this exciting new information, we may be on a different route of resolving acute inflammation and preventing or limiting chronic inflammation that is so rampant in all chronic degenerative diseases.

Here's where the lymphatic system comes in: The lymphatic system is integral to the transmission of immune cells, information, and substances that create a healthy inflammatory reaction and a quick reversal to an anti-inflammatory state. Patients with chronic inflammatory diseases like obesity and diabetes have severely leaky lymphatic vessels that lose IgG, triglycerides, and cells and nutrients that are necessary for a healthy immune system and inter-systemic communication. Keeping those channels open and minimizing transported substances and cell loss will optimize wellness.

INFLAMMATION AND COVID

However, there are some issues when we consider SARS2 infection, commonly known as Covid 19. The cause, timing and treatment of the symptoms of Covid-19 are actually quite different. Symptoms such as loss of smell, fever, chills, sweating, diarrhea, sore throat and cough occur a few days after the patient is infected with SARS2 virus. After a week or so, the respiratory symptoms become worse with shortness of breath, oxygen desaturation and generalized inflammation.

In the first week or two, the virus is multiplying and invading the cells of the body. This varies from patient to patient depending on how disabled they are. Patients with diabetes and obesity are at higher risk because they already have an inflamed constitution.[51]

During the first phase of this disease, I believe the best treatment is to eradicate or prevent the virus from multiplying early. This can be done with monupivir, colchicine, hydroxychloroquine, Ivermectin, zinc, or Remdesivir, monoclonal antibodies, fluvoxamine and nasal spray.[52–59] Sometimes there is an overlap between the two phases that would require both the antiviral and the steroid.

After a week or two, the symptoms of respiratory distress and general debilitation are due to an overabundance of inflammatory substances or a "cytokine storm." This is not the virus, but our own body overproducing substances that create lung fluid, blood clotting, generalized debilitation and shock.[61] Multiple studies of patients during this cytokine storm have reported both high viral counts and low viral counts and particles, leading one to consider that treating the virus infection at that stage may not be as effective as steroids like dexamethasone are.

However, one observation that is common in this disease is T cell depletion.[60-62] T cells are lymphocytes that can produce inflammation, but specifically can also decrease inflammation and repair tissue if they are a specific T cell called a CD4 T regulatory cell. It is my belief that the T cell deficiency in this stage of the infection is of the CD4 T regs, so the inflammation increases and goes wild, and monocytes become macrophages and are attracted to the endothelium of the lymphatics and the blood vessels, and thus cause poor transportation and communication in the lymph vessels, fluid in the lungs and thrombosis and hemorrhage in the blood vessels.

LYMPH AND CHRONIC INFLAMMATION

The lymphatic system is integral to the transmission of immune cells, information and substances that create a healthy inflammatory reaction and a quick reversal to an anti-inflammatory state. Patients with chronic inflammatory diseases like obesity and diabetes have severely leaky lymphatic vessels that lose substances that are necessary for a healthy immune system and inter-systemic communication.[41-48]

Keeping those channels open and minimizing transported substances and cell loss will optimize wellness.

We can then see why a healthy lymphatic system is so important in avoiding chronic degenerative disease by maintaining good lymphatic clearance and messaging from vital tissues in order to respond to chronic inflammation. Examining the lymphatic involvement in arteriosclerosis can enable us to create an overarching concept for atherogenesis.

LIFESTYLE PLUS EPIGENETICS

Inflammation can be counterbalanced by the lifestyle changes made affecting the individual's epigenetic pattern.

Epigenetics is a recent scientific theory that states that the DNA in a cell is not a predetermined outcome creator, but more like an engineer's blueprint filing cabinet that relies on opening up the cabinet to express proteins and peptides that will change the direction of the cell metabolism. These blueprints are selected by lifestyle choices, such as diet, exercise, stress modification, and spirituality. Lesson:

Our external decisions can make dramatic changes in our internal metabolism based on what we choose to incorporate into our life.

This then ties in beautifully with the reverse cholesterol transport concept of lymphatic involvement:

- All choices that improve lymphatic flow decrease the incidence of arteriosclerosis.
- All choices that increase the incidence of arteriosclerosis cause lymphatic dysfunction.

So, we can see how important it is to create a lifestyle that incorporates exercise, stress modification and diet. Exercise is essential for the movement of lymph fluid. Deep breathing, muscular contraction, arterial pulsation and gravity are all important factors for getting the lymph to the liver via the venous system. Stress modification controls the release of cortisol and epinephrine, both of which cause lymphatic constriction and sclerosis. Meditation, yoga, tai chi and Eastern exercise activities all help massage the internal organs and create proper lymphatic function.[37-39]

Diet and supplementation are very important because vegetables and fruits contain polyphenols and flavonoids,[62] which increase lymphatic flow, decrease inflammatory substances and lead to resolution of inflammation.[24,28-30] Besides eating the proper diet, it is vital to drink pure water in large quantities to keep the lymph volume and consistency in the right amounts to maintain good lymphatic flow.[63-67] Some key areas are as follows:

Fiber: Fiber could be labeled as a food. Fiber is found in the plant cell wall as long-chained polysaccharides. Bacteria, through a fermentation process, can digest this cell wall to become a source of energy.[68,69] Fifteen percent of our total caloric intake and 50% of the calories absorbed by the colon are from the breakdown of soluble fiber metabolized by the 400 species of beneficial gut bacteria (5 pounds!).[69] Soluble fibers can bind ingested elements and toxic components, whether from the outside or created as an intermediate product of the metabolism of our own body. It's been recently shown that in the gastrointestinal system from the mouth to colon, bacteria are living with us symbiotically, breaking down indigestible foods into short-chain fatty acids such as acetic, butyric or propionic acid. The compounds and nutrients produced by this fermentation can be absorbed by the gastrointestinal system and circulated around the body as an energy supply or signaling molecules to upregulate or suppress enzymatic systems of our body. Soluble fiber sources have been shown to be beneficial in reducing the incidence of some types of cancer, reducing blood cholesterol levels, obesity, diabetes, cardiovascular disease, and numerous gastrointestinal disorders including inflammatory bowel disease, ulcerative colitis, Crohn's disease and colon cancer.[68,72–75]

Insoluble fiber is derived from plant foods but is not water-soluble and isn't digested or absorbed in the small intestine but is then subjected to bacterial attack in the large intestine; 30 g of fiber or more a day is recommended which induces cell death of human colon tumors and decreases tumor necrosis factors, along with inflammatory cytokines such as IL-6 and IL-1.[75] Conversely, catalyzed by *pathogenic* intestinal bacteria, amino acids may be transformed into nitrosamines which are highly carcinogenic. You can see how important and truly active the role of fiber has in our diet.[69] It's also apparent to see the role of our diet has on keeping a good environment for healthy intestinal bacteria to flourish and live symbiotically with us, keeping our body supplied with the food, proteins, amino acids, fatty acids and energy that we need.

Supplements: It is wise to periodically get a metabolic profile to see if there are any vitamin, fat or protein deficiencies. Several supplements are necessary and notoriously insufficient. For example, 50% of the population has inadequate magnesium intake and 70% of the people aged 65 and over are deficient, which is necessary in over 300 metabolic processes.[70,71] Vitamin D is a pro-hormone that is necessary not only for creation of metabolites, but is also anti-inflammatory and seems to be effective in diminishing Covid infections when found at higher levels in the population.[76,77] Pterostilbene, a substance similar to resveratrol and quercetin (only much more absorbable and effective), is an active ingredient in blueberries that promotes health.[78] Since targeted nutritional supplementation is widely discussed in this textbook, any personal queries should be explored and discussed with your healthcare provider to help support your health.

REFERENCES

1. Cookson, F.B. 1971. The origin of foam cells in atherosclerosis. *Br. J. Exp. Pathol.* 52(1):62–69.
2. Lemole, G. 1981. The Role of Lymphstasis in atherogenesis. *Ann. Thorac. Surg.* 31(3):290–293.
3. Small, D.M. 1988. Mechanisms of reversed cholesterol transport. *Agents Actions Suppl.* 26:26136–26146.
4. Drayna, D, Jarnagin, A.S., McLean, J., Henzel, W., Kohr, W., Fielding, C., Lawn, R. 1987. Cloning and sequencing of human cholesteyl ester transfer protein cDNA. *Nature* 327(6123):632–634. Doi: 10.1038/327532a0.
5. Rudra, D.N., Myant, N.B., Pflug, J.I., Reichl, D. 1984. The distribution of cholesterol and apoprotein a – 1 between the lipoprotein and peripheral plasma and peripheral lymph from normal human subjects. *Atherosclerosis* 53(3):297–308.
6. Nordestgaard, B.G., Hjelms, E., Stender, S., Kjeldsen, K. 1990. Different efflux pathways for high and low density lipoproteins from porcine aortic intima. *Arteriosclerosis* 10(3):477–486.
7. Martel, C., Li, W., Fulp, B., Platt, A.M., Gautier, E.L., Westerterp, M., et al. 2013. Lymphatic vasculature mediates macrophage reverse cholesterol transport in mice. *J. Clin. Invest.* 123(4):1571–1579.
8. Randolph, G., 2008. Emigration of monocyte – derived cells to lymph nodes during resolution of inflammation and its failure in atherosclerosis. *Curr. Opin. Lipidol.* 19(5):462–468.
9. Martel, C., Randolph, G. 2013. Atherosclerosis and transit of HDL through the lymphatic vasculature. *Curr. Atheroscler. Rep.* 15:354.
10. Lemole, G., 2016. Atherogenesis and lymphstasis…Connecting the Dots. *Lymphology* 49:8–14.

11. Lecerfa, J.M., de Lorgeril, M., 2016. Dietary cholesterol: from physiology to cardiovascular risk. *Br. J. Nutr.* 106(1):6–14.

12. Kleinstreuer, C., Hyun, S., Buchanan, J.R. Jr., Longest, P.W., Archie, J.P. Jr., Truskey, G.A. 2001. Hemodynamic parameters and early intimal thickening in branching blood vessels. *Crit. Rev. Biomed. Eng.* 29(1):1–64.

13. Dabagh, M., Jalali, P., Tarbell, J.M., 2009. The transport of LDL across the deformable arterial wall: the effect of endothelial cell turnover and intimal deformation under hypertension. *Am. J. Physiol. Heart. Circ. Physiol.* 297(3):H983–H996.

14. Pfenniger, A., Chanson, M., Kwak, B.R. 2013. Connexins in atherosclerosis. *Biochim. Biophys. Acta.* 1828(1):157–166.

15. Davies, M.J., Woolf, N., Rowles, P.M., Pepper, J. 1988. Morphology of the endothelium over atherosclerotic plaques in human coronary arteries. *Br. Heart J.* 60(6):459–464.

16. Lamarche, B., St-Pierre, A.C., Ruel, I.L., Cantin, B., Dagenais, G.R., Després, J.P. 2001. A prospective, population-based study of low density lipoprotein particle size as a risk factor for ischemic heart disease in men. *Can. J. Cardiol.* 17(8):859–865.

17. Park, Y.M., Febbraio, M., Silverstein, R.L., 2009. CD36 modulates migration of mouse and human macrophages in response to oxidized LDL and may contribute to macrophage trapping in the arterial intima. *J. Clin. Invest.* 119(1):136–145.

18. Rohatgi, A., Khera, A., Berry, J.D., Givens, E.G., Ayers, C.R., Wedin, K.E., et al. 2014. Cholesterol efflux capacity and incident cardiovascular events. *N. Engl. J. Med.* 371(25):2383–2393.

19. Lemole, G.M. 2000. Unifying concept of arteriosclerosis (Table 4.14) an integrative approach to cardiac care. *Medtronic* 46.

20. Gerszten, R.E., Tager, A.M. 2012. The monocyte in atherosclerosis–should I stay or should I go now? *N. Engl. J. Med.* 366:1734–1736.

21. Wanschel, A., Seibert, T., Hewing, B., et al. 2013. Neuroimmune guidance cue Semaphorin 3E is expressed in atherosclerotic plaques and regulates macrophage retention. *Arterioscler. Thromb. Vasc. Biol.* 33:886–893.

22. Llodrá, J., Angeli, V., Liu, J., et al. 2004. Emigration of monocyte-derived cells from atherosclerotic lesions characterizes regressive, but not progressive, plaques. *Proc. Natl. Acad. Sci. USA* 101:11779–11784.

23. Pietzsch, J., Lattke, P., Juilius, U. 2000. Oxidation of apoliopoprotein B-100 in ciuculating LDL is related to LDL residence time in vivo insights from stable-isotope studies. *Arterioscler. Thromb. Vasc Bio.* 20:E63–E67.

24. Ginter, E., Simko, V. 2015. Recent data on Mediterranean diet, cardiovascular disease, cancer, diabetes and life expectancy. *Bratisl. Lek. Listy.* 116:346–348.

25. Yves von der Weid, P., Zawieja, D.C. 2004. Lymphatic smooth muscle: the motor unit of lymph drainage. *Int. J. Biochem. Cell. Biol.* 36(7):1147–1153. Doi: 10.1016/j.biocel.2003. 12.008.

26. Mignini, F., Sabbatini, M., Coppola, L. 2013. Analysis of nerve supply pattern in human lymphatic vessels of young and old men. *Lymphat. Res. Biol.* 10(4):189–197. Doi: 10.1089/lrb.2012.0013.

27. Vuorio, T, Nurmi, H., Moulton, K., et al. 2014. Lymphatic vessel insufficiency in hypercholesterolemic mice alters lipoprotein levels and promotes atherogenesis. *Arterioscler. Thromb. Vasc. Biol.* 34:1162–1170.

28. Fung, T., Hu, F. 2003. Plant-based diets: what should be on the plate? *Am. J. Clin. Nutr.* 78:357–358.

29. Willett, W.C. 1994. Diet and health: what should we eat? *Science* 264:532–537.

30. Chainani-Wu, N, Weidner, G., Purnell, D.M., et al. 2011. Changes in emerging cardiac biomarkers after an intensive lifestyle intervention. *Am. J. Cardiol.* 108:498–507.

31. Takeda, M, Yamashita, T., Sasaki, N., et al. 2010. Oral administration of an active form of vitamin D3 (calcitriol) decreases atherosclerosis in mice by inducing regulatory T cells and immature dendritic cells with tolerogenic functions. *Arterioscler. Thromb. Vasc. Biol.* 30:2495–2503.

32. Riek, A.E., Oh, J., Sprague, J.E., et al. 2012. Vitamin D suppression of endoplasmic reticulum stress promotes an antiatherogenic monocyte/macrophage phenotype in type 2 diabetic patients. *J. Biol. Chem.* 287:38482–38494.

33. Geffken, D.F., Cushman, M., Burke, G.L., et al. 2001. Association between physical activity and markers of inflammation in a healthy elderly population. *Am. J. Epidemiol.* 153:242–250.

34. Desai, P., Williams Jr, A.G., Prajapati, P., et al. 2010. Lymph flow in instrumented dogs varies with exercise intensity. *Lymphat. Res. Biol.* 8:143–148.

35. Rader, D. 2011. The Role of HDL-C in the management of atherosclerosis. *Med. Roundtable (Cardiovasc Ed).* 3:27–37. Roundtable ID: CV11538.

36. Marcondes, M.C., Zhukov, V., Bradlow, H., et al. 2011. Effects of chronic mental stress and atherogenic diet on the immune inflammatory environment in mouse aorta. *Brain Behav. Immun.* 25:1649–1657.

37. Schmidt, D., Reber, S.O., Botteron, C., et al. 2010. Chronic psychosocial stress promotes systemic immune activation and the development of inflammatory Th cell responses. *Brain Behav. Immun.* 24:1097–1104.

38. Cohen, L.M., McChargue, D.E., Collins, F.L. 2003. *The Health Psychology Handbook: Practical Issues for the Behavioral Medicine Specialist*, 1st Edition. SAGE publications, ISBN-13: 978-0761926146 ISBN-10: 0761926143, pp. 171–172.

39. Selye, H. 1975. *The Stress of Life*, Revised Edition, McGraw-Hill, New York, pp. 22–23.

40. Sinzinger, H., Kaliman, J., Oguogho, A. 2000. Eicosanoid production and lymphatic responsiveness in human cigarette smokers compared with non-smokers. *Lymphology* 33:24–31.

41. Nanjee, M.N., Cooke, C.J., Wong, J.S., et al. 2001. Composition and ultrastructure of size subclasses of normal human peripheral lymph lipoproteins: quantification of cholesterol uptake by HDL in tissue fluids. *J. Lipid Res.* 42:639–648.

42. Card, C.M., Yu, S.S., Swartz, M.A. 2014. Emerging roles of lymphatic endothelium in regulating adaptive immunity. *J. Clin. Invest.* 124:943–952.

43. Aebischer, D., Iolyeva, M., Halin, C. 2014. The inflammatory response of lymphatic endothelium. *Angiogenesis* 17:383–393.

44. Lim, H.Y., Rutkowski, J.M., Helft, J., et al. 2009. Hypercholesterolemic mice exhibit lymphatic vessel dysfunction and degeneration. *Am. J. Pathol.* 175:1328–1337.

45. Wilhelm, A.J., Zabalawi, M., Grayson, J.M., et al. 2009. Apolipoprotein A-I and its role in lymphocyte cholesterol homeostasis and autoimmunity. *Arterioscler. Thromb. Vasc. Biol.* 29:843–849.

46. Liao, S., Cheng, G., Conner, D.A., et al. 2011. Impaired lymphatic contraction associated with immunosuppression. *Proc. Natl. Acad. Sci. USA.* 108:18784–18789.

47. Bobryshev, Y.V., Lord, R.S. 1998. Mapping of vascular dendritic cells in atherosclerotic arteries suggests their involvement in local immune-inflammatory reactions. *Cardiovasc. Res.* 37:799–810.

48. Reiss, A.B., Wan, D.W., Anwar, K., et al. 2009. Enhanced CD36 scavenger receptor expression in THP-1 human monocytes in the presence of lupus plasma: linking autoimmunity and atherosclerosis. *Exp. Biol. Med.* 234:354–360.

49. Kraft, J.D., Blorgran, R., et al. 2021. Specializing Pro resolving mediators and the lymphatic system. *Int. J. Mol. Sci.* 22(5):2750.

50. Johnson, L.A. In sickness and in health: 2021 the immunological roles of the lymphatic system. *Int. J. Mol. Sci.* 22(9):4458. Doi: 10.3390/ijims22094458.

51. Salman, A., Mohammad, A., Al-Youha, S, Jamal, M, Almazeedi, S. 2020. COVID-19: impact of obesity and diabetes on disease severity. *Clin Obes.* 10(6):e12414. Doi: 10.1111/cob.12414.

52. Vrachatis, D.A., Giannopoulos, G.V., Giotaki, S.G., Raisakis, K., Kossyvakis, C., Iliodromitis, K.E., Reimbers, B., Tousoulis, D., Cleman, M., Stefanadis, C., Lansky, A., Deftereos, S. 2020. Impact of colchicine on mortality in patients with COVID 19: a meta-analysis. *Hellenic J. Cardiol.* PMID:33421583 PMCID: PMC7833703. Doi: 10.1016/ J. HJC. 2020.11.012.

53. Lopes, M.I., Bonjorno, L.P., Giannini, M.C., Amaral, N.B., Menezes, P.I., Dib, S.M., Gigante, S.L., Benatti, M.N., Rezek, U.C., Emrich-Filho, L.L., Sousa, B.A.A., Almeida, S.C., et al. 2021. Beneficial effects of colchicine for moderate to severe COVID-19: a randomized, double-blinded, placebo-controlled clinical trial. *RMD open* 7(1):e001455.

54. 2020 Ivermectin for COVID-19: Real-time meta analysis of 58 studies. COVID Analysis, Nov 26, 2020 (Version 88), June 7, 2021.

55. Padhy, B.M., Mohnaty, R.R., Das, S., Meher, B.R. 2020. Therapeutic potential of ivermectin as add on treatment in COVID 19: a systematic review and meta-analysis. *J. Pharm. Pharm. Sci.* 23:462–469. PMID:33227231. Doi: 10.18433/jpps31457.

56. Hussain, N., Chung, E., Heyl, J.J., Hussain, B., Oh, M.C., Pinon, C., Boral, S., Chus, D., Babu, B. 2020. A Meta-Analysis on the Effects of Hydroxychloroquine on COVID -19. *Cureus.* Doi: 10.7759/Cureus.10005.

57. Beigel, J.H., Tomashek, K.M., Dodd, L.E., Mehta, A.K., Zingman, B.S., Kalik, A.C., Hohmann, E., Chu H.Y., Luetkemeyer, A., Kline, S., de Catilla, D.L., Finberg, R.W., et al., for the ACTT-1 Study Group Members. 2020. Remdesivir for the Treatment of Covid-19- Final Report. A preliminary version of this article was published on May 22, 2020 at NEJM.org. This article was published on October 8, 2020, and updated on October 9, 2020 NEJM.org.

58. Diao, B., et al. 2020. Reduction and functional exhaustion of T cells in patients with coronavirus disease 2019 (COVID-19). *Front. Immunol.* 11:827.

59. Laing, A.G., et al. 2020. A consensus Covid-19 immune signature combines immune-protection with discrete sepsis-like traits associated with poor prognosis. Preprint at *medRxiv*. Doi: 10.1101/2020.06.0820125112.; Hoertel, N., Sánchez Rico, M., Vernet, R. et al. 2021. Association between SSRI antidepressant use and reduced risk of intubation or death in hospitalized patients with coronavirus disease 2019: a multicenter retrospective observational study. *Mol Psychiatry*. Sep; 26(9):5199–5212. Doi: 10.1038/s41380-021-01021-4. Epub Feb 4 2021. PMID: 33536545.

60. Tan, L., et al. 2020. Lymphopenia predicts disease severity of COVID-19: a descriptive and predictive study. *Signal. Transduct. Target. Ther.* 5:33.

61. Chen, G., et al. 2019. Clinical and immunological features of severe and moderate coronavirus disease 2019. *J. Clin Invest.* 130:2620–2629.

62. Vogel, G., Ströcker, H. 1966. The effect of drugs–especially flavonoids and aescin–on the lymph flow and the permeability of the intact plasma-lymph barrier of rats for fluid and defined macromolecules. *Arzneimittelforschung* 16:1630–1634.

63. Shaïkemeleva, U.S. 1983. [Effect of rutin on the cholesterol content of the lymph, blood and tissues of the dog] Biull. *Eksp. Biol. Med.* 95:35–37.

64. Cotonat, A, Cotonat, J. 1989. Lymphagogue and pulsatile activities of Daflon 500 mg on canine thoracic lymph duct. *Int. Angiol.* 8:15–18.

65. Labrid, C. 1994. Pharmacologic properties of Daflon 500 mg. *Angiology* 45:524–526.

66. Labrid, C. 1995. A lymphatic function of Daflon 500 mg. *Int. Angiol.* 14:36–38.

67. Friesenecker, B., Tsai, A.G., Intaglietta, M. 1996. Cellular basis of inflammation, edema and the activity of Daflon 500 mg. *Int. J. Microcirc. Clin. Exp.* 15:17–21.

68. Molska, M., Regula, J. 2019. Potential mechanisms of probiotics action in the prevention and treatment of colorectal cancer. *Nutrients.* 11(10):2453.

69. Increasing fiber intake. https//www.ucsfhealth.org/educations/increasing-fiber-intake.

70. DiNicolantonio, J.J., O'Keefe, J.H., Wilson, W. 2018. Subclinical magnesium deficiency: a principal driver of cardiovascular disease and a public health crisis. *Open Heart* 5(1):e000668. Doi: 10.1136/openhrt-2017-000668.

71. Food and Nutrition Board, Institute of Medicine. 1997. *Magnesium. Dietary Reference Intakes: Calcium, Phosphorus, Magnesium, Vitamin D, and Fluoride.* National Academy Press, Washington DC, pp. 190–249.

72. Zhao, L., et al. 2018. Gut bacteria selectively promoted by dietary fibers alleviate type 2 diabetes. *Science* 359(6380):151–156. Doi: 10.1126/scienc.aao5774.

73. Davenport, E.R., Sanders, J.G., Song, S.J., Amato, K.R., Clark, A.G., Knight, R. 2017. The human microbiome in evolution. *BMC Biol* 15:1–2.

74. Why the Gut Microbiome Is Crucial for Your Health. Healthline April 2021.

75. Tan, J., McKiezie, C., Potamitis, M., Thorburn, A.N., Mackay, D.R., Macia, L. 2014. Chapter Three – The role of short-chain fatty acids in health and disease. *Adv. Immunol.* 121:91–124. Doi: 10.1016/B978-0-2-800100-4.00003-9.

76. Biesalski, H.K. 2020. Vitamin D deficiency and co-morbidities in COVID-19 patients – A fatal relationshsip? *NFS J.* 20:10–21. Doi: 10.2016/J.nfs.2020.06.001.

77. Callahan, A. 2018. Do I get Enough Vitamin D in the Winter? *NY Times* Feb 16 2018.

78. Wcislo, G. 2014. Chapter 95 – Resveratrol inhibitory Effects against a Malignant Tumor: a molecular introductory review. In *Polyphenols in Human Health and Disease*, Volume 2, pp. 1269–1281.

17 Vitamin G. Grounding as Energetic Nutrition and Its Role in Oxidative Defense and Cardiovascular Disease

Stephen T. Sinatra

Gaetan Chevalier

Drew Sinatra

CONTENTS

Blood Pressure Considerations 360
Grounding and the Immune System 363
Grounding and Energy...365
Summary...366
References...367

In 1977, Dr. Stephen Sinatra became a board-certified cardiologist and Dr. Peter Mitchell won the Nobel Prize a year later on energy transfer and coenzyme Q10 (CoQ10). As a practicing cardiologist for over 40 years, writing dozens of peer-reviewed articles, books, and chapters in medical textbooks, Dr. Sinatra reflected on his greatest discoveries about being a physician. Indeed, it was the utilization of Coenzyme Q10 in his patients as well as the cardiovascular implications of grounding – also known as earthing the body. These two discoveries shared common ground in that grounding and Coenzyme Q10 essentially share electron donor capabilities. This chapter is a testimony to the incredible discovery of grounding and how it transfers the natural electric charge of the planet to the body.

It was almost 15 years ago at an American College of Cardiology conference when Dr. Sinatra met Clint Ober in San Diego. Clint introduced to him the theory of grounding, and it made a lot of sense. Although he was excited about the entire concept, as well as trying to take it to a higher level, like anything else in medicine, the theory behind grounding needed intensive research. Since that encounter with Mr. Ober, more than 20 peer-reviewed articles on the benefits of grounding have become available to mainstream medicine. It took more than a decade of research and clinical investigations to validate the remarkable benefits of grounding.

Over the past four decades, Dr. Sinatra has treated hundreds of patients with acute coronary syndrome and unstable angina, as well as acute myocardial infarction. Although the utilization of thrombolytic therapies, percutaneous transluminal coronary angioplasty (PTCA), stents, and statin medications are crucial in the care of these patients, the grounding phenomena also needs to be recognized as a possible supportive therapy as our research and subsequent publications have clearly

DOI: 10.1201/9781003137849-17

demonstrated the cardiovascular benefits. This chapter will discuss the supportive cardiovascular implications such as blood pressure control, improving heart rate variability, and blood thinning. All these crucial elements reduce cardiovascular risk.

BLOOD PRESSURE CONSIDERATIONS

Although most doctors are privy to pathological situations in raising blood pressure such as coarctation of the aorta, adrenal tumors, thyroid storm, and acute renal shutdown to name a few, most hypertensive situations are of an idiopathic nature requiring pharmaceutical and lifestyle changes for appropriate control.

Over the years, Dr. Sinatra used a non-pharmaceutical approach in many of his patients utilizing Mediterranean-type diets, mind/body techniques, targeted nutritional supplements, detoxification, and low-level exercise programs. Fortunately, high blood pressure in most cases is an easy situation to control without pharmaceutical support. However, in any patient with moderate to severe hypertension with any involvement of renal insufficiency, aggressive pharmaceutical therapy needs to be considered. In many patients, simple weight loss of a mere 5–10 lbs can be therapeutic, especially when taking targeted nutraceutical supplements.

Over the past decade or so, our research group has encountered multiple anecdotal reports of patients sleeping grounded or walking barefoot on the earth who appreciated subsequent blood pressure lowering. In many of Dr. Sinatra's patients who were borderline hypertensives, sleeping grounded assuaged higher blood pressure numbers. Many other physicians reported similar results with their own patients. Although his colleagues were seeing anecdotal results, a clinical investigation needed to be done to assess blood pressure numbers with grounding methodology.

A small pilot study was performed by one of his cardiovascular colleagues, and all ten patients in the study had remarkable blood pressure lowering at the end of the trial period and several were able to discontinue their pharmaceutical medications.[1] Systolic levels decreased over this time, ranging individually from 8.6% to 22.7% with an average decrease of 14.3%. The reasons why earthing can have such a profound impact on blood pressure lowering is that it reduces inflammation and pain,[2] calms and attenuates an overactive sympathetic nervous system,[3] while simultaneously improving the electrodynamics of blood viscosity.[4] Earthing may be the easiest possible way to lower blood pressure. The most recent pilot study, combined with our clinical experience, demonstrates that people with mild to moderate hypertension can normalize with grounding interventions. In patients with moderate to severe hypertension, the reduction in pharmaceutical support has also been realized when grounding the patient. In addition to blood pressure lowering, many of Dr. Sinatra's patients commented that arrhythmia awareness was attenuated as well.

Premature ventricular contractions (PVCs) may be seen in the hypertensive individual as well as in patients who consume too much caffeine, alcohol, and even sugar. Although PVCs are generally harmless in patients with normal left ventricular function, they can create undue stress and worry for many. Several patients who slept grounded, who also had PVCs, reported sleeping better with life-changing attitudes. Perhaps that improvement in PVC awareness was related to a reduction in sympathetic tone and attenuation of the "stress response."

For example, we conducted a study of 27 patients. Grounded participants had improvements in HRV (heart rate variability) that went beyond basic relaxation (Figure 17.1).[3]

HRV refers to beat-to-beat alterations in heartrate. During resting conditions, the electrocardiogram (ECG) in normal individuals demonstrates periodic variation in R-R intervals (the R peak is the most visually obvious peak of the ECG). To simplify, "fixed" heart rates without any variation are detrimental to the cardiovascular system. Variable heart rates provide reliable, non-invasive information on the autonomic nervous system (ANS) including its sympathetic and parasympathetic components. HRV is an important indicator of the status of autonomic balance, as well as stress on the cardiovascular system.[5] A decrease in HRV indicates autonomic dysfunction and is a predictor of not only stress on the cardiovascular system, but sudden cardiac death (SCD) and progression

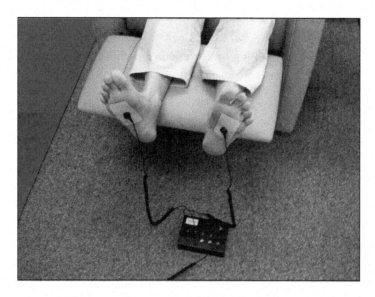

FIGURE 17.1 Grounding system showing patches, wires, and box connecting to a ground rod planted outside through a switch (not shown) and a fuse (not shown). Similar patches and wires from the hands were also connected to the box to ground the hands.

of coronary artery disease as well. The positive effects of grounding on HRV suggest that simple grounding supports the cardiovascular system. Excessive sympathetic stimulation and/or diminished vagal tone are markers of a stressed cardiovascular system. There are multiple situations that contribute to sympathetic activities including physical, emotional, behavioral, and pharmaceutical factors (Table 17.1).

Simply stated, when one grounds to the electron-enriched earth, an improved balance of the ANS occurs. Improvements in HRV can support patients with emotional stress, anxiety, fear, and any other symptoms of autonomic dystonia.

Negative emotions such as anxiety,[6] depression,[7] hostility,[8] and panic[9] have all been demonstrated to reduce HRV. Grounding has the potential to support HRV, reduce excessive sympathetic overdrive, balance the ANS, and thus attenuate the stress response. This has important prognostic considerations, especially because an association between depression and increased risk of cardiovascular events has repeatedly been observed in both the healthy population and those with established cardiovascular disease.[7] The premature infant can also benefit from earthing.

A 2017 study performed at the Pennsylvania State Children's Hospital Neonatal Intensive Care Unit in Hershey revealed that grounding premature infants produced immediate and significant improvements in measurements of the ANS.[10] Grounding improves vagal tone and may support resilience to stress which could lower the risk of neonatal mortality in preterm infants.

Grounding the babies, from 5 to 60 days of age, increased HRV indicating improved vagal tone. Grounding was achieved by adhering a grounding patch on the skin of the babies, while in their incubators or cribs, and connecting the patch wire to the hospital's grounding system. Among the babies tested, grounding raised parasympathetic tone which may enhance vagal nerve transmission and thereby improve the stress and inflammatory regulatory mechanisms in the preterm infants.

Recent research has revealed that the vagus nerve plays a major role in the so-called "anti-inflammatory reflex," a mechanism controlling basic immune responses and inflammation during pathogen invasion and tissue injury. Among other things, the nerve's actions help to inhibit excessive production of pro-inflammatory chemicals.[11,12]

Grounding, indeed, has tremendous therapeutic potential to support those in need.[13] In fact, it is perhaps the most common intervention to improve autonomic function (Table 17.2).

TABLE 17.1

Factors Contributing to Chronic Sympathetic Activation

Air pollution – ambient particulate matter <10 micron (PM (10))
Obesity
Insulin resistance, diabetes, or metabolic syndrome
Hypertension
Depression, anxiety
Congestive heart failure
Sleep apnea
Psychosocial and behavioral conditions
    Chronic stress
    Social isolation and loneliness
    Hostility, anger, or rage
    Smoking
    Sleep deprivation
    Sugar-laden diet
    Sedentary lifestyle
    Abuse of stimulants
Pharmaceutical drugs
    Short-acting calcium channel blockers
    B-agonist bronchodilators
    Peripheral alpha blockers

TABLE 17.2

Interventions to Improve Autonomic Function

Grounding to the Earth

Lifestyle modifications
    Exercise
    Social support
    Religiosity or faith
    Meditation, yoga, tai chi, qi gong
    Restoration of normal sleep
    Weight loss
    Smoking cessation
    Stress reduction, biofeedback
Medications
    B-blockers
    Angiotensin-converting enzyme inhibitors
    Omega-3 fatty acids

Revised and reprinted with permission from Curtis and O'Keefe, Jr.

But how do we explain this healing, energetic phenomenon? It is well known that the earth possesses a slightly negative charge, the result of countless lightning strikes powered by solar radiation. This planetary attribute is based on a limitless, renewable reservoir of free electrons which are negatively charged sub-atomic particles.[14,15]

The earth's charge and storehouse of electrons represent a major natural resource for health and healing. Research on biological grounding suggests that this very same electric charge on the planet's surface plays a nurturing role for both the animal and plant kingdoms. This form of electric nutrition appears to have the potential to restore and stabilize the internal environment of the human body's bioelectric systems that supervise the functions of organs, tissues, cells, and biological rhythms.[16,17]

The Schumann resonance at 7.83 Hz is an electromagnetic "vibration" in the atmosphere and a "humming" of the energetic surface of the earth. Whenever we are in contact with the earth's electron-enriched field, a transfer of electrons results in an instant and significant physiological change in the body. This Schumann resonance or the electric field of the earth is not uniform but varies from moment to moment in a rhythm that affects the motion of the electrons in the surface of the earth. Thus, the surface of the earth is electronically active and dynamic.

Behind the world that we can see and feel with our senses lies a powerful web of invisible energies and forces that affect us continuously which can be referred to as *geophysical fields*.[18] These invisible energies of the earth's gravity, magnetism, electricity, and electromagnetism have consumed centuries of human knowledge in the scientific fields of biology, physics, astronomy, astrophysics, and cosmology.

Relationships with these geophysical rhythms are vital for health. Human physiology has more than 100 biological rhythms that are timed and coordinated with rhythms in the environment.[18]

The Schumann resonance, one of the key frequencies in the grounding phenomenon (with the circadian rhythm), is a standing wave made of electromagnetic fields, vibrating at 7.83 Hz – vibrating roughly at eight times per second. Higher frequencies, produced by lightning strikes throughout the world, have also been determined by physicists and astrophysicists.

Cloud-to-earth lightning bolts pump energy into the atmosphere, creating electromagnetic waves that travel around the earth at the speed of light. The frequency of the Schumann resonance varies as the ionosphere "breathes" in and out due to atmospheric tides. Scientists have also recognized the similarity of the Schumann signal and the alpha brain wave measured with an electroencephalogram. It has been suggested that the Schumann resonance has been engrained into all life. Biologists have concluded that the frequency overlap of such resonances and biological fields is not an accidental phenomenon.[18]

GROUNDING AND THE IMMUNE SYSTEM

Scientists believe that our immune system evolved during millions of years of barefoot contact with the surface of the earth. One can assume that protective antioxidant and anti-inflammatory electrons from the earth were readily obtained by previous cultures during this vast stretch of time as a result of ordinary existence. Life involved direct contact with the earth, which is no longer the case. Something changed in our environment which disconnected us from the natural healing energy of the earth's surface.

An interesting phenomenon has occurred over the last 60 or so years with the parabolic growth of synthetic sole shoes and the growth of diabetes.[17]

Figure 17.2 demonstrates a relationship between the shoe-driven disconnection from the earth's natural electric charge and the inflammation-related disease diabetes. It is an interesting phenomenon in which sales of shoes with synthetic soles have increased in the United States since the 1950s. The curve of walking on synthetic shoes is similar to the curve of diabetes mellitus. As an antidote, Dr. Sinatra can remember when he was 8 years old walking to third-grade elementary school on leather shoes. That was approximately 66 years ago. Before the mid-1950s, 95% of the shoes were made with leather soles, many of which were conducting the Schumann resonance. Currently, 95% or more of shoes have synthetic, non-conductive, mostly rubber-like soles. The interesting question, observation, or perhaps coincidence arises. Is there a correlation between us being ungrounded walking on non-conductive shoes and the alarming increase in the rise of diabetes, as well as other inflammatory conditions? Could the combination of foods which are laden with sugar and other high-fructose corn syrup sweeteners, in combination with a lack of exercise and being ungrounded, perhaps create the perfect storm for diabetes to emerge? Obviously, physicians have documented

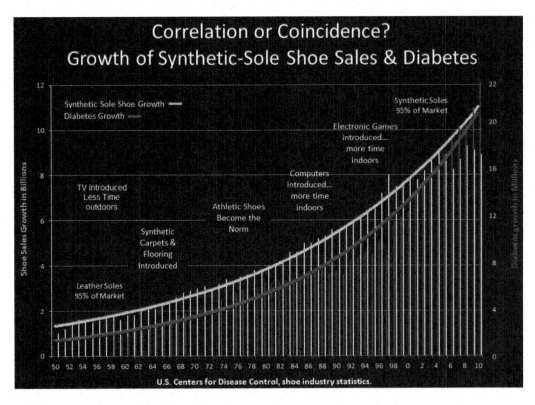

FIGURE 17.2 U.S. Centers for Disease Control, shoe industry statistics.

the profound connection of heart disease and the diabetic relationship. Although diabetes with high blood sugar concentrations is a significant risk factor for cardiovascular disease, perhaps the diabetic connection of a less optimal blood viscosity is an even more meaningful risk factor to consider.

The electrophoretic activity of red blood cells is a function of net negative charge or zeta potential. In other words, the more the net negative charge on red blood cells, the more they repel each other, and the more robust the zeta potential.[4]

In a study of 50 patients with occlusive arterial disease and 50 control counterparts ($N = 100$), the migration time of red cells (seconds) was longer, and the electrophoretic mobility was less in the patients with occlusive disease than in the healthy controls. This study on electrophoretic mobility suggested differences in RBC surface charge (zeta potential). The researchers concluded that patients with occlusive arterial disease have one or more factors in their plasma and RBCs that reduce the net negative charge zeta potential – of the cells, thereby facilitating RBC aggregation.[19] This finding supports the notion that there are many factors that can reduce zeta potential, thereby increasing blood viscosity and increasing RBC aggregation, both of which play a major role in the pathogenesis of arteriosclerosis.

A meta-analysis evaluating the connection between blood viscosity and cardiovascular disease (CVD) demonstrates clearly that the risk of major cardiovascular events increases with higher blood-viscosity levels.[20] In the Edinburgh Artery Study, a population of 4,860 men 45–59 years of age was observed for 5 years. The 20% of men with the highest blood viscosity had a 3.2 times greater risk for cardiac events, compared with the 20% of men with the lowest blood viscosity. 55% of major cardiovascular events occurred in the highest blood-viscosity group versus only 4% in the lowest blood-viscosity group.[21]

The role of increased blood viscosity in the pathogenesis of occlusive arterial disease was clearly and succinctly described by Kensey.[22] Endothelial dysfunction, mechanical shear forces, and alterations in blood flow mechanics at arterial bifurcations and areas of low blood flow eddies are correlated with plaque progression in the coronary vasculature. Similarly, blood viscosity is known to increase in numerous clinical situations, such as hypertension, smoking, lipid disorders, advancing age, and diabetes mellitus.

A 2008 study was the first to report on the zeta potential of red blood cells in patients with diabetes.[23] Researchers from the University of Calcutta described a "remarkable alteration" in the electrodynamics of RBCs – a progressive deterioration of the zeta potential and hypercoagulability among patients with diabetes, which was even worse among those who also had CVD. The researchers also indicated that high blood sugar levels are associated with significant alterations in the electrodynamics of an RBC's outer membrane and may increase the potential for RBC clumping. It was concluded that zeta potential could and should be used as an indicator of cardiovascular disease in patients who have diabetes.[23]

On the basis of a randomized placebo-controlled primary prevention trial (the West of Scotland Coronary Prevention Study), researchers suggested that pravastatin therapy may lower the risk for coronary heart disease and mortality partially by lowering both plasma viscosity and blood viscosity.[24] Many subsequent investigations have demonstrated the pleiotropic effects of statins on blood rheology, including reductions in plasma viscosity,[25] whole-blood viscosity, RBC deformities, and RBC aggregation.[26]

Attenuating inflammation and reducing blood viscosity will help physicians address primary and secondary prevention issues. Blood viscosity can be modified through numerous recognized primary prevention strategies. Moderate exercise, dietary adjustments (low sodium and sugar intake, and no trans fats), smoking cessation, and blood donation all have a positive impact on viscosity as do specific blood viscosity-modifying supplements, such as omega-3 essential fatty acids and pharmaceutical drugs (statins).

Grounding to the earth represents yet another invention that lowers blood viscosity by raising zeta potential, which results in a decrease in RBC aggregation.[4] The earth's surface is electrically conductive and is maintained at a negative potential by a global electrical circuit. This circuit has three main generators: the solar wind entering the **magnetosphere**, the ionospheric wind, and thunderstorms. An estimated 1,000–2,000 thunderstorms are continually active around the globe, emitting thousands of lightning strikes per minute. This creates a constant current of thousands of amperes transferring positive charge to the upper atmosphere and negative charge to the surface of the earth.[27] The earth's surface is therefore an abundant source of free electrons. As soil electrons are conducted to the human body, the grounded body assumes favorable physiologic and electrophysiologic changes. Attenuation of the inflammatory response and a favorable impact on blood viscosity and RBC aggregation have been the most significant findings.

Increased blood viscosity in the general population may be a predictor of cardiovascular events because of its influences on hypertension, thrombogenesis, ischemia, and atherogenesis. Unfortunately, blood viscosity has become a forgotten risk factor and is rarely measured in clinical practice.[28] Interventions that reduce blood viscosity and RBC aggregation are important. Statins appear to be effective for modulating blood viscosity but can have serious side effects, including death. Moreover, many patients have some degree of statin intolerance.[29]

GROUNDING AND ENERGY

The search for evidence-based improvements without significant risk will continue in the healing arts. It has been suggested that a system-wide network or electronic living matrix, a semi-conductor network capable of rapid charge transfer throughout the body, will someday be recognized in the healing profession.[30]

Connective tissues, myofascial, tendons, cell membranes, and cellular cytoskeletal networks belong to this electronic infrastructure. The multiple pathways of this living matrix facilitate the influx of free electrons to reach and neutralize free radicals that are the hallmark of chronic inflammation. Not only that, but this arrangement also helps explain why many grounded individuals feel better and more energized. It seems logical to suggest that the influx of electrons from the earth saturates their mitochondrial electron transport chains that generate adenosine triphosphate (ATP), the energy molecule that powers all of life's activities.

We believe in the energetic nature of the contribution of adenosine triphosphate (ATP) providing the vital energy source for life. As a cardiologist, Dr. Sinatra utilized ATP-supporting ingredients such as D-ribose, coenzyme Q10, L-carnitine, and magnesium as a way of biochemically driving ATP in a preferential direction. It is a simple concept, whenever you promote the body's energy source (ATP), you are optimizing the energy production in the heart as well as the body. Although the nutritional approach to improve the bioenergetics of the nutrient-starved heart has been life-saving for many of his patients, the concept of grounding also has provided relief. Earthing provides another primary source of cellular restoration and energy by supporting the mitochondria, microscopic power plants that literally provide energy to the cell.

Inside the mitochondrial complex, electrons are passed along through an assembly line of enzymes creating ATP. When the body becomes in contact with the electrons from the Mother Earth, the limitless supply of energy is absorbed into the body. Earthing may perhaps be a way to transfer electrons and fortify mitochondria, thus contributing to optimum levels of ATP production in all our cells. The heart is all about ATP, and effective healing in any form of cardiovascular disease requires the restoration of the heart's ATP production. Sick hearts leak out and lose vital ATP. Any cardiac condition such as angina, heart failure, silent ischemia, mitral valve prolapse, and diastolic dysfunction can also result in some form of ATP deficit. The Mother Earth's energy may indeed come to the rescue of vulnerable heart cells.

Grounding or earthing is virtually harmless while having incredible health implications at the same time. Blood pressure lowering, supportive HRV, and thinning the blood are significant contributions in reducing cardiovascular risk including heart attack and even SCD. One caveat of grounding is to exercise caution in anyone taking Coumadin-like blood thinners as the combination of pharmaceutical blood thinning and grounding can virtually make the blood too thin. Cardiologists have seen such cases of excessive blood thinning in their patients. When patients take Coumadin-like derivatives, it is imperative that they discuss earthing or grounding with their doctor to avoid the possibility of any complications.[4]

SUMMARY

New research indicates that grounding the body generates broad, beneficial, and significant physiological changes. The source of these effects is believed to be the mobile electrons omnipresent on the surface of the earth, which are responsible for the planet's negative charge. Lifestyle changes have disconnected most humans from this primordial health and healing resource, creating what may be an unrecognized electron deficiency in the body, an overlooked cause or contributor to chronic inflammation and common chronic and degenerative diseases. High blood pressure, disturbed HRV, and hyperviscosity are cardiovascular situations that can be improved with grounding.

When the earth connection is restored through grounding, electrons flood throughout the body, reducing inflammation and oxidative stress while also reinforcing the body's own defense mechanisms. Electron transfers are the basis of virtually all antioxidant and anti-inflammatory activities. And the earth may very well be the ultimate supplier! When the supply is restored, humans have the potential to thrive.[4]

Earthing or grounding may someday become one of the everyday tools of the conventional cardiologist as well as the everyday healers that see patients on a day-to-day basis. In 2021, it is still in its infancy and more research is presently being done. When physicians recommend evidence-based, harmless, and simple therapeutic natural interventions to reduce human suffering and improve quality of life, we have done our job in the interest of the patient. Almost a century ago, Dr. Peabody stated that "The most important aspect in the care of the patient is the care of the patient."[31] Indeed, grounding with its many profound effects will become not only instrumental but also vital in the care of the patient.

REFERENCES

1. Elkin HK, Winter A. 2018. Grounding patients with hypertension improves blood pressure: A case history series study. *Altern Therapies* 24(6):46–50.
2. Ghaly M, Teplitz D. 2004. The biological effects of grounding the human body during sleep, as measured by cortisol levels and subjective reporting of sleep, pain, and stress. *J Altern Complement Med* 10(5):767–776.
3. Chevalier G, Sinatra ST. 2011. Emotional stress, heart rate variability, grounding and improved autonomic tone: Clinical applications. *Integ Med* 10(3):16–21.
4. Chevalier G, Sinatra ST, Oschman JL, et al. 2013. Earthing (grounding) the human body reduces blood viscosity – a major factor in cardiovascular disease. *J Altern Complement Med* 19(2):102–110.
5. Kleiger RE, Bigger JT, Bosner MS, et al. 1991. Stability over time of variables measuring heart rate variability in normal subjects. *Am J Cardiol* 68(6):626–630.
6. Kawachi I, Colditz GA, Asherio A, et al. 1994. Prospective study of phobic anxiety and risk of coronary heart disease in men. *Circulation* 89(5):1992–1997.
7. Carney RM, Freedland KE. 2009. Depression and heart rate variability in patients with coronary heart disease. *Cleve Clin J Med* 76(Suppl 2):S13–S17.
8. Sloan RP, Shapiro PA, Bigger JT Jr, et al. 1994. Cardiac autonomic control and hostility in healthy subjects. *Am J Cardiol* 74(3):298–300.
9. Yeragani VK, Pohl R, Berger R. 1993. Decreased heart rate variability in panic disorder patients: A study of power-spectral analysis of heart rate. *Psychiatry Res* 46(1):89–103.
10. Passi R, Doheny KK, Gordin Y, et al. 2017. Electrical grounding improves vagal tone in preterm infants. *Neonatology* 112(2):187–192.
11. Thayer J. 2009. Vagal tone and the inflammatory reflex. *Cleve Clin J Med* 76(suppl 2):S23–S26.
12. Schoemaker R, Eisel U. 2015. Chapter 5: Cross Talk between the brain and inflammation. In: Blankesteijn M, Altara R, eds. *Inflammation in Heart Failure*. Boston, MA, Academic Press. pp. 81–91.
13. Sokal K, Sokal P. 2011. Earthing the human body influences physiologic processes. *J Altern Complement Med* 17(4):301–308.
14. Williams E, Heckman S. 1993. The local diurnal variation of cloud electrification and the global diurnal variation of negative charge on the Earth. *J Geophys Res* 98(D3):5221–5234.
15. Anisimov S, Mareev E, Bakastov S. 1999. On the generation and evolution of aeroelectric structures in the surface layer. *J Geophy Res* 104(D12):14359–14367.
16. Oschman J. 2008. Perspective: Assume a spherical cow: The role of free or mobile electrons in bodywork, energetic and movement therapies. *J Bodywork Movement Ther* 12:40–57.
17. Sinatra ST, Oschman JL, Chevelier G, et al. 2017. Electric nutrition: The surprising health and healing benefits of biological grounding (earthing). *Altern Ther* 23(5):8–16.
18. Palmer JD. 2002. *The Living Clock: The Orchestrator of Biological Rhythms*. Oxford, United Kingdom: Oxford University Press.
19. Begg TB, Wade IM, Bronte-Stewart B. 1966. The red cell electrophoretic mobility in atherosclerotic and other individuals. *J Atheroscler Res* 6:303–312.
20. Danesh J, Collins R, Peto R, et al. 2000. Haematocrit, viscosity, erythrocyte sedimentation rate: Meta-analysis of prospective studies of coronary heart disease. *Eur Heart J* 21:515–520.
21. Lowe GD, Lee AJ, Rumley A, et al. 1997. Blood viscosity and risk of cardiovascular events: The Edinburgh Artery Study. *Br J Haematol* 96:168–173.
22. Kensey KR. 2003. Rheology: An overlooked component of vascular disease. *Clin Appl Thromb/ Hemostasis* 9:93–99.
23. Adak S, Chowdhury S, Bhattacharyya M. 2008. Dynamic and electrokinetic behavior of erythrocyte membrane in diabetes mellitus and diabetic cardiovascular disease. *Biochim Biophys Acta* 1780:108–115.
24. Lowe G, Rumley A. Norrie J, et al. 2001. Blood rheology, cardiovascular risk factors, and cardiovascular disease: The West of Scotland Coronary Prevention Study. *Thromb Haemost* 85:946.
25. Doncheva NI, Nikolov KV, Vassileva DP. 2006. Lipid-modifying and pleiotropic effects of gemfibrozil, simvastatin, and pravastatin in patient in patients with dyslipidemia. *Folia Med (Plodiv)* 48(3–4):56–61.
26. Muravyov AV, Yakusevick VV, Surovaya L, et al. 2004. The effect of simvastatin therapy on hemorheological profile in coronary heart disease (CHD) patients. *Clin Hemorheol Microcirc* 31:251–256.

27. Christian HJ, Blakeslee RJ, Boccippio DJ, Boeck WL, Dennis E. Buechler DE et al. Global frequency and distribution of lightning as observed from space by the optieal transient detector. *J Geophys Res* 2003; 108:(D1):4-1–4-15.
28. Kesmarky G, Kenyeres P, Rabai M, et al. 2008. Plasma viscosity: A forgotten variable. *Clin Hemorheol Micro* 39(1–4):243–246.
29. Golomb BA, Evans MA. 2008. Statin adverse effects: a review of the literature and evidence for a mitochondrial mechanism. *Am J Cardiovasc Drugs* 8:373–418.
30. Oschman J. 2009. Charge transfer in the living matrix. *J Bodywork Movement Ther* 13:215–228.
31. Peabody FW. 1927. The care of the patient. *JAMA* 88(12):877–882.

18 The Role of Botanicals in Cardiovascular Health

Tieraona Low Dog

CONTENTS

Introduction...370
Cardiovascular Tonics..370
    Khella Dried Ripe Fruit and Seed (*Ammi visnaga* L.)...370
    Arjuna Tree Bark (*Terminalia arjuna* Roxb. ex DC.)...370
    Hawthorn Berry, Flower, and Leaf (*Crataegus* spp.)..370
    Garlic (*Allium sativum* L.)..371
    Grape Seed (*Vitis vinifera* L.)..372
Anti-Hypertensives...372
    Hibiscus Calyces (*Hibiscus sabdariffa* L.)..373
    Beetroot (*Beta vulgaris* L.)..373
Nervine Relaxants...374
    Lemon Balm Leaf (*Melissa officinalis* L.)..374
    Motherwort Herb (*Leonurus cardiaca* L.)..374
Vascular Tonics...375
    Horse Chestnut (*Aesculus hippocastanum* L.)..375
    Pycnogenol..375
Quality of Botanical Products...376
Summary..376
References..376

INTRODUCTION

Botanical medicine, also referred to as herbal medicine or phytotherapy, utilizes plants, plant parts, and preparations made from them for therapeutic and/or preventive purposes. The role of plants in the management of cardiovascular disease has been a long and distinguished one. Thousands of years ago, it was noted that lily-of-the-valley (*Convallaria majalis* L.), sea squill (*Drimia maritima* (L.) Stearn), and foxglove (*Digitalis purpurea* L.) could ease the suffering from dropsy, an older term for congestive heart failure (CHF), due to the presence of cardioactive glycosides. Hawthorn (*Crataegus* spp.) was noted to benefit the aging heart centuries ago. Foxglove would eventually serve as the source for standardized digitalis, a drug still in use today (Norn 2004). Our first truly effective antihypertensive drug, reserpine, was extracted from *Rauwolfia serpentina*, a plant with a long history of use in Ayurveda, the traditional medicine of India, for the treatment of anxiety, insanity, and venomous bites (Griebenow et al. 1997).

Other significant advances in plant research include the finding that plant sterols and stanols can lower LDL-cholesterol. These are often added to food products as part of a "heart-healthy" dietary approach. The monounsaturated fat in olive oil and multiple constituents in garlic and grape seed have been shown to be beneficial for the cardiovascular system when consumed as part of a healthy diet. Hibiscus and beetroot lower blood pressure. From the broad to the narrow, from crude plant to highly refined extracts, the field of botanical medicine has much to offer for the promotion of cardiovascular wellbeing.

It is beyond the scope of this chapter to cover all the botanicals that could be considered when discussing cardiovascular health. Instead, we will focus on the dominant plants that fall into four key categories: cardiac tonics, anti-hypertensives, nervine relaxants, and vascular tonics. We will conclude with a brief discussion of botanical quality.

CARDIOVASCULAR TONICS

While there is no exact western pharmaceutical equivalent, cardiac tonics were traditionally used to strengthen the aging heart and treat mild forms of CHF, with more severe cases treated with plants rich in cardioactive glycosides (e.g., foxglove, squill). These tonics were considered mild in action and intended to be taken over time. There are three botanicals that stand out across the globe: from the European tradition is hawthorn; from Ayurveda, arjuna bark; and khella from the Middle East/ Mediterranean region. Based upon modern clinical research, garlic and grape seed should also be included in this category, as their cardiovascular effects are mild, health promoting, and relatively broad.

KHELLA DRIED RIPE FRUIT AND SEED (*AMMI VISNAGA* L.)

Papyrus writings from Egypt describe the ancient use of the dried ripe fruit and seeds of khella dried ripe fruit for alleviating renal colic, angina, abdominal pain, and bronchial asthma. These effects are due primarily to the constituents visnadin, visnagin, and khellin. Visnagin acts as a calcium channel blocker, inhibiting vascular smooth muscle contraction, dilating coronary vessels, and increasing coronary circulation (Bhagavathula et al. 2015). Khellin facilitates the passage of kidney stones, relieving renal colic (Khalil et al. 2020), while the asthma drug cromolyn is a synthetic derivative of khellin (Mali and Dhake 2011). While this plant has a long history of use and modern preclinical evidence supports many of its historical uses, there are no clinical trials evaluating its efficacy in cardiovascular disease.

ARJUNA TREE BARK (*TERMINALIA ARJUNA* ROXB. EX DC.)

Arjuna has been used to treat angina and heart failure for more than 2,500 years (Narayana and Kumaraswamy 1996). It is rich in bioactive triterpenoids and flavonoids. Preclinical evidence and small clinical trials confirm that this plant has anti-atherogenic, hypotensive, inotropic, anti-inflammatory, antithrombotic and antioxidant activities (Kapoor et al. 2014). A systematic review of five randomized studies evaluated the use of arjuna bark alone, or in combination with conventional therapies, in patients with stable angina. The dose used in most studies was 500 mg of the bark taken twice daily. Overall, the studies were of poor methodology, and the reviewers concluded that "currently the evidence is insufficient to draw any definite conclusions in favor of or against *Terminalia arjuna* in patients of chronic stable angina" and called for larger, more rigorous clinical trials (Kaur et al. 2014). There is also some research that demonstrates mild hypotensive and hypolipidemic activities. No serious side effects have been noted with arjuna, but long-term safety has not been determined (Dwivedi and Chopra 2014).

HAWTHORN BERRY, FLOWER, AND LEAF (*CRATAEGUS* SPP.)

By far the most familiar and popular cardiac tonic is hawthorn, a flowering shrub in the rose family, treasured by physicians and herbalists for more than two thousand years for strengthening the aging heart, and as a relaxant and sleep aid. Hawthorn is widely accepted in Europe as a treatment for CHF. Hawthorn berries, leaves, and flowers have all been used medicinally, and research shows that they are phytochemically similar in composition, differing primarily in the ratio of specific fla-vonoids and procyanidins (Tassell et al. 2010). Some products contain only one of these three plant parts; sometimes two or all three are combined.

Preclinical data demonstrates that hawthorn extract increases the release of nitric oxide (NO) from the endothelium and potentially inhibits its degradation. Chronic administration has been shown to lead to a dose-dependent increase in myocardial blood flow, as well as reducing smooth muscle cell migration and proliferation (Holubarsch et al. 2018).

There have been numerous clinical studies evaluating the benefit of hawthorn in CHF. The SPICE trial was the largest, being conducted in 13 European countries. Researchers randomized 2,681 patients with New York Heart Association (NYHA) class II–III heart failure and a left-ventricular ejection fraction (LVEF) < 35% to receive either 900 mg/day of hawthorn extract (WS 1442, 4–6.6:1 dry extract of hawthorn flowers and leaves, containing 17.3%–20.1% oligomeric procyanidins) or placebo as an add-on therapy for 2 years (Holubarsch et al. 2007). Patients continued taking their medications with 90% of participants taking at least three concomitant cardioactive drugs: ~85% of the patients in each group were taking diuretics, 83% were taking angiotensin-converting enzyme (ACE) inhibitors, 64% were being treated with β-blockers, and 56% were administered digitalis or nitrates; concomitant antiarrhythmics were used by about 22% of the study participants.

Overall, no beneficial effect was noted between the two groups in any of the primary outcomes. However, in a prospectively planned subgroup analysis, those in the WS1442 group with an LVEF of 25%–35% had a lower cumulative risk of cardiac mortality and sudden cardiac death, suggesting a potential antiarrhythmic and/or anti-ischemic effect, effects observed in animal models. In this trial, almost 50% of the study subjects were diagnosed with NYHA class III heart failure. Given the dose-dependent effects of hawthorn, one must question if the dose of 900 mg/day was adequate.

After reviewing the randomized, double-blinded, placebo-controlled trials of hawthorn extract for CHF, including the aforementioned study, Cochrane reviewers concluded that when taken in totality, the evidence "suggests that there is a significant benefit in symptom control and physiologic outcomes from hawthorn extract as an adjunctive treatment for chronic heart failure" (Pittler et al. 2008). Given its excellent safety profile and lack of interaction with cardiac medications, hawthorn extracts may play a particularly beneficial role for those with milder forms of CHF with an LVEF of 25%–40% (Holubarsch et al. 2018). Given the extensive research on the special extract WS1442, clinicians should consider its use.

GARLIC (*ALLIUM SATIVUM* L.)

Garlic is widely consumed in cuisines around the globe. This member of the *Allium* family, which includes onions and leeks, is also a very popular herbal supplement being promoted for both immune and cardiovascular health. The evidence suggests that garlic in various forms (e.g., aged garlic, garlic powder) treats mild hypertension (Alali et al. 2017), reduces low-grade systemic inflamma-tion (Quesada et al. 2020), and possesses anti-atherosclerotic properties (Orekhov et al. 2013). Two key constituents have been identified in garlic, allicin and γ-glutamyl-*S*-allylcysteine (GSAC), both exerting angiotensin II-inhibiting and vasodilating effects (Hamal et al. 2020).

Garlic has been studied for its impact on blood pressure. The hypotensive activity is likely due to its interaction with hydrogen sulfide- and NO-signaling pathways (Ried and Fakler 2014). A meta-analysis of randomized controlled trials (RCTs) reported a significant effect of garlic on blood pressure, with an average decrease in systolic blood pressure (SBP) of 8.6 mmHg and diastolic blood pressure (DBP) of 6.1 mmHg in participants with hypertension ($n=14$ trial arms, $n=468$ partici-pants) (Ried 2016).

Arterial stiffness contributes to hypertension and is an important predictor of cardiovascular risk. In 2018, a 12-week, double-blind, randomized, placebo-controlled trial of 49 participants with uncontrolled hypertension reported that aged-garlic-extract (Kyolic: 1.2 g/day containing 1.2 mg S-allylcysteine) significantly reduced SBP by 10 ± 3.6 mmHg and DBP by 5.4 ± 2.3 mmHg, compared to placebo. Garlic also significantly reduced central blood pressure, pulse pressure, and arterial stiffness ($p<0.05$). Interestingly, this study also noted that the garlic extract increased microbial diversity in the gut, with a marked increase in *Lactobacillus* and *Clostridia* species (Ried et al. 2018).

The AMAR (Atherosclerosis Monitoring and Atherogenicity Reduction) was a double-blinded, placebo-controlled study that randomized 196 asymptomatic men aged 40–74 to receive 150 mg twice daily of time-released garlic powder (Allicor, INAT-Farma) or placebo for 2 years to evaluate the progression of carotid atherosclerosis. The mean rate of carotid intima-media thickness (IMT) changes in the garlic-treated group (-0.022 ± 0.007 mm/year) was significantly different ($P=0.002$) from the placebo group in which there was a moderate progression of 0.015 ± 0.008 mm. These results suggest that long-term consumption of time-released garlic powder may have a direct anti-atherosclerotic effect on carotid atherosclerosis (Orekhov et al. 2013).

Garlic is very well tolerated in clinical trials. There have been a small number of case reports of postoperative bleeding in patients taking garlic prior to surgery (Wang et al. 2015); however, in 2017, a systematic review failed to note any change in warfarin pharmacokinetic or pharmacodynamics with garlic (Choi et al. 2017). Most of these studies were conducted using aged garlic extracts, and results may not apply to other forms of garlic supplements.

GRAPE SEED (*VITIS VINIFERA* L.)

Grapes, especially grape seeds, are a rich source of potent polyphenol antioxidants that may have a beneficial effect on numerous risk factors involved in the metabolic syndrome such as hyperlipidemia, hyperglycemia, and hypertension (Akaberi and Hosseinzadeh 2016). Grape seed oil is growing in popularity as a heart-healthy cooking oil. Some research shows that, compared to sunflower seed oil, grape seed oil modestly improves insulin resistance and reduces C-reactive protein in overweight/obese women (Irandoost et al. 2013). Preclinical research shows that grape seed extract (GSE) can reduce the development of obesity and its altered metabolic pathways by improving adipokine secretion and oxidative stress (Junsong et al. 2014). GSE also inhibits lipid digestion and absorption, which has a beneficial effect on lipids (Adisakwattana et al. 2010).

Two randomized, placebo-controlled studies suggest that 300 mg/day of GSE (standardized to 90%–95% procyanidins) is beneficial for improving inflammatory mediators and reducing visceral adiposity and LDL-cholesterol lipids in overweight and obese individuals (Parandoosh et al. 2020, Yousefi et al. 2021). This beneficial effect on lipids has been demonstrated in numerous studies. A meta-analysis of 11 randomized, controlled trials ($n=536$ participants) found that GSE significantly reduced LDL-cholesterol and triglycerides (Anjom-Shoae et al. 2020).

Studies show that GSE can lower blood pressure in pre- and stage 1 hypertension. GSE increases prostacyclin (PGI2) and endothelium-derived NO, leading to vasodilation (Pons et al. 2016). A meta-analysis of 16 clinical trials ($n=810$ participants) found GSE supplementation led to significant reductions in SBP (WMD$=-6.077$; $P=0.011$) and DBP (WMD$=-2.803$; $P=0.001$), particularly in overweight/obese participants and those with metabolic syndrome (Zhang et al. 2016).

Grape seed extracts appear to be well tolerated. There is a theoretical risk of bleeding if taken with anticoagulant or antiplatelet medications. A study of nine commercial GSE products found that there is little to no interaction with CYP3A4, and adverse effects are not likely to occur if GSE is taken concomitantly with drugs metabolized by this enzyme system (Wanwimolruk et al. 2014).

ANTI-HYPERTENSIVES

There are numerous plants that have been studied for their hypotensive activity. Research confirms that some commonly used botanicals act as diuretics. For example, parsley seed (*Petroselinum crispum* Mill.) reduces the activity of Na^+–K^+ ATPase in the renal cortex and medulla, leading to a reduction in sodium and potassium, resulting in osmotic water flow into the lumen and diuresis

(Kreydiyyeh and Usta 2002). Celery seed (*Apium graveolens* L.) was shown in a rat model to reduce BP, via diuresis and inhibition of intracellular calcium influx (Moghadam et al. 2013).

Other botanicals appear to lower blood pressure via calcium channel blockade, inhibition of angiotensin-converting enzyme (ACE-I), and/or acting as vasodilators via NO pathways. As we've discussed the hypotensive activity of garlic and GSE, let's turn our attention to hibiscus and beetroot.

HIBISCUS CALYCES (*HIBISCUS SABDARIFFA* L.)

Hibiscus is consumed in the Middle East, Central and South America, India, and other parts of the world, as both a tasty beverage and herbal medicine. The ruby red-colored hibiscus calyces (outer parts of the flower) are sour in taste, hence its other common name, sour tea (Asgary et al. 2016). The calyces are a rich source of polyphenols, anthocyanins, and flavonoids – compounds with beneficial effects on the cardiovascular system (Aziz et al. 2013).

Hibiscus inhibits calcium influx and ACE, while reducing inflammation (Beltrán-Debón et al. 2015). A review of ten clinical trials found a significant decrease in SBP ranging from 6.3 to 31.9 mmHg and a decrease in DBP ranged from 1.1 to 19.7 mmHg. In comparative studies, a standardized hibiscus extract (9.62 mg of total anthocyanins/dose/day) was as effective as captopril and hydrochlorothiazide (HCTZ), but less effective than lisinopril (Walton et al. 2016). Heterogeneity in trial design precluded combination of the results.

Given that hibiscus is widely consumed as a beverage, researchers have examined the antihypertensive activity when taken as a tisane (herbal tea). A randomized, double-blind, placebo-controlled clinical trial involving 65 pre- and mildly hypertensive adults (30–70 years) not taking blood pressure-lowering medications, found that three 240 mL servings per day of brewed hibiscus tea (1.25 g hibiscus per 240 mL) lowered SBP compared with placebo (-7.2 ± 11.4 vs. -1.3 ± 10.0 mm Hg; $P = 0.030$). Participants with higher SBP at baseline showed a greater response to hibiscus treatment ($r = -0.421$ for SBP change; $P = 0.01$). Researchers concluded that hibiscus tea in an amount readily incorporated into the diet lowers BP in pre- and mildly hypertensive adults (McKay et al. 2010).

Hibiscus has a long-standing traditional use as a beverage and is considered safe. A review of the toxicology studies suggest that doses of 200 mg/kg should be safe and data from preclinical and clinical studies failed to provide substantiated evidence of any therapeutically relevant drug interaction potential of commonplace teas or beverages containing hibiscus and its preparations (Da-Costa-Rocha et al. 2014).

BEETROOT (*BETA VULGARIS* L.)

Beetroot is gaining popularity for its purported benefits on cardiovascular function and athletic performance. In fact, the global market for beetroot juice is increasing by 5% per year and shows no signs of slowing (Zamani et al. 2021). Beetroots, like spinach, lettuce, chard, and radishes, are a rich source of inorganic nitrates. Approximately 25% of the nitrate that enters the circulation from the gut becomes concentrated in the salivary glands through active uptake by the sialin transporter, and the rest is excreted by the kidneys (Gee and Ahluwalia 2016). Upon interaction with oral bacteria, nitrate is reduced to nitrite, swallowed, and absorbed, increasing plasma nitrite levels. Endogenous nitrite reductases reduce plasma nitrite to the bioactive nitric oxide (NO), which acts as a vasodilator (Lundberg et al. 2008). Of interest, antiseptic mouthwashes may eliminate up to 94% of the oral commensal bacteria that reduce nitrate to nitrite. Clinical trials show that the effects of antihypertensive drugs are inhibited (totally or partially) in subjects using this type of mouthwash (Oliveira-Paula et al. 2019).

A meta-analysis of placebo-controlled, double-blind, randomized, controlled trials found that beetroot juice consumption (daily doses ranging from 321 to 2,790 mg) is associated with dose-dependent changes in SBP with a mean reduction of 4.4 mmHg ($P < 0.001$) (Siervo et al. 2013).

Another review of nine crossover trials and three parallel trails found that both inorganic nitrate and beetroot consumption are associated with an improvement in vascular function (Lara et al. 2016).

There are no safety issues with consumption of beetroot, beetroot juice, or powdered beets. Beeturia, a reddish hue in the urine, occurs in roughly 10%–14% of the population who consume beets; it is harmless (Watts et al. 1993).

NERVINE RELAXANTS

Nervine relaxants are those herbs that have a calmative effect. As chronic stress and depression have both been associated with increased risk of cardiovascular disease, practitioners of herbal medicine often include a nervine relaxant in their treatment protocol. There are many to choose from such as linden (*Tilia europaea* L.), passionflower (*Passiflora incarnata* L.), and valerian (*Valeriana officinalis* L.). However, there are two that are highly specific to the cardiovascular system: lemon balm and motherwort.

Lemon Balm Leaf (*Melissa officinalis* L.)

Lemon balm, a lovely aromatic member of the mint family, is a rich source of polyphenols, flavonoids, monoterpenes, and sesquiterpenes. It has a very long history of medicinal use, stretching back more than 2,000 years. Known by names such as "heart's delight" and the "gladdening herb", the renowned Persian physician Avicenna (980–1037 CE) praised its calming, uplifting, and beneficial effects upon the heart. It was said to calm the heart, easing palpitations. Preclinical data demonstrate antiarrhythmogenic, negative chronotropic and dromotropic, hypotensive, vasorelaxant, and infarct size-reducing effects (Draginic et al. 2021).

A randomized, doubled-blinded, placebo-controlled study found that patients taking 1000 mg two times daily of lemon balm freeze-dried aqueous extract reduced episodes of heart palpitations by 36%, compared to a 4.2% reduction in the placebo group ($P < 0.0001$). No side effects or changes in laboratory parameters were reported (Alijaniha et al. 2015).

Three additional randomized, double-blinded, placebo-controlled trials conducted in patients with type 2 diabetes reported improvement in various cardiovascular outcomes including HDL-C, triglycerides, high-sensitivity C-reactive protein (hs-CRP), SBP, and DBP (Asadi et al. 2018, 2019, Nayebi et al. 2019). One open-label study in 28 healthy Japanese adults (31–65 years) reported significant reductions in brachial-ankle pulse wave velocity, suggesting a beneficial effect on arterial stiffness (Yui et al. 2017).

There are no significant safety concerns associated with lemon balm. The dose used in most studies was 700–1,000 mg of lemon balm taken twice daily, generally as an aqueous extract.

Motherwort Herb (*Leonurus cardiaca* L.)

Motherwort, a member of the mint family, has long been valued for its beneficial effects upon the heart, hence the species name "*cardiaca*." It has been used as a condiment in various vegetable soup recipes, particularly lentil and split pea, and in flavoring beer and tea. Motherwort remains popular for those with nervous palpitations or hypertension with a nervous, anxious component. Alkaloids in motherwort, stachydrine and leonurine, are mildly sedating, relaxing vascular smooth muscle tone via the inhibition of calcium influx and release of intracellular Ca^{2+} (Chen and Kwan 2001). Lavandulifolioside, another constituent in motherwort, has been shown to have negative chronotropic and hypotensive effects (Miłkowska-Leyck et al. 2002). Based upon long-standing use, the European Medicines Agency states that motherwort preparations can be used to relieve symptoms of nervous tension and nervous conditions of the heart such as palpitations, after serious conditions have been excluded by a medical doctor (EMA 2019a).

A 4-week open prospective study enrolled 50 patients (aged 18–75) with stage 1 or 2 arterial hypertension accompanied by anxiety and insomnia. The researchers examined the effects of motherwort administered in two 300 mg soft gel capsules (1:10 extract in soybean oil; 0.15 mg iridoids) taken twice daily. A statistically significant decrease in SBP and DBP was reported. A significant improvement in the symptoms of anxiety and depression was observed in 32% of patients, a moderate improvement in 48%, a weak effect in 8%, while 12% did not respond to the therapy. A tendency to a decrease in heart rate (from 81.7 to 75.4 beats per minute) was observed but was not statistically significant (Shikov et al. 2011). While the study suffers from lack of blinding and placebo arm, it is consistent with the historical use of motherwort.

There are no significant safety concerns associated with motherwort; however, it is contraindicated in pregnancy due to possible uterine stimulation. The total daily of motherwort is 3–10 g/day of the dried herb as tea. Tincture (1:5) dosing is 2–6 mL taken three times per day (EMA 2019a).

VASCULAR TONICS

Botanicals have long been used to relieve the discomfort of chronic venous insufficiency (CVI), a condition that affects millions of people, particularly women. They are often preferred over compression stockings, particularly in hot and humid weather. While there are numerous vascular tonics including bilberry (*Vaccinium myrtillus*) and ginkgo leaf (*Ginkgo biloba*); horse chestnut seed extract and pycogenol are most popular.

HORSE CHESTNUT (*AESCULUS HIPPOCASTANUM* L.)

The seeds and bark of the horse chestnut tree have been used as traditional medicines in Europe for at least four centuries. The seed was used for the treatment of varicose veins, hemorrhoids, bruising, and various rheumatic complaints. The primary active constituent found in horse chestnut seed extract is aescin – most horse chestnut seed extracts are standardized to this compound.

The beneficial effect of horse chestnut seed extract in CVI is due to its anti-edematous and anti-inflammatory activities. The evidence from a 2012 systematic review of 17 studies concluded that horse chestnut seed extract is an efficacious and safe short-term treatment for CVI (Pittler and Ernst 2012). The European Medicines Agency recognizes this traditional herbal medicinal product for the relief of symptoms of discomfort and heaviness of legs related to minor venous circulatory disturbances. They also state that at least 4 weeks of treatment may be required before beneficial effects are observed (EMA 2019b).

The most common dose used in clinical trials was 300 mg twice daily of horse chestnut seed extract standardized to provide a daily dose of 100 mg of aescin. The standardized extracts are quite safe; however, the *raw* seeds, bark, flowers, and leaves of horse chestnut are unsafe due to the presence of esculin, a toxic compound removed when preparing the extract. The safety of the extract during pregnancy and lactation has not been established and is not recommended. Topical preparations containing 2% aescin are also used to relieve CVI, as well as sprains and bruising.

PYCNOGENOL

Pycnogenol® (trademark of Horphag Research) is a bioflavonoid-rich extract made from the bark of the French maritime pine (*Pinus pinaster* Aiton, ssp. *atlantica*). This proprietary extract has been the subject of more than 100 clinical trials for a variety of health conditions. Preclinical data show that pycnogenol has potent antioxidant, vasodilatory, antithrombotic, collagen stabilizing and anti-inflammatory activities, making it of particular interest for CVI (Gulati 2014). In a 2014 literature review of clinical trials, it was reported that pycnogenol can reduce lower leg edema in CVI, reduce the incidence of deep venous thrombosis during long haul flights, and enhance the healing of venous ulcers and hemorrhoids with topical application and/or oral administration (Gulati 2014).

A 2019 8-week study found that pycnogenol significantly improved capillary filtration (RAS), which is directly associated with swelling, as well as oxidative stress, in those taking 150 mg/day of the extract, compared to a group using compression stockings alone (Cesarone et al. 2019). However, a 2020 review concluded that no definitive conclusion could be made for the effect of pycnogenol in CVI due to small sample sizes, limited number of RCTs, and variation in outcome measurements (Robertson 2020).

The dose range used in clinical trials for CVI is 150–360 mg/day. Pycnogenol was classified as generally recognized as safe by an independent group of toxicologists based upon clinical safety and preclinical toxicology data (American Botanical Council 2019). Pycnogenol does not affect international normalized ratio (INR) in patients taking aspirin (Pella 2005). No drug interaction studies have been published. As a precaution, most authorities recommend that pycnogenol not be given to children under 6 years of age or during the first trimester of pregnancy.

QUALITY OF BOTANICAL PRODUCTS

Botanical products are very popular in the United States with sales exceeding $8 billion in 2017, an 8.5% increase over the previous year (Smith et al. 2018). In the United States and abroad, people cite numerous reasons for using natural remedies including easy access, cost, the perception they are "safer" than pharmaceuticals, and a belief that they promote health. Clinicians express both interest in botanical medicines and concerns about their efficacy, quality, safety, and potential for herb-drug interactions (Ekor 2013).

While it is beyond the scope of this chapter to discuss quality, clinicians should be cognizant of the tremendous variability that exists for botanical products in the marketplace. Products that have been studied in controlled clinical trials are generally of higher quality and should be recommended when possible. Using clinically tested products also allows clinicians to recommend an effective dose based upon study results.

Clinicians' concern about the concomitant use of botanicals with prescription or over-the-counter medications, particularly in children, pregnant/breastfeeding women, elders, and those with diminished renal or hepatic function, is justified. It is difficult to predict pharmacokinetic interactions. There are numerous herb-drug interaction checkers online: this author uses Natural Medicines Comprehensive Database (www.naturalmedicines.therapeuticresearch.com). Clinicians can input medications, botanicals, and other supplements, and potential interactions will be displayed, the strength of the risk rated, and links to the primary research provided. Potential risks should be explained to patients and documented in the chart. If monitoring drug levels or serum tests (e.g., liver function tests) would help mitigate risk, this should be offered in partnership with the patient.

SUMMARY

The first line of the prevention of cardiovascular disease is lifestyle modification. As part of that lifestyle modification, clinicians may consider the use of numerous clinically researched botanicals as a primary and/or adjunctive therapy. If products contain botanicals with diuretic properties, clinicians should consider occasionally monitoring serum electrolytes. Clinicians should always guide patients toward high-quality products, monitor the effectiveness of the therapy, and be observant for potential adverse effects.

REFERENCES

Adisakwattana S, Moonrat J, Srichairat S, Chanasit C, et al. Lipid-Lowering mechanisms of grape seed extract (*Vitis vinifera* L) and its antihyperlidemic activity. *J Med Plants Res* 2010;4(20):2113–2120.

Alali FQ, El-Elimat T, Khalid L, Hudaib R, Al-Shehabi TS, Eid AH. Garlic for cardiovascular disease: prevention or treatment? *Curr Pharm Des* 2017;23(7):1028–1041.

Alijaniha F, Naseri M, Afsharypuor S, Fallahi F, Noorbala A, Mosaddegh M, et al. Heart palpitation relief with *Melissa officinalis* leaf extract: double blind, randomized, placebo-controlled trial of efficacy and safety. *J Ethnopharmacol* 2015;164:378–384.

Akaberi M, Hosseinzadeh H. Grapes (*Vitis vinifera*) as a potential candidate for the therapy of the metabolic syndrome. *Phytother Res* 2016 Apr;30(4):540–556. doi: 10.1002/ptr.5570.

American Botanical Council. Scientific and clinical monograph for Pycnogenol (French maritime pine bark extract) *Pinus pinaster Aiton* subsp. atlantica [Fam. Pinaceae]. 2019. https://www.herbalgram.org/media/13292/pycnog_fullmono012019-cc2020.pdf. Accessed June 17, 2021.

Anjom-Shoae J, Milajerdi A, Larijani B, Esmaillzadeh A. Effects of grape seed extract on dyslipidaemia: a systematic review and dose-response meta-analysis of randomised controlled trials. *Br J Nutr* 2020;124;121–134.

Asadi A, Shidfar F, Safari M, Hosseini AF, Fallah Huseini H, Heidari I, et al. Efficacy of *Melissa officinalis* L. (lemon balm) extract on glycemic control and cardiovascular risk factors in individuals with type 2 diabetes: a randomized, double-blind, clinical trial. *Phytother Res* 2019;33:651–659.

Asadi A, Shidfar F, Safari M, Malek M, Hosseini AF, Rezazadeh S, et al. Safety and efficacy of *Melissa officinalis* (lemon balm) on ApoA-I, Apo B, lipid ratio and ICAM-1 in type 2 diabetes patients: a randomized, double-blinded clinical trial. *Complement Ther Med* 2018;40:83–88.

Asgary S, Soltani R, Zolghadr M, Keshvari M, Sarrafzadegan N. Evaluation of the effects of roselle (*Hibiscus sabdariffa* L.) on oxidative stress and serum levels of lipids, insulin and hs-CRP in adult patients with metabolic syndrome: A double-blind placebo-controlled clinical trial. *J Complement Integr Med* 2016;13(2):175–180.

Aziz Z, Wong SY, Chong NJ. Effects of *Hibiscus sabdariffa* L. on serum lipids: a systematic review and meta-analysis. *J Ethnopharmacol* 2013;150(2):442–450.

Beltrán-Debón R, Rodríguez-Gallego E, Fernández-Arroyo S, et al. The acute impact of polyphenols from *Hibiscus sabdariffa* in metabolic homeostasis: an approach combining metabolomics and gene-expression analyses. *Food Funct* 2015 Sep;6(9):2957–2966.

Bhagavathula AS, Al-Khatib AJM, Elnour AA, Al Kalbani NMS, Shehab A. *Ammi Visnaga* in treatment of urolithiasis and hypertriglyceridemia. *Pharmacognosy Res* 2015 Oct–Dec;7(4):397–400.

Cesarone MR, Belcaro G, Agus GB, Ippolito E, Dugall M, Hosoi M, et al. Chronic venous insufficiency and venous microangiopathy: management with compression and Pycnogenol®. *Minerva Cardioangiol* 2019 Aug;67(4):280–287.

Chen CX, Kwan CY. Endothelium-independent vasorelaxation by leonurine, a plant alkaloid purified from Chinese motherwort. *Life Sci.* 2001 Jan 12;68(8):953–960.

Choi S, Oh DS, Jerng UM. A systematic review of the pharmacokinetic and pharmacodynamic interactions of herbal medicine with warfarin. *PLoS One* 2017;12(8):e0182794.

Da-Costa-Rocha I, Bonnlaender B, Sievers H, Pischel I, Heinrich M. *Hibiscus sabdariffa* L. – a phytochemical and pharmacological review. *Food Chem.* 2014 Dec 15;165:424–443.

Draginic N, Jakovljevic V, Andjic M, Jeremic J, Srejovic I, Rankovic M, et al. *Melissa officinalis* L. as a nutritional strategy for cardioprotection. *Front Physiol* 2021;12:661778.

Dwivedi S, Chopra D. Revisiting *Terminalia arjuna* – an ancient cardiovascular drug. *J Tradit Complement Med* 2014 Oct–Dec;4(4):224–231.

Ekor M. The growing use of herbal medicines: issues relating to adverse reactions and challenges in monitoring safety. *Front Pharmacol* 2013;4:177.

EMA. European Medicines Agency Motherwort (*Leonurus cardiaca* L.) summary. March 15, 2019a. https://www.ema.europa.eu/en/documents/herbal-summary/motherwort-summary-public_en.pdf. Accessed July 5, 2021.

EMA. European Medicines Agency. European Union herbal monograph on *Aesculus hippocastanum* L., semen. March 15, 2019b. https://www.ema.europa.eu/en/documents/herbal-monograph/draft-european-union-herbal-monograph-aesculus-hippocastanum-l-semen-revision-1_en.pdf. Accessed July 7, 2021.

Gee LC, Ahluwalia A. Dietary nitrate lowers blood pressure: epidemiological, pre-clinical experimental and clinical trial evidence. *Curr Hypertens Rep* 2016;18:17.

Griebenow R, Pittrow DB, Weidinger G, Mueller E, Mutschler E, Welzel D. Low-dose reserpine/thiazide combination in first-line treatment of hypertension: efficacy and safety compared to an ACE inhibitor. *Blood Press* 1997 Sep;6(5):299–306.

Gulati OP. Pycnogenol in chronic venous insufficiency and related venous disorders. *Phytother Res* 2014;28:348–362.

Hamal S, Cherukuri L, Birudaraju D, Matsumoto S, Kinninger A, Chaganti BT, et al. Short-term impact of aged garlic extract on endothelial function in diabetes: A randomized, double-blind, placebo-controlled trial. *Exp Ther Med* 2020 Feb;19(2):1485–1489.

Holubarsch CJF, Colucci WS, Eha J. Benefit-risk assessment of crataegus extract WS 1442: an evidence-based review. *Am J Cardiovasc Drugs* 2018;18(1):25–36.

Holubarsch CJF, Colucci WS, Meinertz T, et al. Crataegus extract WS 1442 postpones cardiac death in patients with congestive heart failure class NYHA II-III: a randomized, placebo-controlled, double-blind trial in 2681 patients. American College of Cardiology 2007 Scientific Sessions March 27, 2007; New Orleans, LA. Late breaking clinical trials-3, Session 414-5.

Irandoost P, Ebrahimi-Mameghani M, Pirouzpanah S. Does grape seed oil improve inflammation and insulin resistance in overweight or obese women? *Int J Food Sci Nutr* 2013 Sep;64(6):706–710.

Junsong X, Ying W, Xuelin S, Hua W, Jingmin D, Yanping C. Effects of proanthocyanidins on oxidative stress in nutritional obesity rats. *Shipin Kexue* 2014;35:183–186.

Kapoor D, Vijayvergiya R, Dhawan V. *Terminalia arjuna* in coronary artery disease: ethnopharmacology, pre-clinical, clinical & safety evaluation. *J Ethnopharmacol* 2014 Sep 11;155(2):1029–1045.

Kaur N, Shafiq B, Negi H, Pandey A, Reddy S, et al. *Terminalia arjuna* in chronic stable angina: systematic review and meta-analysis. *Cardiol Res Pract* 2014;2014:281483.

Khalil N, Bishr M, Desouky S, Salama O. *Ammi Visnaga* L., a potential medicinal plant: a review. *Molecules* 2020 Jan;25(2):301.

Kreydiyyeh SI, Usta J. Diuretic effect and mechanism of action of parsley. *J Ethnopharmacol* 2002 Mar;79(3):353–357.

Lara J, Ashor AW, Oggioni C, et al. Effects of inorganic nitrate and beetroot supplementation on endothelial function: a systematic review and meta-analysis. *Eur J Nutr* 2016 Mar;55(2):451–459.

Lundberg JO, Weitzberg E, Gladwin MT. The nitrate-nitrite-nitric oxide pathway in physiology and therapeutics. *Nat Rev Drug Discov* 2008;7:156–167.

Mali RG, Dhake AS. A review on herbal antiasthmatics. *Orient Pharm Exp Med* 2011 Aug; 11(2):77–90.

McKay DL, Chen CY, Saltzman E, Blumberg JB. *Hibiscus sabdariffa* L. tea (tisane) lowers blood pressure in prehypertensive and mildly hypertensive adults. *J Nutr* 2010 Feb;140(2):298–303.

Miłkowska-Leyck K Filipek B, Strzelecka H. Pharmacological effects of lavandulifolioside from *Leonurus cardiaca*. *J Ethnopharmacol* 2002 Apr;80(1):85–90.

Moghadam MH, Imenshahidi M, Mohajeri SA. Antihypertensive effect of celery seed on rat blood pressure in chronic administration. *J Med Food*. 2013;16:558–63.

Narayana A, Kumaraswamy R. A medico-historical review of Arjuna. *Bull Indian Inst Hist Med Hyderabad* 1996;26(1–2):1–10.

Nayebi N, Esteghamati A, Meysamie A, Khalili N, Kamalinejad M, Emtiazy M, et al. The effects of a *Melissa officinalis* L. based product on metabolic parameters in patients with type 2 diabetes mellitus: a randomized double-blinded controlled clinical trial. *J Complement Integr Med*. 2019;16:20180088.

Norn S, Kruse PR. Cardiac glycosides: from ancient history through Withering's foxglove to endogenous cardiac glycosides. *Dan Medicinhist Arbog* 2004;119–132 (Article in Danish).

Oliveira-Paula GH, Pinheiro LC, Tanus-Santos JE. Mechanisms impairing blood pressure responses to nitrite and nitrate. *Nitric Oxide* 2019;85:35–43.

Orekhov AN, Sobenin IA, Korneev NV, Kirichenko TV, Myasoedova VA, Melnichenko AA, et al. Anti-atherosclerotic therapy based on botanicals. *Recent Pat Cardiovasc Drug Discov* 2013 Apr;8(1):56–66.

Parandoosh M, Yousefi R, Khorsandi H, Nikpayam O, Saidpour A, Babaei H. The effects of grape seed extract (*Vitis vinifera*) supplement on inflammatory markers, neuropeptide Y, anthropometric measures, and appetite in obese or overweight individuals: a randomized clinical trial. *Phytother Res* 2020 Feb; 34(2):379–387.

Pella D. *Slovak Study*. Geneva: Horphag Research; 2005.

Pittler MH, Ernst E. Horse chestnut seed extract for chronic venous insufficiency. *Cochrane Database Syst Rev* 2012 Nov 14;11(11):CD003230.

Pittler MH, Guo R, Ernst E. Hawthorn extract for treating chronic heart failure. *Cochrane Database Syst Rev* 2008 Jan 23;1:CD005312.

Pons Z, Margalef M, Bravo Fl, Arola-Arnal A, Muguerza B. Acute administration of single oral dose of grape seed polyphenols restores blood pressure in a rat model of metabolic syndrome: role of nitric oxide and prostacyclin. *Eur J Clin Nutr* 2016 Mar;55(2):749–758. doi: 10.1007/s00394-015-0895-0.

Quesada I, de Paola M, Torres-Palazzolo C, Camargo A, Ferder L, Manucha W, Castro C. Effect of garlic's active constituents in inflammation, obesity and cardiovascular disease. *Curr Hypertens Res* 2020 Jan 10;22(1):6.

Ried K. Garlic lowers blood pressure in hypertensive individuals, regulates serum cholesterol, and stimulates immunity: an updated meta-analysis and review. *J Nutr* 2016 Feb;146(2):389S–396S.

Ried K, Fakler P. Potential of garlic (*Allium sativum*) in lowering high blood pressure: mechanisms of action and clinical relevance. *Integrat Blood Press Control* 2014;7:71–82.

Ried K, Travica N, Sali A. The effect of Kyolic aged garlic extract on gut microbiota, inflammation, and cardiovascular markers in hypertensives: the GarGIC trial. *Front Nutr* 2018;5:122.

Robertson NU, Schoonees A, Brand A. Visser J. Pine bark (*Pinus* spp.) extract for treating chronic disorders. *Cochrane Database Syst Rev* 2020 Sep 29;9(9):CD008294.

Shikov AN, Pozharitskaya ON, Makarov VG, Demchenko DV, Shikh EV. Effect of *Leonurus cardiaca* oil extract in patients with arterial hypertension accompanied by anxiety and sleep disorders. *Phytother Res* 2011 Apr;25(4):540–543.

Siervo M, Lara J, Ogbonmwan I, Mathers JC. Inorganic nitrate and beetroot juice supplementation reduces blood pressure in adults: a systematic review and meta-analysis. *J Nutr* 2013;143:818–826. doi: 10.3945/jn.112.170233.

Smith T, Kawa K, Eckl V, Morton C, Stredney R. Herbal supplement sales in US increased 8.5% in 2017, topping $8 billion. *HerbalGram* 2018;119:62–71.

Tassell MC, Kingston R, Gilroy D, Lehane M, Furey A. Hawthorn (*Crataegus* spp.) in the treatment of cardiovascular disease. *Pharmacogn Rev.* 2010 Jan–Jun;4(7):32–41.

Walton R, Whitten DL, Hawrelak JA. The efficacy of *Hibiscus sabdariffa* (rosella) in essential hypertension: a systematic review of clinical trials. *Austr J Herb Med* 2016;28(2):48–51.

Wang HP, Yang J, Qin LQ, Yang XJ. Effect of garlic on blood pressure: a meta-analysis. *J Clin Hypertens (Greenwich).* 2015 Mar;17(3):223–231.

Wanwimolruk S, Phopin K, Prachayasittikul V. Cytochrome P450 enzyme mediated herbal drug interactions (Part 2). *EXCLI J* 2014;13:869–896.

Watts AR, Lennard MS, Mason SL, Tucker GT, Woods HF. Beeturia and the biological fate of beetroot pigments. *Pharmacogenetics* 1993;3(6):302–311.

Yousefi R, Parandoosh M, Khorsandi H, Hosseinzadeh N, et al. Grape seed extract supplementation along with a restricted-calorie diet improves cardiovascular risk factors in obese or overweight adult individuals: a randomized, placebo-controlled trial. *Phytother Res* 2021 Feb;35(2):987–995.

Yui S, Fujiwara S, Harada K, Motoike-Hamura M, Sakai M, Matsubara S, et al. Beneficial effects of lemon balm leaf extract on in vitro glycation of proteins, arterial stiffness, and skin elasticity in healthy adults. *J Nutr Sci Vitaminol (Tokyo)* 2017;63:59–68.

Zamani H, de Joode MEJR., Hossein IJ, Henckens NFT, Guggeis MA, Berends JE, de Kok TMCM, van Breda SJG. The benefits and risks of beetroot juice consumption: a systematic review. *Crit Rev Food Sci Nutr* 2021;61:788–804.

Zhang H, Liu S, Li L, Liu S, Liu S, Mi J, Tian G. The impact of grape seed extract treatment on blood pressure changes: a meta-analysis of 16 randomized controlled trials. *Medicine (Baltimore).* 2016 Aug;95 (33):e4247. doi: 10.1097/MD.0000000000004247.

19 Depression, Anxiety, Stress, and Spirituality in Cardiovascular Disease

Erminia Guarneri and Shyamia Stone

CONTENTS

Depression...382
Anxiety...383
    Overlap between Anxiety and Depression...383
    Defining Anxiety...384
    Stress...384
        Stressors...385
Pathophysiology..385
Biological Mechanisms...385
    Inflammation..385
    Platelet Activation...386
    Autonomic Dysfunction..386
    HPA Axis Dysfunction..386
    Endothelial Dysfunction...386
    Cardiovascular Reactivity...387
    Acute Emotional Effects...387
Behavioral Mechanisms..387
Prevention and Screening..387
    Conventional Treatment..388
    Integrative Treatment..388
        Diet 389
        Gut Health...390
        Nutritional Supplements 390
Herbal Therapies...392
    Herbal Anxiolytics..392
    Herbal Adaptogens..393
Light Therapy..393
Mind-Body Techniques...393
    Heart Rate Variability 393
    Breathing..394
    Meditation..394
Lifestyle 394
    Exercise..394
    Yoga...395
    Social Support and Compliance..395
Spirituality..396

DOI: 10.1201/9781003137849-19

Summary 396
Challenges 396
Take Away Messages 397
References 397

DEPRESSION

Depression in its broadest reach may be understood as a state of being that spans from a fleeting emotional experience or mood, to that of a more long-term pathological state.

According to the Diagnostic and Statistical Manual of Mental Disorders (DSM-5), depression as a disorder may be classified as Disruptive Mood Dysregulation Disorder, Major Depressive Disorder, Persistent Depressive Disorder (Dysthymia), or Depressive Disorder Due to Another Medical Condition.[8] The most commonly studied clinical diagnosis of depression related to CVD is Major Depressive Disorder (MDD). Diagnostic criteria for MDD can be found in Table 19.1.

While the DSM-5[8] is the gold standard in diagnosis of depressive disorders and is utilized by mental health professionals, depression is often identified in medical offices through a variety of self-report measures (Table 19.2).

The PHQ-9, for example, is an easy-to-use, validated tool for identifying the severity of depression. These instruments provide information about severity of depressive symptoms based upon frequency, severity, and impact on quality of life. Each of these measures simplifies DSM criteria and provides an estimated guideline of the level of depression that may include categories such as normal/not depressed, mild, borderline, moderate, and severe depression.[9–12] A measure specifically for cardiac patients has been developed that also assesses specific presentations of depression that may occur after a cardiovascular incident, including concern about health and recovery, fear of impending health issues or dying, and loss of independence or function.[13]

It is important to recognize symptoms of depression in individuals even if they do not fit the criteria for diagnosis of MDD. It is not necessary for a patient to have MDD to be at risk for depressive symptoms contributing to CVD, as depressive symptoms in themselves have been correlated with adverse cardiac outcomes.[14,15]

From an etiological standpoint, studies have determined that patients with depression have twice the risk of developing new-onset CVD.[16] Depression is also correlated with greater mortality in patients with a history of acute myocardial infarction (MI), with depressed patients having three times greater incidence of mortality post-MI than patients that are not depressed.[16] These outcomes are not only related to the presence or absence of depression, but the 5-year mortality rate has also been correlated with severity of depression.[17] Interestingly, MDD is noted as the second leading cause of disability in America, behind ischemic heart disease, which ranks number one,[18] though arguably, these could be varying manifestations of related disease processes, which will be discussed in the pathophysiology section.

Depression exists on a continuum from normal emotion to pathology, with variations in clinical presentation. The etiology of depression is still being discovered, as differing mechanisms may be at work in each of the presenting criteria.[19] Perhaps the most comprehensive view is the biopsychosocial model of depression, which shows a multifactorial etiology including genetics,[19] biochemistry, cognition, personality traits, environmental factors, trauma,[20] and social interactions.[21] Pathophysiological features of depression can include structural and functional brain changes as witnessed through neuroimaging studies,[22,23] specifically showing a reduction of dopamine network responses in the brain.[22] Overall, MDD is thought to be due to deficiencies of dopamine, serotonin, and/or norepinephrine, that may occur concurrently or may lead into one another.[24]

TABLE 19.1

DSM Criteria for Relevant Depressive and Anxiety Disorders

Disorder	DSM V Criteria[8]
Major depressive disorder (MDD)	Depressed mood or loss of interest or pleasure in activities for most of the day nearly every day for at least 2 weeks, accompanied by five of the following: • Unintentional weight loss or weight gain (5% of body weight in one month), or increased or decreased appetite • Insomnia or hypersomnia • Psychomotor agitation or retardation • Fatigue or loss of energy • Feeling guilty or worthless • Decreased concentration or decisiveness • Increased thoughts of death or suicidality

Generalized anxiety disorder (GAD)	Over the course of 6 months, occurring more days than not:
	• Excessive anxiety and worry for a variety of events/activities
	• Difficulty controlling the worry
	• Anxiety/worry is associated with three or more of the following:
	  • Restlessness
	  • Fatigue
	  • Difficulty concentrating
	  • Irritability
	  • Muscle tension
	  • Sleep disturbance
	• Symptoms cause distress or impairment in important areas of functioning

Panic disorder (PD)	Recurrent panic attacks, which consist of a sudden surge of intense fear or discomfort, and is accompanied by: • Heart palpitations or tachycardia • Sweating • Trembling • Shortness (or sensation of shortness) of breath • Sensation of choking • Chest pain/discomfort • Nausea or abdominal pain • Dizziness or light-headedness • Chills or hot flashes • Numbness or tingling sensations • Detached feelings (derealization or depersonalization) • Fear of losing control • Fear of dying An attack must also be followed with a month or more of worry about additional attacks, or change in behavior to avoid having panic attacks

ANXIETY

OVERLAP BETWEEN ANXIETY AND DEPRESSION

There is a high level of comorbidity between depression and anxiety, even in their clinical forms of MDD and Generalized Anxiety Disorder (GAD). In fact, it has been postulated that MDD and GAD may be different presentations of the same disorder.[25] Comorbidity rates between MDD and GAD range from 40% to 98%, with 67% of individuals with GAD reporting MDD at some point in their lives, and 20% of individuals with MDD reporting GAD in the past.[26] In addition to common features, there also appears to be shared etiological factors, including similar genetics,[27] and the

---

TABLE 19.2

Screening Measures for Depression and Anxiety

Depression	Patient health questionnaire (PHQ-9)[9]
	Beck depression inventory (BDI)[11]
	Hospital anxiety depression scale (HADS)
	Center for Epidemiologic Studies Depression scale-10 (CES-10)[10]
	Cardiac depression scale[13]
Anxiety	Generalized anxiety disorder (GAD-7) questionnaire[31]
Depression and anxiety	Patient health questionnaire anxiety and depression scale (PHQ-ADS)[32]

---

trait of neuroticism that predisposes for both depression and anxiety.[26] However, it is possible that comorbidity is due to overlap in the diagnostic criteria for disorders such as MDD and GAD.[28] Both depression and anxiety have been shown to be correlated with CVD.

DEFINING ANXIETY

Anxiety exists on a spectrum from that of a mental-emotional state, or a trait, to that of a psychological disorder.[29] A *state* of anxiety is fleeting, and is experienced as a momentary sense of fear of a potential threat.[30] This heightened emotional state can be a healthy part of the human experience, leading to motivation and vigilance when situationally necessary. Anxiety can also be in response to a positive event, manifesting as the stimulation of excitement.

Anxiety disorders as outlined in the DSM-5 include separation anxiety disorder, phobias, social anxiety disorder, panic disorder (PD), agoraphobia, and GAD. The two disorders that have been the most extensively studied in conjunction with cardiovascular disease are GAD and PD.[8] Diagnostic criteria for these disorders can be found in Table 19.1.

Trait forms of anxiety may be screened in a clinical setting through use of self-report measures, which has primarily consisted of the Generalized Anxiety Disorder (GAD-7) questionnaire.[31] However, recently, a combined measure of the Patient Health Questionnaire Anxiety and Depression Scale (PHQ-ADS) has been created in order to combine PHQ-9 and GAD-7 into one measure.[32] Although the PHQ-ADS is still in its initial validation phase, it shows promise as an initial screening tool due to the overlap between anxiety and depression.

Some individuals with anxiety show genetic predisposition for dysregulation of serotonin[33] and glutamic acid decarboxylase.[34] Disturbances of neurotransmitters norepinephrine, serotonin, and gamma aminobutyric acid (GABA) have also been associated with GAD.[22] While there are widely varying experiences of anxiety that are reflected in the spectrum of state, trait, or disorder, fMRI data has shown similar neurological networks in the brain that are activated across all forms of anxiety.[30] Areas of activation correspond with heightened amygdala responses and overall greater emotional responsiveness.[35] Additional environmental risk factors associated with development of GAD include a greater incidence of trauma throughout life and adverse childhood events.[36]

Clinical presentation of anxiety may appear with classic emotional complaints that can be assessed through the above DSM-5 criteria or GAD-7 assessment. However, anxiety may also present as physical symptoms such as sleep disturbance, fatigue, difficulty relaxing, muscle tension, and recurrent headaches.[37]

STRESS

Psychological stress is defined as a perceived tension or worry that impacts an individual's behaviors and ability to cope.[38]

Stressors

The term "stress" has also been used to describe stressors themselves, those things that one encounters that incite a stressful response. Stressors may exist in any of these arenas, thereby increasing the stress put on the body's systems to come back to a point of balance, which has been termed "allostasis".[39] The concept of allostasis illustrates the way in which the body has an active regulatory process to maintain physiological balance and adapt to changing needs utilizing physiological responses such as hormones, temperature changes, and blood pressure.[40] Therefore, it is possible to see that stressors have a direct impact on physiology through the body's mechanisms to perceive these events, react, and then compensate in attempt to preserve balance. However, there are times when balance is unable to be achieved, and this is referred to as "allostatic load" – a state wherein the normal balancing processes are overtaxed or fail to act, leading to a lack of adaptation and dysregulation of the physiological systems that are in flux in response to stressors.[41] These systems include the hypothalamic-pituitary-adrenal (HPA) axis, the sympathetic nervous system, and the immune system.[41]

Stressors may be acute or chronic and may vary between individuals based upon their perceptions of what is and isn't stress. Acute stressors are encountered on a daily basis in small doses, such as having to complete tasks of daily living. They may also come in response to unexpected life changes in health, family, home, or livelihood. Acute stressors can negatively impact individuals, though chronic stressors appear to have a greater cumulative burden on the body's ability to allostatically adjust. Chronic stressors have been shown to include low social support, low socioeconomic stress, occupational stress, marital or relationship stress, and caregiver strain.[15]

PATHOPHYSIOLOGY

There is considerable overlap in the underlying processes of depression, anxiety, and stress. There is a twofold interaction between the mental-emotional states of depression, anxiety, and stress, with the physical manifestation of CVD, including both biological and behavioral mechanisms.

BIOLOGICAL MECHANISMS

INFLAMMATION

Inflammation is a complex process that involves the immune system's response to potentially harmful stimuli, which triggers the signaling of various cytokines and chemokines to create protective responses within the body.[42] However, when inflammatory processes are systemic, the risk of cardiovascular disease is increased.

Various reviews have shown inflammation as a major underlying causal factor for depression,[43,44,169] anxiety,[45] and CVD.[46,169] Xiong and colleagues found that patients with MDD and congestive heart failure (CHF) had statistically significant higher levels of inflammatory markers than patients without MDD and CHF. Elevated serum markers in depression included cytokines IL-1, IL-4, IL-6, IL-17, IFN-gamma, MIP-1, and TNF-alpha.[44] The Third National Health and Nutrition Examination Study had also revealed a higher serum CRP in patients with MDD,[47] a marker that is highly correlated with CVD risk.[48] Elevated pro-inflammatory cytokines have also been found in patients with anxiety, as Godbout and Glaser[38] found increased levels of IL-6 and CRP in patients who were experiencing chronic stress. Inflammatory cytokines have been found to increase autonomic imbalance, stimulate the sympathetic nervous system, cause electrical instability in the myocardium, depress cardiac function, lead to endothelial dysfunction, cause vasoconstriction, and generate atherosclerosis.[46,169]

Interestingly, Steenkamp and colleagues[49] evaluated oxidative stress levels (measured by F2-isoprostanes and oxidized glutathione) in patients with MDD and found that the symptoms of anxiety that the patients experienced were more closely correlated with oxidative stress than the symptoms of depression. Oxidative stress negatively impacts cell membranes, proteins, nucleic acids, and lipids[49] and has also been correlated with exacerbation of symptoms of anxiety and hypertension.[45] Depression has been induced in mice through lipopolysaccharides (LPS), thereby showing that inflammation and oxidative stress cause decreased mitochondrial function in the hippocampus, which also leads to depression.[169] Mitochondrial function may be restored through utilizing antioxidants, which have been shown to decrease oxidative stress, depression, and CVD.[169]

PLATELET ACTIVATION

Increased inflammation may also be correlated with greater platelet activation that is found in depressed patients with CVD, leading to increased risk of coronary artery occlusion.[50] Depression has also been associated with a hyperactive platelet 5-HT2A receptor signal transduction system, which leads to increased thrombosis.[29] Chronic stress, depression, and anxiety symptoms have also been associated with pronounced platelet activation.[51]

AUTONOMIC DYSFUNCTION

Depression and anxiety may also be correlated with CVD through their influence on altering autonomic vascular tone. This has been most directly studied through the concept of heart rate variability (HRV). HRV is a measurement of R-R intervals and the cyclic variation that reflects autonomic balance between sympathetic and parasympathetic nervous system activity.[52] Autonomic nervous system imbalance with increased sympathetic nervous system activation and decreased vagal tone has been correlated with CVD and risk of adverse cardiac events,[52,169] through such mechanisms as triggering atherosclerosis and/or platelet aggregation, and leading to changes in lipid metabolism.[53] Low HRV is related to poor cardiac outcomes and increased risk of post-MI mortality,[54] and is correlated with sudden cardiac death even in those that have not been diagnosed with CVD.[55]

HPA AXIS DYSFUNCTION

Since HRV is a description of the sympathetic and parasympathetic nervous system balance, it is no surprise that we would see a connection between depression, anxiety, and the HPA axis. Various studies have shown increased levels of cortisol in individuals with both depression,[53,55,56] and anxiety[38] illustrating a correlation between HPA axis activation and emotional disorders.

Elevated cortisol leads to an increased risk of insulin resistance, central obesity, and hyperlipidemia, which are well-known risk factors for CVD.[29,53] Other catecholamines such as norepinephrine have also been shown to be increased in depression[57,58] and chronic stress.[51] Increased catecholamine levels have been found to cause damage to cardiac myocytes,[59] and lead to apoptosis of ventricular myocytes,[60] thereby increasing risk of adverse cardiac outcomes.[57] Chronic HPA axis activation has also been shown to decrease immune function and impact susceptibility to infection, as well as increasing pro-inflammatory cytokines, feeding back into the inflammatory cycle.[29]

ENDOTHELIAL DYSFUNCTION

Endothelial dysfunction is the earliest indicator of vascular disease leading to atherosclerosis and adverse cardiac events including aneurysm, ischemia, and infarction. A study by van Sloten and colleagues[61] illustrates a much greater level of endothelial dysfunction in elderly individuals with depression after adjusting for those with CVD. On the other hand, a study by Stillman and colleagues[62] showed that anxiety decreased endothelial function and vascular smooth muscle function in individuals with atherosclerosis, even in the absence of depression. Inflammation is a unifying etiology for both mental health challenges and cardiovascular events including reduced endothelial function.

CARDIOVASCULAR REACTIVITY

Upon encountering stressors, the cardiovascular system has various compensatory mechanisms to increase perceived need. Anxiety and chronic stress have been hypothesized to increase cardiac reactivity resulting in alteration of cardiovascular mechanisms. For example, individuals with anxiety have increases in resting heart rate, dysfunction in the baroreflex, and variability in ventricular repolarization.[29] All of these mechanisms increase the risk of cardiovascular events.

ACUTE EMOTIONAL EFFECTS

Individuals with underlying coronary artery disease may experience adverse effects from hemodynamic stress including disrupting an atherosclerotic plaque that leads to thrombus.[29] While another phenomenon that may occur in patients without known cardiovascular disease is intense, sudden emotional stress triggering the onset of myocardial stunning.[63,64] This phenomenon has been thought to be related to increased activation of the sympathoneural and adrenomedullary systems, and has been termed acute myocardial stunning, LV apical ballooning syndrome, takotsubo cardiomyopathy, or broken heart syndrome.[64] An increase in cardiac events was seen following the terrorist attack on the World Trade Center (WTC) on September 11, 2001. On the date of this event, intakes at the New York Methodist Hospital Telemetry and Coronary Care units reported significantly higher rates of acute MI (4.3% elevation) and tachyarrhythmia (6.3% elevation).[65] A review by Bazoukis and colleagues[66] also demonstrated an increase in acute coronary syndrome after several large-scale earthquakes including Christchurch, Great East Japan, Niigata-Chuetsu, Northridge, Great Hanshin-Awaji, Sichuan, Athens, Armenia, and Noto Peninsula.

BEHAVIORAL MECHANISMS

While there are known biological correlates between depression, anxiety, chronic stress, and CVD, these emotional states have many effects on behaviors. In a study performed by Ziegelstein and colleagues,[67] it was found that within a hospital setting, patients who were found to have depression (spanning from mild depression to MDD or dysthymia) showed lower adherence to treatment protocols including low-fat diet, exercise, stress reduction, and increasing social support. Additionally, those patients who had MDD took prescribed medications less consistently.[67]

There are also additive behaviors of self-medication that serve as risk factors for CVD, such as cigarette smoking, excess alcohol consumption,[68] and overeating.[69]

PREVENTION AND SCREENING

In patients with known cardiovascular disease, it is important to perform screenings for emotional disorders of depression, anxiety, and chronic stress. It is possible to utilize the self-report screening measures mentioned previously (i.e., PHQ-9, BDI, CED-S, GAD-7), or work in collaboration with a mental health professional to determine patient risk. While these measures may provide information regarding a patient's emotional state, they can be impersonal, and due to the stigma of mental health concerns, patients are not always forthcoming in this format. It is important to develop a positive relationship with the patient to facilitate trust and openness, while allowing the practitioner to attend to underlying emotional concerns.

It is debatable whether psychotherapy and pharmacotherapy for depression and anxiety help to mitigate CVD risk, and over-treatment may result in adverse cardiovascular side effects.[70,71] It is therefore very important to aim for prevention through integrative therapies, which are described in detail below.

CONVENTIONAL TREATMENT

For many CVD patients, signs of depression and anxiety go unnoticed until after they have experienced a cardiac event. One method of treatment of depression and anxiety in CVD involves planned collaborative care, which includes screening for mental health disorders in cardiac patients, and subsequent provision of adjunctive care between cardiologists and mental health professionals or nurses.[72,73] Several trials of this method have showed significant reductions in depression, as well as other cardiac risk factors (e.g., low-density lipoprotein cholesterol, blood pressure).[72-74] Most of the studies done on this setting have focused on depression as it is the most highly correlated with adverse cardiac outcomes, but very few have looked specifically at anxiety or chronic stress. There are potential barriers to screening anxiety in this setting since many anxiety symptoms can be cardiac in nature, such as heart palpitations, tachycardia, and chest pressure.[29] Some patients having panic attacks may also perceive that they are having an MI, as it is suspected that up to 25% of patients presenting to the emergency department for symptoms of a heart attack may be experiencing a panic attack, though it's rarely diagnosed.[75]

Conventional mental health treatment that is used in the collaborative care setting is a combination of psychotherapy and pharmacotherapy. Psychotherapy generally takes place in the form of Cognitive Behavioral Therapy (CBT) performed by a mental health professional, which focuses on identifying and altering thoughts and behaviors that lead to depression and/or anxiety,[58] or Interpersonal Therapy (IPT), which involves identifying problematic social situations and developing increased social skills to mitigate depression or anxiety.[76] While considered safe and effective, there is the risk that symptoms may increase through increasing awareness of negative thoughts,[58] but this form of therapy is still considered standard of care in treatment of depression and anxiety, and safe for those with comorbid CVD.

It has been recommended that pharmacotherapy for individuals with CVD should start with first-line selective serotonin receptor inhibitors (SSRIs) such as citalopram or sertraline.[58] While effectiveness of SSRIs is similar across types, citalopram and sertraline have fewer interactions with cytochrome p450 and subsequently are less likely to cause pharmacokinetic interactions with cardiac medication.[58] However, SSRIs are contraindicated when used in conjunction with other medications that lead to QT interval prolongation.[77] In a review by Von Ruden[78] and colleagues evaluating association between SSRIs and cardiovascular risk, it was found that of 13 studies evaluated, 5 showed decreased cardiovascular morbidity or mortality, 2 showed worsened prognosis with SSRI use, and 6 found no association. One of the few positive studies, Sertraline Against Depression and Heart Disease in Chronic Heart Failure (SADHART) specifically evaluated the use of sertraline as an antidepressant agent and its impact on CHF. Results ultimately found that of the 44.3% of patients with remittance of depression, there were significantly fewer cardiovascular events in comparison to the 41.4% that did not achieve remission, though the latter group was determined to have a greater severity of depression at baseline.[79] Lamictal, commonly used for mood stability, now carries a black box warning for the potential of causing high-degree heart block. We recommend 7 days of arrhythmia monitoring in all patients treated with lamictal.

Other pharmaceutical agents may also be employed; for example, bupropion may be an effective alternative in patients who are sensitive to side effects of SSRIs or who are attempting smoking cessation.[58] However, tricyclic antidepressants have been associated with adverse cardiac events and should be avoided in patients with CVD.[58] For individual's needing medication, we strongly recommend pharmacogenetic testing. Sequencing a patient's DNA helps to select safe and effective pharmacological treatment avoiding both undesirable side effects and need for multi-drug therapies.[80]

INTEGRATIVE TREATMENT

There are a myriad of options to target common etiological factors of depression, anxiety, and CVD as well as interventions to prevent progression of CVD due to depression, anxiety, or chronic stress. These range from nutrition to supplements and herbs, and lifestyle change.

Diet

Depression has been specifically correlated with anhedonia, or inability to experience pleasure. Subsequently, the dopaminergic reward pathways that are often associated with changing behaviors are not activated, resulting in much lower motivation to exert extra effort for little-to-no feeling of reward.[22] Interestingly, despite this inability to feel pleasure, when given sucrose solutions, depressed patients show enjoyment and preference for sweets, indicating that the pleasure response is still possible.[22]

Correspondingly, anxiety processes also impact reward processing through different mechanisms. Individuals with anxiety who are experiencing acute stress or feelings of threat show blunted responses to reward.[22] Brain imaging studies have shown that acute stress causes a reduction in neural reward responses, thus altering reward circuitry.[22]

While dietary changes are certainly difficult to enact for patients with depression and anxiety, they are very important to mitigate the progression of these disorders and CVD. It may not come as a surprise that the Western diet consisting of processed/fried foods, refined grains, and sugary products has been shown to increase risk of depression and anxiety.[81–83] Hypoglycemia and poor blood sugar control have also been linked with increased cortisol in anxiety disorders,[84] and a very low carbohydrate diet in certain individuals may potentiate depression.[85]

Studies show the diet that mitigates depression risk most is characteristically anti-inflammatory with an emphasis on whole foods, specifically vegetables rich in folate, olive oil, fish, nuts, and legumes.[81,86] This is essentially the Mediterranean diet, a diet that has been touted for cardiovascular health for many years.[87,88] The idea behind the Mediterranean diet is that it contains foods with anti-inflammatory properties. The anti-inflammatory diet, like the Mediterranean diet, emphasizes macronutrients that are the least inflammatory: increasing omega-3 fatty acids and decreasing omega-6 fatty acids and saturated fats, having lower amounts of high-glycemic carbohydrates in the diet to avoid excess insulin production, and overall consumption of fewer calories.[89] Based upon the common mechanism of inflammation underlying depression, anxiety, chronic stress, and CVD, it would follow that focusing on reduction of inflammation is a large component of reducing cardiac risk.

However, it is clear that diets are not one-size-fits-all. It is possible for the body to develop an immunological response to certain foods, leading to food intolerances and food sensitivities. These reactions have been found to increase inflammation[90] and activate immune cells, such as mast cells.[91] Food sensitivities and intolerances have been linked to a variety of health issues and symptoms that include depression and anxiety.[70,92] While randomized controlled trials (RCTs) performed on food intolerances or sensitivities as correlated with anxiety and depression are limited, clinical experience suggests that an elimination diet impacts symptoms due to a reduction in inflammation. However, with any restrictive diet, it is important to monitor patient anxiety levels, as it is possible that prescribing a restrictive diet may actually exacerbate symptoms of anxiety and depression.

Dietary recommendations should be individualized for patients based upon their level of functioning and motivation. Providing easy recipes and lists of healthful prepared foods from local stores and restaurants can enhance compliance. The use of medical food or meal replacement powders to simplify the threshold of effort required for patients to be successful should be considered. Patient buy-in is extremely important, and allowing them to be a part of creating their plan has been shown to increase outcomes.[73]

An underutilized resource to assist CVD patients in making behavioral changes is secondary prevention programs such as cardiac rehabilitation. Many cardiac rehabilitation programs focus on nutritional education, physician-supervised exercise, stress management, and group support.[93,94] Conventional cardiac rehabilitation programs have the greatest emphasis on exercise which is short sighted. Intensive cardiac rehabilitation programs such as the Ornish Lifestyle Change program and the Pritikin program, which provide a greater focus on lifestyle change, have been shown to influence favorable outcomes such as reducing angina, body mass index, systolic blood pressure, total cholesterol, LDL cholesterol, and blood glucose.[93]

The Ornish program has also been shown to reverse coronary artery disease, demonstrating the tremendous impact of lifestyle change.[93–95]

Gut Health

Research on the "gut-brain axis" is shedding light on the role of the microbiome in health. Changes in the gut microbiome have been linked to metabolic disorders such as obesity and diabetes,[96] depression and anxiety.[97] The gut microbiome composition is dependent on many factors such as inoculation of bacteria at birth, stress, hormone levels, and exposure to various strains of bacteria throughout life. However, the gut microbiome is also closely linked to food choices and responds very quickly to dietary changes.[97] Animal studies have shown that inoculation with Western diets and certain dietary carbohydrates can alter the microbiome within 24 hours after consumption.[96] While this emphasizes the need for a balanced diet, high in anti-inflammatory plant based foods, it also emphasizes the potential benefit of analyzing an individual's gut microbiome. Stool testing allows for sequencing of the microbiome for identification of pathogenic bacterial strains. Stool testing also shows inflammation, detoxification, digestive byproducts, and small intestine function. In functional medicine, there is a gut repair protocol called the "5 R Framework for Gut Restoration", that follows a sequence of steps including remove, replace, repair, reinoculate, and rebalance, in order to heal the gut and the microbiome.[98]

Nutritional Supplements

Depression has been associated with a multitude of nutrient deficiencies including thiamine, riboflavin, niacin, biotin, pantothenic acid, vitamin B6, folic acid, vitamin B12, vitamin C,[70] and vitamin D.[99] Both depression and anxiety have also been correlated with iron-deficiency anemia.[100,101] Subsequently, a general nutrient evaluation should be included in the evaluation of patients with depression and/or anxiety, and CVD. In addition to any nutrients that may be deficient, there are important nutrients that have been shown to work therapeutically to impact depression and anxiety; these are highlighted below. Obtaining a nutrient evaluation allows for the personalization of dietary supplements.

Fatty Acids

Omega-3 fatty acids in concentrations up to 9.6 g/day have been found to reduce symptoms of depression.[102,103] It appears that the eicosapentaenoic acid (EPA) concentration correlates more with mitigation of depression than docosahexaenoic acid (DHA).[104] Smaller doses of omega-3 fatty acids do not appear to have the same benefit for depression, but decreased CVD risk has been associated with doses of 3–4 g/day.[105,106] Just 2 g/day of omega-3 fatty acids significantly reduced symptoms of anxiety.[107] It is important to prescribe high-quality sources of omega-3 fatty acids to ensure they are low in mercury and other toxins. Mercury may exacerbate autonomic nervous system dysfunction,[70,108] further contributing to depression, anxiety, and cardiovascular disease.

Vitamin D

Vitamin D is a fat-soluble vitamin synthesized by exposure to the sun. Vitamin D is crucial for brain function, and a deficiency of vitamin D is associated with an 8%–14% increase in depression and a 50% increase in suicide.[109] Even outside of laboratory-defined deficiency, serum concentration of vitamin D had an inverse correlation with depressive symptoms.[110] Ideal functional laboratory ranges find that levels closer to the middle of the laboratory reference range are protective for a variety of conditions, lower oxidative stress, and decreased LDL levels.[109] The connection between vitamin D and depression may be further elucidated through the vitamin D receptor (VDR) genetic mutation, which predisposes to having lower levels of vitamin D as well as higher rates of depression.[111]

Minerals

Minerals serve as cofactors for a variety of processes that ultimately may contribute to depression. Zinc has been shown to be an antagonist of the N-methyl-D-aspartate glutamate receptor, and levels have been found to be decreased in depressed patients.[112] In a study of patients with MDD, 25 mg of zinc supplementation reduced depressive symptoms in conjunction with SSRIs in comparison to placebo.[112] Additionally, selenium has been found to be reduced in patients with depression, particularly those with comorbid alcoholism, and in higher concentrations has been shown to improve mood.[113] Chromium picolinate at 400 mcg has been found to impact differential outcomes for atypical depression[114] by altering brain serotonin levels[115] and is also correlated with reducing insulin resistance,[116] an outcome that benefits both depression and CVD risk.

Magnesium is an essential cofactor in many biochemical reactions in the body.[117] Magnesium has been shown to decrease hs-CRP and lower blood sugar. Stress hormones trigger extracellular shunting of magnesium, leading to a decrease in serum magnesium concentration.[117] Low serum magnesium has in turn been shown to increase stress hormones such as catecholamines and cortisol, which perpetuates a cycle of stress and hypomagnesemia.[117] Mitral valve prolapse (MVP) has also been strongly correlated with hypomagnesemia, and symptoms of anxiety, chest pain, weakness, dyspnea, and palpitations can be significantly diminished after supplementation with magnesium.[118] Existing evidence shows a correlation between magnesium supplementation and reduction in anxiety-related symptoms such as perceived stress and insomnia.[117] While there are not many studies on magnesium as a monotherapy and anxiety as a disorder, there are numerous studies that show benefits of magnesium for anxiety in combination with other nutrients such as vitamin B6 and anxiolytic herbs.[117,119]

B Vitamins

Several B-vitamin deficiencies have been correlated with depression, including thiamine, riboflavin, niacin, biotin, pantothenic acid, B6, folic acid, and B12.[70] A well-rounded, high-quality B-complex vitamin may serve to assist in mitigating these deficiencies. However, several of these have been studied for their effects at higher therapeutic doses.

Vitamin B6 (pyridoxine) exerts a modulatory effect on serotonin and GABA, and has been shown to reduce blood pressure, reduce homocysteine levels, and downregulate glucocorticoid receptors.[120] Vitamin B6 may be used therapeutically in doses of 100–300 mg daily to incite these effects, thereby decreasing anxiety and depression.[120] It can also be combined with magnesium for a synergistic effect on anxiety.[117]

Folic acid in doses of 500 mcg has been found to improve depression symptoms when added to an SSRI.[121] Folic acid supplementation has been the subject of much nutritional research due to its varying bioavailability in certain forms based upon genetic polymorphisms. If an individual has a heterozygous or homozygous mutation at the methylenetetrahydrofolate reductase (MTHFR) gene, it suggests an inability to methylate B-vitamins, thus requiring supplementation with forms of B-vitamins that are already methylated, specifically L-methylfolate and methylcobalamin.[122] The MTHFR C677T polymorphism has also been associated with increased risk of depression,[122,123] as well as cardiovascular risk factors such as increased blood pressure.[124] Currently, there are no studies linking MTHFR polymorphism to anxiety; however, there are other related polymorphisms that should be taken into consideration, such as catechol-o-methyltransferase (COMT). A COMT polymorphism, especially at the met158 allele, is linked to higher anxiety levels,[125,126] indicating an over-active methylation pathway. In these patient's supplementation with B-vitamins, particularly methylfolate may cause anxiety. Subsequently, it is recommended that a patient's MTHFR polymorphisms are tested, and they are supplemented according to their need for 5-methyltetrahydrofolate (L-methylfolate or 5-MTHF) or folinic acid.

SAMe has also been studied in the treatment of depression. One mechanism of its action may be linked to the MTHFR polymorphism as it is a universal methyl donor. SAMe in doses of 150 mg/day to 400 mg three times per day has been found to be equally or more effective than tricyclic antidepressants for the treatment of MDD.[127] It is important to note that SAMe should be avoided in individuals with anxiety or bipolar disorder, as it may contribute to mania and anxiety. SAMe can also enhance SSRI effects.[128] SAMe should also be avoided in individuals with a homozygous COMT polymorphism as this may increase risk of anxiety.

Amino Acids

L-Tryptophan and *5-hydroxytryptamine (5-HTP)* have been used to increase levels of serotonin, in lieu of SSRI medication for depression and anxiety. L-Tryptophan intake at a dose of 2 g three times per day was studied in the 1970s and found to have equivalent outcomes with TCAs.[129] Since this time, it has become more controversial due to its potential interaction with SSRIs and development of serotonin syndrome. In addition, eosinophilic myalgia syndrome was linked to a contaminant in tryptophan supplements. However, if no serotonin-producing drugs are being utilized, tryptophan and 5-HTP can serve to potentiate serotonin and decrease depressive or anxious symptoms, provided that a source made to pharmaceutical grade is utilized. A study performed by Lu and colleagues found that in an animal model, a post-MI population had lower 5-HTP levels in the hippocampus, suggesting this as a potential mechanism of post-cardiac event depression.[130] A proposed mechanism of low tryptophan in depression is based upon HPA axis regulation of tryptophan.[131] Since HPA axis dysregulation in itself is a mechanism of correlation between depression and CVD, targeting HPA axis regulation is also an area of treatment.

L-Lysine and L-arginine are additional amino acids that serve to impact stress and anxiety. L-Lysine has been shown to act as a partial serotonin receptor 4 antagonist, and a partial benzodiazepine agonist.[132] While there is not much research available for the use of L-lysine as a monotherapy, when L-lysine is used in combination with L-arginine, they reduce subjective trait and stress-induced state anxiety, as well as levels of stress hormones such as cortisol.[132,119]

HERBAL THERAPIES

Many herbal therapies exist that can serve to mimic actions of pharmaceuticals, or mitigate underlying mechanisms that link depression, anxiety, and CVD.

One of the most widely used herbal antidepressants and anxiolytics is *Hypericum perforatum* or St. John's Wort. This is an acceptable treatment for depression or anxiety to reduce CVD risk; however, it is also a strong inducer of cytochrome P450 3A4 (CYP3A4) enzyme, thereby reducing plasma concentrations of drugs metabolized in this pathway.[133] Since many CVD patients are on a polypharmacy regimen, *H. perforatum* is not recommended unless close consideration of herb-drug interactions has taken place and is being monitored.

HERBAL ANXIOLYTICS

Several herbs have been well studied for their anxiolytic properties and used across various cultures to treat anxiety.

Passiflora incarnata or passionflower has been used for hundreds of years and considered an acceptable treatment for restlessness and nervousness. It has been studied in comparison to benzodiazepines for the treatment of chronic anxiety, and one study showed passionflower to be as effective as benzodiazepines in managing symptoms of anxiety.[134] Perhaps the greatest differences noted were that benzodiazepines had a faster onset, and passionflower did not incite the adverse effect of performance impairment found with benzodiazepines.[134] There are few adverse effects that are rarely noted with passionflower, but they may include dizziness, drowsiness, and confusion.[119]

Piper methysticum is commonly known as kava and has been used for centuries as a drink to decrease anxiety, restlessness, and insomnia.[119] Kava has been found to inhibit norepinephrine and dopamine reuptake as well as MAOB, and enhance GABA binding.[119] This combination of actions allows kava to have unique properties in that it is anxiolytic, but not sedative like benzodiazepines. There have been controversies about the safety of kava in the past due to reports of hepatotoxicity; however, the rarity of these claims suggests potential poor supplement quality or overuse as a recreational beverage.[119]

HERBAL ADAPTOGENS

Herbal adaptogens serve to mitigate stress and help normalize HPA axis function.[135] Deviations from the normal cortisol rhythm throughout the day can cause symptoms of anxiety and depression. Normalization of this rhythm can be accomplished through the utilization of herbal adaptogens. Salivary and urine metabolite testing over a 24-hour period can offer a snapshot of an individual's HPA axis functioning. When cortisol is suppressed, it is helpful to utilize stimulating adaptogenic herbs such as *Eleutherococcus senticosus* and *Rhodiola rosea*.[135]

R. rosea has also been studied for its antidepressant properties.[76] *Ginkgo biloba*, which may also be particularly beneficial in elderly patients through increasing cerebrovascular blood flow,[136] has been used as an herb to support cardiovascular health, as its actions include antioxidant activity, free-radical scavenging, vasodilation, vascular protection, membrane stabilization, inhibition of platelet-activating factor, and regulation of metabolism.[136] Of course, the use of *Gingko* in combination with blood thinners such as warfarin and the newer direct oral anti-coagulants is not recommended.

Some adaptogenic herbs can have a more equalizing effect on the cortisol rhythm and can be utilized when a patient's cortisol rhythm is unknown. These modulating adaptogens include *Schisandra chinensis* and *Withania somnifera* (ashwagandha). Ashwagandha has been researched as an anxiety treatment and has shown significant improvements in subjective anxiety and stress.[137] One study demonstrated better outcomes with the use of ashwagandha and naturopathic care versus psychotherapy in the form of CBT and placebo.[138] Ashwagandha has also been shown to decrease oxidative stress and offers neuroprotection when under chronic stress.[139]

LIGHT THERAPY

Seasonal affective disorder (SAD) refers to depression that occurs when light exposure is limited. This has led to research exploring the impact of light on depression and serotonin synthesis,[140] which has implications for all types of depression. While light therapy is a highly accepted form of treatment for SAD, it has also been studied as a noninvasive modality to treat non-seasonal depression.[141–143] A review by Zhao and colleagues[144] illustrates the efficacy of utilizing light therapy in the morning within 30 minutes of waking to combat depression in various populations including geriatric populations, individuals with MDD, and those with minor depression. A significant decrease in depressive symptoms was found across various treatment conditions, though the greatest results were found when white or pale blue light is administered at an intensity of 5,000 lux for 50 minutes within 30 minutes of waking for a duration of 2–4 weeks.[144] Light therapy is noninvasive, with no reported adverse effects, and additional benefits of increasing sleep efficacy and evening melatonin production.[145] Where possible, light therapy could also be incorporated with exercise, by encouraging patients to go for a 50–60 minute walk in the sun every morning upon waking.

MIND-BODY TECHNIQUES

HEART RATE VARIABILITY

Autonomic dysfunction is a risk factor for CVD that is perpetuated through states of depression and anxiety, and it can be measured through HRV. Low HRV is linked to poor cardiovascular outcomes. HRV can be measured and utilized to help foster self-awareness and facilitate control of physiological processes such as heart rate and breathing.[146] Performing HRV training assists in increasing resting HRV[146] as well as increasing parasympathetic tone in the face of stressors,[147] thus leading to lower anxiety and lower risk of CVD. HRV training may be performed with comprehensive biofeedback software, or with HRV-specific software, which is readily available for home use.[147,148]

BREATHING

There are many mind-body techniques that impact the autonomic nervous system and overall health.[170] Breathing exercises are among the simplest, most accessible, and efficacious. The SPRINT trial showed that in patients with stage 1 non-medicated hypertension, performing guided breathing and meditation exercises over 12 months reduced resting systolic blood pressure,[170] resting diastolic blood pressure,[170] and perceived stress levels.[170,171] Making exhalation a few seconds longer than inhalation stimulates the parasympathetic nervous system and promotes relaxation. Some patients may want to utilize smartphone applications, though instructions for breathing exercises can easily be given to patients after illustrating the practice in office, and should be encouraged on a daily basis as well as during stressful periods and before bed to promote relaxation.

MEDITATION

Mindfulness and meditation techniques have been found to impact CVD through modulation of the autonomic nervous systems.[93] Transcendental meditation (TM) is a practice that focuses the mind on silent repetition of a mantra in the form of a word or phrase.[149] Twenty minutes twice daily of TM has been shown to decrease anxiety and PTSD symptoms,[149] as well as decreasing systolic and diastolic blood pressures.[93,150] TM has been shown to decrease major adverse cardiac events by 48% over a period of 5 years in African Americans with hypertension.[93,150] Mindfulness-Based Stress Reduction (MBSR), based on the Buddhist form of meditation, has been shown to improve telomerase activity, improve immune response, and decrease anxiety.[151] In fact, one study showed that even a single mindfulness-based meditation session could decrease morning systolic blood pressure in patients.[171] Both TM and MBSR are easy to learn, and training is readily available. For individuals that prefer guided meditations, there are many mobile phone applications and programs that can be utilized to help develop and maintain a meditation practice.

LIFESTYLE

While behavioral change is one of the most challenging treatments when it comes to depression and CVD, it can also be the most impactful. For example, eating an anti-inflammatory diet while eliminating tobacco use and alcohol consumption is necessary for both cardiovascular health and depression. Nicotine increases adrenal hormone secretion, raising cortisol levels and leading to the HPA axis dysfunction that is underlying depression and CVD.[70] Cortisol elevation decreases levels of tryptophan, serotonin, and melatonin in the brain, and also desensitizes serotonin receptors.[70] Cigarette smoking generates an abundance of free radicals, causes oxidative stress, and reduces levels of antioxidants in the body that are protective against both depression and CVD.[70] Alcohol is a well-known chemical depressant, which also increases adrenal hormone secretion, alters brain function, disrupts sleep cycles, leads to reactive hypoglycemia, and depletes nutrients that are necessary for mood stabilization.[70] Patients should be strongly encouraged to undergo addiction treatment to remove these barriers to health.

EXERCISE

Exercise is perhaps the most beneficial treatment for both depression and cardiovascular health.[152] Regular exercise works to prevent obesity, a risk factor for both depression and CVD, and to lower systemic inflammation.[70] Exercise has been shown to decrease cortisol levels and increase levels of mood-boosting beta-endorphins.[153] Recent research on exercise has elucidated the ability of exercise to increase brain-derived neurotrophic factor (BDNF), a growth factor responsible for cell growth and regeneration, synaptic remodeling and plasticity, while also impacting hypothalamic pathways of homeostasis, central metabolism, and regulation of angiogenesis and muscle regeneration.[154] A study performed by Zembron-Lacny and colleagues[154] showed that individuals who were more active had higher BDNF and better lipoprotein profiles with less oxidative stress and inflammation.

YOGA

Yoga is a practice that literally means "union", as its purpose is to unite the body and mind. It is a practice that incorporates both breathing techniques and physical exercise. Yoga has been shown to impact stress levels positively, leading to greater resilience of both body and mind. The practice of yoga has also been shown to decrease episodes of angina and atrial fibrillation,[93] as well as cardiovascular risk factors including lowering blood pressure,[155] decreasing cortisol and inflammatory markers,[93] decreasing LDL and triglycerides, and increasing HDL cholesterol.[156] Additionally, yoga may help to mitigate some of the connections between depression/anxiety/stress and CVD through increasing HRV,[157] and normalizing autonomic function.[158] The Ornish program for reversing heart disease combined yoga and meditation with vegetarian diet, group support, and exercise. The result of this integrative health approach in the secondary prevention of cardiovascular disease was a 91% reduction in angina and evidence coronary disease reversal.[93–95]

SOCIAL SUPPORT AND COMPLIANCE

Lack of social support and loneliness are recognized risk factors for cardiovascular disease. Social support whether through family, friends, or the cardiac rehabilitation team is critical to success especially with lifestyle change. Utilizing motivational interviewing to generate a collaborative treatment plan allows patients to have some control over what therapies are included in their treatment regimen.

Individuals with chronic disease are much more likely to practice self-care with support from friends and family to assist them in making the necessary lifestyle changes and in remaining compliant with medications and/or supplements.[159] While a therapist should certainly be a part of the team, it is also important for a depressed or anxious individual to have regular social interactions. Cardiac rehabilitation, for example, provides an excellent and safe social support network and instills confidence, especially with exercise.

In our modern society, we are often physically isolated from one another; however, technology has provided novel ways to help patients who are depressed. There are online communities of individuals who have experienced similar health concerns, and people can gain validation through reading about these experiences on message boards, from telling their stories, from being heard. There are also several mobile phone applications that may serve to fill in the gaps for some people with mental-emotional concerns. There are apps with daily reminders to eat, drink water, take medications, shower, and seek social interaction – all things that are difficult for depressed or anxious individuals to do.[160] There are mindfulness and meditation apps to help individuals relax and cope with stress through guided imagery or progressive relaxation. There is even an automated messaging system that employs methods from CBT to provide guidance through a text message conversation, allowing for on-demand support.[161] While lifestyle changes may be difficult, there are many ways to make them more accessible and achievable for patients. As practitioners, we just have to be willing to think outside the box. Cardiac rehabilitation provides a safe environment for individuals to learn lifestyle change and connect with others having similar health challenges.[93]

SPIRITUALITY

Spirituality is often used as a term to encompass many matters of belief including religion, secular belief systems, and a general sense of meaning.[162] This broad understanding of the term creates a situation wherein patients are able to define spirituality for themselves. Some individuals may adopt spiritual practices that are in line with an existing doctrine, while others may find a unique connection with something such as a higher power or nature.[21]

Spirituality is associated with positive health outcomes including decreased physical symptoms such as pain and fatigue, increased quality of life,[163] and even greater longevity.[164] Patients with religious involvement or spiritual practices have better coping skills, and less anxiety and depression.[164] A review by Lucchese and colleagues[162] analyzed the relationship between religion, spirituality, and cardiovascular disease, concluding that religion and spirituality have a multifaceted impact on CVD by manifesting positive emotions while decreasing depression, anxiety, and substance abuse. Several studies have better cardiovascular outcomes in individuals with a religious practice,[165–167] including decreased odds of MI[165] decreased risk of mortality from coronary heart disease,[166] or secondary to elective cardiovascular surgery.[167]

Spirituality may help to create resilience both physically and psychologically, to mitigate the impact of chronic stress, depression, and anxiety on cardiovascular health. Subsequently, it is important for practitioners to be willing to engage in discussions with patients about spiritual practices, and encourage patients to find a path to inner peace that is in keeping with their belief system. Spirituality may include religious practices, service, or practices such as meditation, mindfulness, prayer, and gratitude.[168] The practices of service, forgiveness, gratitude, and appreciation are fundamental to the spiritual path, and are medicine for the heart.

SUMMARY

Cardiovascular disease is not simply a disease of the cardiovascular system. Cardiovascular disease is a reflection of the health of the whole human being including biochemical states, emotional states, social connectedness, and spirituality. If practitioners focus solely on the classic cardiovascular disease risk factors such as tobacco use, diabetes, and hypertension, they will miss the important comorbidities of depression, stress, and anxiety and the opportunity to treat these important root causes.

Depression, perceived stress, and anxiety have direct physiological impacts on cardiovascular health, through mechanisms as inflammation, autonomic dysfunction, HRV, platelet activation, and cardiac reactivity. It is no mystery that depression, stress, and anxiety have biochemical impacts on various body systems, both directly and through alteration of behavioral practices. Subsequently, treatment of an individual with cardiovascular disease must not only address the structural and physiological pathology, but must also look beyond that pathology for triggers that are psychological. Utilizing integrative therapies such as nutrition, botanicals, mind-body medicine, spirituality, and lifestyle counseling assists patients with CVD to truly heal their hearts and develop resilience.

CHALLENGES

The research presented in this chapter shows the breadth of exploration that has been done in correlating depression, anxiety, stress, and cardiovascular disease. Unfortunately, the standard of care of CVD does not provide screening or treatment recommendations for this prominent comorbidity. It has been argued that screening may lead to over-treatment with pharmaceutical therapy for patients who show signs of depression and anxiety. However, if the tools presented in this chapter are utilized to mitigate depression, anxiety, and stress in patients with CVD in lieu of over-medicalization of the mental-emotional concerns, it is possible to treat the underlying causes of the comorbidity. There are opportunities to explore these connections further, to evaluate outcomes of patients that are treated with an integrative approach that involves prevention, nutritional therapies, lifestyle change, counseling, and spirituality. At a minimum, it is exceptionally important to listen to CVD patients, provide heart-centered care, and normalize the emotions of sadness, stress, and anxiety.

TAKE AWAY MESSAGES

- Mental-emotional states such as depression, anxiety, and stress negatively impact cardiovascular health and outcomes.
- Extensive research has shown the correlation between depression and CVD as well as post-MI mortality rates. However, the overlap between depression and anxiety shows that there are likely many of the same pathways at work.
- Inflammation and oxidative stress are triggers for depression, stress, and anxiety.
- Depression, anxiety, and CVD are connected through a variety of mechanisms including inflammation, oxidative stress, platelet activation, autonomic dysfunction, HPA axis dysfunction, endothelial dysfunction, cardiovascular reactivity, and behavioral mechanisms. While these connections exist, it is difficult to determine the directionality of causation, and thus there is room for intervention on all sides through prevention of CVD, prevention of depression/anxiety, lowering of stress, and mitigating every stage of the pathogenesis by focusing on the mechanisms listed above.
- Patients with CVD should be screened for depression and anxiety to allow for secondary prevention of adverse cardiac events and outcomes.
- Treatment should be individualized, collaborative, and integrative.
- Patients should be tested for any root cause risk factors and treated for these using appropriate treatment modalities.
- Treatments should include an appropriate combination of psychotherapy or counseling, mind-body modalities, lifestyle changes, herbal or nutritional antidepressants/anxiolytics, and/or pharmaceuticals such as SSRIs when indicated.
- Pharmacogenomics and genetics can personalize treatment.
- Practitioners should strongly consider comprehensive programs such as cardiac rehabilitation. It is also possible to use patient social support systems and technology to assist in patient motivation and compliance.

REFERENCES

1. Maciocia G. 2015. *The Foundations of Chinese Medicine*. 3rd ed. London: Elsevier Health Sciences.
2. Davidson KW, Alcántara C, Miller GE. 2018. Selected psychological comorbidities in coronary heart disease: challenges and grand opportunities. *Am Psychol*. 73(8):1019–1030.
3. Malzberg B. 1937. Mortality among patients with involution melancholia. *Am J Psychiatry*. 93:1231–1238.
4. Bulka CM, Daviglus ML, Persky VW, et al. 2018. Association of occupational exposures with cardiovascular disease among Hispanics/Latinos: results from the Hispanic community health study/study of Latinos. *Heart* 0:1–10.
5. Alissa EM, Ferns GA. Heavy metal poisoning and cardiovascular disease. *J Toxicol*. 2011;2011:870125. doi:10.1155/2011/870125.
6. Alissa EM, Ferns GA. Heavy metal poisoning and cardiovascular disease. *J Toxicol*. 2011;2011:870125. doi:10.1155/2011/870125.
7. Ignarro LJ, Balestrieri ML, Napoli C. 2007. Nutrition, physical activity, and cardiovascular disease: an update. *Cardiovasc Res*. 73:326–340.
8. Joseph MS, Konerman MA, Zhang M, et al. 2018. Long-term outcomes following completion of a structured nutrition and exercise lifestyle intervention program for patients with metabolic syndrome. *Diabetes Metab Syndr Obes Targets Ther*. 11:753–759.
9. American Psychiatric Association. 2013. *Diagnostic and Statistical Manual of Mental Disorders*. 5th ed. Washington, DC: American Psychiatric Association.

10. Kroenke K, Spitzer RL. 2002. The PHQ-9: a new depression diagnostic and severity measure. *Psychiatr Ann.* Sep 1;32(9):509–515.

11. Radloff LS. 1977. The CES-D scale: a self-report depression scale for research in the general population. *Appl Psychol Meas.* Jun;1(3):385–401.

12. Beck AT, Steer RA, Brown GK. 1996. *Beck Depression Inventory-II.* San Antonio, TX. Vol. 78(2): 490–8.

13. Steer RA, Brown GK, Beck AT, et al. 2001. Mean Beck depression inventory-II scores by severity of major depressive episode. *Psychol Rep.* 88(3 Pt 2):1075–6.

14. Hare DL, Davis CR. 1996. Cardiac depression scale: validation of a new depression scale for cardiac patients. *J Psychosom Res.* Apr 1;40(4):379–86.

15. Nicholson A, Kuper H, Hemingway H. 2006. Depression as an aetiologic and prognostic factor in coronary heart disease: a metaanalysis of 6362 events among 146 538 participants in 54 observational studies. *Eur Heart J.* 27(23):2763–74.

16. Rozanski A, Blumenthal JA, Davidson KW, et al. 2005. The epidemiology, pathophysiology, and management of psychosocial risk factors in cardiac practice: the emerging field of behavioral cardiology. *J Am Coll Cardiol.* 45:637–51.

17. Hare DL, Toukhsati SR, Johansson P, et al. 2014. Depression and cardiovascular disease: a clinical review. *Eur Heart J.* 35(21):1365–72.

18. Lesperance F, Frasure-Smith N, Talajic M, et al. 2002. Five-year risk of cardiac mortality in relation to initial severity and one-year changes in depression symptoms after myocardial infarction. *Circulation* 105:1049–53.

19. Montgomery SA. 2008. The under-recognized role of dopamine in the treatment of major depressive disorder. *Int Clin Psychopharmacol.* 23(2):63–9.

20. Hasler G. 2010. Pathophysiology of depression: do we have any solid evidence of interest to clinicians? *World Psychiatry.* 9(3):155–61.

21. Heim C, Newport DJ, Mletzko T, et al. 2008. The link between childhood trauma and depression: insights from HPA axis studies in humans. *Psychoneuroendocrinology.* 33(6):693–710.

22. Oberg E. 2014. Wellness, lifestyle and preventive medicine. In Wardle J, Sarris J, eds. *Clinical Naturopathy: An Evidence-Based Guide to Practice.* 2nd ed. Chatswood: Elsevier Health Sciences.

23. Dillon DG, Rosso IM, Pechtel P, et al. 2014. Peril and pleasure: an RDOC-inspired examination of threat responses and reward processing in anxiety and depression. *Depress Anxiety.* 31(3):233–49.

24. Singh MK, Gotlib IH. 2014. The neuroscience of depression: implications for assessment and intervention. *Behav Res Ther.* 62:60–73.

25. Dunlop BW, Nemeroff CB. 2007. The role of dopamine in the pathophysiology of depression. *Arch Gen Psychiatry.* 64(3):327–37.

26. Blanco C, Rubio JM, Wall M, et al. 2014. The latent structure and comorbidity patterns of generalized anxiety disorder and major depressive disorder: a national study. *Depress Anxiety.* 31(3):214–22.

27. Zbozinek TD, Rose RD, Wolitzky-taylor KB, et al. 2012. Diagnostic overlap of generalized anxiety disorder and major depressive disorder in a primary care sample. *Depress Anxiety.* 29(12):1065–71.

28. Roy MA, Neale MC, Pedersen NL, et al. 1995. A twin study of generalized anxiety disorder and major depression. *Psychol Med.* 25(5):1037–49.

29. Sunderland M, Mewton L, Slade T, et al. 2010. Investigating differential symptom profiles in major depressive episode with and without generalized anxiety disorder: true co-morbidity or symptom similarity? *Psychol Med.* 40(7):1113–23.

30. Thurston RC, Rewak M, Kubzansky LD. 2013. An anxious heart: anxiety and the onset of cardiovascular diseases. *Prog Cardiovasc Dis.* 55(6):524–37.

31. Takagi Y, Sakai Y, Abe Y, et al. 2018. A common brain network among state, trait, and pathological anxiety from whole-brain functional connectivity. *Neuroimage.* 172:506–16.

32. Spitzer RL, Kroenke K, Williams JB, et al. 2006. A brief measure for assessing generalized anxiety disorder: the GAD-7. *Arch Intern Med.* May 22;166(10):1092–7.

33. Chilcot J, Hudson JL, Moss-morris R, et al. 2018. Screening for psychological distress using the patient health questionnaire anxiety and depression scale (PHQ-ADS): initial validation of structural validity in dialysis patients. *Gen Hosp Psychiatry.* 50:15–9.

34. You JS, Hu SY, Chen B, et al. 2005. Serotonin transporter and tryptophan hydroxylase gene polymorphisms in Chinese patients with generalized anxiety disorder. *Psychiatr Genet.* 15(1):7–11.

35. Unschuld PG, Ising M, Specht M, et al. 2009. Polymorphisms in the GAD2 gene-region are associated with susceptibility for unipolar depression and with a risk factor for anxiety disorders. *Am J Med Genet B Neuropsychiatr Genet.* 150B(8):1100–9.

36. Nitschke JB, Sarinopoulos I, Oathes DJ, et al. 2009. Anticipatory activation in the amygdala and anterior cingulate in generalized anxiety disorder and prediction of treatment response. *Am J Psychiatry.* 166(3):302–10.

37. Safren SA, Gershuny BS, Marzol P, et al. 2002. History of childhood abuse in panic disorder, social phobia, and generalized anxiety disorder. *J Nerv Ment Dis.* 190(7):453–6.

38. Baldwin D. 2018. Generalized anxiety disorder in adults: epidemiology, pathogenesis, clinical manifestations, course, assessment, and diagnosis. In Stein MB, Hermann R, eds. *UpToDate.* Waltham, MA: UpToDate; www.uptodate.com. Accessed October 10, 2018.

39. Godbout JP, Glaser R. 2006. Stress-induced immune dysregulation: implications for wound healing, infectious disease and cancer. *J Neuroimmune Pharmacol.* 1:421–7.

40. Sterling P, Eyer J. 1988. Allostasis: a new paradigm to explain arousal pathology. In Fisher S, Reason J, eds. *Handbook of Life Stress, Cognition, and Health.* New York: John Wiley & Sons; 629–49.

41. Logan JG, Barksdale DJ. 2008. Allostasis and allostatic load: expanding the discourse on stress and cardiovascular disease. *J Clin Nurs.* 17(7B):201–8.

42. Schulkin J. 2004. *Allostasis, Homeostasis, and the Costs of Physiological Adaptation.* New York: Cambridge University Press.

43. Antonelli M, Kushner I. 2017. It's time to redefine inflammation. *FASEB J.* 31(5):1787–91. https://faseb.onlinelibrary.wiley.com/doi/full/10.1096/fj.201601326R.

44. Zuzarte P, Duong A, Figueira ML, et al. 2018. Current therapeutic approaches for targeting inflammation in depression and cardiovascular disease. *Curr Drug Metab.* 19(8):674–87.

45. Xiong GL, Prybol K, Boyle SH, et al. 2015. Inflammation markers and major depressive disorder in patients with chronic heart failure: results from the sertraline against depression and heart disease in chronic heart failure study. *Psychosom Med.* 77(7):808–15.

46. Salim S, Asghar M, Taneja M, et al. 2011. Potential contribution of oxidative stress and inflammation to anxiety and hypertension. *Brain Res.* 1404:63–71.

47. Smykiewicz P, Segiet A, Keag M, et al. 2018. Proinflammatory cytokines and ageing of the cardiovascular-renal system. *Mech Ageing Dev.* 175:35–45.

48. Ford DE, Erlinger TP. 2004. Depression and C-reactive protein in US adults: data from the Third National Health and Nutrition Examination Survey. *Arch Intern Med.* 164:1010–4.

49. Dong Y, Wang X, Zhang L, et al. 2018. High-sensitivity C reactive protein and risk of cardiovascular disease in China-CVD study. *J Epidemiol Community Health.* Dec 7:jech-2018.

50. Steenkamp LR, Hough CM, Reus VI, et al. 2017. Severity of anxiety-but not depression-is associated with oxidative stress in Major Depressive Disorder. *J Affect Disord.* 219:193–200.

51. Serebruany VL, Glassman AH, Malinin AI, et al. 2003. Enhanced platelet/endothelial activation in depressed patients with acute coronary syndromes: evidence from recent clinical trials. *Blood Coagul Fibrinolysis.* 14(6):563–7.

52. Aschbacher K, Mills PJ, Von Känel R, et al. 2008. Effects of depressive and anxious symptoms on norepinephrine and platelet P-selectin responses to acute psychological stress among elderly caregivers. *Brain Behav Immun.* 22(4):493–502.

53. Cygankiewicz I, Zareba W. 2013. Heart rate variability. In Buijs RM, Swaab DF, eds. *Autonomic Nervous System.* Vol. 117. Edinburgh: Elsevier.

54. Zhang Y, Chen Y, Ma L. 2018. Depression and cardiovascular disease in elderly: current understanding. *J Clin Neurosci.* 47:1–5.

55. Carney RM, Blumenthal JA, Stein PK, et al. 2001. Depression, heart rate variability, and acute myocardial infarction. *Circulation.* 104(17):2024–8.

56. Kubzansky LD, Kawachi I, Weiss ST, et al. 1998. Anxiety and coronary heart disease: a synthesis of epidemiological, psychological, and experimental evidence. *Ann Behav Med.* 20(2):47–58.

57. Otte C, Marmar CR, Pipkin SS, et al. 2004. Depression and 24-hour urinary cortisol in medical outpatients with coronary heart disease: the Heart and Soul Study. *Biol Psychiatry.* 56(4):241–7.

58. Otte C, Neylan TC, Pipkin SS, et al. 2005. Depressive symptoms and 24-hour urinary norepinephrine excretion levels in patients with coronary disease: findings from the Heart and Soul Study. *Am J Psychiatry.* 162(11):2139–45.

59. Whooley MA. 2006. Depression and cardiovascular disease: healing the broken-hearted. *JAMA.* 295(24):2874–81.

60. Mann DL, Kent RL, Parsons B, et al. 1992. Adrenergic effects on the biology of the adult mammalian cardiocyte. *Circulation.* 85(2):790–804.

61. Communal C, Singh K, Pimentel DR, et al. 1998. Norepinephrine stimulates apoptosis in adult rat ventricular myocytes by activation of the beta-adrenergic pathway. *Circulation.* 98(13):1329–34.

62. Van sloten TT, Schram MT, Adriaanse MC, et al. 2014. Endothelial dysfunction is associated with a greater depressive symptom score in a general elderly population: the Hoorn Study. *Psychol Med.* 44(7):1403–16.

63. Stillman AN, Moser DJ, Fiedorowicz J, et al. 2013. Association of anxiety with resistance vessel dysfunction in human atherosclerosis. *Psychosom Med.* 75(6):537–44.

64. Wittstein IS, Thiemann DR, Lima JAC, et al. 2005. Neurohumoral features of myocardial stunning due to sudden emotional stress. *N Engl J Med.* 352:539–48.

65. Wittstein IS. 2007. The broken heart syndrome. *Cleve Clin J Med.* 74:S17–22.

66. Feng J, Lenihan DJ, Johnson MM, et al. 2006. Cardiac sequelae in Brooklyn after the September 11 terrorist attacks. *Clin Cardiol.* 29(1):13–7.

67. Bazoukis G, Tse G, Naka KK, et al. 2018. Impact of major earthquakes on the incidence of acute coronary syndromes – a systematic review of the literature. *Hellenic J Cardiol.* 59(5):262–7.

68. Ziegelstein RC, Fauerbach JA, Stevens SS, et al. 2000. Patients with depression are less likely to follow recommendations to reduce cardiac risk during recovery from a myocardial infarction. *Arch Intern Med.* 160:1818–23.

69. Antonogeorgos G, Panagiotakos DB, Pitsavos C, et al. 2012. Understanding the role of depression and anxiety on cardiovascular disease risk, using structural equation modeling; the mediating effect of the Mediterranean diet and physical activity: the ATTICA study. *Ann Epidemiol.* 22:630–7.

70. Goossens L, Braet C, Bosmans G. 2010. Relations of dietary restraint and depressive symptomatology to loss of control over eating in overweight youngsters. *Eur Child Adolesc Psychiatry.* 19(7):587–96.

71. Bongiorno P, Murray M. 2013. Affective disorders. In Pizzorno J, Murray M, eds. *Textbook of Natural Medicine.* 4th ed. St. Louis, MS: Elsevier; 1162–77.

72. Hansen RA, Khodneva Y, Glasser SP, et al. 2016. Antidepressant medication use and its association with cardiovascular disease and all-cause mortality in the reasons for geographic and racial differences in stroke (REGARDS) study. *Ann Pharmacother.* 50(4):253–61.

73. Huffman JC, Mastromauro CA, Beach SR, et al. 2014. Collaborative care for depression and anxiety disorders in patients with recent cardiac events: the management of sadness and anxiety in cardiology (MOSAIC) randomized clinical trial. *JAMA Intern Med.* 174(6):927–35.

74. Katon WJ, Lin EH, Von Korff M, et al. 2010. Collaborative care for patients with depression and chronic illnesses. *N Engl J Med.* 363:2611–20.

75. Katon W, Russo J, Lin EH, et al. 2012. Cost-effectiveness of a multicondition collaborative care intervention: a randomized controlled trial. *Arch Gen Psychiatry* 69:506–14.

76. Katon WJ, Von Korff M, Lin E. 1992. Panic disorder: relationship to high medical utilization. *Am J Med.* 92:S7–11.

77. Sarris J. 2014. Depression. In Wardle J, Sarris J, eds. *Clinical Naturopathy: An evidence-Based Guide to Practice.* 2nd ed. Chatswood: Elsevier Health Sciences.

78. Angermann CE, Ertl G. 2018. Depression, anxiety, and cognitive impairment: comorbid mental health disorders in heart failure. *Curr Heart Fail Rep.* 15(6):398–410.

79. Von ruden AE, Adson DE, Kotlyar M. 2008. Effect of selective serotonin reuptake inhibitors on cardiovascular morbidity and mortality. *J Cardiovasc Pharmacol Ther.* 13(1):32–40.

80. Jiang W, Krishnan R, Kuchibhatla M, et al. 2011. Characteristics of depression remission and its relation with cardiovascular outcome among patients with chronic heart failure (from the SADHART-CHF study). *Am J Cardiol.* 107(4):545–51.

81. Perlis RH, Mehta R, Edwards AM, et al. 2018. Pharmacogenetic testing among patients with mood and anxiety disorders is associated with decreased utilization and cost: a propensity-score matched study. *Depress Anxiety.* 35(10):946–52.

82. Jacka FN, Pasco JA, Mykletun A, et al. 2010. Association of western and traditional diets with depression and anxiety in women. *Am J Psychiatry.* 167(3):305–11.

83. Bakhtiyari M, Ehrampoush E, Enayati N, et al. 2013. Anxiety as a consequence of modern dietary pattern in adults in Tehran–Iran. *Eat Behav.* 14(2):107–12.

84. Yannakoulia M, Panagiotakos DB, Pitsavos C, et al. 2008. Eating habits in relations to anxiety symptoms among apparently healthy adults. A pattern analysis from the ATTICA Study. *Appetite.* 51(3):519–25.

85. Jezova D, Vigas M, Hlavacova N, et al. 2010. Attenuated neuroendocrine response to hypoglycemic stress in patients with panic disorder. *Neuroendocrinology.* 92(2):112–9.

86. Brinkworth GD, Buckley JD, Noakes M, et al. 2009. Long-term effects of a very low-carbohydrate diet and a low-fat diet on mood and cognitive function. *Arch Intern Med.* 169(20):1873–80.

87. Sanhueza C, Ryan L, Foxcroft DR. 2013. Diet and the risk of unipolar depression in adults: systematic review of cohort studies. *J Hum Nutr Diet.* 26(1):56–70.

88. Estruch R, Ros E, Salas-salvadó J, et al. 2018. Primary prevention of cardiovascular disease with a Mediterranean diet supplemented with extra-virgin olive oil or nuts. *N Engl J Med*. 378(25):e34.

89. Ros E, Martínez-González MA, Estruch R, et al. 2014. Mediterranean diet and cardiovascular health: teachings of the PREDIMED study. *Adv Nutr*. May 6;5(3):330S–6S.

90. Sears B. 2015. Anti-inflammatory diets. *J Am Coll Nutr*. 34(Suppl 1):14–21.

91. Ohtsuka Y. 2015. Food intolerance and mucosal inflammation. *Pediatr Int*. 57(1):22–9.

92. Theoharides TC, Tsilioni I, Patel AB, et al. 2016. Atopic diseases and inflammation of the brain in the pathogenesis of autism spectrum disorders. *Transl Psychiatry*. 6(6):e844.

93. Brostoff J, Gamlin L. 2000. *Food Allergies and Food Intolerance: The Complete Guide to Their Identification and Treatment*. Rochester, VT: Healing Arts Press.

94. Freeman AM, Taub PR, Lo HC, et al. 2019. Intensive cardiac rehabilitation: an underutilized resource. *Curr Cardiol Rep*. 21(4):19.

95. Silberman A, Banthia R, Estay IS, et al. 2010. The effectiveness and efficacy of an intensive cardiac rehabilitation program in 24 sites. *Am J Health Promot*. 24(4):260–6.

96. Ventegodt S, Merrick E, Merrick J. 2006. Clinical holistic medicine: the Dean Ornish program ("opening the heart") in cardiovascular disease. *Sci World J*. 6:1977–84.

97. Delzenne NM, Neyrinck AM, Bäckhed F, et al. 2011. Targeting gut microbiota in obesity: effects of prebiotics and probiotics. *Nat Rev Endocrinol*. 7(11):639–46.

98. Luna RA, Foster JA. 2015. Gut brain axis: diet microbiota interactions and implications for modulation of anxiety and depression. *Curr Opin Biotechnol*. 32:35–41.

99. Institute of Functional Medicine. The 5R framework for gut restoration. Presented at: *Applying Functional Medicine in Clinical Practice*, in Baltimore, MD; September 2016.

100. Spedding S. 2014. Vitamin D and depression: a systematic review and meta-analysis comparing studies with and without biological flaws. *Nutrients*. Apr;6(4):1501–18.

101. Peuranpää P, Heliövaara-Peippo S, Fraser I, et al. 2014. Effects of anemia and iron deficiency on quality of life in women with heavy menstrual bleeding. *Acta Obstet Gynecol Scand*. Jul 1;93(7):654–60.

102. Benton D, Donohoe RT. 1999. The effects of nutrients on mood. *Public Health Nutr*. 2(3A):403–9.

103. Su KP, Huang SY, Chiu CC, et al. 2003. Omega-3 fatty acids in major depressive disorder: a preliminary double-blind, placebo-controlled trial. *Eur Neuropsychopharmacol*. Aug 1;13(4):267–71.

104. Jazayeri S, Tehrani-doost M, Keshavarz SA, et al. 2008. Comparison of therapeutic effects of omega-3 fatty acid eicosapentaenoic acid and fluoxetine, separately and in combination, in major depressive disorder. *Aust N Z J Psychiatry*. 42(3):192–8.

105. Martins JG. 2009. EPA but not DHA appears to be responsible for the efficacy of omega-3 long chain polyunsaturated fatty acid supplementation in depression: evidence from a meta-analysis of randomized controlled trials. *J Am Coll Nutr*. 28(5):525–42.

106. Mozaffarian D, Wu JH. 2011. Omega-3 fatty acids and cardiovascular disease: effects on risk factors, molecular pathways, and clinical events. *J Am Coll Cardiol*. 58(20):2047–67.

107. REDUCE-IT™ Cardiovascular Outcomes Study of Vascepa® (icosapent ethyl) Capsules Met Primary Endpoint [Press release]. Bedminster, NJ. Amarin Corporation; September 24, 2018. https://investor.amarincorp.com/node/15741/pdf. Accessed October 8, 2018.

108. Su KP, Tseng PT, Lin PY, et al. 2018. Association of use of omega-3 polyunsaturated fatty acids with changes in severity of anxiety symptoms: a systematic review and meta-analysis. *JAMA Netw Open*. 1(5):e182327.

109. Milioni ALV, Nagy BV, Moura ALA, et al. 2017. Neurotoxic impact of mercury on the central nervous system evaluated by neuropsychological tests and on the autonomic nervous system evaluated by dynamic pupillometry. *Neurotoxicology*. 59:263–9.

110. Sepehrmanesh Z, Kolahdooz F, Abedi F, et al. 2016. Vitamin D supplementation affects the beck depression inventory, insulin resistance, and biomarkers of oxidative stress in patients with major depressive disorder: a randomized, controlled clinical trial. *J Nutr*. 146(2):243–8.

111. Hoogendijk WJ, Lips P, Dik MG, et al. 2008. Depression is associated with decreased 25-hydroxyvitamin D and increased parathyroid hormone levels in older adults. *Arch Gen Psychiatry*. 65(5):508–12.

112. Minasyan A, Keisala T, Lou YR, et al. 2007. Neophobia, sensory and cognitive functions, and hedonic responses in vitamin D receptor mutant mice. *J Steroid Biochem Mol Biol*. 104(3–5):274–80.

113. Nowak G, Szewczyk B. 2002. Mechanisms contributing to antidepressant zinc actions. *Pol J Pharmacol*. 54(6):587–92.

114. Finley JW, Penland JG. 1998. Adequacy or deprivation of dietary selenium in healthy men: clinical and psychological findings. *J Trace Elem Exp Med*. 11:11–27.

115. Davidson JR, Abraham K, Connor KM, et al. 2003. Effectiveness of chromium in atypical depression: a placebo-controlled trial. *Biol Psychiatry.* 53(3):261–4.
116. Attenburrow MJ, Odontiadis J, Murray BJ, et al. 2002. Chromium treatment decreases the sensitivity of 5HT2A receptors. *Psychopharmacology.* 159:432–6.
117. Anderson RA. 1998. Chromium, glucose intolerance and diabetes. *J Am Coll Nutrition.* 17:548–55.
118. Pouteau E, Kabir-ahmadi M, Noah L, et al. 2018. Superiority of magnesium and vitamin B6 over magnesium alone on severe stress in healthy adults with low magnesemia: a randomized, single-blind clinical trial. *PLoS One.* 13(12):e0208454.
119. Lichodziejewska B, Kłoś J, Rezler J, et al. 1997. Clinical symptoms of mitral valve prolapse are related to hypomagnesemia and attenuated by magnesium supplementation. *Am J Cardiol.* 79(6):768–72.
120. Lakhan SE, Vieira KF. 2010. Nutritional and herbal supplements for anxiety and anxiety-related disorders: systematic review. *Nutr J.* 9:42.
121. Mccarty MF. 2000. High-dose pyridoxine as an 'anti-stress' strategy. *Med Hypotheses.* 54(5):803–7.
122. Coppen A, Bailey J. 2000. Enhancement of the antidepressant action of fluoxetine by folic acid: a randomised, placebo controlled trial. *J Affect Disord.* 60(2):121–30.
123. Jha S, Kumar P, Kumar R, et al. 2016. Effectiveness of add-on l-methylfolate therapy in a complex psychiatric illness with MTHFR C677 T genetic polymorphism. *Asian J Psychiatr.* Aug 1;22:74–5.
124. Rai V. 2014. Genetic polymorphisms of methylenetetrahydrofolate reductase (MTHFR) gene and susceptibility to depression in Asian population: a systematic meta-analysis. *Cell Mol Biol* (Noisy-le-grand). 60(3):29–36.
125. Rashed L, Abdel Hay R, Alkaffas M, et al. 2017. Studying the association between methylenetetrahydrofolate reductase (MTHFR) 677 gene polymorphism, cardiovascular risk and lichen planus. *J Oral Pathol Med.* 46(10):1023–9.
126. Woo JM, Yoon KS, Yu BH. 2002. Catechol O-methyltransferase genetic polymorphism in panic disorder. *Am J Psychiatry.* 159(10):1785–7.
127. Pooley EC, Fineberg N, Harrison PJ. 2007. The met(158) allele of catechol-O-methyltransferase (COMT) is associated with obsessive-compulsive disorder in men: case-control study and meta-analysis. *Mol Psychiatry.* 12(6):556–61.
128. Papakostas GI, Cassiello CF, Iovieno N. 2012. Folates and S-adenosylmethionine for major depressive disorder. *Can J Psychiat.* Jul;57(7):406–13.
129. Abeysundera H, Gill R. 2018. Possible SAMe-induced mania. *BMJ Case Rep.* Jun 27;2018:bcr-2018.
130. Lindberg D, Ahlfors UG, Dencker SJ, et al. 1979. Symptom reduction in depression after treatment with L-tryptophan or imipramine. Item analysis of Hamilton rating scale for depression. *Acta Psychiatr Scand.* 60(3):287–94.
131. Lu X, Wang Y, Liu C, et al. 2017. Depressive disorder and gastrointestinal dysfunction after myocardial infarct are associated with abnormal tryptophan-5-hydroxytryptamine metabolism in rats. *PLoS One.* 12(2):e0172339.
132. Sorgdrager FJH, Doornbos B, Penninx BWJH, et al. 2017. The association between the hypothalamic pituitary adrenal axis and tryptophan metabolism in persons with recurrent major depressive disorder and healthy controls. *J Affect Disord.* 222:32–9.
133. Smriga M, Torii K. 2003. L-Lysine acts like a partial serotonin receptor 4 antagonist and inhibits serotonin-mediated intestinal pathologies and anxiety in rats. *Proc Natl Acad Sci USA.* 100(26):15370–5.
134. Komoroski BJ, Zhang S, Cai H, et al. 2004. Induction and inhibition of cytochromes P450 by the St. John's wort constituent hyperforin in human hepatocyte cultures. *Drug Metab Dispos.* May 1;32(5):512–8.
135. Akhondzadeh S, Naghavi HR, Vazirian M, et al. 2001. Passionflower in the treatment of generalized anxiety: a pilot double-blind randomized controlled trial with oxazepam. *J Clin Pharm Ther.* 26(5):363–7.
136. Panossian A. 2005. Stimulating effect of adaptogens: an overview with particular reference to their efficacy following single dose administration. *Phytother Res.* 19:819–38.
137. Tian J, Liu Y, Chen K. 2017. *Ginkgo biloba* extract in vascular protection: molecular mechanisms and clinical applications. *Curr Vasc Pharmacol.* Jan 1;15:532–48.
138. Pratte MA, Nanavati KB, Young V, et al. 2014. An alternative treatment for anxiety: a systematic review of human trial results reported for the Ayurvedic herb ashwagandha (*Withania somnifera*). *J Altern Complement Med.* 20(12):901–8.
139. Cooley K, Szczurko O, Perri D, et al. 2009. Naturopathic care for anxiety: a randomized controlled trial ISRCTN78958974. *PLoS One.* 4(8):e6628.
140. Durg S, Dhadde SB, Vandal R, et al. 2015. *Withania somnifera* (ashwagandha) in neurobehavioural disorders induced by brain oxidative stress in rodents: a systematic review and meta-analysis. *J Pharm Pharmacol.* 67(7):879–99.

141. Lambert GW, Reid C, Kaye DM, et al. 2002. Effect of sunlight and season on serotonin turnover in the brain. *Lancet.* 360(9348):1840–2.
142. Martiny K. 2017. Novel augmentation strategies in major depression. *Dan Med J.* 64(4):B5338.
143. Mårtensson B, Pettersson A, Berglund L, et al. 2015. Bright white light therapy in depression: a critical review of the evidence. *J Affect Disord.* 182:1–7.
144. Wirz-justice A, Bader A, Frisch U, et al. 2011. A randomized, double-blind, placebo-controlled study of light therapy for antepartum depression. *J Clin Psychiatry.* 72(7):986–93.
145. Zhao X, Ma J, Wu S, et al. 2018. Light therapy for older patients with non-seasonal depression: a systematic review and meta-analysis. *J Affect Disord.* 232:291–9.
146. Lieverse R, Van Someren EJ, Nielen MM, et al. 2011. Bright light treatment in elderly patients with nonseasonal major depressive disorder: a randomized placebo-controlled trial. *Arch Gen Psychiatry.* 68(1):61–70.
147. Goessl VC, Curtiss JE, Hofmann SG. 2017. The effect of heart rate variability biofeedback training on stress and anxiety: a meta-analysis. *Psychol Med.* 47(15):2578–86.
148. Whited A, Larkin KT, Whited M. 2014. Effectiveness of emWave biofeedback in improving heart rate variability reactivity to and recovery from stress. *Appl Psychophysiol Biofeedback.* 39(2):75–88.
149. McCraty R, Atkinson M, Tomasino D, et al. 2006. The coherent heart: heart-brain interactions, psychophysiological coherence, and the emergence of system-wide order. Retrieved from http://www.heartmath.org/research/publications.html.
150. Lang AJ, Strauss JL, Bomyea J, et al. 2012. The theoretical and empirical basis for meditation as an intervention for PTSD. *Behav Modif.* 36(6):759–86.
151. Schneider RH, Grim CE, Rainforth MV, et al. 2012. Stress reduction in the secondary prevention of cardiovascular disease: randomized, controlled trial of transcendental meditation and health education in Blacks. *Circ Cardiovasc Qual Outcomes.* 5(6):750–8.
152. Lengacher CA, Reich RR, Kip KE, et al. 2014. Influence of mindfulness-based stress reduction (MBSR) on telomerase activity in women with breast cancer (BC). *Biol Res Nurs.* 16(4):438–47.
153. Summers KM, Martin KE, Watson K. 2010. Impact and clinical management of depression in patients with coronary artery disease. *Pharmacotherapy.* 30(3):304–22.
154. Lobstein DD, Rasmussen CL, Dunphy GE, et al. 1989. Beta-endorphin and components of depression as powerful discriminators between joggers and sedentary middle-aged men. *J Psychosom Res.* 33(3):293–305.
155. Zembron-lacny A, Dziubek W, Rynkiewicz M, et al. 2016. Peripheral brain-derived neurotrophic factor is related to cardiovascular risk factors in active and inactive elderly men. *Braz J Med Biol Res.* 49(7):e5253.
156. Patel C, North WR. 1975. Randomised controlled trial of yoga and bio-feedback in management of hypertension. *Lancet.* 2(7925):93–5.
157. Bijlani RL, Vempati RP, Yadav RK, et al. 2005. A brief but comprehensive lifestyle education program based on yoga reduces risk factors for cardiovascular disease and diabetes mellitus. *J Altern Complement Med.* 11(2):267–74.
158. Satyapriya M, Nagendra HR, Nagarathna R, et al. 2009. Effect of integrated yoga on stress and heart rate variability in pregnant women. *Int J Gynaecol Obstet.* 104(3):218–22.
159. Bernardi L, Sleight P, Bandinelli G, et al. 2001. Effect of rosary prayer and yoga mantras on autonomic cardiovascular rhythms: comparative study. *BMJ.* 323(7327):1446–9.
160. Won MH, Son YJ. 2017. Perceived social support and physical activity among patients with coronary artery disease. *West J Nurs Res.* 39(12):1606–1623.
161. Aloe Bud. 2018. Self-care companion. *Aloebud.com.* https://aloebud.com/. Accessed October 10, 2018.
162. Woebot. 2018. Your charming robot friend who is here for you, 24/7. *Woebot.io.* https://woebot.io/. Accessed October 10, 2018.
163. Lucchese FA, Koenig HG. 2013. Religion, spirituality and cardiovascular disease: research, clinical implications, and opportunities in Brazil. *Rev Bras Cir Cardiovasc.* 28(1):103–28.
164. Boudreaux ED, O'Hea E, Chasuk R. 2002. Spiritual role in healing. An alternative way of thinking. *Prim Care* 29: 439–54, viii.
165. Mueller PS, Plevak DJ, Rummans TA. 2001. Religious involvement, spirituality, and medicine: implications for clinical practice. *Mayo Clin Proc.* 76(12):1225–35.
166. Friedlander Y, Kark JD, Stein Y. 1986. Religious orthodoxy and myocardial infarction in Jerusalem – a case control study. *Int J Cardiol.* 10(1):33–41.
167. Goldbourt U, Yaari S, Medalie JH. 1993. Factors predictive of long-term coronary heart disease mortality among 10,059 male Israeli civil servants and municipal employees. A 23-year mortality follow-up in the Israeli Ischemic Heart Disease Study. *Cardiology.* 82(2–3):100–21.

168. Oxman TE, Freeman DH, Manheimer ED. 1995. Lack of social participation or religious strength and comfort as risk factors for death after cardiac surgery in the elderly. *Psychosom Med.* 57(1):5–15.
169. Guarneri M, Bradley R. 2015. Be the willow: stress, resiliency, and diseases of the heart. In Sinatra S, Houston MC. *Nutritional and Integrative Strategies in Cardiovascular Medicine.* Boca Raton, FL: CRC Press; 318–37.
170. Pope B, Wood, S. 2020. Advances in understanding mechanisms and therapeutic targets to treat comorbid depression and cardiovascular disease. *Neurosci Biobehav Rev.* 116:337—349.
171. Chandler J, Sox L, Diaz V, et al. 2020. Impact of 12-month smartphone breathing meditation program upon systolic blood pressure among non-medicated stage 1 hypertensive adults. *IJERPH.* 17(6):1955.

Index

Note: **Bold** page numbers refer to tables and *italic* page numbers refer to figures.

acetaminophen 226
acetyl–L-carnitine 161–2
acupuncture 60–2, **62**
acute emotional effects 387
acute inflammation 145, 352–3
adenosine diphosphate (ADP) 195, *195*
adenosine monophosphate (AMP) 196
adenosine triphosphate (ATP) 190, 192, 366
    cellular concentration of 196, *197*
    chemical energy in 195
    free energy of hydrolysis of 194
    in heart cells 196
ADMA *see* asymmetric dimethyl L-arginine (ADMA)
advanced glycation end products (AGEs) 14, 49, 133–4
AIM-HIGH study 117–19
airborne transmission, COVID-19 339
air pollution 285–6, **286**
alcohol 17–18
Alexander DD 80
    Mayo Clinic Proceedings 81
algae 78–9
alpha-gliadin 256
alpha-linolenic acid (ALA) 4, 77, 79
alpha lipoic acid (ALA) 153, 158
alternate-day intermittent fasting (ADF) 17
amino acids 392
AMP-activated protein kinase (AMPk) 41, 53
anatomical, sex differences 218
angiotensin-converting enzyme (ACE) 12
angiotensin-converting enzyme inhibitors (ACEI) **167,** 269
angiotensin II (A-II) 147
angiotensin receptor blockers **167**
animal protein diets 15
    fish 15–16
    soy protein 15
The Annals of Thoracic Surgery 351
antacids 135
antibiotics, use of 134–5
anti-cytokine therapy 305
anti-hypertensives 372–3
    beetroot (*Beta vulgaris* L.)373–4
    hibiscus calyces (*Hibiscus sabdariffa* L.) 373
anti-inflammatory reflex 361
anxiety disorders
    defined as 384
    DSM criteria for **383**
    overlap between depression and 383–4
    screening measures for **384**
    stress 384–5
arjuna tree bark (*Terminalia arjuna*) 370
arterial stiffness 2–3, *5*
artichokes
    health benefits 37
    nutritional benefits of 36–7
astaxanthin 39–40
    from krill 88–9

A Study of Cardiovascular Events in Diabetes (ASCEND) 83
asymmetric dimethyl L-arginine (ADMA) 135
atherosclerosis 2–3, *5,* 50–1, 270
    as inflammatory process 298, *299*
Atherosclerosis Monitoring and Atherogenicity Reduction
    (AMAR) 372
atherosclerotic plaque formation 2, *3, 101*
ATP and the Heart (Ingwall) 194
Aung T 81
autography 40–1
autonomic dysfunction 386
autonomic nervous system (ANS)360, 361

bacterial colonization 266
BaleDoneen Method 319–21
barrier function 51
B-cell immunity 339–40, **340**
beetroot (*Beta vulgaris* L.)373–4
beetroot juice and extract 160–1
behavioral mechanisms 387
beneficial SCFAs 274, 275
berberine 53, 122
bergamot 54, **54**
Bernard C 349
beta-blockers **167**
bifidobacteria 275
bioavailability, of n-3 supplements 86
biofeedback 59
biological mechanisms
    acute emotional effects 387
    autonomic dysfunction 386
    cardiovascular reactivity 387
    endothelial dysfunction 386
    HPA axis dysfunction 386
    inflammation 385–6
    platelet activation 386
bisphenols 287–8
black tea 161
Black women 219, 220, 226
blood clotting 51
blood pressure (BP) 85, 360–3, *361,* **362**
    ; *see also* hypertension
blood sugar 49–50
blood viscosity 365
blueberry 57
botanical medicine 369–70
    anti-hypertensives 372–3
        beetroot (*Beta vulgaris* L.)373–4
        hibiscus calyces (*Hibiscus sabdariffa* L.) 373
    cardiovascular tonics 370
        arjuna tree bark (*Terminalia arjuna*) 370
        garlic (*Allium sativum* L.)371–2
        grape seed (*Vitis vinifera* L.) 372
        hawthorn (*Crataegus* spp.)370–1
        khella dried ripe fruit and seed
            (*Ammi Visnaga* L.) 370

Cooley D 349
coronary artery calcium (CAC) score 14
coronary artery disease 31–3
    body heals itself 41–2
    lycopene 37
        tomato nutrition 37–8
    mTOR 41–2
    nattokinase and lumbrokinase 38–9
        astaxanthin 39–40
        NMN/autography/mTOR 40–1
        omega-3 essential fatty acids 40
    olive oil 34–5
        adulteration in 35–6
        artichoke health benefits 37
        nutritional benefits of artichokes 36–7
        selection of 36
    polyphenols 33
        cocoa and dark chocolate 33–4
Coronary Drug Project (CDP) 118
coronary heart disease (CHD) 2
    dyslipidemia
        combination therapies 122
        FUNGENUT Study 105
        GEMINAL Study 105
        nutraceutical supplements for treatment 123, **123**
        nutrients and dietary supplements 115–22
        nutrition 102–5
        pathophysiology 98–100
        PREDIMED Study 105–6
        specific foods, nutrients, and dietary supplements
            106–15
        treatment 100–2
    mediterranean diet 3–5, 7
    nutrition and 3, **6–7**
    treatment of 2
COVID-19 335–6, 345
    endothelium 337–8, *338*
    inflammation and 353–4
    integrative approach to prevent and care patients
        342–3
    pathophysiology of 337
    strategies to boost immunity 343–4, *345*
    structural components 336, *336*
    tests to define prognosis and status
        D-dimer 342
        PULS Cardiac test 341–2, *342*
    transmission of 338–9
    variants **336,** 336–7, **337**
    viral replication and immune responses
        antigen tests and limitations 341
        incubation periods and impact on PCR testing
            strategies 339
        period of infectivity 339
        serology and B-cell immunity 339–40, **340**
        T-cell responses to 340, *341*
curcumin 116, 136–7, 275
CVD *see* cardiovascular disease (CVD)
cytokines 305
cytokine storm 337, 344

dark chocolate 33–4, 159
DASH diets *see* dietary approaches to stop hypertension
        (DASH) diets
D-dimer 342
DeBakey M 349

dehydroepiandrosterone (DHEA) 237, 240
depression 382
    DSM criteria for 382, **383**
    screening measures for 382, **384**
detoxification, in cardiovascular system 64
Device-Guided-Breathing-Exercises (DGBE) 60
DHA *see* docosahexaenoic acid (DHA)
diabetes mellitus (DM) 98, 99, 296
diastolic dysfunction (DD) 198
    in women 221–3
dichlorodiphenyltrichloroethane (DDT) 64
diet 56, 389–90
Diet And Reinfarction Trial (DART) 80, 81
dietary acid load 16
dietary and nutritional components 16
Dietary Approaches to Stop Hypertension (DASH) diet
        7–8, 57, 133
dietary fats, omega 3 fatty acids 8–9
dietary interventions, to decrease endotoxemia 275
dietary nitrates 160–1
dietary sodium 19–20
dietary TFA 11
Diet Heart Hypothesis 99
diet-induced dysbiosis 272, **272**
direct renin inhibitors **168**
direct vasodilators **168**
diuretics **168**
docosahexaenoic acid (DHA) 78, 275
    cardiometabolic mechanisms and biomarkers related
        to 84–5
    from genetically modified plants 79
double blind randomized placebo controlled trial
        (DBRPC) 153
doxycycline 305
D-ribose (ribose) 191, *195,* 199–201
droplets/aerosols, COVID-19 338
drug-induced side effects 100
drug therapy, for hypertension 164–6
dysbiosis 266
    diet-induced 272, **272**
dyslipidemia
    combination therapies 122
    FUNGENUT Study 105
    GEMINAL Study 105
    nutraceutical supplements for treatment 123, **123**
    nutrients and dietary supplements 115–16
        berberine 122
        citrus bergamot 116
        curcumin 116
        guggulipids 116
        lycopene 116
        niacin (vitamin B3) 116–19
        pantethine 119
        plant sterols (phytosterols) 119–20
        policosanol 120
        red yeast rice 121
        resveratrol 121
        tocotrienols 120–1
        vitamin C 121–2
    nutrition
        Framingham Heart Study 102
        Indian Heart Study 104–5
        Lyon Diet Heart Study 104
        Mediterranean diet 104
        nutrigenomics 105

dyslipidemia (*cont.*)
    OmniHeart Trial 103
    Ornish diet 102–3
    Portfolio diet 104
    Pritikin diet 102
    Seven Countries Study 102
    Therapeutic Lifestyle Changes diet 103
  pathophysiology 98–100, *100, 101*
  PREDIMED Study 105–6
  specific foods, nutrients, and dietary supplements
    flax seeds 114
    garlic 114
    green tea 114–15
    monounsaturated fats 114
    omega-3 fatty acids 106, 111–13
    orange juice 115
    pomegranate seeds and juice 115
    sesame seeds 115
    soy 115
  treatment 100, 102

Earth Biogenome Project 41, 42
earthing *see* grounding
eggs 12–13
eicosapentaenoic acid (EPA) 78, 275
  cardiometabolic mechanisms and biomarkers related
      to 84–5
  from genetically modified plants 79
electromagnetic forces 39
electromagnetic radiation (EMR) 68–9
electron transport chain 202
emotional stress 361, 387
endocrine system 265
endothelial-derived relaxing factor (EDRF) 65
endothelial dysfunction 2–3, *5,* 386
endothelial function, role of 52–3
endothelial NO synthase (eNOS) 134, 136
endothelial progenitor cells (EPCs) 147
endothelium 337–8, *338*
  functions of 51–2
energy, grounding system and 365–6
energy starvation, in failing heart 196, *198,* 198–9
enteric nervous system (ENS) 265
environmental toxins 281
  air pollution 285–6, **286**
  bisphenols 287–8
  effects on blood pressure 64–5
  lead **283,** 283–5
  persistent organic pollutants 286–7
  systemic approaches 288
    gamma glutamyl transferase 288
    sauna 289
Environmental Working Group 66
eosinophilic protein X (EPX) 274
epigallocatechin gallate (EGCG) 114
epigenetics, lifestyle plus 354–5
estradiol 232–4
etanercept 305
ethyl esters *vs.* triglycerides 86–7
European Heart Journal 40
European Prospective Investigation into Cancer and
      Nutrition (EPIC) study 154
exercise 58–9, **169,** 243, 354, 394–5
exocrine pancreatic insufficiency (EPI) 273

expanded lipid profiles 99, *100*
extended-release niacin (ERN) 118
extra virgin olive oil (EVOO) 104, 154
  coronary artery disease 34–5
    adulteration in 35–6
    artichoke health benefits 37
    nutritional benefits of artichokes 36–7
    selection of 36

Fasano, Alessio 49
fasting 62–3
fasting mimicking diet (FMD) 17
fatty acids 390
fecal fat 274
fecal-oral transmission, COVID-19 339
fermented foods and drinks 67
fiber 162, 354–5
fibrinolysis 51
fight-or-flight hormones 59
Finkle W D 240
fish 15–16
  allergies to 89–90
fish body oil 78
fish oil 78
  krill oil *vs.* 87–8
  oxidation 90
  quality control issues of 90
flavonoids 156–7
  alpha lipoic acid 158
  coenzyme Q10 157–8
  garlic 158
  lycopene 157
  pycnogenol 158
  seaweed 159
flax seed 114, 344
Flock M R 80
fluids 57–8
folic acid 391
food choices 61
food patterns 135–6
food source 50
14-hour overnight fasting 17
*Fourth National Report on Human Exposure to
      Environmental Chemicals* 281, *282*
Framingham Heart Study (FHS) 102
French paradox 33
Functional Genomics and Nutrition (FUNGENUT)
      Study 105
functional medicine 251
Functional Medicine Model of Precision Medicine 252
functional, sex differences 218
Fusobacterium nucleatum 297

gamma glutamyl transferase (GGTP) 288
gamma tocopherol 155
garlic (*Allium sativum* L.) 53–4, 61, 114, 158, 371–2
gastrointestinal metabolic markers 274
gastrointestinal supportive foods 67
GEMINAL Study 105
gender differences 219–20
generalized anxiety disorder (GAD)383, **383,** 384
Generalized Anxiety Disorder (GAD-7) questionnaire 384
geophysical fields 363
gestational diabetes 220

GGTP *see* gamma glutamyl transferase (GGTP)
Ginkgo biloba 393
GISSI-prevention trial 81, 106
gliadorphin 256
Global Burden of Diseases, Injuries, and Risk Factors
    Study (GBD 2017) 250
glutathione deficiency 344, *345*
gluten 18, 89
glycine propionyl L-carnitine (GPLC) 208
glycosaminoglycans (GAGs) 50–1
grape seed (*Vitis vinifera* L.) 372
grape seed extract (GSE) 160, 372
grape seed oil 372
green tea 114–15, 161, 311
ground flaxseeds 56
grounding 63, 360–1, *361,* 366–7
    and energy 365–6
    and immune system 363–5, *364*
    interventions to improve autonomic function
        361, **362**
guggulipids 116
Gundry S 256
Gut-Associated Lymphoid Tissue (GALT) 344
gut-derived hormones 269
gut health 390
gut microbiome 277
    clinical presentation of CVD 272–4
    dietary components effects on 271–2, **272**
    hypertension and 269
    metabolic endotoxemia 267–9
    metabolic functions of 265–6
    pathophysiology of CVD 266–7
    periodontal disease 269–70
    prevention and treatment strategies 274–6
    specific microbial species and microbiota composition
        270–1

hawthorn (*Crataegus* spp.)370–1
hawthorn extract 163
health care 55
Health-Related Quality of Life (HRQoL) protocols 251
heart failure (HF)
    defined as 190
    energy depletion in 196
heart rate 85
heart rate variability (HRV)360, 361, 386, 393–4
Heart Sense for Women 220
herbal adaptogens 393
herbal anxiolytics 392–3
herbal medicine *see* botanical medicine
herbal therapies 392
    herbal adaptogens 393
    herbal anxiolytics 392–3
hesperidin 162
hibiscus calyces (*Hibiscus sabdariffa* L.) 373
high blood pressure, recommendations for 63–4
high carbohydrate intake 310
high-density lipoprotein (HDL) cholesterol 53–4, 62, 85
high-fiber 66–7
high-sensitivity C-reactive protein (hs-CRP) 205
Honolulu Heart Program 79
hormonal, sex differences 218
hormone therapy
    is good for every woman 236–7

    methods of 237
    risk of 235–6
horse chestnut (*Aesculus hippocastanum* L.) 375
HPS2-THRIVE 118, 119
human ACE2 (hACE2) receptor 337
hunter-gatherer diet *see* Paleolithic diet
hydrogen peroxide solution 308
hydrolysis 307
5-hydroxytryptamine (5-HTP) 392
hydroxytyrosol (HT) 34
hyperbaric oxygen 308
hypertension 144
    balance of 147–8, *148, 149*
    beetroot juice and extract 160–1
    calcium 151
    clinical considerations 166, **167–70**
    cocoa 159
    dietary nitrates and nitrites 160–1
    diet, lifestyle, and 56
    drug therapy for 164–6
    epidemiology and pathophysiology 145, *145*
    exercise and 58–9
    fasting and 62–3
    fiber 162
    finite vascular responses 145, *146,* 147, *147*
    flavonoids 156–7
        alpha lipoic acid 158
        coenzyme Q10 157–8
        garlic 158
        lycopene 157
        pycnogenol 158
        seaweed 159
    fluids, salt, and 57–8
    grape seed extract 160
    grounding and 63
    and gut microbiome 269
    hawthorn extract 163
    hesperidin 162
    inflammation 145, *146,* 147, *147*
    integrative approach to treatment of **169–70**
    L-arginine 152–3
    L-carnitine and acetyl– L-carnitine 161–2
    magnesium 151
    melatonin 159–60
    MUFA 154
    N-acetylcysteine 162–3
    naturopathic approach 54–6
    omega-3 fats and omega-6 fats 153–4
    oxidative stress 145, *146,* 147, *147*
    potassium 150–1
    probiotics 163–4
    protein 151–2
    quercetin 163
    sesame 162
    sodium 150
    stress, breathing, and 59–60
    targeted nutritional supplements, botanical medicines,
        and acupuncture 60–2, **62**
    taurine 153
    teas 161
    treatment with nutrition and nutritional supplements
        148–50
    vascular immune dysfunction 145, *146,* 147, *147*
    vitamin B6 (pyridoxine) 156

hypertension (*cont.*)
  vitamin C 154–5
  vitamin D 155–6
  vitamin E 155
  in women 223–4
  zinc 151
  ; *see also* blood pressure (BP)
hypertensive disorders, of pregnancy 220
hypothalamic-pituitary-adrenal (HPA) axis dysfunction 386

Ile-Pro-Pro (IPP) 12
immune system 265
  grounding system and 363–5, *364*
immunology 274
Indian Heart Study 104–5
inflammation 49–51, 145, *146,* 147, *147,* 385–6
  acute 352–3
  atherosclerosis 298, *299*
  biological resolution of 305
  and blood viscosity 365
  chronic 352, 354
  and COVID 353–4
  and immunology 274
inflammatory biomarkers 85–6
inflammatory coronary heart disease/diabetes 205
Ingwall J
  ATP and the Heart 194
inorganic phosphate (Pi) 195, *195*
insoluble fibers 355
integrative treatment 388
  diet 389–90
  gut health 390
  nutritional supplements 390
    amino acids 392
    B vitamins 391–2
    fatty acids 390
    minerals 391
    vitamin D 390
interleukin-1 (IL-1) gene 300
International Heart Journal 202
International Journal of Molecular Medicine 39
intestinal permeability 267, 268
iron 311–12

JAMA Cardiology 81
Japan Collaborative Cohort (JACC) study 20
Japan EPA Lipid Intervention Study (JELIS) 82, 111
Journal of Hypertension Research 223
Journal of the American College of Cardiology
      204, 208, 238

Kapil V 134
Katz, Sandor Ellix
  Wild Fermentation 67
kava *(Piper methysticum)* 392–3
Kensey KR 364
Khatta M 203
khella dried ripe fruit and seed (*Ammi Visnaga* L.) 370
Korean National Health and Nutrition Examination
      Surveys 19
kosher 89
krill oil 78
  vs. fish oil 87–8
Kuopio Ischaemic Heart Disease Risk Factor Study 13

labeling issues, omega-3 products 90
LaPlace's law 198
L-arginine 132, *134,* 152–3, 344, 392
Lausche E 350
lead **283,** 283–5
leaky gut 267
left ventricular hypertrophy 198
lemon balm leaf (*Melissa officinalis* L.) 374
levocarnitine (L-carnitine/carnitine) 161–2, 191, 206–9
lifestyle 56, 394
  exercise 394–5
  social support and compliance 395
  yoga 395
lifestyle optimization 46
lifestyle plus epigenetics 354
  fiber 354–5
  supplements 355
light therapy 393
Lindeberg, Staffan 48
lipid-lowering effect 53, 54
lipid-storage disease 250
lipopolysaccharides (LPS) 267, 268, 275
lipoprotein particle size 85
liver supportive foods 67
L-lysine 392
long-chain fatty acids (LCFA) 10, 12
long-chain polyunsaturated fatty acids (LCPUFA)
      77–8, 86
Long-Term Outcomes Study to Assess Statin Residual
      Risk with Epanova in High Cholesterol
      Risk Patients with Hypertriglyceridemia
      (STREGTH) 83–4
low-density lipoprotein (LDL) cholesterol 51, 62, 84,
      85, 351
low-fat diets 47
low hydrochloric (HCl) acid 273
L-tryptophan 392
Lucchese FA 396
lumbrokinase
  coronary artery disease 38–9
    astaxanthin 39–40
    NMN/autography/mTOR 40–1
    omega-3 essential fatty acids 40
lycopene 116, 157, 311
  coronary artery disease 37
    tomato nutrition 37–8
lymphatic dysfunction 350
lymphatics 352
  and chronic inflammation 354
Lyon Diet Heart Study (LDHS) 104

macronutrients **169**
magnesium (Mg^{++}) 19–20, 61, 191, 311, 391
  hypertension 151
  in mitral valve prolapse 225
  switching on energy enzymes 209
magnetosphere 365
Major Depressive Disorder (MDD) 382, **383**
major vascular events (MVE) 118
marine collagen peptides (MCPs) 152
marine-derived omega-3 fatty acids 77–8
  delivery forms for supplementation 79
  sources of 78–9, 89
Mayo Clinic meta-analysis 112, 113

Index

McCully K 249
meditation 394
Mediterranean diet (MedDiet) 3–5, 7, 32, 42, 47–8, 104,
    154, 208, 276–7, 310
medium-chain fatty acids (MCFA) 10, 12
melatonin 311
    hypertension 159–60
men, CVD in 237–8, 244
    dehydroepiandrosterone 240
    exercise 243
    low testosterone and 238–9
    natural supplements 243
    non-pharmaceutical approaches 243
    testosterone replacement therapy **239,** 239–41
        methods of **242,** 242–3
        standard work-up 241–2
menopausal hormone therapy 234
menopause 224
metabolic cardiology 191, 192
    cell, secrets of 193–6, *195, 197*
    coenzyme Q10 190–2
        and heart *202,* 202–4
        inflammatory coronary heart disease/diabetes 205
        tissue deficiencies and low serum blood levels of 203
        ubiquinone, ubiquinol and MITOQ 205–6
    D-ribose 199–201
    energy starvation in failing heart 196, *198,* 198–9
    levocarnitine (L-carnitine/carnitine) 206–9
    magnesium 191
        switching on energy enzymes 209
    taurine 209
metabolic endotoxemia 267–9
metabolic syndrome 226
methylmercury 16
microbial diversity 266
micronutrients 310
milk 12
milk chocolate 33
milk products 12
mind-body techniques
    breathing exercises 394
    heart rate variability 393–4
    meditation 394
mind-body therapies 59
Mindfulness-Based Stress Reduction (MBSR) 394
minerals 391
Mitchell P 359
mitochondrial dysfunction 190
MITOQ 205–6
mitral valve prolapse (MVP) 391
    in women 224–5
monounsaturated fatty acids (MUFA) 9, 10, 114
    hypertension 154
motherwort herb (*Leonurus cardiaca* L.)374–5
mouthwash, use of 134–5
mTOR 40–2
mushrooms 344
mussels 78
myocardial infarction (MI) 2, 201, 218, 249, 382
myocardial performance index (MPI) 251
MyPerioPath test 301–2, *302,* 314, *314, 315, 317*

N-acetylcysteine (NAC) 162–3
National Cholesterol Education Program (ATP III) 103

National Health and Nutrition Examination Survey
    (NHANES) 80
National Heart, Lung, and Blood Institute (NHLBI) 103
National Lipid Association (NLA) 118
nattokinase
    coronary artery disease 38–9
        astaxanthin 39–40
        NMN/autography/mTOR 40–1
        omega-3 essential fatty acids 40
natural therapies 193
" nature's biological response modifiers" 52
naturopathic approach, hypertension 54–6
naturopathic doctors (NDs) 46
nausea 218
Neo40 137
nervine relaxants 374
    lemon balm leaf (*Melissa officinalis* L.) 374
    motherwort herb (*Leonurus cardiaca* L.)374–5
nervous system 265
New England Journal of Medicine 82
niacin (vitamin B3) 116–19
nicotinamide mononucleotide (NMN) 40–1
nitric oxide (NO) 131–2
    antacids inhibit 135
    clinical benefits of 138, **138**
    curcumin 136–7
    diet and lifestyle habits
        standard American diet 133–4, *134*
    food patterns 135–6
    loss of production 132, *133*
    resveratrol 136
    supplements 137
    use of mouthwash and antibiotics 134–5
nitrites 160–1
nonalcoholic fatty liver disease (NAFLD) 13
non-alcoholic steatohepatitis (NASH) 37
non-celiac gluten sensitivity (NCGS) 253
non-gluten proteins 256
non-high-density lipoprotein (non-HDL) cholesterol 85
nonsteroidal anti-inflammatory drugs (NSAIDs) 223
nonsurgical periodontal disease management 306
nutraceuticals 123, **123**
nutrients and dietary supplements
    dyslipidemia 115–16
        berberine 122
        citrus bergamot 116
        curcumin 116
        guggulipids 116
        lycopene 116
        niacin (vitamin B3) 116–19
        pantethine 119
        plant sterols (phytosterols) 119–20
        policosanol 120
        red yeast rice 121
        resveratrol 121
        tocotrienols 120–1
        vitamin C 121–2
nutrigenomics 105
nutrition 303
    and coronary heart disease 3, **6–7**
    dyslipidemia
        Framingham Heart Study 102
        Indian Heart Study 104–5
        Lyon Diet Heart Study 104

nutrition (*cont.*)
    Mediterranean diet 104
    nutrigenomics 105
    OmniHeart Trial 103
    Ornish diet 102–3
    Portfolio diet 104
    Pritikin diet 102
    Seven Countries Study 102
    Therapeutic Lifestyle Changes diet 103
  host modulation using 309–12
  role of 52–3
nutritional supplements
  amino acids 392
  B vitamins 391–2
  fatty acids 390
  minerals 391
  vitamin D 390
nuts 18–19

Ober C 359
oleic acid 154
oleuropein (OL) 34
olive leaf extract (OLE) 154
olive oil 57, 154
omega-3 fatty acids 8–11, 40, 79–80, 90–1, 106,
    111–13, 390
  allergies to fish and shellfish related to products 89–90
  astaxanthin from krill 88–9
  cardiometabolic mechanisms and biomarkers related to
    EPA and/or DHA 84–5
  CVD intervention studies using 80–2
    ASCEND 83
    REDUCE-IT 82
    STRENGTH 83–4
    VITAL 82–3
  ethyl esters *vs.* triglycerides 86–7
  fish oil
    krill oil *vs.* 87–8
    quality control issues of 90
  hypertension 153–4
  inflammatory biomarkers and specialized
    pro-resolving mediators 85–6
  LDL, HDL and non-HDL cholesterol 85
  long-term supplementation with 112
  omega-3 index and CVD risk 80
omega-6 fatty acids 35
  hypertension 153–4
omega-9 fatty acids 154
omega-3 index (O-3I) 80
Optimal Macronutrient Intake for Heart Health Trial
    (OmniHeart Trial) 103
oral bacteria 297
oral biofilm 295
  managing of 306–9
  in periodontal disease, caries and periapical disease
    295–6
oral L-arginine 152
orange juice 115
organic fruits 66–7
Ornish diet 102–3
Ornish Lifestyle Change program 389, 390, 395
Oxford Vegetarian Study 47
oxidation-reduction (REDOX) chemical reactions 202
oxidative damage 68–9

oxidative phosphorylation 198–9, 202
oxidative stress, hypertension 145, *146,* 147, *147*
oxygen 308
ozone 309

Paleolithic diet 47–8
pancreatic elastase 1 (PE1) 273
pancreatic elastase treatment 275
panic disorder (PD) **383**
pantethine 54, 119
parenteral L-arginine 152
particulate matter (PM) 285
Passiflora incarnata 392
passionflower *(Passiflora incarnata)* 392
Patient Health Questionnaire Anxiety and Depression
    Scale (PHQ-ADS) 384
Patient-Reported Outcome Measurement Information
    System (PROMIS) 252
pattern recognition receptors (PRR) 145
PCBs *see* polychlorinated biphenyls (PCBs)
PCR-swab tests 339
Peabody FW 366
PEACE trial 222
peptides 12
periapical disease, oral biofilm in 295–6
periapical infections 294
periodontal disease 269–70, 294, 296
  and atherosclerosis as inflammatory process 298, *299*
  biofilm elimination over long term 312–15, *313–15*
  and cardiovascular disease 297–8
  causes of 294–5
  collaboration between physician and dentist 315–16
  collaborative inflammation and biofilm treatment
    CIMT results 318, *318,* 319
    FidaLab post-treatment report 318, *320*
    initial disease diagnosis (FidaLab)316, *317,* 318
    initial periodontal charting 316, *316*
    MPO lab information 318, *318*
    MyPerioPath test 316, *317,* 318, *319*
  diagnosing of 299–303, *301, 302*
  host modulation 305–6
    using nutrition 309–12
  managing oral biofilm 306–9
  microbiological stability 314, *314*
  oral biofilm in 295–6
  pre- and post-treatment results 303, *304*
  treatment and maintenance 303–4
periodontal infection 297–8
peripheral artery disease (PAD) 225–6
Permanetter B 203
peroxide value (PV) 90
persistent organic pollutants (POPS)286–7
pharmacotherapy 388
phenylacetylglutamine (PAG) 269
5-phosphoribosyl-1-pyrophosphate (PRPP) 196, *197,* 200
phytonutrient-rich 66–7
Piper methysticum 392–3
plant-based nutrition 14–15
plant sterols (phytosterols) 119–20
plaque 295, 296
platelet activation 386
policosanol 120
polychlorinated biphenyls (PCBs) 64–5, 286–7
polycyclic aromatic hydrocarbons (PAHs) 285

polymerase chain reaction (PCR) 300
polyphenol-rich foods 276
polyphenols 33
    cocoa and dark chocolate 33–4
polyunsaturated fatty acids (PUFA) 77
pomegranate (*Punica granatum* L.)
    alpha lipoic acid 158
    coenzyme Q10 157–8
    garlic 158
    lycopene 157
    pycnogenol 158
    seaweed 159
pomegranate seeds and juice 115
POPS *see* persistent organic pollutants (POPS)
Porphyromonas gingivalis 270, 297
Portfolio diet 104
potassium 19–20
    hypertension 150–1
PPIs *see* proton pump inhibitors (PPIs)
precision medicine 251
PREDIMED diet 3–5, 7, 9, 10, 32
PREDIMED study 48
    dyslipidemia 105–6, **107–11**
pregnancy 224
    hypertensive disorders of 220
premature ventricular contractions (PVCs) 360
Prevention with Mediterranean Diet (PREDIMED)
        trial 154
Pritikin diet 102
Pritikin program 389
probiotics 269, 276, 344
    hypertension 163–4
protease insufficiency 274
protein
    dietary acid load and 16
    hypertension 151–2
    vegetarian diets and plant-based nutrition 14–15
proton pump inhibitors (PPIs) 135
psychological stress 384–5
psychotherapy 388
PULS Cardiac test 341–2, *342*
PVCs *see* premature ventricular contractions (PVCs)
pycnogenol 158, 375–6

Q-SYMBIO study 204
quercetin 275
    hypertension 163

racial disparities 220
randomized controlled clinical trials (RCCTs) 9, 10, 117
Reduction of Cardiovascular Events with Icosapent Ethyl-
        Intervention Trial (REDUCE-IT) 82
red yeast rice (RYR) 121
re-esterified triglycerides (rTG) fish oil product 87
refined carbohydrates 13–14
refined sugar 48–9
relative-risk reduction (RRR) 111
resveratrol 121, 136, 275
    alpha lipoic acid 158
    coenzyme Q10 157–8
    garlic 158
    lycopene 157
    pycnogenol 158
    seaweed 159

reverse cholesterol transport 351
Rhodiola rosea 393
risk factors, in women 219
Roberts J 191

Saeed A 218
saliva 300
salivary testing 303
salt 57–8
salt sensitivity 150
SAMe 391–2
sardine muscle protein 152
saturated fatty acids (SFA) 9–11, 99
sauna therapy 65–6, 289
Schumann resonance 363
seasonal affective disorder (SAD) 393
seaweed 159
selenium 391
serology 339–40, **340**
Sertraline Against Depression and Heart Disease in
        Chronic Heart Failure (SADHART) 388
serum fatty acids 87
sesame seeds 115, 162
Seven Countries Study (SCS) 102
severe acute respiratory syndrome coronavirus 2
        (SARS-CoV-2) *see* COVID-19
sex differences 218–19
SFA *see* saturated fatty acids (SFA)
shellfish, allergies to 89–90
short-chain fatty acid (SCFA) 10, 269
        beneficial 274, 275
        putrefactive 273
Sinatra ST 224, 225, 359, 360, 363, 366
Singapore Academy of Medicine 339
Singh RB 207
skin brushing 68
Slots J 308
small intestinal bacterial overgrowth (SIBO) 273
sodium (Na+) 150
sodium hypochlorite (NaOCl) 307–8
sodium–potassium ratio 19
soluble fibers 355
soy 115
soy protein 15
Spain 32
special foods, to lower blood pressure 56–7
specialized pro-resolving mediators (SPMs) 85–6,
        305, 353
spirituality 396
spore-forming probiotics 276
SPRINT trial 223, 394
standard American diet (SAD) 133–4, *134*
standard Western diet 48–9
statin drugs 202, *202*
statin treatment, side effects with 221
Steenkamp LR 385
Streptococcus mutans 297
Streptococcus viridians 297
stress 59–60, 218, 384–5
stressors 385
Study of Women Across the Nation (SWAN) 219
sudden cardiac death (SCD) rate 8
sugars 13–14
sugar substitutes 13–14

sulforaphane 275
supplements 355
surface transmission, COVID-19 339
sustainability issues 89

targeted nutraceuticals 40, 55, 360
targeted nutrition 3
targeted nutritional supplements 60–2, **62**
taurine 209
    hypertension 153
T-cell responses, to COVID-19340, *341*
teas, hypertension 161
testosterone 238–9
testosterone replacement therapy (TRT) **239,** 239–41
    methods of **242,** 242–3
    standard work-up 241–2
TFA *see* trans fatty acids (TFA)
therapeutic fasting 68
Therapeutic Lifestyle Changes (TLC) diet 103
Thompson D 312, 314, 318
thrombosis 51
"timing" hypothesis 236
tissue inflammation 250
tocotrienols 120–1
toll-like receptors (TLRs) 9
tomato nutrition 37–8
Total Mouth Disinfection method 312–14, 318
TOTOX value 90
Traditional Mediterranean Diet (TMD) 3–5, 7
traditional risk factors 217, 219
transcendental meditation (TM) 60, 394
trans fatty acids (TFA) 11, 99
Treatment of Preserved Cardiac Function Heart Failure
        (TOPCAT) trial 222
triglyceride (TG)-lowering effect 84
triglycerides (TG) *vs.* ethyl esters 86–7
trimethylamine-N-oxide (TMAO) 208
trimethylamine N-oxide (TMAO) 267
type 2 diabetes mellitus (T2DM) 13, 14, 53, 199

ubiquinol 205–6
ubiquinone 205–6
U-shaped curve 17

Val-Pro-Pro (VPP) 12
vascular immune dysfunction 145, *146, 147, 147*
    hypertension 145, *146, 147, 147*
vascular lining 51–2
vascular receptors, biochemical and biomechanical insults
        interact with *4*
vascular salt sensors 150

vascular tonics 375
    horse chestnut (*Aesculus hippocastanum* L.) 375
    pycnogenol 375–6
vegetables 66–7, 161
vegetarian diet 47–8
vegetarian diets plant-based nutrition 14–15
vegetarian/vegan 89
Vigen R 239
vitamin B6 (pyridoxine) 156, 391
vitamin C 121–2, 154–5
vitamin D 155–6, 311, 390
Vitamin D and Omega-3 Trial (VITAL) 82–3
vitamin E 155
vomiting 218

wakame seaweed *(Undaria pinnatifida)* 159
wheat (gluten) 49–50
wheat-related disorder (WRD)249–50
    causes of wheats' immunogenicity 256–9, *258*
    diversity of 255, *255*
    frequency of *254,* 254–5
    immune response to wheat 255–6
    mechanisms of cardiac involvement in 251
whey protein 12
Wi-Fi 68–9
Wild Fermentation (Katz) 67
women, CVD in 226–7, 232
    defining problem in 220–1
        diastolic dysfunction 221–3
        hypertension 223–4
        mitral valve prolapse 224–5
        peripheral artery disease 225–6
    estradiol and 232–3
    hormones and metabolism 234
        critical window/"timing" hypothesis 236
        hormone therapy 235–7
        menopausal hormone therapy effects 234
    low estradiol and 233–4
    mortality in 217
    with nausea and vomiting 218
Women's Health Initiative (WHI) 103

yoga 395

Zembron-lacny A 395
Zhao X 393
zinc (Zn++)311, 391
    hypertension 151
zonulin 18, 49
Zou L 308
Zutphen Elderly Study 36–7, 41